Second Edition

Advanced
Sports Nutrition

Dan Benardot
PhD, RD, FACSM

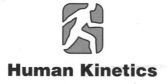

Human Kinetics

Library of Congress Cataloging-in-Publication Data

Benardot, Dan, 1949-
  Advanced sports nutrition / Dan Benardot. -- 2nd ed.
    p. cm.
  Includes bibliographical references and index.
  ISBN-13: 978-1-4504-0161-6 (soft cover)
  ISBN-10: 1-4504-0161-9 (soft cover)
  1. Athletes--Nutrition. I. Title.
  TX361.A8B45 2011
  613.2'024796--dc23

                            2011031137

ISBN-10: 1-4504-0161-9 (print)
ISBN-13: 978-1-4504-0161-6 (print)

Copyright © 2012, 2006 by Dan Benardot

This publication is written and published to provide accurate and authoritative information relevant to the subject matter presented. It is published and sold with the understanding that the author and publisher are not engaged in rendering legal, medical, or other professional services by reason of their authorship or publication of this work. If medical or other expert assistance is required, the services of a competent professional person should be sought.

The web addresses cited in this text were current as of October 2011, unless otherwise noted.

Acquisitions Editor: Laurel Plotzke Garcia; **Managing Editor:** Anne Cole; **Assistant Editor:** Elizabeth Evans; **Copyeditor:** Patricia L. MacDonald; **Indexer:** Nan Badgett; **Permissions Manager:** Martha Gullo; **Graphic Designer:** Joe Buck; **Graphic Artist:** Julie L. Denzer; **Cover Designer:** Keith Blomberg; **Photographer (cover):** © Christophe Schmid (left), © Lario Tus (middle), © Human Kinetics (right); **Photo Asset Manager:** Laura Fitch; **Visual Production Assistant:** Joyce Brumfield; **Photo Production Manager:** Jason Allen; **Art Manager:** Kelly Hendren; **Associate Art Manager:** Alan L. Wilborn; **Illustrations:** © Human Kinetics, unless otherwise noted; **Printer:** Versa Press

Printed in the United States of America   10 9 8 7 6 5 4 3 2

The paper in this book is certified under a sustainable forestry program.

Human Kinetics
Website: www.HumanKinetics.com

United States: Human Kinetics
P.O. Box 5076
Champaign, IL 61825-5076
800-747-4457
e-mail: humank@hkusa.com

Canada: Human Kinetics
475 Devonshire Road Unit 100
Windsor, ON N8Y 2L5
800-465-7301 (in Canada only)
e-mail: info@hkcanada.com

Europe: Human Kinetics
107 Bradford Road
Stanningley
Leeds LS28 6AT, United Kingdom
+44 (0) 113 255 5665
e-mail: hk@hkeurope.com

Australia: Human Kinetics
57A Price Avenue
Lower Mitcham, South Australia 5062
08 8372 0999
e-mail: info@hkaustralia.com

New Zealand: Human Kinetics
P.O. Box 80
Torrens Park, South Australia 5062
0800 222 062
e-mail: info@hknewzealand.com

E5292

To Robin

Contents

Foreword   viii   ◆   Preface   ix   ◆   Acknowledgments   xii

Part I   Nutrition Sources for Athletes   1

1   Energy Nutrients 2

Get the facts on the energy substrates (carbohydrate, protein, and fat), how their differential intakes affect the athletic endeavor, and how the recommended intakes can optimize your performance.

2   Vitamins and Minerals 43

Exercise increases vitamin and mineral requirements. Learn the best ways to ensure sufficient vitamin and mineral intakes as well as the possible outcomes of inadequate or excessive intakes.

3   Fluids and Electrolytes 83

Maintaining fluid balance is critically important for sustaining athletic performance. This chapter helps you learn hydration strategies that will optimize your physical activity capacity.

4   Ergogenic Aids 110

Ergogenic aids are substances *intended* to improve athletic performance, but few actually work as advertised. Learn about the metabolic bases for these aids, how they can work, and why they may cause more problems than they resolve.

Part II   Nutrition Aspects of Optimal Performance   131

5   GI Function and Energy Delivery 132

The gastrointestinal tract is responsible for processing all the foods and beverages you consume and for delivering the resulting nutrients to the blood for transport to tissues. This chapter discusses normal GI function, common problems experienced by athletes, and possible solutions.

6 Nutrient and Fluid Timing. 153

Both nutrient and fluid balance are critical for achieving optimal body composition, weight, and athletic performance. This chapter discusses the importance of timing nutrient and fluid intake in a way that dynamically matches need so that tissue requirements are satisfied in real time.

7 Oxygen Transportation and Utilization 180

The delivery of oxygen to working muscles is critically important for performance. This chapter reviews issues related to oxygen transport and utilization and the many parts of the oxidative system where nutrients are involved.

8 Strategies for Anti-Inflammation and Muscular Health. 189

Exercise is an inflammatory event that can interfere with training. This chapter provides recommendations for specific foods and nutrients and when they should be consumed to reduce inflammation and improve muscle recovery.

Part III Factors Affecting Nutrition Needs   197

9 Travel. 198

Athletes inevitably travel to competitions, and some trips take them across multiple time zones to unfamiliar food cultures. This chapter reviews the strategies athletes can follow to reduce the risk of compromised performance.

10 High Altitude. 208

Many athletes choose to live or train at high altitude, with the goal of improving red blood cell concentration and oxygen-carrying capacity. This chapter reviews the nutrition strategies that can help athletes optimize their training and performance at high altitude.

11 Gender and Age 218

Male, female, younger, and older athletes have different nutrition requirements. This chapter presents age- and gender-specific information to help male and female athletes of all ages meet their nutrition needs.

12 Body Composition and Weight 231

Athletes must achieve both an ideal weight and body composition to be successful, regardless of the sport. This chapter reviews the strategies athletes can follow to safely achieve an ideal competitive weight and body composition.

Part IV Nutrition Strategies for Specific Energy Systems   257

13 Anaerobic Metabolism for High-Intensity Bursts and Power 258

High-intensity activity requires a level of energy production that exceeds the body's capacity to derive all of this energy through oxidative metabolism. This chapter helps athletes involved in primarily anaerobic activities understand the best ways to satisfy their nutrition needs.

14 Aerobic Metabolism for Endurance 288

Endurance athletes must find ways to consume enough of the right fuels to enable high-level performance over long periods. This chapter provides strategies to help endurance athletes meet their nutrition needs.

15 Metabolic Needs for Both Power and Endurance 313

Many athletes must have both power and endurance. This chapter discusses the nutrition needs of athletes requiring a combination of power and endurance as well as gives training and game-time nutrition strategies for satisfying these needs.

Part V Nutrition Plans for Specific Sports 333

16 Sports Requiring Power and Speed 334

This chapter includes seven sample eating plans for intakes of 2,100, 2,300, 2,700, 3,100, 3,400, 3,700, and 4,600 calories for a variety of speed and power sports. The plans include differently timed practice sessions to help athletes understand the dynamic interaction between energy utilization and requirements.

17 Sports Requiring Endurance 350

This chapter includes five eating plans for intakes of 1,900 (lacto-ovo vegetarian), 2,000 (gluten free), 2,300, 2,800, and 4,500 calories. The plans use different endurance sports with multiple training schedules to help athletes understand how to best meet nutrition requirements for a variety of schedules.

18 Sports Requiring Combined Power and Endurance 362

This chapter includes five eating plans for intakes of 2,300, 2,500, 2,400 (injury recovery), 2,800, and 3,800 calories. These plans use different sports requiring a combination of power and endurance to illustrate different training schedules and the eating strategies to meet nutrition needs.

Appendix: Institute of Medicine's Dietary Reference Intakes for Macronutrients   374

Endnotes   382   ◆   Index   406   ◆   About the Author   411

Foreword

Elite athletes all over the world know Dr. Dan Benardot. They seek his guidance because they know his sage advice may be the difference between a gold medal and the rest of the field. Institutions of higher learning from just about every continent invite him to visit their classrooms and laboratories. They want their students to learn from the best. At Georgia State University, we simply know him as Dan—a remarkable friend, a superb colleague, a devoted husband, and dad to the greatest kids on the planet.

The first edition of *Advanced Sports Nutrition* was wildly successful. It was used in countless classrooms as well as by athletes of all sizes, shapes, and skill. It was used by elite athletes and not-so-elite athletes. It became required reading of sport nutritionists and exercise science students as they learned about appropriate nutrition for human performance. And it became the source of choice for coaches who would then counsel athletes on how to get the edge on their competition. But like every book that is successful, it needed some revision and updating. That is precisely why *Advanced Sports Nutrition, Second Edition* is so vital.

This second edition includes a new chapter on GI distress in physical activity and a new chapter on reducing exercise-induced inflammation. There have been major reference updates throughout the book, and more sport-specific examples have been added in parts IV and V. Dr. Benardot's own work in the Georgia State University Laboratory for Elite Athlete Performance (LEAP) emphasizes not only energy delivery and use but also the timing of nutrient ingestion, which then optimizes energy utilization. Because of the importance of within-day energy balance, Dr. Benardot has added many more diet examples to keep athletes in energy balance. Within-day energy balance was something Dan was working on nearly two decades ago; today everyone is talking about it. The procedure of tracking energy consumption and energy expenditure throughout the day (and not at the end of a period of time such as 24 hours) has now become commonplace for not only improved athletic performance but for structured weight loss programs as well. For athletes, the timing of energy intake before, during, and after training or competition is more important than ever. Within-day energy balance is not limited to elite athletes, whether able bodied (Olympic Games) or physically impaired (Paralympic Games). Athletes of all ages, both genders, and all skill levels should pay more attention to their energy intake. *Advanced Sports Nutrition, Second Edition* addresses these (and many more) issues and how they relate to sport performance.

Socrates once said, "Worthless people live only to eat and drink; people of worth eat and drink only to live." That was quite the observation he made way back around 450 BC. But it was also proverbial in the sense that this same observation can be made of athletes today. Thanks to Dr. Benardot, the mystery of how to fuel athletes for exercise has now become manifest in this second edition.

Walter R. Thompson, PhD, FACSM, FAACVPR
Regents Professor
Department of Kinesiology and Health in the College of Education
Division of Nutrition, School of Health Professions in the Byrdine F. Lewis
School of Nursing and Health Professions
Georgia State University

Preface

Serious athletes push the envelope of human capacity to become stronger and faster. The athletes who learn how to do this correctly by dynamically matching energy and nutrient needs with difficult training schedules are ultimately the ones who succeed and who can stay at the top of their game. The second edition of *Advanced Sports Nutrition* has maintained its original intent of serving as a comprehensive guide to nutrition for athletes, coaches, and the sports medicine professionals who work with them, but it includes even more information than the original. The ultimate purpose of this book, therefore, is to help athletes and those who work with them understand what it takes to become supremely conditioned for their specific sport *and* to do so in a way that lowers common activity-associated health and injury risks. Episodic injuries and illnesses are so common among athletes that many consider these problems a normal part of the athletic endeavor. But this need not be the case, and athletes who can avoid these setbacks progress more steadily toward their goals. Making the right nutrition choices results in athletes with happier, healthier, longer, and more successful careers.

This edition has been updated with new references and information in every chapter, but it also includes chapters that are entirely new. For example, many athletes face chronic or acute GI problems that interfere with training and performance. Included in this edition is information to help athletes understand the possible causes of GI distress and strategies for alleviating these problems. Chapter 5 includes material on gluten intolerance (celiac disease), which is increasingly prevalent in both athlete and nonathlete groups. This new edition also includes evidenced-based research findings on nutrition strategies for reducing muscle soreness, an area that has recently received a great deal of scientific attention but for which there remains an enormous amount of misinformation.

Additionally, all the diet plans have been updated and now use a unique methodology that visually illustrates the interaction between energy expenditure and energy intake during the day. These diet plans have been created to help athletes understand how to satisfy energy and nutrient needs with different frequencies and intensities of energy expenditure. A primary goal of these diet plans is to help athletes understand the *patterns* of eating that are needed to satisfy different training schedules.

There is an almost constant expansion of professional and Olympic sports, and the number of athletes who can function at the elite level is on the rise. There is also an ever-increasing group of people who, although not elite athletes, are certainly enthusiastically committed to regular involvement in their sports. This book has been written with this group in mind, providing information in a way that enables the reader to readily access nutrition principles so they can be appropriately applied, regardless of the sport or level of the participating athlete. To make it easier for readers to connect with their specific sport, this edition has increased the number of sports described, with information on the sport-specific nutrition concerns and strategies for each of them.

Endurance events have a burgeoning following, with virtually all age groups represented in competitions that now pepper the landscape in practically all medium and large cities. Even a casual observer can see a large group of older-than-60 competitors participating in half marathons and marathons around the country. Ultraendurance events have also seen an increase in participation, with huge numbers of participants in Ironman events and multiday running events. While a wonderful thing to witness, the activity in first aid tents at these events also appears to be increasing, raising the serious question about whether participants fully understand the stresses of such long-endurance competitions and the strategies that can and should be followed to reduce risk of dehydration, hyponatremia, and heat illness. Without overlooking the critical importance of conditioning prior to participating in such events, this book provides these competitors with both the desired strategies and the scientific basis for why these strategies make sense. And these strategies may differ for males, females, and different age groups because every group has different nutrition needs that should be well understood and satisfied to diminish exercise-associated risks. This book provides important information that is specific to different genders and ages to help competitors—and those in their support system—know what to do.

Many people begin exercise programs for the expressed purpose of improving weight and body composition. Depending on how this is done, and whether a solid nutrition plan is integrated into the exercise program, this could be a good or a bad thing. Far too many people substitute exercise for eating with the hope that this will lower weight. Yes, weight is likely to be lowered, but there is good evidence to suggest that the *wrong* weight is lowered. In this book I provide many examples of a simple rule: The body's reaction to an inadequate energy intake is to lower the tissue that needs energy. You will learn why severe energy deficits are counterproductive to health, weight, and performance. This book also includes information that will help you understand common body-composition assessment techniques and how they can be used to achieve the desired body profile.

A substantial amount of misinformation exists regarding optimal strategies for achieving peak athletic performance and health. This is especially true about "nutritional" products sold under the pretense that they hold the secret to enhancing performance. The placebo effect is certainly at play with these products, so there may be some perceived improvement from their consumption, but they typically lack the research to back their claims, and the sports medicine literature is filled with cases of athletes who have used such products with negative unintended consequences. Investigations show that commonly marketed ergogenic aids frequently include banned substances that can put both the health and eligibility of athletes at risk. Compounding the potential for problems is the tendency for many beginning athletes to attempt improvement in their athletic capabilities too quickly, with training programs and dietary supplements that are intended to emulate the regimens of highly conditioned professionals. This is a formula for disaster that can result in overtraining injuries, malnutrition, and psychological stress—all of which have the potential to take talented young athletes out of a sport. Given the realities of athletic competition and the enormous rewards available to those who reach the pinnacle of their sports, it may be difficult for athletes to be wholly rational about the proper nutrition strategies that will help them best achieve their desired goals, and advertisers for nutritional products know that athletes are susceptible targets. Even when the connection between odd dietary intakes and optimal athletic performance are shown to be false, athletes and coaches persist in advancing the dietary myths. The truth is that most of the money spent on special products is making someone richer but isn't making athletes any better. There is no substitute for matching good food intake with nutrition needs. A good starting point for athletes to consider is that *food* (not supplements or ergogenic aids) is the basic unit in nutrition science.

The scientific information in the field of sport nutrition is expanding rapidly. More highly trained researchers are now doing investigations in this area, and an ever-increasing number of articles in scientific journals focus on the relationship between nutrition and athletic performance. As a result of this expanding knowledge base, old beliefs are clarified and new beliefs are created. To some extent, everyone involved in sports must keep their minds open enough to question old paradigms and allow new ones to settle in. Position papers dealing with sport nutrition from the American Dietetic Association and the American College of Sports Medicine are much more specific than they once were about the nutrition factors that enhance performance, because much more specific information is known. Health and injury risks related to the potential malnutrition faced by many athletes are now an integral part of the science of sport nutrition and are emphasized in these position papers. In simple terms, the science has evolved from the philosophy that doing the wrong thing nutritionally *may* hurt you to understanding that doing the wrong thing nutritionally *will* hurt you.

If athletes follow a sound training and nutrition program, they are likely to be successful and healthy, but seemingly minor mistakes could result in injuries that might take talented athletes out of the only Olympic cycle they could ever hope to compete in. Exercise and involvement in a sport can, should, and usually does lead to wonderful things. The underlying philosophy of this book is that involvement in sports should lead to a lifetime enhancement of health rather than a lifetime of problems, and good eating habits help make this happen.

Acknowledgments

As a member of a robust academic community, I realized long ago that nothing I do occurs in a vacuum. Conversations over coffee, ideas shared informally in meetings, and information provided during student presentations all fill me with ideas that I am quite certain have infiltrated this book. So, to all my colleagues and students, I say thank you for making my life so invigorating and full. In particular, I want to mention by name three colleagues who share my love of academe and all it has to offer and who are overflowing with a never-ending stream of *good* ideas. These colleagues, Dr. Walt Thompson, Dr. Sid Crow, and Dr. George Pierce, make all the work feel interesting and worth it.

I am pleased to have an ongoing association with a number of sports governing bodies and have particularly enjoyed my work with U.S. Figure Skating and the outstanding sports medicine professionals they have brought together to care for the talented national-team athletes. Central to this effort is Mitch Moyer, senior director of athlete high performance. Mitch has been willing to do whatever it takes—including thinking outside the box to change some traditional nutrition paradigms—to help make American figure skaters stronger, healthier, and better athletes. People such as Mitch advance the science of sport in ways that few people adequately appreciate.

It is also important for me to mention my wife, Robin, who is a nutrition scientist and practitioner, and whom I constantly rely on for advice and feedback. Her insights are invaluable and appear everywhere in this book.

Nutrition Sources for Athletes

Energy Nutrients

A key feature of physical activity is that it increases the rate of energy (i.e., caloric) expenditure. Athletes therefore have a greater need for energy nutrients (carbohydrate, protein, and fat) than do nonathletes, and much research focuses on the best strategies for meeting these energy requirements while ensuring optimal distribution of the energy substrates to support exercise of various intensities and durations. It is clear that the higher the exercise intensity, the greater the proportionate reliance on carbohydrate as a fuel, and many studies provide valuable insights on the best consumption patterns for optimizing glycogen stores, ensuring adequate carbohydrate availability during training and competition, and reducing muscle soreness and enhancing muscle recovery. The contribution of protein to muscle function and recovery is much better understood now than in the recent past, and there is considerable information about how carbohydrate, protein, and fat influence mental and muscle function.

The recent popularity of higher-protein, higher-fat, and lower-carbohydrate diets has serious and potentially negative implications for athletic performance. Nevertheless, their popularity may be better understood if viewed in the context of food intolerances and food sensitivities rather than their potential for directly influencing performance. It is important that athletes and coaches understand how the appropriate energy intake and energy substrate distribution help optimize both mental and muscle function. This chapter presents the essential elements of carbohydrate, protein, and fat metabolism in exercise, along with a critical scientific view on how these substrates contribute to optimal athletic performance (see table 1.1; see appendix A for the Institute of Medicine's dietary reference intakes for macronutrients).

In physics, the term *calorie* is a measure of energy, with 1 calorie representing the amount of energy required to raise the temperature of 1 gram of water by 1 degree Celsius. In nutrition, the term *calorie* is 1,000 times this amount, so it is referred to as a *kilocalorie (kcal)*. Despite this difference, when discussing matters of nutrition, it is commonly understood that reference to a *calorie* is really a *kilocalorie.* In this book references to *calorie* or *calories* is used interchangeably with *kilocalorie* or *kilocalories.*

CARBOHYDRATE

In the minds of many athletes, carbohydrate often plays second fiddle to protein. This is partly due to misinformation about how truly important carbohydrate is to the athletic endeavor, but it may also be due to common misunderstandings about what carbohydrate is. Table 1.2, which covers common carbohydrate terms, clarifies some of the complexities associated with carbohydrate. Some athletes go so far as stating they avoid carbohydrate, but when asked what they eat, the first things they mention are fruits and vegetables, which are almost entirely composed of carbohydrate. There are, in fact, various types of carbohydrate, and our bodies react differently to each type. Glucose and bran, for instance, are both carbohydrate, but they are on opposite ends of the energy-provision spectrum. Glucose enters the bloodstream relatively quickly and initiates a fast and high insulin response, but the potential energy in bran never manifests itself as a source of energy in the bloodstream because of its indigestibility, and it tends to mediate the insulin response by slowing the rate at which other energy sources enter the bloodstream. These within-carbohydrate differences mandate that athletes not consider all carbohydrate foods as having the same outcomes and carefully consider the best type of carbohydrate to consume before, during, and after exercise.

Glucose is the main fuel for the creation of muscular energy, which is in the form of adenosine triphosphate (ATP). A failure to sustain glucose delivery to working muscles results in cessation of high-intensity activity (commonly referred to as "hitting the wall"). Therefore, understanding how to avoid glucose depletion should be a major focus of an athlete's nutrition practices. Sustaining carbohydrate sufficiency is problematic because, unlike either protein or fat, humans have a limited storage capacity for carbohydrate.

Blood sugar (i.e., blood glucose) is the primary fuel for the brain. When blood sugar becomes low, mental fatigue sets in, and mental fatigue results in muscular fatigue regardless of how much energy is stored in muscles. If liver glycogen and blood glucose were the sole source of energy for working muscles, you could continue to exercise for approximately 18 minutes (16 minutes from liver glycogen and 2 minutes from blood sugar) before achieving mental (and therefore muscular) fatigue. Luckily, liver glycogen and blood sugar are not the sole source of energy for physical activity, but higher intensity activities use blood

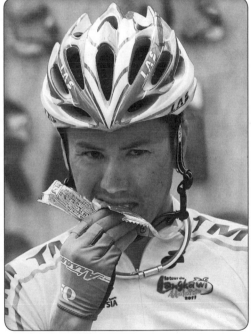

The right snack at the right time aids performance.

sugar and liver glycogen more rapidly. This fact alone should encourage athletes to adopt carbohydrate intake strategies that prevent depletion.

Carbohydrate adequacy is most critical at higher levels of exercise intensity because there is a greater reliance on carbohydrate as a source of muscular fuel. Higher-intensity training regimens, therefore, may require more frequent intakes of carbohydrate to satisfy need (see figure 1.1). Despite years of research confirming the importance of maintaining carbohydrate availability for sustaining muscular endurance and mental function, many athletes still believe protein is the single most critical nutrient for achieving athletic success. Although protein should not be diminished in its importance, delivering the right amounts of carbohydrate at the right times optimizes the limited carbohydrate stores, ensures better carbohydrate delivery to the brain, reduces the possibility of depleting the limited stores, and sustains athletic performance at a high level. Although protein is critically important to health and most certainly plays a role in sustaining and enlarging muscle mass, reducing muscle soreness, and improving muscle recovery, consuming excessively large doses of protein does little to improve athletic performance when it replaces carbohydrate.

Table 1.1 Basic Functions of the Energy Substrates

Carbohydrate (4 kcal/g)	• Fuel for working muscles (from starch, sugars, and glycogen) • Cholesterol and fat control (from dietary fiber) • Digestion assistance (from dietary fiber) • Nutrient and water absorption (from sugars) • Maintenance of blood sugar (all digestible carbohydrates; important for mental function and delayed fatigue)
Protein (4 kcal/g)	• Energy source (if carbohydrates are depleted) • Delivery of essential amino acids (amino acids the body needs but can't make) • Essential for developing new tissue (important during growth and injury repair) • Essential for maintaining existing tissue (helps control normal wear and tear) • Basic substance in the manufacture of enzymes, antibodies, and hormones • Fluid balance (helps control water level inside and outside cells) • Carrier of substances in the blood (transports vitamins, minerals, and fat to and from cells)
Fat (9 kcal/g)	• Delivery of fat-soluble vitamins (vitamins A, D, E, and K) • Delivery of essential fatty acids (fatty acids the body needs but can't make) • Energy and muscular fuel (for low-intensity activity) • Satiety control (helps make you feel satisfied from eating) • Substance in many hormones

Table 1.2 Common Carbohydrate Terms

Term	Definition
Glucose	A simple monosaccharide (sugar) with a molecular formula of $C_6\text{-}H_{12}\text{-}O_6$. It is a principle source of energy for cellular metabolism and the primary fuel for the central nervous system (brain). Glucose is a building block for larger carbohydrate molecules such as sucrose (a disaccharide) as well as cellulose, starch, and glycogen (polysaccharides). Plants produce glucose during photosynthesis.
Glycogen	A polysaccharide representing the main storage form of glucose in the body, primarily found in the liver and muscles. When carbohydrate energy is needed, muscle glycogen is converted into glucose for use by the muscle cells, and liver glycogen is converted into glucose for use throughout the body, including the central nervous system.
Glycolysis	A metabolic process that breaks down glycogen and glucose aerobically (with oxygen) or anaerobically (i.e., without oxygen) through a series of reactions to either pyruvic acid or lactic acid and releases energy for the body in the form of ATP. This is the primary energy source for intense exercise for short periods.
Gluconeogenesis	The metabolic process that results in the generation of glucose from non-carbohydrate substances, such as lactate, glycerol, and glucogenic amino acids.
Monosaccharide	Monosaccharides represent the most basic units of carbohydrates. A monosaccharide is a single-sugar molecule. The 3 primary monosaccharides in human nutrition are glucose, fructose, and galactose. Other common monosaccharides include ribose and xylose.
Disaccharide	Any of a variety of carbohydrates that consist of two monosaccharides held together with a bond. The common disaccharides include sucrose (table sugar), which is composed of glucose and fructose; lactose (milk sugar), which is composed of glucose and galactose; and maltose (grain sugar), which is composed of 2 molecules of glucose.
Polysaccharide	A polysaccharide is a complex molecule containing many repeating sugar units ($\geq$10) in long polymer chains. The most common sugar unit is glucose. Common polysaccharides are starch, glycogen, and cellulose. Some polysaccharides are digestible (e.g., starch), while others are not (e.g., fiber). The type of bond holding the monosaccharides together determines digestibility.
Carbohydrate polymer	Commonly used in sports gels, carbohydrate polymers typically include simple sugars and long-chain carbohydrate polymers and glucose polymers (maltodextrins, rice syrup, polysaccharides, oligosaccharides). The goal of sports gels is to pack more energy in a small package than can be delivered in a sports beverage, without negatively affecting gastric emptying.
Dietary fiber	Often referred to as roughage, dietary fiber consists of both soluble (dissolves in water) and insoluble (does not dissolve in water) polysaccharide that is not digestible. It comes from the portion of plant foods that is indigestible (i.e., we get no energy from it), but it aids in digestion and promotes regularity. Diets high in dietary fiber are associated with lower risk for many chronic diseases, including cancer and diverticulosis.
Insoluble fiber	Insoluble fiber adds bulk to the diet, helps maintain intestinal health by absorbing many times its own weight in water, and is mainly found in vegetables and the bran layer of grains. Consisting mainly of cellulose and hemicellulose, wheat bran is an example of insoluble fiber.
Soluble fiber	Soluble fiber dissolves easily in water and takes on a soft, gel-like texture in the intestines. Mainly pectin, gum, and mucilage, soluble fiber is found in oat bran, beans, peas, and most fruits. It is associated with lower blood sugar levels, reducing the risk of hyperinsulinemia, obesity, and cancer.

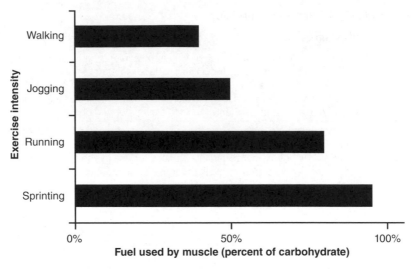

Figure 1.1 Exercise intensity and carbohydrate fuel usage.

Carbohydrate Types

Not all types of carbohydrate have the same form, function, and health impact. The basic unit of all carbohydrates is the monosaccharide, or single-molecule carbohydrate. The common monosaccharides all have six carbons and, while they vary only slightly in hydrogen–oxygen configuration, these subtle variations account for important metabolic differences. The basic metabolic unit for human cells is the monosaccharide glucose, and the other monosaccharides have biochemical pathways that enable them to be converted to glucose. The number of monosaccharides bonded together provides the main basis for classifying carbohydrate (see table 1.3).

Each of the three most common dietary monosaccharides (glucose, fructose, and galactose) has different characteristics of solubility, sweetness, and reactivity with the food environment in which it is found. With the exception of fructose, which is present in an increasingly wide variety of processed foods that contain high-fructose (corn) sweetener, most monosaccharides are delivered in the food supply as breakdown products of disaccharides (i.e., sugars composed of two connected monosaccharides). It should be understood that the distribution of glucose and fructose in high-fructose corn syrup is similar to that of sucrose (table sugar), but it contains a higher proportion of *free* fructose that is not bound to glucose. This difference may lead to difficulty in some athletes with fructose sensitivity, who may experience diarrhea from consumption of free fructose. There is also some indication that free fructose may result in a higher uric acid production, which results in gout-like joint pain.

There are three main disaccharides—sucrose, lactose, and maltose—each containing a different combination of monosaccharides (see table 1.4). Together, the monosaccharides and disaccharides are referred to as simple carbohydrates, or sugars, while the polysaccharides are commonly referred to as complex carbohydrates. The indigestible carbohydrates are also complex carbohydrates, but they are commonly referred to as dietary fiber. The sugars (the mono- and disaccharides) have different sweetness characteristics, with fructose tasting the sweetest, followed by sucrose, glucose, and lactose (the least sweet). However, the

Table 1.3 Carbohydrate Classification

Simple carbohydrates	**Sugars**	Monosaccharides (1-molecule carbohydrates)	Glucose (also called dextrose) Fructose (also called levulose, or fruit sugar) Galactose	Some sugars, or simple carbohydrates, may cause a fast rise in blood sugar, thereby stimulating excess insulin production, which causes a fast drop in blood sugar. Glucose and maltose have the highest glycemic effect.
		Disaccharides (2-molecule carbohydrates)	Sucrose Lactose Maltose	
Complex carbohydrates	**Partially digestible polysaccharides**	Oligosaccharides (3- to 20-molecule carbohydrates)	Maltodextrins Fructo-oligosaccharides Raffinose Stachyose Verbascose	Partially digestible polysaccharides are commonly found in legumes and, although they may cause gas and bloating, are considered healthy carbohydrates.
	Polysaccharides	Digestible polysaccharides (20-plus-molecule starch carbohydrates)	Amylose Amylopectin Glucose polymers	These complex carbohydrates should provide the main source of carbohydrate energy. Glucose polymers are made from starch and are often used in sports drinks and athlete gels.
		Indigestible polysaccharides (20-plus-molecule nonstarch carbohydrates)	Cellulose Hemicellulose Pectins Gums Mucilages Algal polysaccharides Beta-glucans Fructans	These complex carbohydrates provide fiber, which is important for GI tract health and disease resistance.
	Other	Other carbohydrates	Mannitol Sorbitol Xylitol Glycogen Ribose (a 5-carbon sugar)	Mannitol, sorbitol, and xylitol (sugar alcohols) are nutritive sweeteners that do not contribute to tooth decay. They are commonly used in products because of their moisture retention and food-stabilizing characteristics, but they are digested slowly and are known to cause GI distress if consumed in high amounts. Glycogen is the main carbohydrate storage form in animals, while ribose is part of the genetic code (deoxyribonucleic acid, or DNA).

sugars also differ in mouth feel and solubility (e.g., fructose is less soluble than sucrose), all of which influence food manufacturers in their choice of sugars in food preparation. Athletes now have a wide array of sports beverages and gels from which to choose, and each contains various proportions of the mono- and disaccharides and, with sports gels, different types of

Table 1.4 Relationship Between Monosaccharides and Disaccharides

Disaccharide	Contains these monosaccharides
Sucrose (cane or beet sugar)	Glucose Fructose
Lactose (milk sugar)	Glucose Galactose
Maltose (malt sugar)	Glucose Glucose

carbohydrate polymers. Each formulation is attempting to achieve the best combination of flavor, mouth feel, gut tolerance, gastric emptying, electrolyte replacement, energy delivery to working muscles, and, ultimately, superior performance outcomes.

Carbohydrate Metabolism

Humans can store approximately 350 grams (1,400 kilocalories) in the form of muscle glycogen, an additional 90 grams (360 kilocalories) of glycogen in the liver, and a small amount of circulating glucose in the blood (~5 grams, or about 20 kilocalories). The larger the muscle mass the greater the potential glycogen storage, but also the greater the potential need for glycogen.

In addition, greater glycogen storage is associated with greater fluid storage, with a ratio of 1 gram of glycogen resulting in 3 grams of additional water storage. In some sports this higher glycogen-associated fluid storage is considered advantageous (e.g., imagine a marathoner on a hot day who needs excess body water to sustain sweat rate), but in other sports it might be considered a problem (e.g., imagine a gymnast who needs the highest possible strength-to-weight ratio to do a tumbling routine—the extra water weight could be a problem, but the glycogen is needed to quickly create muscular ATP energy). Clearly, athletes should optimize glycogen storage in a way that is best for their particular sport.

We have systems for maintaining blood glucose within a relatively narrow range (70 to 110 milligrams per deciliter) by recruiting insulin and glucagon. Insulin and glucagon are pancreatic hormones that work synergistically to control blood glucose. Excess production of insulin can result in hypoglycemia (low blood sugar), with a resultant excess production of fat; inadequate insulin production or ineffective insulin results in hyperglycemia (high blood sugar) and diabetes. See figure 1.2 for an illustration of how pancreatic hormones normalize blood glucose.

Insulin is secreted by the beta cells of the pancreas, whereas glucagon is secreted by the alpha cells of the pancreas. The stimulus for insulin secretion is high blood glucose (the higher the glucose, the higher the insulin response), but the pancreas is constantly secreting a small amount of insulin even when blood glucose is in the normal range, causing a steady flow of glucose to the cells of the brain and muscles. Insulin lowers blood glucose by affecting the cell membranes of muscle and fat cells, thereby allowing glucose from the blood to enter the cell. This action causes a transfer from blood glucose to cell glucose and explains the blood-glucose-lowering effect of insulin; it also enables cells to receive a needed source of energy. See figure 1.3 for an illustration of the possible pathways taken by blood glucose.

With low blood glucose, which may occur between meals and during exercise, glucagon is secreted to break down liver glycogen and migrate the resultant free glucose into the

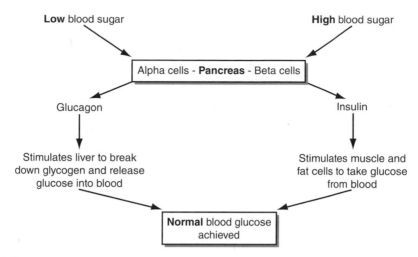

Figure 1.2 The impact of the pancreas on normalizing the blood glucose level.

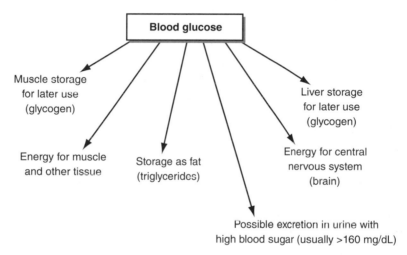

Figure 1.3 Possible pathways taken by blood glucose.

blood. Lower levels of blood glucose result in greater glucagon production. Glucagon may also stimulate gluconeogenesis (the manufacture of glucose from nonglucose substances). During gluconeogenesis, for instance, the amino acid alanine is derived from skeletal protein and is converted to glucose by the liver. About 60 percent of the glucose released by the liver to sustain blood sugar is from liver glycogen stores, but the remainder is from glucose synthesized from lactate, pyruvate, glycerol, and amino acids that include alanine.[1] The rate of liver glucose infused into the blood during exercise is a function of exercise intensity, with higher-intensity exercise causing a faster rate of liver glucose release.[2] The combination of lower blood insulin and higher epinephrine (i.e., adrenalin) and glucagon during long-duration activity stimulates liver glucose release.

Besides insulin and glucagon, two other hormones also influence blood glucose. Epinephrine is a stress hormone that initiates an extremely rapid breakdown of liver glycogen to quickly increase blood glucose levels. Cortisol, which is secreted from the adrenal gland, is also a stress hormone that promotes muscle protein catabolism. This protein breakdown makes certain glucogenic amino acids[3] available for gluconeogenesis, ultimately resulting in an increase in blood glucose. Both epinephrine and cortisol are released as a result of exercise-related stress, and both can be mediated through maintenance of blood glucose. Controlling epinephrine production helps preserve liver glycogen, and controlling cortisol helps preserve muscle protein. This is a strong argument for athletes to consume carbohydrate during exercise. This is also a strong argument for coaches to remain calm before and during competitions, since a stressful behavior directed toward an athlete may increase the athlete's psychological stress, which is associated with higher epinephrine production and, therefore, a faster decrease in liver glycogen.

The glucose circulating in the blood is derived mainly from dietary carbohydrate, with starches constituting the major food source. Complex carbohydrates (starches) are digested into monosaccharides (glucose, fructose, and galactose) for absorption into the blood. Some people have inadequate lactase to break down the milk sugar lactose into its component monosaccharides (glucose and galactose), causing the lactose to go indigested in the gut. Referred to as *lactose intolerance*, this leads to bloating, abdominal pain, diarrhea, and dehydration. Excess glucose in the liver and muscle is stored as glycogen, but only up to the glycogen saturation point. The liver has a maximum glycogen storage capacity of approximately 87 to 100 grams (348 to 400 kilocalories), while the muscles can store an average of approximately 350 grams (1,400 kilocalories) or more in larger persons. Providing additional glucose to cells when glycogen stores are saturated leads to the excess being stored as fat (in both muscle and fat cells). The liver glycogen is primarily responsible for stabilizing blood glucose, while the muscle glycogen is mainly responsible for providing an energy source to working muscles that can be metabolized both aerobically and anaerobically.

Blood sugar is not easily maintained when liver glycogen is depleted, even when muscle glycogen stores are full. Blood glucose is the primary fuel source for the central nervous system. Low blood sugar results in depressed central nervous system (CNS) activity, coupled with increased irritability and a lower capacity to concentrate. For athletes, low blood sugar may be related to mental fatigue, which results in muscle fatigue. Because liver glycogen and blood glucose stores are easily depleted during even short-duration activities, the intake of carbohydrate during activity is a critical factor in maintaining mental function and, ultimately, muscle function. In simple terms, athletes who allow blood sugar to drop below normal experience a drop in athletic performance because of compromised CNS function, even if the muscles are full of fuel.

Glycolysis

Adenosine triphosphate (ATP) is the high-energy compound for cells. Tissues have a limited storage capacity of immediately available ATP, so it must be generated quickly during exercise. Humans are inefficient at converting burned fuel to mechanical force, with approximately 60 to 80 percent of all burned fuel (ATP) lost as heat and only 20 to 40 percent actually involved in moving muscle. Since we cannot acquire additional metabolic heat (i.e., body temperature cannot rise significantly), storage of readily available ATP (as phosphocreatine) is limited. Were it not, we could produce so much heat so rapidly that cooling would be impossible, resulting in rapid overheating and death. Limited storage of readily available ATP could, therefore, be considered a self-preservation mechanism. The higher the exercise intensity, the faster the ATP must be regenerated. In steady-state, low-intensity activity, ATP can be adequately produced aerobically from the oxidation of carbohydrate and fat. However, as exercise intensity increases, athletes need a level of ATP production that cannot be fully supplied aerobically.[4,5] See table 1.5 for a summary of the energy metabolic systems.

Glycolysis is the process through which a high volume of ATP can be produced through the rapid breakdown of glycogen to glucose, resulting in ATP from glucose. Glycolysis can occur in the presence of oxygen (aerobic glycolysis) or without oxygen (anaerobic glycolysis), making glycogen a highly flexible fuel. Aerobic glycolysis has the capacity to produce more ATP than anaerobic glycolysis and, unlike anaerobic glycolysis, can do so without producing lactic acid. For this reason, anaerobic glycolysis is also referred to as the lactic acid system. In activities where the intensity exceeds the capacity to bring sufficient oxygen into the system to meet energy demands, anaerobic glycolysis becomes the major pathway for ATP production. However, extremely high-intensity anaerobic activities are self-limiting because the lactic acid buildup permits activity to continue for a maximum of only 1.5 to 2 minutes. It is typical for high-intensity sports to have opportunities for recovery. For instance, the artistic gymnastics floor routine is 1.5 minutes long, after which the gymnast can rest and recover to prepare for the next high-intensity event; and hockey players are substituted frequently (a hockey player almost never skates continuously for more than 2 minutes) to allow for muscle recovery.

Table 1.5 Energy Metabolic Systems

System	Characteristics	Duration
Phosphocreatine system (PCr)	Anaerobic production of ATP from stored phosphocreatine	Used for maximum-intensity activities
Anaerobic glycolysis (lactic acid system)	Anaerobic production of ATP from the breakdown of glycogen; the by-product of this system is the production of lactic acid	Used for extremely high-intensity activities that exceed the athlete's capacity to bring in sufficient oxygen; can continue producing ATP with this system no more than 2 min
Aerobic glycolysis	Aerobic production of large amounts of ATP from the breakdown of glycogen	Used for high-intensity activities that require a large volume of ATP but that are within the athlete's capacity to bring sufficient oxygen into the system
Oxygen system (aerobic metabolism)	Aerobic production of ATP from the breakdown of carbohydrate and fat	Used for lower-intensity activities of long duration that can produce a substantial volume of ATP but without the production of system-limiting by-products

The lactic acid produced in anaerobic glycolysis can best be considered a form of stored energy, just waiting for sufficient oxygen to reenter the system. When exercise intensity is reduced and the athlete has enough oxygen in the system for aerobic metabolic processes, the lactic acid is converted back to pyruvic acid and used to produce ATP aerobically. *Note:* A high production of lactic acid from extremely intense activity is more likely to negatively affect a dehydrated athlete than a well-hydrated athlete because the pool of fluid (blood volume) that accepts the lactic acid leaving cells is larger and, therefore, more resistant to pH change (i.e., change in relative acidity). In common parlance, "the solution to pollution is dilution."

Gluconeogenesis

Gluconeogenesis refers to the process of making glucose from noncarbohydrate substances. Blood glucose is critical for central nervous system function, aids in the metabolism of fat, and supplies fuel to working cells. However, because of its limited storage capacity, a minimum level of glucose is always available through the manufacture of glucose from noncarbohydrate substances. There are three primary systems for gluconeogenesis:

1. Triglycerides are the predominant storage form of fat in the human body and consist of three fatty acids attached to a glycerol molecule. The breakdown of triglycerides results in free glycerol (a three-carbon substance), and the combination of two glycerol molecules in the liver results in the production of one glucose molecule (a six-carbon substance). Glycerol is the only simple lipid (fat) in human nutrition that can ultimately be metabolized like a carbohydrate.

2. Catabolized muscle protein results in an array of free amino acids that were the building blocks of the muscle. Several amino acids are glucogenic (i.e., capable of creating glucose) and can be converted by the liver to form glucose. After only 40 minutes of strenuous activity, free alanine (a glucogenic amino acid) can increase by 60 to 96 percent, even more if work occurs under conditions of low blood sugar.[6] This strongly suggests that muscle breakdown can occur quickly if an athlete allows blood sugar to drop during physical activity.

3. In anaerobic glycolysis, lactate is produced and removed by the cell as a means of maintaining cellular pH. This lactate can be converted back to pyruvic acid for the aerobic production of ATP, or two lactate molecules can combine in the liver to form glucose. The conversion of lactate to glucose is referred to as the Cori cycle (lactate removed from the muscle and glucose returned to the muscle). Lactate (often used synonymously with lactic acid) should not be thought of as a bad, because it helps to preserve cellular function and can be used as fuel.

Carbohydrate Utilization During Exercise

Low carbohydrate levels result in exercise fatigue. Since carbohydrate stores (i.e., glycogen stores) and available free glucose are in limited supply (~350 kilocalories of glycogen in the liver; ~1,400 kilocalories of glycogen in muscles; about 40 kilocalories of glucose in blood), athletes should consider how to initiate exercise with sufficient glycogen stores to sustain activity at the desired intensity or should establish a routine that keeps glycogen stores from becoming depleted. Even if muscle glycogen stores are adequate, low liver glycogen stores will result in hypoglycemia and mental fatigue, and mental fatigue leads to muscle fatigue.

The higher the exercise intensity, the more athletes rely on carbohydrate as an energy substrate. However, even low-intensity (i.e., mainly aerobic) exercise that derives most of its fuel from fat still requires some level of carbohydrate for the complete combustion of fat and to maintain blood glucose. Therefore, all modes of physical activity have some degree of carbohydrate dependence. Several factors influence the proportionate contribution of carbohydrate to total fuel requirements during exercise. Factors that increase the reliance on carbohydrate include the following:

- High-intensity activity
- Long-duration activity
- Exercise in hot and cold temperature extremes
- Exercise at high altitude
- Age (higher in young boys than in men)

Factors that decrease the relative energy expenditure from carbohydrate include the following:

- Endurance training
- Good aerobic conditioning
- Temperature adaptation
- Gender

There is a common misconception that low-intensity activity (up to ~65 percent $\dot{V}O_2$max) is the most efficient means of fat loss. In fact, many popular exercise programs have been organized around the idea that a greater amount of fat is most efficiently "burned" with low-intensity aerobic exercise (see figure 1.4). However, the proportion of fat burned should not be confused with the volume of fat burned. While you're sitting reading this sentence, you are very likely deriving the vast majority of your energy requirements from fat. However, the total volume of fat being burned is extremely low. (If this were not so, sitting in front of a TV would be a terrific means of initiating a fat-loss program.) When exercise intensity is increased, the proportion of energy derived from fat is decreased, and the proportion of energy derived from carbohydrate is increased, but some level of fat is always being burned. The total caloric requirement per unit of time is much greater in high-intensity activity than in low-intensity activity, and the volume of fat burned is greater in high-intensity activity (despite a lower proportion of fat meeting total energy requirements). Therefore, athletes should work as intensely as possible within a given time frame to increase fat loss and optimize body composition (see chapter 12).

Here is an example:

- Joe does low-intensity (i.e., aerobic) activity for 60 minutes and burns 300 kilocalories, of which 80 percent (240 kilocalories) comes from fat.
- Jack does higher-intensity activity for 60 minutes and burns 500 kilocalories, of which 60 percent (300 kilocalories) comes from fat.

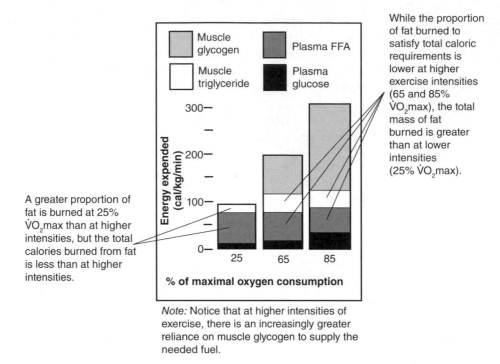

Figure 1.4 Energy substrate requirement at different levels of exercise intensity.

Adapted from J.A. Romijn, E.F. Coyle, L.S. Sideossis, et al., 1993, "Regulation of endogenous fat and carbohydrate in relation to exercise intensity and duration," *American Journal of Physiology: Endocrinology and Metabolism* 265(3): E380-391. Used with permission of the American Physiological Society.

- Jack burned 200 more total calories and 60 more fat calories than Joe, even though Joe burned a higher proportion of fat calories.

Carbohydrate is a critical fuel for athletes because we can more efficiently create energy per unit of oxygen from carbohydrate than from any other fuel. One liter of oxygen can yield approximately 5 calories from carbohydrate but only 4.7 calories from fat. In addition, aerobic glycolysis can produce ATP for muscular work in a larger quantity and at a faster rate than the oxidation of fat can produce it. The increased energy efficiency of carbohydrate helps explain the muscular fatigue that quickly occurs during high-intensity activities when muscle glycogen is nearly depleted. An athlete simply cannot supply sufficient ATP to working muscles to maintain the workload.

Central Nervous System Fatigue Theories

The conversion rate of adenosine diphosphate (ADP) to ATP is a critical step in the supply of energy to working muscles. Inadequate carbohydrate availability lowers the rate of ADP to ATP conversion, making it impossible for muscles to continue exercise at a high intensity level. In addition, the failure to convert ADP to ATP causes a buildup of ADP that also contributes to muscle fatigue.[7]

Other factors involving the central nervous system also cause muscle fatigue.[8] Collectively referred to as central fatigue theory, these factors involve mechanisms that cause more than the usual amount of the amino acid tryptophan to pass the blood–brain barrier, which stimulates an increase in the amount of serotonin (5-HT) that is produced. A neurotransmitter, 5-HT causes people to feel relaxed and, if enough is produced, to feel sleepy and lethargic. For the athlete, this could translate into muscular fatigue because mental fatigue leads to muscle fatigue.

- **Factor 1:** Blood sugar is the primary fuel for the brain, which must continue to function. If blood sugar becomes low, the brain stimulates the production of new blood sugar in a process called gluconeogenesis (i.e., the creation of new glucose from nonglucose substances). With low blood sugar and low muscle glycogen stores, muscle breakdown becomes an important source of substrate for gluconeogenesis. This results in an increased catabolism of branched-chain amino acids (BCAAs), which causes a reduction in circulating blood BCAAs.[9] BCAAs and tryptophan compete for the same receptor carriers that enable their passage through the blood–brain barrier. When BCAAs are high, the tryptophan passage to the brain is controlled. However, when the BCAA blood level is low (as happens when they are catabolized for energy), tryptophan can sequester more of the receptor carrier, and more tryptophan enters the brain. Tryptophan stimulates the formation of 5-HT. To prevent this from happening, blood and muscle glucose levels must be maintained to avoid gluconeogenesis.
- **Factor 2:** Consumption of foods high in tryptophan (such as turkey or milk) can increase the volume of tryptophan passing the blood–brain barrier, causing an increase in 5-HT production. The increase in 5-HT results in premature fatigue.[10]
- **Factor 3:** Fats compete for the same protein carrier in the blood as tryptophan. High fat intakes preferentially compete for this protein carrier, leaving a higher proportion of free tryptophan that can cross the blood–brain barrier. This causes an increase in 5-HT production, which may lead to premature fatigue.[10]

Although it may be logical that the intake of both BCAAs and carbohydrate could reduce 5-HT production and, therefore, inhibit both mental and physical fatigue, studies have not been conclusive because of the difficulty differentiating between brain and muscle effects.[11] In addition, there may be interference from compounds such as caffeine, the ingestion of which has been shown to delay fatigue by temporarily stimulating the central nervous system.[12] (Information on caffeine and its impact on performance is included in chapter 4 on ergogenic aids.)

Carbohydrate Requirements

The Institute of Medicine recommends 130 grams (520 kilocalories) of carbohydrate per day, which is the average minimal usage of glucose by the brain.[11] The desirable range of carbohydrate intake is 45 to 65 percent of total caloric intake (also referred to as the acceptable macronutrient distribution range, or AMDR), and the daily value (DV) for carbohydrate on food labels is based on a recommended intake of 60 percent of total caloric consumption. These recommendations also generally advise that no more than 25 percent of carbohydrate intake be derived from sugars (mono- and disaccharides).[13,14]

Dietary fiber consumption (from indigestible and partially digestible polysaccharides) should be at the level of 38 grams per day for adult men and 25 grams per day for adult women. Adequate fiber consumption aids in the maintenance of normal blood sugar (by controlling the absorption rate), reduces heart disease risk, and lowers constipation risk. The difference between genders in recommended fiber consumption is based on the lower total food mass and calories typically consumed by women.

It has been suggested that our only true requirement for carbohydrate is for vitamin C, a six-carbon, glucose-like substance that most animals can derive through an enzyme conversion of glucose. There is some historical evidence that our human ancestors consumed very little carbohydrate and survived. However, when considering athletes and the mountain of research demonstrating that carbohydrate is clearly the limiting substrate in athletic performance, it becomes clear that human survival and human performance are entirely different matters. Athletes need carbohydrate, regardless of where the athletic endeavor lies on the anaerobic to aerobic continuum. Athlete requirements for carbohydrate are based on several factors. Athletes must consume enough carbohydrate to

- provide energy to satisfy the majority of caloric needs;
- optimize glycogen stores;
- allow for muscle recovery after physical activity;
- provide a well-tolerated source of energy during practice and competition;
- provide a quick and easy source of energy between meals to maintain blood sugar; and
- provide an energy source to sustain blood sugar during physical activity.

The traditional guideline for determining caloric intake has been to consider the amount of carbohydrate to be consumed as a proportion of total caloric intake. The recommendation for the general population is that carbohydrate should supply 50 to 55 percent of total calories, and the dietary reference intake (DRI) is 130 grams per day (520 calories per day) for male and female adults. However, the amount typically recommended for athletes is between 55 and 65 percent of total calories, assuming an adequate total caloric intake. Another, and clearly better, way of determining carbohydrate requirement is by taking into consideration the amount of carbohydrate to be consumed (in grams) per kilogram of body mass. The carbohydrate intake recommendations for endurance-trained athletes range from between 7 and 8 grams (with some recommendations up to 10 grams) of carbohydrate per kilogram of body weight per day.[17,18] The current recommendations for carbohydrate consumption in athletes include the following:

- Athletes should consume sufficient carbohydrate to meet the majority of fuel requirements for their training programs and to optimize the restoration of muscle glycogen stores between bouts of physical activity.
- Immediately after and up to 4 hours after exercise, athletes should consume, at frequent intervals, 1.0 to 1.2 grams of carbohydrate per kilogram of body mass per hour. (Example: A 150-pound [70 kg] athlete wishing to consume 1.2 grams of carbohydrate per kilogram per hour for 4 hours after exercise would consume 1,344 calories from carbohydrate during the 4 hours after physical activity: 70 kg × 1.2 g × 4 hr × 4 cal/g = 1,344 cal.)
- For daily recovery from moderate-duration low-intensity training, athletes should consume 5 to 7 grams of carbohydrate per kilogram of body mass per day. (Example:

A 70 kg athlete wishing to consume 6 grams of carbohydrate per kilogram would consume 1,680 calories from carbohydrate: 70 kg × 6 g × 4 cal/g = 1,680 cal.)

- For daily recovery from moderate to heavy endurance training, athletes should consume 7 to 12 grams of carbohydrate per kilogram of body mass per day. (Example: A 70 kg athlete wishing to consume 10 grams of carbohydrate per kilogram would consume 2,800 calories from carbohydrate: 70 kg × 10 g × 4 cal/g = 2,800 cal.)

- For daily recovery from an extremely intensive exercise-training bout that has a duration of 4 to 6 (or more) hours per day, athletes should consume 10 to 12 grams of carbohydrate per kilogram of body mass per day. (Example: A 70 kg athlete wishing to consume 12 grams of carbohydrate per kilogram would consume 3,360 calories from carbohydrate: 70 kg × 12 g × 4 cal/g = 3,360 calories.)

These recommendations should be adjusted for individual athlete requirements, which are at least partially based on state of conditioning, duration of the activity, and intensity of the activity. Note that glycogen replenishment is more difficult if the athlete is not in a well-hydrated state.

It is also important to choose recovery foods that contain a wide variety of nutrients besides carbohydrate.[18] Protein, for instance, is an important component of recovery intake because it aids glycogen recovery. Athletes who have less than 8 hours between exercise bouts should optimize available eating time by snacking on high-carbohydrate, nutrient-rich foods immediately after the first workout session. Longer periods between exercise bouts afford greater flexibility in the eating pattern. Studies of carbohydrate consumption of several athlete groups have found differences in carbohydrate intakes. See table 1.6 for a summary of carbohydrate intakes—often inadequate—of athletes involved in different sports.

These data indicate that an athlete typically consumes between 5 and 10 grams of carbohydrate per kilogram of body mass, or between 20 and 40 kilocalories of carbohydrate per kilogram of body mass. A hypothetical 155-pound (70 kg) athlete would consume between 1,400 and 2,800 calories from carbohydrate, which represents far greater carbohydrate consumption than the DRI of 520 calories. Assuming this represents approximately 60 percent of total calories from carbohydrate, this athlete would consume a total of 2,300 to 4,700 kilocalories per day. Following the same logic, a 300-pound (136 kg) lineman on a football

Table 1.6 Carbohydrate Intakes of Different Athlete Groups*

Study reference	Sport	Moderate intake (g/kg)	High intake (g/kg)
Costill et al. 1988	Swimming	5.3	8.2
Lamb et al. 1990	Swimming	6.5	12.1
Kirwan et al. 1988	Running	3.9	8.0
Sherman et al. 1993	Running	5.0	10.0
Simonsen et al. 1991	Rowing	5.0	10.0
Sherman et al. 1993	Cycling	5.0	10.0

*Based on grams of carbohydrate per kilogram of body mass.

Adapted, by permission, from L.M. Burke, 2000, Dietary carbohydrates. In *Nutrition in sport*, edited by R.J. Maughan (Oxford: Blackwell Science), 82.

team would require 2,700 to 5,400 kilocalories just from carbohydrate each day, an amount that would be difficult to consume because carbohydrate has a relatively low energy density (i.e., only 4 kilocalories per gram). The generally recommended carbohydrate intake is based on the intensity and duration of exercise, with a higher requirement for greater duration and greater intensity. This should not be interpreted to mean it is acceptable for athletes involved in exercise of shorter duration and lower intensity to consume lower-carbohydrate diets. It is clear from a large body of evidence that, regardless of exercise discipline, all athletes do better when they routinely consume a relatively high-carbohydrate diet. See table 1.7 for examples of how much carbohydrate athletes should consume to optimize performance and recovery.

Most carbohydrates are derived from cereals, legumes, fruits, and vegetables. There is no discernible amount of carbohydrate in meats and only a small amount of carbohydrate in milk and cheese. A number of dairy products have sugars added (yogurt, ice cream) to make them more widely acceptable as sources of carbohydrate.

Table 1.7 Carbohydrate Requirement for Athletes

Activity or timing	Recommended intake	Example
Immediate recovery (0 to 4 hr) after exercise	1.2 g of carbohydrate per kg of body weight per hour (consumed at frequent intervals)	A 155 lb (70 kg) athlete would consume 70 g of carbohydrate (280 kcal) immediately after exercise, followed by an additional 70 g each hour for 4 hr.
Daily recovery from a moderate-duration, low-intensity training program	5 to 7 g of carbohydrate per kg of body weight per day	A 155 lb (70 kg) athlete would consume 350 to 490 g of carbohydrate (1,400 to 1,960 kcal) over the course of an entire day. (This amount includes the amount consumed for recovery immediately after exercise.)
Daily recovery from a moderate to heavy endurance training program	7 to 12 g of carbohydrate per kg of body weight per day	A 155 lb (70 kg) athlete would consume 490 to 840 g of carbohydrate (1,960 to 3,360 kcal) over the course of an entire day. (This amount includes the amount consumed for recovery immediately after exercise.)
Daily recovery from an extreme exercise program that includes 4+ hr per day	10 to 12 g of carbohydrate (or more) per kg of body weight per day	A 155 lb (70 kg) athlete would consume 700 to 840 g of carbohydrate (2,800 to 3,360 kcal) over the course of an entire day. (This amount includes the amount consumed for recovery immediately after exercise.)

Glycemic Index and Glycemic Load

The glycemic index is a numerical measure of how quickly consumed carbohydrates manifest themselves as blood glucose. Foods are compared with the ingestion of glucose, which enters the blood quickly because it requires no digestion and is readily absorbed. The higher the glycemic index number, the greater the blood sugar response to eating that food; the lower the glycemic index number, the lower the blood sugar response to eating that food. Glucose has a glycemic index score of 100, which is the basis of comparison for other foods. Foods are compared on an isocaloric basis (i.e., all providing the same number of calories), which is logical but is also the cause of some of the confusion associated with the glycemic index. For instance, carrots have a high glycemic index (>85), but the amount of carrots typically consumed is so low that the total calories of glucose from carrots entering the blood would be small.

Some foods have a surprisingly high glycemic index, while others are surprisingly low. Corn Flakes cereal, for instance, has a much higher glycemic index (84) than table sugar (65). When you assess the carbohydrate makeup of these two foods, however, it makes sense. The cereal grain in Corn Flakes is mainly composed of the disaccharide maltose, which is made of two glucose molecules. Table sugar, on the other hand, is made of sucrose, which is composed of one molecule of glucose and one molecule of fructose. The fructose must be converted by the liver to glucose, and this extra conversion slows the speed with which it manifests itself as blood glucose.

Because the volume of glucose and the speed at which it enters the blood can influence the amount of insulin produced, it is generally desirable for people to consume carbohydrate foods that have a medium to low glycemic index. (Glycemic index foods of ≥70 are considered high; 56 to 69 is considered medium; and ≤55 is considered low.) However, there are times, such as during and immediately after exercise, when high-glycemic foods might be better for athletes. See table 1.8 for examples of carbohydrate foods and their glycemic index and glycemic load.

Generally speaking, carbohydrate foods higher in fiber have a lower glycemic index, so they are good choices for athletes. However, dietary fiber may be a source of gas and distention, making them poor choices for consumption just before or during competition. Soluble fiber foods may create less of a problem, but athletes should experiment to determine which foods are most easily tolerated. See table 1.9 for a list of foods high in soluble and insoluble fiber. Athletes often find that starchy carbohydrates with low fiber concentrations, such as pasta, are the most easily tolerated and deliver the high volume of carbohydrates athletes require.

The amount of carbohydrate consumed also affects blood glucose levels and insulin responses. To account for this, the glycemic load of a food is calculated by multiplying the glycemic index by the amount of carbohydrate in grams provided by the food and dividing the total by 100. The dietary glycemic load represents the sum of the glycemic loads for all foods consumed in the diet.

Carbohydrates and Physical Activity

Because physical activity dramatically increases the rate of energy expenditure, athletes must strategize to best supply the needed energy to achieve success. It is critical for athletes to obtain sufficient energy intake to support total energy requirements, including

Table 1.8 Glycemic Index and Glycemic Load of Commonly Consumed Foods

Food	Typical food serving size	Glycemic index from 50 g (200 calories) of carbohydrate	Glycemic load (per typical serving)
Dates (dried)	2 oz (60 g)	103	42
Corn Flakes	1 cup	81	21
Jelly beans	1 oz (30 g)	78	22
Puffed rice cakes	3 cakes	78	17
Baked Russet potato	1 medium potato	76	23
Doughnut	1 medium doughnut	76	17
Soda crackers	4 crackers	74	12
White bread	1 large slice	73	10
Table sugar	2 tsp	68	7
Pancake	1 pancake, 6 in (15 cm) in diameter	67	39
White rice	1 cup	64	23
Brown rice	1 cup	55	18
White spaghetti	1 cup	44	18
Whole-wheat spaghetti	1 cup	37	14
Orange, raw	1 medium orange	42	5
Apple, raw	1 medium apple	38	6
All-Bran cereal	1 cup	38	9
Kidney beans, dried and boiled	1 cup	28	7
Pearled barley, boiled	1 cup	25	11
Peanuts	1 oz (30 g)	14	1

Note that table sugar has both a lower glycemic index and glycemic load than Corn Flakes, white bread, a baked potato, and rice cakes even though it is generally considered more of a problem in human health. This should not encourage people, however, to eat table sugar freely since it has no vitamins or minerals associated with it.

Adapted, by permission, from J. Higden, 2007, *An evidence-based approach to dietary phytochemicals* (New York: Thieme), 197. © Thieme Medical Publishers, Inc.

Table 1.9 Foods High in Soluble and Insoluble Fiber

Good sources of soluble fiber	Good sources of nonsoluble fiber
Bananas	Barley
Barley	Beets
Beans and legumes	Brussels sprouts
Carrots	Cabbage
Citrus fruits	Cauliflower
Oat bran	Fruits and vegetables with skin
Oatmeal	Rice (except for white rice)
Peas	Turnips
Rice bran	Wheat bran
Strawberries	Wheat cereal
Sweet potatoes	Whole-wheat breads

those for normal tissue maintenance, growth (in children and adolescents), tissue repair, and the energy requirements of the activity itself. It is impossible to discuss the ideal distribution of energy substrates without first conceptualizing how to best meet total energy needs. Although this may seem a logical and simple act, virtually all surveys have found that athletes fail to consume sufficient energy to fully satisfy their needs. This is much like planning to take a Ferrari on a 100-mile trip, and you appropriately put high-octane gas in the fuel tank—but only enough of it to go 80 miles. Despite the high quality of the fuel, the Ferrari just won't get there, and poorly fueled athletes will also have difficulties doing what's required to be optimally competitive. Once a strategy has been established for obtaining sufficient energy, then athletes and coaches can reasonably consider how to parse the energy into the optimal array of energy substrates: carbohydrate, protein, and fat. It is generally accepted that athletes should consume sufficient carbohydrate to meet the majority of their exercise-related energy needs and to restore muscle glycogen stores between exercise sessions.[18]

Ideally, athletes should consume complex carbohydrates (i.e., nonsugar carbohydrates) when possible but may consume simple carbohydrates during and immediately after exercise. Other energy substrates (protein and fat) should also be consumed to fulfill total nutrient requirements, but carbohydrate should remain the predominant energy source. The relatively low caloric density of carbohydrate (only 4 calories per gram compared with 9 calories per gram from fats) makes it difficult for athletes to consume sufficient energy and carbohydrate unless there is a well-established plan to do so. Athletes would do well to remember that training alone, without a sound and dynamically linked nutrition plan to support the training, will be self-limiting.

FAT

Fat is a highly concentrated source of energy, providing 9 calories per gram compared with carbohydrate and protein, which both provide 4 calories per gram. A small volume of fat, therefore, goes a long way toward increasing caloric delivery. There exists literature espousing the benefits of high fat intakes (i.e., intakes of 30 percent or more of total calories from fat), but there is no evidence to suggest that dietary fat does anything to improve athletic performance, body composition, or weight when consumed in excess. The adult AMDR for total fat intake is 20 to 35 percent of total calories, and there is no scientific information suggesting that more than 25 percent of total calories from fat is generally better for athletes. However, for athletes who have difficulty sustaining weight because of a massive energy expenditure (such as cross-country skiers) or because they must sustain high weights (such as football linemen and sumo wrestlers), higher fat intakes (up to the AMDR limit of 35 percent) may be useful for satisfying energy needs. Few Americans consume less than 35 percent of total calories from fat, so consumption of less fat is not easy, and unless steps are taken to provide sufficient energy from other substrates (mainly from more complex carbohydrates) to replace the eliminated fat, athletes may place themselves in an energy-deficit state that is, in itself, detrimental to performance. Therefore, while a reduction in fat intake is generally useful because it allows more carbohydrate and protein to be consumed to satisfy energy needs, a conscious effort should be made to provide enough total energy when fat intake is reduced. Since fat has more than twice the caloric concentration of either protein or carbohydrate, more than twice the volume of food must be consumed to make up the difference in reduced fat volume.

Cholesterol, oils, butter, and margarine are all fats, or lipids, but each has slightly different characteristics. The one common attribute shared by lipids is that they are soluble in organic solvents but not soluble in water. (Anyone who has tried to mix Italian dressing knows this to be true. The oil in the dressing eventually rises to the top, no matter how hard the bottle is shaken.) The term *fat* is usually applied to lipids that are solid at room temperature, and the term *oil* is applied to lipids that are liquid at room temperature. The most commonly consumed form of lipid is triglyceride, which consists of three fatty acids and one glycerol molecule (thus the name triglyceride). Despite the numerous forms of lipids, we can obtain them all from the food supply, and we are also capable of making many types of lipids by combining carbon units from other substances. Nearly every cell in the body has the capacity to make cholesterol, which is why a person can have a high blood cholesterol level even when on a low-cholesterol diet. In fact, blood cholesterol is more closely associated with fat intake than cholesterol intake for the following reason: The greater the fat consumed (regardless of type), the greater the emulsifying agent that must be produced to digest and absorb it. This emulsifying agent (bile) is 50 percent cholesterol, and this cholesterol is absorbed with the consumed fat, increasing the body's pool of cholesterol. Besides our ability to manufacture cholesterol, we can also manufacture phospholipids, triglycerides, and oils. In fact, it is this ability to effectively manufacture different types of lipids that limits the necessity to consume large amounts of dietary lipids.

Fat Functions

A certain amount of fat, between 20 and 35 percent of total consumed calories, is necessary to ensure a sufficient energy and nutrient intake. The fat-soluble vitamins—vitamins A, D, E, and K—must be delivered in a fat package. Linoleic acid, an essential fatty acid, is needed for specific body functions and must be consumed because we are incapable of synthesizing it. Some dietary fat is also needed to give us a feeling of satiety during a meal, creating the important physiological signal that it is time to stop eating. Dietary fats have a longer gastric emptying time than do carbohydrates, which contributes to the feeling of satiety with dietary fats. Of course, fat also makes foods taste good.

Different types of fats deliver different kinds of fatty acids. Linoleic acid (an omega-6 fatty acid, meaning the double bond in the carbon chain is at the sixth carbon) and omega-3 fatty acids (the double bond is at the third carbon) contribute to good health when they are in a ratio of 3 to 1 (omega-6 to omega-3). Omega-3 fatty acids have certain attributes that may be beneficial to athletes by reducing muscle and joint inflammation (more on this later in the chapter).

Lipid Structure

Lipids have different levels of saturation, a term that refers to the number of double bonds in the carbon chain. Fatty acids with no double bonds are saturated, those with one double bond are monounsaturated, and those with more than one double bond are polyunsaturated. Single bonds are stronger and less chemically reactive than double bonds, so the greater the number of double bonds, the greater the opportunity for the fatty acid to react with its chemical environment. It is this differential reactive capacity that makes the number of double bonds an important factor in human nutrition.

Saturated fatty acids are most prevalent in fats of animal origin, palm kernel oil, and coconut oil. Monounsaturated fats are highest in olive oil and canola oil but are also present in fats of animal origin. Polyunsaturated fats are highest in vegetable oils (with the exception of olive oil, which is more than 75 percent monounsaturated). For reducing health risks, it is desirable to consume more polyunsaturated and monounsaturated fatty acids than saturated fatty acids. Saturated fats are associated with higher cholesterol levels, so they should be minimized when possible. This is most easily achieved by reducing the consumption of animal fats, chocolate candies (often high in saturated tropical oils), fried foods, and high-fat dairy products. Modifying the source of fats while sustaining a high intake of fats does not have a desirable impact on health. Most people, including the vast majority of athletes, would do well to reduce the total intake of fats and, of the fats consumed, have a greater proportion of mono- and polyunsaturated fatty acids. In simple terms this means avoiding most fried foods, high-fat dairy products and other animal fats, and processed meats and consuming more fresh fruits, fresh vegetables, and whole-grain cereals.

Triglycerides

The majority of consumed lipids are triglycerides, which contain three fatty acids and a glycerol molecule (see figure 1.5). Fat is stored in the form of triglycerides, which we manufacture when excess energy is consumed. We store triglycerides in adipose tissues (groups of fat cells) and inside muscle cells (intramuscular triglyceride), both of which are available as an energy source when needed, but the intramuscular triglyceride is more immediately available. When fat is burned as a source of energy, the stored triglycerides are taken out of storage, and each molecule is cleaved into its component fatty acids and glycerol molecule. Each fatty acid can then be broken apart (two carbon units at a time) and thrown into the cellular furnaces (mitrochondria) for the creation of ATP to form heat and provide the energy for muscular work. This process is referred to as the beta-oxidative metabolic pathway because burning fat, besides requiring some carbohydrate for its complete oxidation, also requires oxygen. Unlike carbohydrate, which can be metabolized aerobically (with oxygen) or anaerobically (without oxygen), fatty acids can only be metabolized aerobically.

Glycerol is a unique lipid that is burned like a carbohydrate rather than a fat and is also an effective humectant (it holds water). Some long-endurance athletes have found that adding

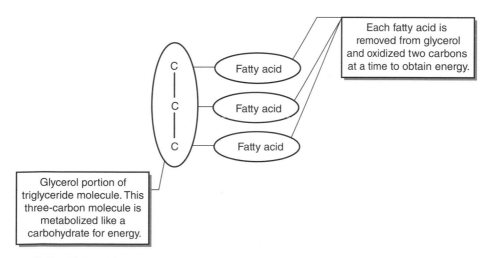

Figure 1.5 Triglyceride structure.

glycerol to water helps them retain more water (i.e., to superhydrate) than if they consumed water alone. In an extremely hot and humid environment, water loss is likely to be higher than the athlete's fluid-replacement capacity, so beginning a competition in a superhydrated state may provide some advantages. In studies of tennis athletes and Olympic-distance triathletes, those who consumed glycerol in water before competition experienced some protective hyperhydration benefits when exercising in high heat.[22,23] However, the World Anti-Doping Agency (WADA) has recently placed glycerol on the prohibited list, so it should not be consumed by athletes competing in sanctioned events. It should also be noted that being superhydrated is likely to impart a degree of discomfort that requires adaptation. Athletes who consume fluids containing glycerol often describe the feeling of holding extra body water as making them feel "like a water bag," "heavy," or "stiff."

Essential Fatty Acids

Linoleic (omega-6) and linolenic (omega-3) fatty acids are the essential fatty acids. As with all nutrients carrying the *essential* label, they are required for metabolic processes but we are incapable of synthesizing them, so they must be consumed in the foods we eat. The omega-6 classification means these fatty acids, which are polyunsaturated, have their final double bond six carbons from the end of the carbon chain. The omega-3 classification means these fatty acids have their last double bond three carbons from the end of the carbon chain. Linoleic acid is an essential part of lipid membranes and is required for normal skin health. Linolenic acid is necessary for neural function and growth. The AMDR for omega-6 fatty acids is 5 to 10 percent of total calories (11 to 22 grams per day); and for omega-3 fatty acids, 0.6 to 1.2 percent of total calories or (1.3 to 2.6 grams per day).[13] Both fatty acids are easily obtained from vegetable oils (e.g., corn, safflower, canola) and the oils of fatty cold-water fish.

Some attention has been given to the potential benefits of omega-3 fatty acids for athletic performance. According to Bucci, these potential benefits include the following:

- Improved delivery of oxygen and nutrients to muscles and other tissues because of reduced blood viscosity
- Improved aerobic metabolism because of enhanced delivery of oxygen to cells
- Improved release of somatotropin (growth hormone) in response to normal stimuli, such as exercise, sleep, and hunger, which may have an anabolic effect or improve postexercise recovery time
- Reduction of inflammation caused by muscular fatigue and overexertion, which may improve postexercise recovery time
- Possible prevention of tissue inflammation

There is also evidence that omega-3 supplementation from fish oil is useful for reducing the severity of exercise-induced bronchoconstriction (EIB) in elite athletes. In general, studies evaluating the effectiveness of omega-3 fatty acids do not show consistent improvements in strength and endurance, nor is there consistent evidence that omega-3 fatty acids reduce muscle soreness.[27-29] The major impact of omega-3 fatty acid consumption appears to be a possible enhancement of aerobic metabolic processes, which is an important factor in both athletic performance and the ability to effectively burn fat as an energy substrate. These oils have also been shown to reduce the ability of red blood cells to congregate, thereby decreasing the chance of unwanted blood clots. This reduces the risk of heart attack, which is most commonly caused by a clot formation in one of the major heart arteries. This should not suggest that an increase in total fat consumption is either desirable or necessary to obtain these benefits. On the contrary, higher fat intakes are typically associated with reduced athletic performance. However, athletes might consider altering the types of fats consumed by including periodic but regular 4- to 5-ounce (125 to 150 gram) servings of salmon, albacore tuna, Atlantic herring, and other cold-water fish in their diets to increase the proportion of omega-3 fatty acids available to them. Even a once-weekly consumption of cold-water fish is sufficient to significantly reduce the risk of heart attack and stroke.[11] Another recommended standard of omega-3 fatty acid intake for athletes is approximately 1 to 2 grams per day.

Ideally, the ratio of omega-6 to omega-3 fatty acids should be 3 to 1. Most Western diets have a ratio of omega-6 to omega-3 fatty acids that is too high and may compromise health. While not evident in the AMDR, there is a generally accepted understanding that improving the ratio of omega-3 to omega-6 fatty acids (with a greater emphasis on the omega-3 fatty acids) may serve to reduce illness risk.

Good food sources of omega-6 fatty acids include the following:

- Sunflower oil
- Safflower oil
- Corn oil
- Sesame oil
- Hemp oil
- Pumpkin oil
- Soybean oil
- Walnut oil
- Wheat germ oil

Omega-3 fatty acids can be obtained from high-fat cold-water fish (EPA, DHA) and also from certain seeds and nuts. Food sources of omega-3 fatty acids include the following:

- Eicosapentaenoic acid (EPA), from fish
- Docosahexaenoic acid (DHA), from fish
- Alpha-linolenic acid (ALA), from
    - seeds and nuts
    - flaxseed and flaxseed oil
    - soybeans and soybean oil
    - walnuts
    - brazil nuts

Fat Requirements

From an exercise standpoint, there is no reason to believe that increasing fat consumption results in improving athletic performance, unless the increase in fat intake is the only reasonable means for the athlete to obtain sufficient energy. For the athlete who needs more than 4,000 calories each day to meet the combined demands of growth, exercise, and tissue maintenance, moderate increases in dietary fat (preferably from plant and fish sources) may be needed. Since fat is a more concentrated form of energy than either carbohydrate or protein, more energy can be consumed in a smaller food package if the foods contain more fat. If an athlete tries to restrict fat completely, a much higher volume would need to be consumed (carbohydrate and protein have less than half the energy density of fat), making it difficult to schedule enough meals or enough time during meals to consume the needed energy. The outcome in this case would be an inadequate energy intake, which has its own set of negative consequences.

Lipids and Physical Activity

Even the leanest, healthiest athletes have a substantial energy pool of stored lipids. The average storage in adipose tissue ranges between 50,000 and 100,000 calories, or enough energy to theoretically walk or run 500 to 1,000 miles (800 to 1,600 kilometers) without a refueling stop. (The typical energy cost of walking or running 1 mile [1.6 km] is approximately 100 calories.) In addition, athletes store approximately 2,000 to 3,000 calories of lipids inside the muscle tissue. These triglyceride lipids are available as a fuel under the proper conditions of oxygen and oxidative enzyme availability. As a percentage of total calories, maximal fat oxidation occurs at 60 to 65 percent of $\dot{V}O_2$max, but a significant proportion of energy utilization from fat remains at even higher levels of $\dot{V}O_2$max.

Triglycerides stored in adipose tissue are cleaved into their component molecules of glycerol and fatty acids and transported to the blood plasma. The glycerol is available to all tissues for energy metabolism, and the free fatty acids are transported to working muscles where they are oxidized for energy. The glycerol can also be burned for energy in the working muscle or can be transported to the blood plasma as a source of energy for other tissues. Glycerol is a unique simple lipid in that it can be converted to sugar by the liver to help sustain blood sugar. It is, in fact, the only lipid that is metabolized like a carbohydrate.

The lower the exercise intensity, the greater the proportion of fat burned to satisfy energy needs. As exercise intensity increases, the proportion of fat burned decreases and the proportion of carbohydrate burned increases. It is this basic reality that explains why so many people perform low-intensity activities to burn fat and lower body-fat levels. However, the proportion of fat burned should not be confused with the total volume of fat burned at different intensities of physical activity. As exercise intensity increases, the total number of calories burned per unit of time also increases. Although there may be a decrease in the proportion of fat burned to satisfy total energy needs in higher-intensity activity, the total volume of fat burned is greater because the total energy requirement is higher (see figure 1.4 on page 14). The takeaway message from this metabolic reality is that athletes interested in lowering body fat should exercise at least as high as 65 percent of $\dot{V}O_2$max for the duration of their workouts to optimize the total mass of fat that is burned. Exercising at lower intensities burns a greater proportion of fat but a lower volume of fat than exercising at higher intensities.

Athlete Conditioning and Metabolizing Fat

Improving athletic endurance through a program of endurance training increases both the size and number of mitochondria (and related oxidative enzymes) inside cells, which increases the capacity of the athlete to use a greater amount of fat during physical activity. Since athletes store far more fat calories than carbohydrate calories, increasing the ability to use fat induces a proportionate reduction of carbohydrate reliance, thereby increasing endurance. Put simply, if you can burn a greater volume of fat at higher exercise intensities, you can make your carbohydrate stores last longer so that your endurance is improved (see figure 1.6).

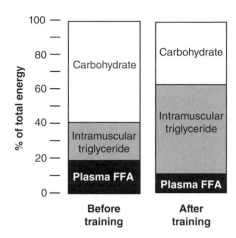

Figure 1.6 Change in fat reliance after endurance training.

Adapted from W.H. Martin, G.P. Dalsky, B.F. Hurley, et al., 1993, "Effect of endurance training on plasma free fatty acid turnover and oxidation during exercise," *American Journal of Physiology: Endocrinology and Metabolism* 265(5): E708-714. Used with permission of the American Physiological Society.

It is important to note, however, that fat oxidation cannot be improved to the point of eliminating the need for carbohydrate (blood sugar, liver glycogen, and muscle glycogen) during intense exercise. Also, a greater ability to metabolize fat for energy should not motivate an athlete to increase the proportionate intake of fat. Assuming an adequate caloric intake, athletes can manufacture and store the fat they need, and higher intakes of dietary fat are a clear risk factor in atherosclerotic heart disease. Even a short-term increase in fat intake with a concomitant decrease in carbohydrate intake for only 3 to 5 days leads to a reduction in endurance performance when compared with a high carbohydrate intake.

Medium-Chain Triglycerides (MCTs)

There is conflicting evidence that medium-chain triglyceride (MCT) oil (triglycerides with fatty acid chains that range from 6 to 12 carbon atoms) may have certain beneficial attributes for athletes. MCT oil is directly absorbed and rapidly catabolized into fatty acids and glycerol. It is easily and quickly oxidized for energy and appears to mimic the effects of carbohydrate metabolism rather than fat metabolism. There is also some evidence that it enhances the movement of fats from storage to be burned as energy, and it may also increase the rate at which energy is burned (i.e., a higher energy metabolism).[33-36] In a study assessing the relative impact of carbohydrate versus carbohydrate plus MCT oil on cycling time-trial performance, carbohydrate improved performance on the 100-kilometer distance, but the addition of MCT oil did not further improve performance. However, another study suggests that the timing of MCT oil consumption is an important factor in endurance performance. Consumption of 400 milliliters (13.5 ounces) of a 3.44 percent MCT oil solution before the time trial, plus a 10 percent glucose solution during the time trial, was associated with improved performance over the time-trial distance. It was concluded that a reduced reliance on glycogen and an enhanced reliance on fat (MCT oil) was responsible for this observed performance enhancement. By contrast, a study of regular MCT oil consumption neither improved endurance nor altered energy metabolism in well-trained male runners.

Importantly, there is some evidence that MCT oil supplementation may adversely alter the blood lipid concentrations, which should be seriously considered in athletes with family histories of heart disease.

MCT oil consumption may offer an advantage for athletes having difficulty sustaining a desirable body composition. Healthy people who consume 5 to 10 grams (45 to 90 calories) of MCT oil experience a greater diet-induced thermogenesis (i.e., energy expenditure) than after the equivalent consumption of long-chain triglycerides (the most common form of fat found in foods), and this higher thermogenesis may stimulate weight loss.[41,42]

Although it does not exist in concentrated amounts in any food, MCT oil is available in many stores and, because it is saturated, it is stable and has a long shelf life. For athletes who find it difficult to consume sufficient total energy, consumption of 2 to 3 tablespoons (30 to 45 ml) of MCT oil may prove to be beneficial. MCT oil is burned differently than other fats, so taking this small amount could, in theory, be a good strategy to ensure that athletes who have difficulty taking in enough calories can meet their needs.

Please note that the maximum consumption of MCT oil for most athletes is 30 grams (270 calories) during a single feeding. Exceeding this amount dramatically increases the risk of developing GI distress, including diarrhea. Another guideline for MCT oil consumption is to not exceed a daily dose of 1.5 grams per kilogram divided into at least three doses to limit the risk of diarrhea. MCT oil, while potentially useful, has some inherent limitations related to its potential contribution to total energy intake.

PROTEIN

Many athletes consider protein to be the key to athletic success. It is difficult to find athletes (especially power athletes) who can resist consuming some form of protein supplement, and of those who do take supplements, most are convinced their successes are substantially attributable to the extra protein. In fact, most athletes consume more protein than they require and, in doing so, may limit the intake of other essential nutrients that are critical to achieving athletic success. In addition, there is increasing evidence that the pattern of protein intake during the day may be an important factor in how well the consumed protein can successfully be used anabolically. Nevertheless, few athletes consider the within-day intake pattern as an important issue. Put simply, eating too much of any nutrient, including protein, translates into eating less of another nutrient that may be equally important; and eating too much of a nutrient at once fails to optimize the nutrient's utilization.

Endurance athletes, who may appear thin and less muscular than power athletes, actually have a protein requirement that is nearly equivalent (per unit of body weight) to that of power athletes. Some studies suggest that endurance athletes have an even higher protein requirement than power athletes (per unit of body weight) because they burn a small amount of protein as part of their normal endurance activities.[45,46] By contrast, power athletes typically consume a great deal more protein than they need and, to make matters worse, many consume protein powders or amino acid supplements to increase protein intake still further. Considering that a single ounce of meat provides about 7,000 milligrams of high-quality amino acids and that a typical amino acid supplement provides between 500 and 1,000 milligrams, few of the protein intake strategies that many athletes follow are logical. Additionally, many of these supplements are far more expensive than the food equivalent.

Protein Functions

Consumed proteins are digested into amino acids, and these amino acids join other amino acids produced by the body to constitute the amino acid pool. (See figure 1.7 for an illustration of amino acid structure.) The tissues take the amino acids from this pool to synthesize the specific proteins the body needs (muscle, hair, nails, hormones, enzymes, and so on). This amino acid pool is also available for use as energy (via a deamination process) to be burned if other fuels (carbohydrate and fat) cannot satisfy energy needs.

The major functions of protein include the following:

1. Protein provides a source of carbon for energy-yielding reactions. Certain amino acids can be converted to glucose and metabolized to provide ATP, and amino acids can also be stored as fat that can subsequently be catabolized to provide ATP.

2. Protein is a critical compound in controlling fluid volume and osmolarity in the blood and body tissues. This function is a major controlling factor in maintaining water balance.

3. Proteins are amphoteric (substances with the capacity to behave as either an acid or a base), with the capacity to buffer both acid and alkaline environments to maintain an optimal blood pH. Antibodies are protein-based substances critical for maintaining health.

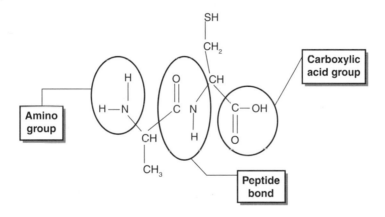

Example: Chemical structure of alanine (Note: Two alanine molecules can be combined with the nitrogen removed to make glucose in the liver via the glucose-alanine cycle. The process of making new glucose is referred to as *gluconeogenesis*).

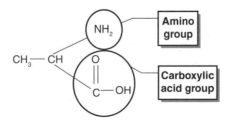

Figure 1.7 Typical structure of amino acids.

4. Proteins form enzymes that are involved in digestive and other cellular processes that create needed chemical end products.

5. Proteins are a critical component of body tissues, including the organs (heart, liver, pancreas, and so on), muscles, and bones.

6. Proteins are "smart" transporters of substances in the blood, moving substances to the correct receptor sites. For instance, transferrin is the protein transporter for iron.

7. Proteins are synthesized into specific hormones (such as insulin) and neurotransmitters (such as serotonin) that control body function.

See table 1.10 for a summary of amino acid and protein functions.

Table 1.10 Amino Acid and Protein Functions

Working proteins (produce hemoglobin, enzymes, and hormones; maintain normal blood osmolarity; form antibodies; used as energy source)	Enzymes
	Antibodies
	Transport proteins
	Hormones
Structural proteins (constitute cell structure; help develop, repair, and maintain tissues)	Muscles, tendons, ligaments
	Skin
	Bone and teeth cores
	Hair and nails

Protein Metabolism

Protein is composed of carbon, hydrogen, oxygen, nitrogen, and, in some cases, sulfur. Protein is the only nutrient that contains nitrogen, a fact that makes it both essential and potentially toxic. Amino acid building blocks constitute the larger molecular structures of protein. Some of these amino acids can be synthesized from other amino acids (referred to as nonessential amino acids), while some must be obtained from the foods we eat (referred to as essential amino acids—that is, it is essential that we get them from our diets). There is widespread confusion about essential and nonessential amino acids because the word *nonessential* suggests that, although they are present, they are not really needed. This, however, could not be further from the truth. Both the essential and nonessential amino acids are equally important in human metabolic processes. See table 1.11 for a list of the essential and nonessential amino acids.

Individual amino acids combine to make larger proteins. The sequence of the amino acids and the secondary and tertiary structures of the protein determine protein function. When dietary protein is consumed, it is digested into polypeptides (small protein molecules) and eventually into individual amino acids. The amino acids are absorbed into the blood and transported to different tissues, where they are manufactured into necessary proteins. Tissues manufacture the proteins that are needed through the amino acids available to them. To ensure that the tissues are capable of manufacturing needed proteins, the essential amino acids must simultaneously be present for protein synthesis to take place. Some

Table 1.11 Nonessential and Essential Amino Acids

Nonessential amino acids (can be synthesized by humans from fragments of other amino acids)		Essential amino acids (cannot be synthesized by humans; must be obtained from consumed foods)	
Amino acid	Abbreviation	Amino acid	Abbreviation
Alanine	Ala	Histidine[a]	His
Arginine[CE]	Arg	Isoleucine[BC]	Ile
Asparagine	Asn	Leucine[BC]	Leu
Aspartic acid	Asp	Lysine	Lys
Cysteine[CE]	Cys	Methionine	Met
Glutamic acid	Glu	Phenylalanine	Phe
Glutamine[CE]	Gln	Threonine	Thr
Glycine[CE]	Gly	Tryptophan	Trp
Proline[CE]	Pro	Valine[BC]	Val
Serine	Ser		
Tyrosine[CE]	Tyr		

BC = branched-chain amino acid.

CE = conditionally essential amino acid (it may be necessary to consume these amino acids under certain metabolic conditions).

[a]Histidine, unlike the other eight essential amino acids, does not induce a protein-deficient state (i.e., negative nitrogen balance) when removed from the diet.

Source: National Academy of Sciences, 2005, *Dietary reference intakes for energy, carbohydrate, fiber, fat, fatty acids, cholesterol, protein, and amino acids (macronutrients)* (Washington, DC: National Academies Press), 591, 593.

people believe that if you want healthy looking hair and nails, you should consume the primary protein that hair and nails are made of (gelatin). Gelatin is a low-quality protein with a poor distribution of the essential amino acids, so it would not encourage an optimal protein synthesis of any needed protein. Put simply, eating hair and nails does not encourage optimal synthesis of hair and nails. The best way to ensure an optimal synthesis of needed proteins is to make all the essential amino acids available to cells at the same time so they are capable of making whatever they need.

The liver is the central processing unit for protein synthesis, continually monitoring protein needs and synthesizing amino acids and proteins to satisfy a variety of needs. This protein synthesis is accomplished through transamination and deamination reactions. In transamination, the nitrogen from one amino acid is used for the manufacture of another amino acid; in deamination, the amino group is removed from an amino acid and converted to ammonia (see figure 1.8). The remaining carbon structure is reconstructed as fat and stored, or converted to glucose (as happens with the amino acids alanine and glutamine), or burned for energy. Once all protein needs are met, the fate of all remaining amino acids is deamination. The ammonia created during deamination is toxic to the body, but enzymes in the liver convert the ammonia to urea. Urea is excreted from the body in the urine. Therefore, the greater the extra protein consumed, the greater the production of ammonia that must be removed from the system (as urea). The majority of the remaining deaminated carbon chains are typically stored as fat.

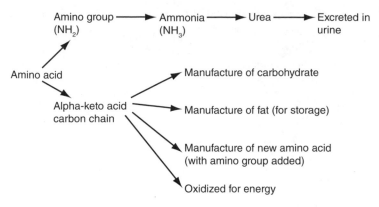

Figure 1.8 Deamination and the reconstruction of the remaining carbon structure.

Several amino acids have specific effects on the central nervous system (see table 1.12). Because of these known effects, single amino acids are sold with the purpose of imparting these known outcomes. Tryptophan, for instance, is sold as an agent that causes relaxation or sleepiness. The dangers, however, of pushing high doses of single amino acids into the system are sufficiently large that this should not be done unless under the careful supervision of a physician. The best strategy is to supply the widest possible array of essential amino acids from food alone, which allows the individual tissues to synthesize the amino acids needed for optimal body function.

Table 1.12 Amino Acids With Neurotransmitter Products and Functions

Amino acid	Product	Function
Tryptophan	Serotonin Melatonin	Mood, pain, food intake, arousal
Tyrosine Phenylalanine	Dopamine Norepinephrine Epinephrine	Motor function, mood, arousal, attention, anxiety
Histidine	Histamine	Food intake, arousal, thermoregulation
Arginine	Nitric oxide	Arousal, anxiety, memory
Threonine	Glycine	Motor function

Protein Quality

Many high-quality proteins contain all the essential amino acids in a distribution that aids cellular protein synthesis (i.e., proteins with a high biological value). The two common methods for determining protein quality are (1) calculating the proportion of nitrogen retained (the greater the proportion of nitrogen retained, the greater the protein utilization and, therefore, the higher the protein quality) and (2) comparing the protein against egg protein (albumin), which is known to have a near perfect distribution of essential amino acids.

The following food lists show protein quality using method 1 (the percentage of nitrogen retained, from most to least) and method 2 (the degree to which the food protein compares to egg protein).[48,49] Both lists are from high to low protein quality.

Percentage of Nitrogen Retained

- Whey protein: 96 percent
- Whole soybean: 96 percent
- Chicken egg: 94 percent
- Soybean milk: 91 percent
- Cow milk: 90 percent
- Cheese: 84 percent
- Rice: 83 percent
- Fish: 76 percent
- Beef: 74.3 percent
- Soybean curd (tofu): 64 percent
- Whole-wheat flour: 64 percent
- White flour: 41 percent

Protein Quality Compared to Whole Egg

- Whey protein concentrate: 104
- Whole egg: 100
- Cow milk: 91
- Beef: 80
- Casein: 77
- Soy: 74
- Wheat gluten: 64

Protein Requirements

Protein yields approximately 4 calories per gram, which is the same energy concentration as carbohydrate. The recommended level of protein intake for the general population is 12 to 15 percent of total calories. Therefore, someone consuming 2,000 calories per day has an energy equivalent of 240 to 300 calories (60 to 75 grams) of protein per day. A better way of predicting protein need is to base the requirement on grams of protein per kilogram of body mass per day (g/kg). Most nonathletes do well with .8 gram of protein per kilogram of body weight. Using this guideline, a 165-pound (75 kg) nonathlete has a protein requirement of 60 grams per day. On a per kilogram basis, athletes typically have a higher protein requirement because of a greater lean mass per unit of weight (i.e., a lower body-fat percentage), a greater need for tissue repair, and the small amount of protein burned as a source of fuel during physical activity. This increases the protein requirement for athletes to approximately double that of nonathletes (approximately 1.5 grams per kilogram, with a typical requirement range of between 1.2 and 1.7 grams per kilogram). Therefore, a 165-pound (75 kg) athlete may have a protein requirement of 120 grams (480 calories) per day. Although 120 grams of daily protein may seem high, it represents a relatively small proportion of total daily calories and is easily obtained by following the Dietary Guidelines for Americans (2010). These guidelines focus on the premise that nutrient needs can and should be met mainly through food consumption. By comparison, the average recommended intake for carbohydrate is about 7.5 grams per kilogram (30 calories of carbohydrate per kilogram of body weight), ranging from 5 to 12 grams per kilogram, so this 165-pound athlete would have a requirement of 2,250 calories from carbohydrate alone. See table 1.13 for the protein content of a typical 2,000-calorie meal plan.

Table 1.13 Protein Content of a 2,000-Calorie Meal Plan

Food	Amount	Calories	Protein (g)
Orange juice	8 oz (240 ml)	112	1.7
Bread, whole-wheat, toasted	2 thick slices	171	9.1
Jam, strawberry	1 tablespoon	56	0.1
Egg, whole, large, boiled	1 large egg	71	6.3
Roast beef sandwich: Roast beef, lean Whole wheat bread Mayonnaise	 2 ounces 2 regular slices 1 tablespoon	 92 138 93	 16.3 7.3 0.1
Milk, 1% fat	8 oz (240 ml)	103	8.2
Apple, raw	1 medium apple	95	0.5
Tossed vegetable salad	3 cups	66	5.2
Ranch salad dressing	1 tablespoon	73	0.2
Chocolate chip cookies	1 ounce (3 small)	120	1.5
Sports beverage	16 oz (480 ml)	127	0.0
Chicken breast, no skin, baked	1/2 breast	138	24.7
Broccoli, boiled	1 medium stalk	63	4.3
Baked potato	1 medium potato	160	4.3
French bread	1 large slice	185	7.5
Ice cream, vanilla	1/2 cup	137	2.3
Totals		**2,000**	**99.6**

Note: A 120-pound athlete requires approximately 1.5 grams of protein per kilogram of body weight. To convert pounds to kilograms, divide pounds by 2.2 (120/2.2 = 55 kg). Then multiply kilograms by 1.5 (55 x 1.5 = 82.5). The protein requirement for this 120-pound athlete is 82.5 grams (330 calories). The protein provided by this 2,000-calorie meal plan provides 99.6 grams of protein, which is almost 17 grams more than this athlete requires.

Athletes require a higher protein intake than nonathletes for a number of reasons:

- Amino acids (from protein) contribute 5 to 15 percent of the fuel burned during exercise. The amount of protein used for energy rises as muscle glycogen decreases. It is generally thought that endurance exercise is more glycogen depleting than power exercise, so endurance activities are likely to result in a higher proportionate usage of protein.
- Exercise may cause muscle damage, which increases the protein requirement for tissue repair.
- Endurance exercise may cause a small amount of protein to be lost in the urine (where there is typically none or very little without exercise).

Despite the increased protein requirement for athletes, most athletes consume much more protein (from food alone) than they require. A look at the protein content of some commonly consumed foods demonstrates this point. Although most athletes have no difficulty consuming sufficient protein, the following groups of athletes should monitor protein intake carefully because it may be difficult for them to get enough:

- Young athletes who have the combined demands of muscular work and growth
- Athletes who are restricting food intake in an attempt to achieve a desirable weight or body profile
- Vegetarian athletes who do not eat meat, fish, eggs, or dairy foods
- Athletes who restrict food intake for religious or cultural reasons

Although we can derive energy (calories) from protein, doing so is a bit like sprinkling the family diamonds on your breakfast cereal because you think it improves the texture. It is a complete waste of valuable resources. Protein is so important for building and maintaining tissues and for making hormones and enzymes that burning it up as a fuel could and should be considered wasteful. To complicate matters, when protein is burned as a fuel, the nitrogen must be removed from the amino acid chains and excreted. This elevated nitrogenous excretion requires a concomitant increase in the amount of water lost as urine. Thus, two undesirable things occur: You waste valuable protein by burning it up, and you increase the risk of dehydration because of the increased volume of water that is lost when nitrogenous wastes are excreted. In addition, high-protein diets are shown to increase the excretion of calcium in the urine, which must be considered a clear health risk for anyone who may already be at risk of bone disease from other causes (e.g., low estrogen, inactivity, inadequate vitamin D, insufficient calcium). Another potential problem is that high-protein diets tend to also be high in fat, which may increase cardiovascular disease risk. Therefore, the best way to make certain your protein needs are met without consuming an excess is to consume a sufficient amount of food that focuses on complex carbohydrates but also contains regularly dispersed amounts of dairy products and meats (or plenty of legumes if you're a vegetarian). See table 1.14 for a list of plant sources of protein.

Table 1.14 Plant Sources of Protein

Source	Examples
Grains	Barley Bulgur Corn Oats Pasta Rice
Legumes	Dried beans Dried peas Lentils Soybeans
Seeds and nuts	Brazil nuts Cashews Peanuts Sesame seeds Walnuts
Vegetables (much poorer source of protein than other sources listed above)	Broccoli Carrots Potatoes Tomatoes

Protein and Physical Activity

Protein utilization is, to a large degree, a function of total energy intake adequacy. An inadequate total energy intake forces athletes to burn protein for energy, making less protein available for other critical functions. Therefore, the protein requirement for athletes (i.e., 12 to 15 percent of total calories or 1.2 to 1.7 grams per kilogram) is based on the assumption that total energy intake is adequate.

A standard tenet in nutrition is that carbohydrate has a protein-sparing effect. This means if you can supply sufficient carbohydrate to the system for fuel, then protein will be spared from being burned so it can be used for more important functions. Studies have generally found that the maximal rate of protein utilization for nonenergy uses is approximately 1.5 grams of protein per kilogram of body weight.[45-47] If this amount is exceeded, body tissues must make some decisions about what to do with the excess. The excess can be stored as fat, or some of the excess can be burned as energy. In either case, nitrogen must be removed from the amino acids, and this nitrogenous waste must be removed from the body. Virtually all studies that have looked at the total energy consumption of athletes indicate that athletes consume less total energy than they should to support the combined needs of activity, growth, and tissue maintenance. Since burning protein causes a large amount of metabolic waste, it would be better to meet the total energy requirement by satisfying much of it through provision of a cleaner-burning fuel—carbohydrate.

A goal for most athletes is to remain in a nitrogen-balanced state in which as much nitrogen is coming into the system as is being excreted. A negative nitrogen balance suggests that more nitrogen is being excreted than is being consumed, a state that will inevitably lead to muscle loss. A positive nitrogen balance suggests that more nitrogen is being retained than is being excreted, a state suggesting that muscle is being gained. The amount of protein required to maintain a nitrogen-balanced state in nonathlete adults has been well studied and established at the level of .8 gram of protein per kilogram of body weight per day, while for athletes an intake of between 1.2 and 1.7 grams of protein per kilogram of body weight per day is needed. Both the athlete and nonathlete recommendations are based on the consumption of a total caloric intake that satisfies energy needs.

The higher protein recommendation for athletes is based on four factors described earlier, including more lean body mass, a greater loss of protein in urine, protein burned for energy, and protein needed for muscle repair.[45-47] Table 1.15 shows the protein requirements of physically active people.

Table 1.15 Protein Requirements of Physically Active People

| Athlete type | Total energy (cal/day) | Protein | | |
		g/kg/day	g/day	Percentage of total cal/day
Endurance[a,b]	3,800	1.2-1.4	84-98	9-10
Strength[a,c]	3,200	1.6-1.7	112-119	14-15

[a]Assumes a resting energy expenditure of 40 cal/kg of body weight per day.

[b]Assumes a male runner who runs 10 miles/day (16 km/day) at a 6 min/mile pace.

[c]Assumes an additional cost of 6 cal/kg of body weight per day for heavy resistance training.

Reprinted, by permission, from M.J. Gibala, 2002, "Dietary protein, amino acid supplements, and recovery from exercise," *GSSI Sports Science Exchange* #87 15(4). [Online]. Available: www.gssiweb.com/Article_Detail.aspx?articleid=602 [June 16, 2011].

The Institute of Medicine has stated that additional protein for healthy adults who exercise regularly is not needed because exercise increases protein retention. Nevertheless, both the American College of Sports Medicine and the American Dietetic Association recommend that protein intakes range between 1.2 and 1.7 grams per kilogram of body weight in physically active people. In reality, most athletes consume far more protein than they require, and typically more than the maximum recommended level of 1.7 grams per kilogram. Some strength and power athletes regularly consume 300 to 775 percent of the recommended level of protein for the general public (.8 gram per kilogram).[53,54] Possible exceptions to high protein intakes may occur among vegetarian athletes and athletes in subjectively judged sports who strive to maintain low body weights (e.g., gymnasts, divers, figure skaters).

Protein oxidation during intense short-term exercise is insignificant, but protein provides from 3 to 5 percent of total energy needs during endurance exercise.[55,56] Protein utilization during exercise will rise to a level greater than 5 percent of total energy needs if glycogen levels are low, blood sugar is low, exercise intensity is high, or exercise duration is long.

High-protein foods have a long gastric emptying time so are not recommended immediately before or during exercise. In addition, there is no evidence that adding protein to a glucose- and sodium-containing sports beverage does anything useful for either endurance or power enhancement. In fact, protein added to a sports beverage that is consumed during competition increases the risk of gastrointestinal distress and may delay the delivery of fluids and carbohydrate to needy muscles. Protein added to a sports beverage reduces the content of what athletes really need: fluid, carbohydrate, and electrolytes. Therefore, the majority of energy in the preexercise meal and during exercise fluid replacement should be from carbohydrate.

An increasing body of evidence suggests that adding small amounts of protein to postexercise food and drink is useful for muscle recovery, although the benefit of protein is reduced if sufficient carbohydrate is ingested postexercise to replenish glycogen stores[53] (see figure 1.9).

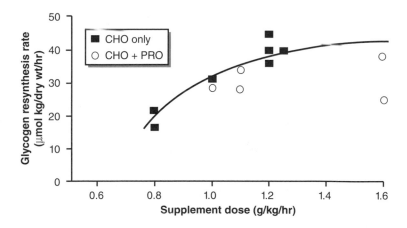

Figure 1.9 Postexercise carbohydrate and protein supplementation on glycogen resynthesis.

Reprinted, by permission, from M.J. Gibala, 2002, "Dietary protein, amino acid supplements, and recovery from exercise," *GSSI Sports Science Exchange* #87 15(4). [Online]. Available: www.gssiweb.com/Article_Detail.aspx?articleid=602 [June 16, 2011].

Protein and Muscle Development

The strength-to-weight ratio is critically important in virtually all athletic endeavors, so athletes are rightly interested in ways to improve or sustain muscle mass. Athletes and their coaches commonly believe the central nutrition strategy for achieving this is to increase protein consumption. However, assuming caloric needs are met, the anabolic maximum for protein is reached at an intake level of approximately 1.5 grams of protein per kilogram of mass. Clearly, if there is a relationship between protein consumption and muscle mass, it must be related to other factors including the type of exercise performed relative to the amount and type of protein consumed, the within-day distribution of protein consumed, and the coingestion of protein with other nutrients. There are, of course, also limitations in how well different populations may hope to enhance musculature, even when optimal nutrition strategies are coupled with appropriate resistance activities. Aging reduces the responses of muscle fibers and the anabolic signaling response to resistance exercise. Although few differences exist between the muscular responses of young women and young men to acute exercise, the muscular responses of older women may be blunted more than in older men.[54]

The timed distribution of protein from food within a day has been assessed, with findings that clearly indicate improved muscle maintenance and enlargement when large peaks and valleys in protein consumption are avoided.[55] Findings suggest that 90 grams of protein (enough to provide 1.5 grams per kilogram for a 60-kilogram, or 132-pound, person) was inadequate to sustain muscle mass when the protein intake (from foods) was postloaded so that most of the protein was consumed during the evening meal. However, when the same amount of protein was evenly redistributed to provide an equal amount (30 grams) of protein at each meal (breakfast, lunch, and dinner), the studied population was able to sustain and, in some cases, even increase muscle mass.[55] The timing of nutrient ingestion also influences the anabolic response of muscle after exercise. Amino acid uptake is greater when free essential amino acids and carbohydrate are ingested before rather than after resistance exercise. However, consumption of whey protein (a whole-food protein) increased amino acid balance from negative to positive regardless of whether it was consumed before or after exercise.[56]

There is a common misunderstanding that extra protein intake alone will support a larger muscle mass, and this theory is the main rationale for the large protein intakes seen in many athletes. In fact, additional total calories are required to support a larger muscle mass, and protein should constitute the same relative proportion of the extra calories consumed. For instance, if a 75-kilogram (165 pound) man wishes to increase his muscle mass by 3 kilograms (6.6 pounds), he would need to consume approximately 1.5 additional grams of protein for each kilogram of muscle mass desired. This amounts to only 4.5 grams of additional protein to support the larger muscle mass. By contrast, 30 grams per kilogram of additional carbohydrate, or 90 grams of additional carbohydrate in total, is required to support the larger muscle mass. Here is the total additional caloric requirement represented by the additional muscle:

- 4.5 grams protein × 4 calories per gram = 18 kilocalories from protein
- 90 grams carbohydrate × 4 calories per gram = 360 kilocalories from carbohydrate
- Total additional calories = 378 calories per day above current requirements to support a 3-kilogram increase in muscle mass

Of course, this athlete would also need to stimulate muscle enlargement by undertaking the appropriate strength-building exercises. Otherwise, the extra calories would manifest themselves as stored fat rather than additional muscle. It is likely that the large amount of protein consumed by so many athletes represents the extra calories they require to maintain or enlarge the muscle mass. Although it is certainly possible to use protein as a primary energy source, it is not the most desirable source because of the nitrogenous wastes produced with protein oxidation. In addition, protein can be an expensive source of calories when provided in supplement form. For instance, eggs (an extremely high-quality source of protein) cost approximately 13 cents per 8 grams of protein, while protein capsules cost approximately $1.20 per 8 grams of protein and may be of questionable quality.

The coingestion of protein and carbohydrate has been assessed to determine if this enhances muscular protein update. One study found that trained men who ingested carbohydrate at the upper end of the recommended level to improve endurance performance (about 8 to 10 grams per kilogram) experienced no enhancement in skeletal muscle energy delivery with the addition of protein.[57] On the other hand, when protein was ingested with carbohydrate during recovery from aerobic exercise, it had the effect of increasing muscle synthesis and improving whole-body net protein balance when compared with an equal caloric load of carbohydrate alone.[58] It has also been demonstrated that an inadequate level of carbohydrate intake compromises skeletal muscle protein utilization and synthesis.[59]

To summarize, building muscle involves more than simply increasing protein and amino acid intakes. It involves the following:

- Addition of resistance activity to provide the physiological motivation (stimulation) to enlarge the muscle mass. It appears that low-load, high-volume resistance activity is superior to high-load, low-volume resistance activity in inducing acute muscle development.[60]

- The maintenance of a sufficient total energy intake to fully satisfy the energy requirement, including the additional requirement of the added resistance activity. The goal is to allow consumed protein to be used for anabolic purposes rather than to be catabolized as a source of energy to help meet energy needs. In addition, it is possible to build muscle only if strategies are followed to reduce muscle breakdown. Sustaining a good energy balance throughout the day helps achieve this goal, enabling an improved potential for muscle building.

- A protein intake of approximately 1.5 grams of protein per kilogram of body mass. With an adequate total energy intake, this level of protein appears to fully satisfy the anabolic requirements of new muscle synthesis.

- A distribution of protein during the day that avoids large peaks and valleys in protein intake. Ideally, the protein consumed should be evenly distributed over multiple meals during the day.

- The consumption of a high-quality protein source (such as whey protein) either before or after exercise. This strategy appears to enhance muscle protein synthesis.

- The consumption of a carbohydrate and protein mixture immediately after exercise. This strategy also appears to enhance muscle protein synthesis. Athletes should avoid consuming only protein after exercise since this is a key opportunity to replenish depleted glycogen stores, and carbohydrate is needed for this purpose.

Protein and Vegetarian Athletes

In the general public, vegetarianism is associated with lower weight, lower fat intake, and lower risk of several chronic diseases, including heart disease, diabetes, high blood pressure, and obesity.[65,66] And it is certainly possible for vegetarian athletes to also perform well and stay healthy, but not without some very careful planning. The problems experienced by vegetarian athletes were well summarized by a former Olympic coach who was a long-time and well-established coach at a major university. During a conversation, he said, "I no longer give scholarships to any athlete who identifies himself or herself as vegetarian. They get injured more often and they are less able to recover quickly from an injury. I end up paying them a scholarship for 4 years, but they compete for the university for less than a single full season. I simply can't afford it." This coach, of course, was simply reacting to a reality gained through years of experience. However, with some simple planning, it is likely that vegetarian athletes can compete well, with an injury risk that is no higher than that of omnivorous athletes. To understand the necessary dietary planning, it is first necessary to accept the very real dietary risks faced by vegans, including a higher risk of inadequate intakes of the following:[63,64]

- Energy
- Protein
- Calcium

- Iron
- Zinc
- Vitamin B_{12}

To a large extent, these dietary weaknesses are associated with the avoidance of high-protein animal-based foods. Therefore, lacto vegetarians (consume milk and other dairy products), ovo vegetarians (consume eggs), pesco vegetarians (consume fish), and lacto-ovo vegetarians (consume both dairy products and eggs) are less likely to suffer the nutrition risks faced by vegans who consume no animal products of any kind. Although vegetarians who consume animal products still face nutrition risks, these are more easily overcome through careful dietary planning and the careful intake of selected nutrients. For instance, dairy products are notoriously poor sources of iron, so a lacto vegetarian may overcome energy and protein inadequacies but still have a high risk of developing iron-deficiency anemia. In fact, it would be hard to find foods that are more efficient delivery vehicles for iron and zinc than meats, so meat avoidance may, without planning, result in a deficiency of both of these nutrients.

A vegan diet is associated with the risk of dysmenorrhea (either oligomenorrhea or amenorrhea) from insufficient energy, which is associated with lower bone density and higher fracture risk; iron-deficiency anemia, which compromises aerobic metabolic processes; pernicious anemia from inadequate vitamin B_{12}, which compromises the body's capacity to generate new red blood cells and, ultimately, lowers oxidative capacity; vitamin D (cholecalciferol) deficiency; and impaired calcium and zinc status. These risks are real and should be accepted as likely in vegan athletes. To illustrate this point, the risk of dysmenorrhea is high in female athletes, and a significant proportion of this risk is due to vegetarian athletes.[65] The energy intake associated with vegetarianism is sufficiently poor that vegetarianism is now considered a risk factor for the development of eating disorders in adolescents.[66] There are also performance-based concerns. Creatine (which is derived from the Greek word for *meat*) has been found to be lower in vegetarian than in non-vegetarian athletes. And it is now known that, although humans are perfectly capable of synthesizing creatine, its synthesis is not adequately compensated for with low meat intakes.

The protein problem faced by vegetarian athletes may be due to an inadequate total energy intake. Even with an adequate total protein consumption, which vegetarian athletes can easily achieve through the combined consumption of legumes, grains, seeds, and nuts, an inadequate energy intake increases the breakdown of protein to satisfy the requirement for energy.[67,68] This protein utilization for energy may result in a de facto protein inadequacy. In simple terms, humans have energy-first systems. The energy requirement must first be satisfied, even through the breakdown of protein, before other anabolic muscle building or muscle recovery processes can occur.

Meats and dairy products provide all the essential amino acids in a single food, but plant sources of protein do not. Therefore, athletes consuming vegetarian meals (i.e., meals with no animal proteins) should be careful to combine foods in ways that optimize essential amino acid availability. The general rule for ensuring a good distribution of all the essential amino acids is to combine cereals and legumes at the same meal. Both cereals and legumes are good sources of valine, threonine, phenylalanine, and leucine. Corn and other cereal grains are poor sources of isoleucine and lysine but are good sources of tryptophan and methionine. By contrast, legumes are good sources of isoleucine and lysine but poor sources of tryptophan and methionine. By combining cereal grains and legumes, the amino acid weakness of one food is complemented by the amino acid strength of the other food to provide a good-quality protein. The same-meal principle is important because the amino acid pool in the body is transient. Eating a low-quality source of protein at one meal and a food with a balancing protein in another meal will not effectively contribute to a high-quality amino acid pool that aids cellular metabolism of protein.

Protein and Postexercise Muscle Recovery

Consuming a drink that contains approximately .1 gram of protein per kilogram (30 calories of protein for a 75-kilogram athlete) after heavy resistance training does appear to improve muscle protein balance.[69] The general guideline is for endurance athletes to consume carbohydrate at the rate of a minimum of 1.2 grams per kilogram of body weight each hour during the first 3 to 5 hours after prolonged exercise. This strategy ensures muscle glycogen replenishment. The addition of some protein in this carbohydrate mix may be useful for muscle recovery, but the majority of postexercise substrate should clearly be from carbohydrate.

Recent studies suggest that milk, which provides the high-quality protein whey, may be a useful postexercise recovery beverage.[70] Work by Shirreffs et al. (2007), in studying 11 young male and female athletes, found that postexercise consumption of a sodium chloride (salt) added to fat-free milk was more effective for hydration recovery than the consumption of a standard sports beverage or plain water.[71] Chocolate milk consumption postexercise has also been found to reduce exercise-associated muscle damage and improve postexercise recovery;[72] team sports athletes who performed exercise to induce acute muscle damage had better recovery when consuming low-fat milk or a low-fat chocolate milkshake than when consuming a pure carbohydrate beverage;[73] and young wrestlers consuming fat-free milk after resistance activity achieved a higher level of muscle mass than those who consumed soy or carbohydrate.[74] Clearly, the combination of a high-quality protein, such as whey, with carbohydrate and fluid enhances muscle recovery better than the individual components alone.

IMPORTANT POINTS

- Only the energy substrates provide energy. Although vitamins and minerals help cells develop energy from the energy substrates, they do not provide energy.

- The distribution of energy substrates should be as follows, with the ranges depending on the individual athlete and the activity: protein, 1.2 to 1.7 grams per kilogram; carbohydrate, 5.0 to 12.0 grams per kilogram; fat, sufficient intake to satisfy total energy requirements once protein and carbohydrate intake is satisfied.

- The intake of energy should be dynamically matched to physiological needs. Many athletes backload energy intake, providing the energy they needed for an activity long after the activity has been completed.

- Athletes should remember that it takes very little intense activity to lower blood sugar, the main fuel for the brain, causing mental fatigue. Mental fatigue causes muscle fatigue, so athletes should have a system for maintaining blood sugar (typically by sipping on a sports beverage at regular intervals) during activity.

- Not all carbohydrates are the same, even though they all fit under the general description of carbohydrate. Consumption of highly digestible starch-based carbohydrate is best before a competition; sugar consumption is fine during a competition; and other carbohydrate foods, including whole grains and vegetables with significant sources of fiber, are good the rest of the time.

- Although the requirement for protein is relatively small, the intake of protein should be evenly spread throughout the day (~30 grams per meal) to optimize protein utilization. Large fluctuations of protein intake (often associated with protein shakes and supplements) do not help the athlete as much as the same amount of protein provided in regular, even units.

- Since fat is a highly concentrated form of energy, it is easy to consume an excess amount. Doing so could limit the required intake of protein and carbohydrate.

- Vegetarian athletes must plan their diets carefully to obtain sufficient energy, protein, iron, zinc, calcium, and vitamin B_{12}.

Vitamins and Minerals

Vitamins and minerals are essential for metabolizing energy substrates, for aiding in tissue building, for fluid balance in the intercellular and extracellular environments, for carrying oxygen and other elements needed for metabolic work, and for removal of metabolic by-products from working tissues. In addition, vitamins and minerals play a role in reducing the exercise-induced oxidative stress experienced by athletes. Because of their higher rates of energy metabolism and higher muscular and skeletal stresses, athletes have a higher need for many of the vitamins and minerals than do nonathletes. The scientific community as a whole is much better versed on the health problems associated with inadequate vitamin and mineral intakes than on the performance issues that may arise from deficiencies. Therefore, the amount of individual vitamins and minerals needed and the optimal delivery systems for ensuring adequate tissue levels are not well understood either by scientists or by most athletes, who often err on the side of providing an excessive vitamin and mineral load through high-dose supplementation. In addition, some companies now include selected vitamins in sports beverages without sufficient thought as to their impact on increasing fluid osmolality[1] and reducing the rate of fluid delivery to working muscles. The end result of this strategy is excess vitamin and mineral intake plus inferior fluid delivery.

Many athletes use high-dose dietary supplements as part of their regular training or competition routine, including about 85 percent of all elite track and field athletes.[2] However, there is increasing evidence that "more than enough is not better than enough" when considering optimal delivery of vitamins and minerals to working tissues. While inadequate vitamin and mineral intakes create health and performance problems, there are increasing examples in the scientific literature of how excess intakes of vitamins and minerals also create human-system difficulties. Although heavy and prolonged training is associated with depressed immune cell function, there is no convincing evidence that high doses of so-called immune-boosting supplements, including antioxidant vitamins, glutamine, zinc, echinacea, and probiotics, prevent exercise-induced immune impairment.[3,4] A study of vitamin E and immunity after the Kona Triathlon World Championship emphasizes this conclusion. This study found that vitamin E intake (800 IU for 1 to 2 months) compared with placebo

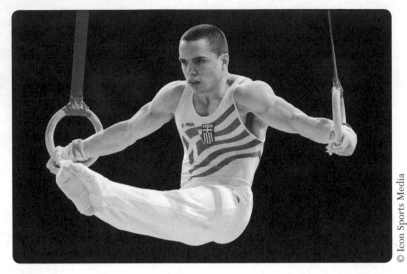

© Icon Sports Media

Optimal performance is not achieved by exceeding vitamin and mineral requirements.

ingestion before the race actually promoted lipid peroxidation and inflammation during exercise rather than helping to diminish it.[5]

To make matters even worse for athletes, many dietary supplements that appear legitimate are laced with undeclared substances prohibited by the International Olympic Committee (IOC) and the World Anti-Doping Agency. Regardless of whether this contamination is purposeful or a result of poor quality control, the otherwise innocent athlete would be removed from competition for having a positive test for any of these unintentionally consumed products. In 2001, 24 percent of all dietary supplement samples tested positive for nandrolone (a banned anabolic steroid) by IOC-accredited laboratories, and there were many countries of origin for these contaminated supplements, including the Netherlands, the United States, the United Kingdom, Austria, Italy, Spain, Germany, and Belgium.[6] Taken together, these findings should make athletes think twice before taking high-dose dietary supplements when there is no diagnosed reason to take them. Although there are a few dietary supplements that, when taken in reasonable doses, may be helpful to athletes who have special needs (particularly when food intakes are restricted), it is increasingly clear that nutrient supplementation should be used only when a real foods are not practical or not available.

This chapter discusses vitamin and mineral requirements for exercise, the functions of these nutrients, and the optimal delivery strategies to ensure athletes obtain what they need without adding to the cellular stress associated with excess or deficiency. Standards for nutrient intake adequacy have been established by the Institute of Medicine (see table 2.1). These standards, referred to as the dietary reference intakes (DRIs), are based on the assessment of the estimated average requirement (EAR), the recommended dietary allowance (RDA), the adequate intake (AI), and the tolerable upper intake level (UL). Although the focus of the recommended dietary allowance (the earlier standard for nutrient intake adequacy) was based on lowering the risk that someone would suffer from a nutrient-deficiency disease, the focus of the DRI is to lower the risk of developing chronic disease by ensuring a properly balanced nutrient intake.

Note: The DRI values for pregnancy may be higher than those listed in the quick guide tables in this chapter. Pregnant women should consult their physicians regarding optimal nutrient intakes.

Table 2.1 Dietary Reference Intakes Definitions

The Dietary Reference Intakes (DRIs) are quantitative estimates of nutrient intakes to be used for planning and assessing diets for healthy people. These values include both recommended intakes and tolerable upper intake levels. The DRIs are determined by the Institute of Medicine, a nonprofit group that provides health policy advice to the National Academy of Sciences. The DRIs are based on the scientific evaluation of the recommended dietary allowance, the adequate intake, the tolerable upper intake level, and the estimated average requirement.

Recommended Dietary Allowance (RDA)	The average daily dietary intake level that is sufficient to meet the nutrient requirement of nearly all healthy people (97 to 98 percent) in a particular life stage and gender group.
Adequate Intake (AI)	A recommended intake value based on observed or experimentally determined approximations or estimates of nutrient intake by a group (or groups) of healthy people that are assumed to be adequate—used when an RDA cannot be determined.
Tolerable Upper Intake Level (UL)	The highest level of daily nutrient intake that is likely to pose no risk of adverse health effects for almost all people in the general population. As intake increases above the UL, the potential risk of adverse effects increases.
Estimated Average Requirement (EAR)	A daily nutrient intake value that is estimated to meet the requirement of half the healthy people in a life stage and gender group—used to assess dietary adequacy and as the basis for the RDA.

VITAMINS

Vitamins are substances needed by cells to encourage specific cellular chemical reactions. Some vitamins (particularly B vitamins) are involved in energy reactions that enable cells to derive energy from carbohydrate, protein, and fat. Since athletes burn more energy than do nonathletes, these vitamins are of particular interest in this book. Other vitamins are involved in maintaining mineral balance. Vitamin D, for instance, encourages greater absorption of dietary calcium and phosphorus. The synergism between vitamins and minerals is a critical factor in understanding their nutrient requirements. The fact that these nutrients have integrated functions should encourage athletes to present the widest possible spectrum of vitamins and minerals to their cells. Single vitamin or single mineral supplementation may, therefore, corrupt nutrient balance and the delicate relationship between these nutrients. Table 2.2 gives some tips for maximizing vitamin intake.

Vitamins are organized into fat-soluble and water-soluble categories. The fat-soluble vitamins require a fat-based environment in which to function, and the water-soluble vitamins require a water-based environment. To one degree or another, we have the capacity to store all vitamins. That is to say, if we ate a meal 2 days ago that contained a large amount of vitamin C but ingested no vitamin C in the foods we consumed yesterday, we wouldn't expect to suffer from symptoms of vitamin C deficiency today. Cells that require vitamin C are able to store more than they need even though there are no clear storage depots where large amounts of the vitamin can be stored. Fat-soluble vitamins, however, do have a relatively large storage capacity. This difference in storage capacity is responsible for the commonly repeated recommendation that water-soluble vitamins should be consumed

Table 2.2 Maximizing Vitamin Intake

To maximize vitamin intake from your diet, try the following:
Eat a wide variety of colorful fruits and vegetables.
When possible eat fresh fruits and vegetables, especially those in season.
Don't overcook vegetables—long cooking times reduce nutrient content.
Steam or microwave your vegetables rather than boil them—nutrients seep out in boiling water, only to be poured down the drain.

every day because they are (supposedly) *not* stored. It has also led to the myth that any excess in water-soluble vitamin intake is without problems because the excess is excreted in the urine. It is true that excess intake of fat-soluble vitamins, especially vitamins D and A, can produce severe toxicity. Even vitamin E, which for many years was considered to have a relatively low toxicity potential, has been found to increase all-cause mortality when taken in doses of 400 international units (IU) per day or more.[7] Taking excess water-soluble vitamins, however, may also lead to difficulties. A prime example of this is peripheral neuropathy (loss of feeling in the fingers), a neurological problem caused by excess intake of vitamin B_6 (500 to 5,000 milligrams per day for 1 to 3 years is enough to create permanent damage).[8] Another problem is that humans are adaptable to intake. Therefore, the greater the volume consumed, the greater the eventual need to obtain the same biological effect.

Water-Soluble Vitamins

A discussion of individual water-soluble vitamins follows. See tables 2.3 through 2.11 for a summary of the functions, sources, and possible problems associated with these vitamins.[9] Figure 2.1 illustrates the multiple relationships between the B vitamins and energy metabolic processes.

Vitamin B_1

Vitamin B_1 (thiamin) is present in a variety of food sources, including whole grains, nuts, legumes (beans and dried peas), and pork. It works in unison with other B vitamins to convert the energy in the foods we consume to muscular energy and heat. Thiamin contributes to this metabolic process by removing carbon dioxide in energy reactions with its active coenzyme thiamin pyrophosphate (TPP), an enzyme that is particularly important in carbohydrate energy metabolism. The daily requirement for vitamin B_1 is closely associated with energy intakes and requirements as well as with increases in the intake of carbohydrate, the presence of infection, and increases in physical activity.

Since thiamin has an important role in energy substrate utilization, it is logical to assume that a deficiency may negatively affect athletic performance. However, although thiamin deficiencies have been found in certain groups of athletes, including gymnasts and wrestlers, there are no associated adverse effects on performance.[10-14] Recent studies on adventure racers and ski mountaineer racers confirm that the risk of thiamin deficiency in physically

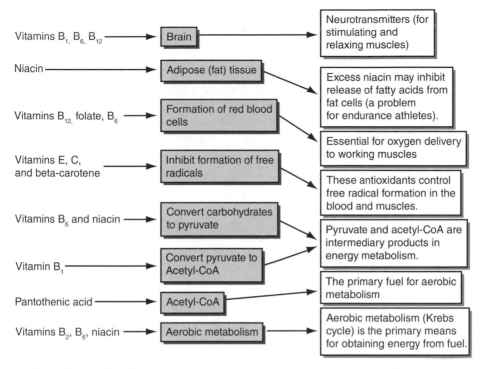

Figure 2.1 The relationship of vitamins to energy metabolism and muscle function.

active people is low.[15,16] The average intake of vitamin B_1 in adventure racers was 3.5 (± 3.2) milligrams in men and 5.2 (± 6.5) milligrams in women. It was determined in this study that 14 of the 18 male subjects had a 100 percent probability of an adequate vitamin B_1 intake, and 3 of the 6 female subject had a 100 percent probability of an adequate vitamin B_1 intake. In the ski mountaineering subjects, the average intake of vitamin B_1 was 163 percent of the recommended level. These and other studies of athletes suggest that thiamin consumption is likely to become an issue only in athletes who are on calorically restrictive intakes.

The DRI for thiamin (1.2 milligrams per day for males, 1.1 milligrams per day for females) may be inadequate for athletes. The actual requirement is based on approximately .5 milligram of thiamin for each 1,000 calories consumed, and athletes often consume more than 3,000 calories (often 5,000 to 6,000 calories). It does appear that the upper limit for thiamin intake would be 3.0 milligrams per day, even for an athlete consuming more than 6,000 calories per day. It is reasonable, therefore, to recommend an intake of two times the DRI (~2.2 to 2.4 milligrams per day) for athletes consuming high levels of energy. Athletes commonly consume high-carbohydrate foods that, because of enrichment and fortification, are good sources of thiamin. This makes it likely that most well-nourished athletes already consume more than the recommended level of thiamin each day.

Table 2.3 Vitamin B₁ Quick Guide

Alternative name	Thiamin
Dietary reference intake (DRI)	Adult males: 1.2 mg/day Adult females: 1.1 mg/day
Recommended intake for athletes	1.5 to 3.0 mg/day, depending on total calories consumed (high calories = more)
Functions	Carbohydrate metabolism, nervous system function
Good food sources	Whole-grain cereals, beans, pork, enriched grains
Deficiency	Confusion, anorexia, weakness, calf pain, heart disease
Toxicity	None known (no safe upper limit established)

Vitamin B₂

Vitamin B₂ (riboflavin) is involved in energy production and normal cellular function through its coenzymes flavin adenine dinucleotide (FAD) and flavin mononucleotide (FMN). These coenzymes are mainly involved in obtaining energy from consumed carbohydrate, protein, and fat. Food sources of riboflavin include dairy products (e.g., milk, yogurt, cottage cheese), dark green leafy vegetables (e.g., spinach, chard, mustard greens, broccoli, green peppers), whole-grain foods, and enriched-grain foods.

No studies suggest that riboflavin-deficiency symptoms are common in athletes. Also, no apparent toxicity symptoms occur from consuming more than the DRI. Several studies have suggested that athletes may have higher requirements than the DRI, which is based on approximately .6 milligram per 1,000 calories. In a series of studies performed on exercising women and women seeking to lose weight, the riboflavin requirement was found to range between .63 and 1.40 milligrams per 1,000 calories.[17-19]

There is some evidence that physical activity increases the requirement to a level slightly higher than .5 milligram per 1,000 calories but not more than 1.6 milligrams per 1,000 calories.[20] However, even with this apparently higher requirement for athletes, no studies clearly demonstrate an improvement in athletic performance with intakes greater than the RDA. Since low-dose supplements of this vitamin induce no apparent toxicity symptoms, athletes could take a supplement delivering 1.6 to 3.0 milligrams of riboflavin as part of a B-complex supplement. This level of intake would serve as an adequate preventive measure to help athletes avoid the symptoms—headache, nausea, weakness—associated with extremely high doses (more than 100 times the RDA).[21]

Vegetarian athletes may be at a higher risk of riboflavin deficiency, particularly if they avoid consumption of good sources of riboflavin, including soy and dairy products.[22] Vegetarian athletes who increase the intensity of their exercise regimens would also be considered at higher risk, particularly if their regular food intakes do not include plant sources of riboflavin (whole-grain and enriched cereals, soy products, almonds, asparagus, bananas, sweet potatoes, and wheat germ).[23]

Table 2.4 Vitamin B$_2$ Quick Guide

Alternative name	Riboflavin
Dietary reference intake (DRI)	Adult males: 1.3 mg/day Adult females: 1.1 mg/day
Recommended intake for athletes	1.1 mg per 1,000 calories
Functions	Energy metabolism, protein metabolism, skin health, eye health
Good food sources	Fresh milk and other dairy products, eggs, dark green leafy vegetables, whole-grain cereals, enriched grains
Deficiency	Inflamed tongue; cracked, dry skin at corners of mouth, nose, and eyes; bright light sensitivity; weakness; fatigue
Toxicity	None known (no safe upper limit established)

Niacin

Niacin, which also refers to nicotinic acid and nicotinamide and is sometimes called vitamin B$_3$, is involved in energy production from carbohydrate, protein, and fat; glycogen synthesis; and normal cellular metabolism through its active coenzymes. These enzymes, nicotinamide adenine dinucleotide (NAD) and nicotinamide adenine dinucleotide phosphate (NADP), are essential for normal muscle function. The niacin-deficiency disease pellagra is well documented in human populations suffering from famine or monotonous intakes of unenriched grain products, but there is no evidence of niacin deficiency in athletes.

Niacin is found in meat, whole or enriched grains, seeds, nuts, and legumes. Body cells have the capacity to synthesize niacin from tryptophan (60 milligrams of tryptophan yields 1 milligram of niacin), an amino acid found in all high-quality protein foods (e.g., meat, fish, poultry). Given the broad spectrum of foods that contain niacin, it is relatively easy for adults to consume the DRI of 14 to 16 milligrams per day, or 6.6 niacin equivalents (NEs) per 1,000 calories. NEs are equal to 1 milligram of niacin or 60 milligrams of dietary tryptophan; you can obtain niacin directly from food or indirectly by consuming the amino acid tryptophan. The NE unit of measure takes both sources into account.

A deficiency of niacin results in muscular weakness, loss of appetite, indigestion, and skin rash. It is possible to produce toxicity symptoms from excess niacin intake; symptoms include gastrointestinal distress and feeling hot (becoming red faced or flushed). It may also result in a tingling feeling around the neck, face, and fingers. These symptoms are commonly reported in people taking large doses of niacin to lower blood lipids.

In studies evaluating the performance effects of niacin supplementation, endurance was reduced because the excess niacin caused a reduction in fat metabolism.[24-26] This resulted in a greater reliance on carbohydrate fuels (glucose and glycogen) to support physical activity. Because glycogen storage is limited, athletes taking niacin supplements had lower endurance. To date, there is no evidence that the requirement for niacin is increased with physical activity.

Table 2.5 Niacin Quick Guide

Alternative names	Niacinamide, nicotinic acid, nicotinamide, vitamin B$_2$
Dietary reference intake (DRI)	Adult males: 16 mg/day Adult females: 14 mg/day
Recommended intake for athletes	14 to 20 mg/day
Functions	Energy metabolism, glycolysis, fat synthesis
Good food sources	Foods high in tryptophan (an amino acid that can be converted to niacin): milk, eggs, turkey, chicken Foods high in niacin: whole-grain foods, lean meat, fish, poultry, enriched grains
Deficiency	Anorexia, skin rash, dementia, weakness, lethargy Disease: pellagra
Toxicity	Tolerable upper intake levels: 10 to 15 mg/day for young children (age 1-8) 20 to 35 mg/day for children and adults (age 9-70+) Symptoms: flushing, burning, and tingling sensations of extremities, hepatitis and gastric ulcers with chronic high intake

Vitamin B$_6$

Vitamin B$_6$ refers to several compounds (pyridoxine, pyridoxal, pyridoxamine, pyridoxine 5-phosphate, pyridoxal 5-phosphate, and pyridoxamine 5-phosphatepyridoxine) that all display the same metabolic activity. Vitamin B$_6$ is most concentrated in meats (especially liver) and is also found in wheat germ, fish, poultry, legumes, bananas, brown rice, whole-grain cereals, and vegetables. Because the function of this vitamin is closely linked to protein and amino acid metabolism, the requirement is linked to protein intake (the higher the protein intake, the higher the vitamin B$_6$ requirement). The proportion of adults who may have intakes below the recommended level (data from the UK) range from 6 percent in males and 10 percent in females.[27]

The adult requirement is based on .016 milligram of B$_6$ per gram of protein consumed each day[9] and is satisfied in those consuming typical protein intakes. When you consider that high-protein foods are also typically high in vitamin B$_6$, those consuming protein from food (regardless of the amount) are most likely to have adequate B$_6$ levels as well. However, many athletes consume additional protein in purified supplemental forms (protein powders, amino acid powders), making it conceivable that athletes with high supplemental protein intakes may have an inadequate B$_6$ intake.

Vitamin B$_6$ functions in reactions related to protein synthesis by aiding in the creation of amino acids and proteins (transamination reactions), and it is also involved in protein catabolism through involvement in reactions that break down amino acids and proteins (deamination reactions). It is involved, therefore, in manufacturing muscle, hemoglobin, and other proteins critical for athletic performance. The major enzyme of vitamin B$_6$, pyridoxal phosphate (PP), is also involved in the breakdown of muscle glycogen for energy through the enzyme glycogen phosphorylase.

A chronic deficiency of vitamin B_6 leads to symptoms of peripheral neuritis (loss of nerve function in the hands, feet, arms, and legs), ataxia (loss of balance), irritability, depression, and convulsions. An excess intake of vitamin B_6, primarily from consumption of supplements, does lead to toxicity symptoms that have been documented in humans. These symptoms are similar to those seen in B_6 deficiency and include ataxia and severe sensory neuropathy (loss of sensation in the fingers). Toxicity symptoms have been documented in women taking supplements that, on average, equal 119 milligrams per day to treat premenstrual syndrome and several types of mental disorders.[28, 29]

There is a theoretical basis for investigating vitamin B_6 and athletic performance. B_6 is involved in the breakdown of amino acids in muscle as a means of obtaining needed energy and in converting lactic acid to glucose in the liver.[30] Vitamin B_6 is also involved in the breakdown of muscle glycogen to derive energy. Other functions of vitamin B_6 that may be related to athletic performance include the formation of serotonin and the synthesis of carnitine from lysine. There is evidence that some athletes may be at risk of inadequate vitamin B_6 status.[31-33] Poor B_6 status reduces athletic performance.[34]

Because many athletes are always looking for that extra edge, there is an understandable attractiveness to natural substances that are legal. Vitamin B_6 is sometimes marketed as one of those natural and legal substances; besides its importance in energy metabolism, it is linked with the production of growth hormone, which can help increase muscle mass.[35] It appears as if the combined effect of exercise and vitamin B_6 on growth hormone production is greater than either of these factors individually.[36, 37]

Before athletes take vitamin B_6 supplements, the following factors should be considered:[31]

- Most athletes have adequate vitamin B_6 intakes and a healthy vitamin B_6 status.
- Those athletes with poor vitamin B_6 status are generally those with inadequate energy intakes.
- A greater proportion of female athletes and athletes participating in sports that emphasize low body weight (gymnastics, wrestling, figure skating) are likely to have inadequate energy and protein intakes and, therefore, inadequate vitamin B_6 intakes.
- High doses of vitamin B_6 have been shown to have toxic effects.
- Although poor B_6 status is associated with reduced athletic performance, there is no good evidence that consuming more than the recommended intake has a beneficial effect on athletic performance.[38]
- Vitamin B_6 supplementation does not appear necessary to enhance athletic performance if a balanced diet with adequate energy is consumed.[39]

All things considered, these factors should encourage athletes to consume an adequate intake of energy substrates rather than resort to supplements of vitamin B_6.

Table 2.6 Vitamin B$_6$ Quick Guide

Alternative names	Pyridoxine, pyridoxal, pyridoxamine
Dietary reference intake (DRI)	Adult males: 1.3 to 1.7 mg/day Adult females: 1.3 to 1.5 mg/day
Recommended intake for athletes	1.5 to 2.0 mg/day
Functions	Protein metabolism, protein synthesis, metabolism of fat and carbohydrate, neurotransmitter formation, glycolysis
Good food sources	High-protein foods (meats), whole-grain cereals, enriched cereals, eggs
Deficiency	Nausea, mouth sores, muscle weakness, depression, convulsions, impaired immune system
Toxicity	Tolerable upper intake levels: 30 to 40 mg/day for young children (age 1-8) 60 to 100 mg/day for children and adults (age 9-70+) Symptoms: peripheral neuritis (loss of sensation in limbs), loss of balance and coordination

Vitamin B$_{12}$

Vitamin B$_{12}$ is the most chemically complex of all the vitamins. It contains the mineral cobalt (thus the name *cobalamin*) and, while essential for all cell function, has a major involvement in red blood cell formation, folic acid metabolism, DNA synthesis, and nerve development.

Dietary sources of this vitamin are mainly foods of animal origin (meats, eggs, dairy products); it is essentially absent from plant foods. Gut bacteria may also produce a small amount of absorbable vitamin B$_{12}$.[39] Vegetarian athletes who avoid all foods of animal origin (i.e., they do not eat meat, nor do they consume eggs or dairy products) would therefore be at risk for vitamin B$_{12}$ deficiency.

B$_{12}$ deficiency results in pernicious anemia, a form of anemia that most commonly occurs in the elderly with compromised stomach function. The stomach normally produces intrinsic factor, which is required for vitamin B$_{12}$ absorption. Without intrinsic factor, even a normal dietary intake of vitamin B$_{12}$ will result in deficiency disease because of malabsorption. Symptoms of deficiency include fatigue, poor muscular coordination (possibly leading to paralysis), and dementia.

Athletes have abused vitamin B$_{12}$ for years. Many athletes are injected with large amounts of vitamin B$_{12}$ (often 1-gram injections) before competitions.[40,41] Despite the commonality of this strategy, there is no evidence that vitamin B$_{12}$ does anything whatsoever to improve performance when taken in excess.[42-44]

It certainly makes sense that athletes consume foods that will help them avoid deficiencies of any kind, including B$_{12}$ deficiency. Anemia caused by a vitamin B$_{12}$ deficiency would clearly affect performance by reducing oxygen-carrying capacity, leading to reduced endurance. Potentially, muscular coordination could also be impaired. Unless someone has a genetic predisposition for B$_{12}$ malabsorption (typically because of an inadequate production

Table 2.7 Vitamin B$_{12}$ Quick Guide

Alternative name	Cobalamin
Dietary reference intake (DRI)	Adult males: 2.4 mcg/day Adult females: 2.4 mcg/day
Recommended intake for athletes	2.4 to 2.5 mcg/day
Functions	Protein metabolism, protein synthesis, metabolism of fat and carbohydrate, neurotransmitter formation, glycolysis
Good food sources	Foods of animal origin (meat, fish, poultry, eggs, milk, cheese) and fortified cereals
Deficiency	Pernicious anemia (more likely caused by malabsorption of the vitamin than by dietary inadequacy, although vegans are at risk) Symptoms: weakness, easy fatigue, neurological disorders
Toxicity	Tolerable upper intake levels not established, although the DV is 6 mcg

of intrinsic factor), there is no basis for taking supplements if a balanced mixed-food diet is consumed. Vegan athletes, on the other hand, have good reason to be concerned about vitamin B$_{12}$ status. It makes good sense for vegan athletes to take a supplement providing the DRI of 2.4 micrograms per day, and also consume foods that are fortified with vitamin B$_{12}$ (such as some soy milk products).

Athletes above the age of 50 may develop difficulty absorbing sufficient vitamin B$_{12}$ because of common age-related changes in gut function, leading to a reduction in intrinsic factor (needed for the absorption of the vitamin). A potentially successful strategy to avoid deficiency in this age group is to take a once-weekly sublingual vitamin B$_{12}$ supplement that is absorbed through the mucosal surface in the mouth (thus avoiding potentially difficult gut absorption). A study assessing the administration of vitamin B$_{12}$ compared the typical oral replacement therapy and the sublingual supplement (500 micrograms of either) and found no difference in serum concentrations of vitamin B$_{12}$ after 4 weeks of administration.[45]

Folate (Naturally Occurring) and Folic Acid (Synthetic)

Folate is widespread in the food supply, with the highest concentrations in liver, yeast, leafy vegetables, fruits, and legumes. The synthetic form, folic acid, is now also fortified in grain products (breads, cereals, spaghetti) within the United States, where fortified foods deliver approximately 140 micrograms of folic acid per 100 grams of food. Folate from fresh foods is easily destroyed through common household food preparation techniques (it is susceptible to high heat, heated acid [e.g., vinegar, lemon juice] solutions, and ultraviolet light) and long storage times, so biological availability of naturally occurring folate is better from fresh and unprocessed foods. The bioavailability of the folic acid from fortified foods appears to be more stable and, therefore, may be a more consistent source of the vitamin than naturally occurring folate.

Folate functions in amino acid metabolism and nucleic acid synthesis (RNA and DNA), and a deficiency leads to alterations in synthesizing cells. Tissues with a rapid turnover are particularly susceptible to folic acid deficiency, including red and white blood cells as well as tissues of the gastrointestinal tract and the uterus. Adequate folate intake 6 to 12 months before and during pregnancy is associated with the elimination of fetal neural tube defects (most notably spina bifida).[46,47] Folic acid is measured in dietary folate equivalents (DFEs), where 1 DFE equals

- 1.0 microgram of food folate;
- .6 microgram of folic acid from fortified food or as a supplement consumed with food; or
- .5 microgram of a folic acid supplement consumed on an empty stomach.

Because folate functions with vitamin B_{12} in forming healthy new red blood cells, a deficiency leads to megaloblastic anemia. Other deficiency problems include gastrointestinal distress (diarrhea, malabsorption, pain) and a swollen, red tongue. Excess folic acid intake may mask vitamin B_{12} deficiency and may also increase cancer risk.[48-50] Folate toxicity from excess intake has not been reported in humans, and no studies have reported on the relationship between folic acid and athletic performance. However, since athletes have an above-normal tissue turnover because of the pounding the body takes in various sports, and with the evidence that red blood cell turnover is faster in athletes than in nonathletes, there is a good reason for athletes to be certain that adequate folic acid intake is satisfied.[51,52] The prudent approach is through the regular consumption of foods, including whole grains (now fortified with folic acid) and fresh fruits and vegetables. If this is not possible, a daily supplement at the level of the DRI (400 micrograms per day) is an effective means of maintaining folate status.

Table 2.8 Folic Acid and Folate Quick Guide

Alternative name	Folate
Dietary reference intake (DRI)	Adult males: 400 mcg/day Adult females: 400 mcg/day
Recommended intake for athletes	400 mcg/day
Functions	Methionine (essential amino acid) metabolism, formation of DNA, formation of red blood cells, normal fetal development
Good food sources	Green leafy vegetables, beans, whole-grain cereals, oranges, bananas
Deficiency	Megaloblastic anemia, neural tube defects (as a result of low intake during pregnancy) Symptoms: weakness, easy fatigue, neurological disorders
Toxicity	Tolerable upper intake levels: 300 to 400 mcg/day for young children (age 1-8) 600 to 1,000 mcg/day for children and adults (age 9-70+) Symptoms: none established

Biotin

Biotin works with magnesium and adenosine triphosphate (ATP) to play a role in carbon dioxide metabolism; new glucose production (gluconeogenesis); carbohydrate metabolism; and synthesis of glycogen, fatty acids, and amino acids.[9] Good food sources of biotin include egg yolks, soy flour, liver, sardines, walnuts, pecans, peanuts, and yeast. Fruits and meats are poor dietary sources of the vitamin. Bacteria in the intestines also synthesize biotin. Because of this intestinal synthesis, a deficiency of this vitamin is rare but can be induced through the intake of large amounts of raw egg whites, which contain avidin, a protein that binds to biotin (20 raw egg whites would be needed to disturb biotin metabolism). When a deficiency does occur, symptoms include loss of appetite, vomiting, depression, and dermatitis. There is no evidence that athletes are at risk for biotin deficiency, and no information exists on the relationship between biotin and athletic performance. Therefore, no recommendation on biotin intake for athletes above the suggested DRI can be made.

Table 2.9 Biotin Quick Guide

Alternative name	None
Dietary reference intake (DRI)	Adult males: 30 mcg/day Adult females: 30 mcg/day
Recommended intake for athletes	30 mcg/day
Functions	Glucose and fatty acid synthesis, gluconeogenesis, gene expression
Good food sources	Egg yolks, legumes, dark green leafy vegetables (also produced by intestinal bacteria)
Deficiency	Rare; if it occurs, due to high egg white intake Symptoms: anorexia, depression, muscle pain, dermatitis
Toxicity	Tolerable upper intake levels not established

Pantothenic Acid

Pantothenic acid is a structural component of coenzyme A (CoA), a compound of central importance in energy metabolic processes. It is involved, through CoA, in carbohydrate, protein, and fat metabolism. Pantothenic acid is widely distributed in the food supply, making it unlikely that an athlete would suffer from a deficiency, particularly with adequate total energy intake. If a rare deficiency does occur, symptoms include easy fatigue, weakness, and insomnia. The highest concentrations of pantothenic acid are found in meat, whole-grain foods, beans, and peas. Supplemental doses of the vitamin are typically 10 milligrams per day (double the DRI of 5 milligrams per day) and, at this level, have not resulted in toxicity. However, few data are available on the potential for pantothenic acid toxicity, so athletes should be cautious about high-dose supplementation with this vitamin.

A possible relationship exists between pantothenic acid supplementation and exercise performance, but more information is needed before a sound recommendation can be made on pantothenate intake for athletes. In studies that have experimented with pantothenic acid supplements to determine a requirement level, the typical dosage has been 10 milligrams per day. At this level of intake, 5 to 7 milligrams per day are excreted in the urine.[6] Therefore, it appears that taking supplements at the level of 10 milligrams per day is excessive.

Table 2.10 Pantothenic Acid Quick Guide

Alternative name	Pantothenate
Dietary reference intake (DRI)	Adult males: 5 mg/day Adult females: 5 mg/day
Recommended intake for athletes	4 to 5 mg/day
Functions	Energy metabolism as part of coenzyme A, gluconeogenesis, synthesis of acetylcholine
Good food sources	Present in all *but* processed and refined foods
Deficiency	Unknown in humans
Toxicity	Tolerable upper intake levels not established, although the DV is 10 mg Symptoms: unknown

Vitamin C

Vitamin C functions as an antioxidant and is also involved in reactions that form collagen, a connective tissue protein. It also has clear functions that can potentially influence athletic performance, including the following:[53]

- Aids in the synthesis of carnitine, which is a transport molecule that carries fatty acids into mitochondria for energy metabolism
- Aids in the production of epinephrine and norepinephrine, which are neurotransmitters that can rapidly degrade glycogen to make glucose available to working muscles
- Aids in the transportation and absorption of nonheme iron (mainly from fruits and vegetables) in the intestines (typically, nonheme iron is not well absorbed; since iron deficiency is a major problem for athletes, any way of improving iron availability from foods is desirable)
- Aids in the synthesis of cortisol, which is a powerful catabolic hormone
- Aids in the resynthesis of vitamin E to its active antioxidant state

Fresh fruits and vegetables are the best sources of vitamin C. Meats and dairy products are low in vitamin C, and cereal grains contain none (unless fortified). Vitamin C is easily destroyed by cooking (heat) and exposure to air (oxygen). It is also highly water soluble, making it easily removed from foods cooked in water. The deficiency disease scurvy is almost nonexistent today. Toxicity from regular high supplemental intakes of the vitamin is rare, but it may include a predisposition to developing kidney stones and a reduction in tissue sensitivity to the vitamin. Doses of 100 to 200 milligrams per day will saturate the body with vitamin C,[54] yet many people take supplemental doses of 1,000 to 2,000 milligrams per day, well above the 75 to 90 milligrams per day of the DRI.

A number of studies have evaluated the relationship between vitamin C intake and athletic performance, although the results are inconsistent. Part of the problem with many of these studies is poor standardization between subjects and a general lack of comparative controls. Nevertheless, according to a review of studies that used controls and provided vitamin C supplements at or below 500 milligrams per day (remember that the DRI is 75 milligrams for adult women and 90 milligrams for adult men), there was no measurable benefit to athletic performance.[55] One study noted that when a 500-milligram dose of vitamin C was provided shortly (4 hours) before testing, there was a significant improvement in strength and a significant reduction in maximal oxygen consumption, but no impact on muscular endurance.[56] When subjects were provided with the same amount for 7 days, the result was an improvement in strength but a decrease in endurance. When these same subjects were provided with 2,000 milligrams each day for 7 days, the athletes' $\dot{V}O_2$max was lowered, but no change was evident in endurance performance.

Athletes involved in concussive sports—where muscle soreness occurs or an injury requires more collagen formation—may benefit from a slightly higher level of vitamin C. Studies on animals suggest that vitamin C improves the healing process, and inadequate vitamin C inhibits healing.[57] It has also been suggested that muscle soreness may be more rapidly relieved when consuming moderate supplemental doses of vitamin C and other antioxidants.[58]

It is difficult to make a rational recommendation on vitamin C and performance, but athletes should keep the safe upper limit (2,000 milligrams per day) of this vitamin in mind before investing in supplements. Because some studies demonstrate that high doses may cause endurance problems, the intake level should be kept below the point of causing performance deficits.

Vitamin C is known to enhance iron absorption. In 1993, there were three reported deaths due to iron overload, and the people who died were taking large daily doses of vitamin C.[59] Also consider that many athletes already consume more than 250 milligrams of vitamin C each day from food alone because of their high intake of fresh fruits and vegetables. A reasonable recommendation is to eat an abundant amount of fresh fruits and vegetables (wonderful sources of carbohydrate and many other nutrients besides vitamin C). If that's not possible, a reasonable strategy is to take a moderate daily supplement containing the DRI (between 75 and 90 milligrams per day). Except for athletes chronically consuming diets that are inadequate in energy, athletes meet the DRI and consume more vitamin C than the general nonathlete population.[60] Even someone consuming a low but regular intake of fruits and vegetables is likely to meet the DRI for vitamin C, but a low-level supplement may provide an appropriate safety buffer.

Table 2.11 Vitamin C Quick Guide

Alternative names	Ascorbic acid, ascorbate, dehydroascorbate, L-ascorbate
Dietary reference intake (DRI)	Adult males: 90 mg/day Adult females: 75 mg/day
Recommended intake for athletes	200 mg/day
Functions	Collagen formation, iron absorption, epinephrine formation
Good food sources	Fresh fruits (particularly citrus and cherries) and vegetables
Deficiency	Rare; if it occurs, results in scurvy Symptoms: bleeding gums, deterioration of muscles and tendons, sudden death
Toxicity	Tolerable upper intake levels: 400 to 650 mg/day for young children (age 1-8) 1.2 to 2.0 g/day for children and adults (age 9-70+) Increased risk of kidney stone formation with chronic intake of 1g/day or more

Fat-Soluble Vitamins

Fat-soluble vitamins are carried in a fat solute and represent an important reason why athletes should not consume a diet excessively low (i.e., below 20 percent of calories) in fat. There are four fat-soluble vitamins—A, D, E, and K—and each is effectively stored to be used as needed. See tables 2.12 through 2.15 for a summary of the functions, sources, and possible problems associated with these vitamins.[61,62] There are limits to the storage capacity of fat-soluble vitamins, so chronically high intakes may lead to serious disease states resulting from toxicity. To emphasize this point, the two most potentially toxic substances in human nutrition are vitamins A and D. Achieving toxic-level doses of these vitamins is difficult if consuming the usual foods, but toxic doses may be easily obtained from a regular supplemental intake of these vitamins. Generally speaking, however, our storage capacity for these vitamins eliminates the need for supplemental intake.

Vitamin A

The active form of vitamin A is retinol, which we obtain from foods of animal origin, including liver, egg yolks, fortified dairy products (e.g., vitamin A and D milk), margarine, and fish oil. The DRI ranges between 700 retinol activity equivalents (RAE) for women and 900 RAE for men. One RAE equals

- 1 microgram of retinol,
- 12 micrograms of beta-carotene,
- 24 micrograms of alpha-carotene, or
- 24 micrograms of beta-cryptoxanthin.

Vitamin A has a well-established relationship with normal vision; helps keep bones, skin, and red blood cells healthy; and is also needed for the immune system to function normally. There is no evidence that taking extra vitamin A aids athletic performance. Since the vitamin has clearly toxic effects when taken in excess (the maximum upper limit that poses the risk of adverse effects is 3,000 RAE for women and men), athletes should be cautioned against taking supplemental doses. Toxicity of vitamin A manifests itself in several ways, including dry skin, headache, irritability, vomiting, bone pain, and vision problems. Excess vitamin A intake during pregnancy is associated with an increase in birth defects.

The carotenoids (mainly beta-carotene) are referred to as precursors for vitamin A since they can be converted to vitamin A by cells. Serum vitamin A appears to reflect relatively well-maintained body stores, but beta-carotene appears to fluctuate more because it varies with recently consumed carotenoids.[23] Consuming foods containing beta-carotene is an indirect way of obtaining vitamin A. Beta-carotene is found in all red, orange, yellow, and dark green fruits and vegetables (carrots, sweet potatoes, spinach, apricots, cantaloupes, tomatoes, and so on). It is a powerful antioxidant, protecting cells from oxidative damage that could lead to cancer, and it can be converted to vitamin A as we need it. Unlike preformed vitamin A (retinol), beta-carotene does not exhibit the same clear toxic effects if excess doses are consumed. However, a consistently high intake of carrots, sweet potatoes, and other foods high in beta-carotene may cause a person to develop a yellowish skin tone as the beta-carotene accumulates in subcutaneous fat.

Athlete surveys suggest that different sports have different vitamin A and beta-carotene risks. Young wrestlers, gymnasts, and ballet dancers had average intakes that were below 70 percent of the recommended intake, while other male and female athletes appeared to have typical intakes that meet the recommended level.[63-66] The difference may be the food restriction common in the sports with lower intakes.

It is conceivable that beta-carotene may, as an antioxidant, prove to be effective in reducing postexercise muscle soreness and may aid in postexercise recovery. However, this is a theoretical connection only; no study makes a direct link between beta-carotene intake and reduced soreness and improved recovery. One study found that beta-carotene reduced exercise-induced asthma, and another found it was a useful antioxidant for reducing DNA damage in humans.[67,68] Given these limited findings and its relatively low toxicity potential, the U.S. Olympic Committee (USOC) has recognized beta-carotene's potential as an antioxidant.[69]

Table 2.12 Vitamin A Quick Guide

Alternative name	Retinol (precursor: beta-carotene)
Dietary reference intake (DRI)	Adult males: 900 mcg/day Adult females: 700 mcg/day
Recommended intake for athletes	700 to 900 mcg/day
Functions	Maintaining healthy epithelial (surface) cells, eye health, immune system health
Good food sources	Retinol: liver, butter, cheese, egg yolks, fish liver oils Beta-carotene: dark green and brightly pigmented fruits and vegetables
Deficiency	Dry skin, headache, irritability, vomiting, bone pain, night blindness, increased risk of infection, blindness
Toxicity (high toxicity potential)	Tolerable upper intake levels: 600 to 900 mcg/day for young children (age 1-8) 1.7 to 3.0 mg/day for children and adults (age 9-70+) Symptoms: liver damage, bone malformations, death

Vitamin D

The requirement for vitamin D has received a great deal of scientific scrutiny recently, and studies have concluded that vitamin D plays a more significant role in human health than previously believed. We can obtain the vitamin in an inactive form from food and sunlight exposure (see figure 2.2). Ultraviolet radiation (sunlight) exposure of the skin transforms a cholesterol derivative (7-dehydrocholesterol) into an inactive form of vitamin D called cholecalciferol (D_3). To be functional, the inactive form of vitamin D must be activated by the kidneys. Therefore, kidney disease may be the cause of vitamin D–related disorders. Dietary sources of vitamin D include eggs, fortified milk, liver, butter, and margarine. Cod liver oil, which was once given commonly as a supplement, is a concentrated source of the vitamin. Mushrooms and certain plant foods also provide a form of vitamin D called ergocalciferol (D_2). A limited number of foods may also be fortified with vitamin D, including cereal flours, milk and milk products, and calcium-fortified fruit juices.

The DRI for vitamin D is 15 micrograms (600 IU) per day for all teenagers and adults below the age of 70 and 20 micrograms (800 IU) for those 70 years old and above. The upper limit for this vitamin has recently been increased to a level of 100 micrograms per day (4,000 IU) for all teenagers and adults.

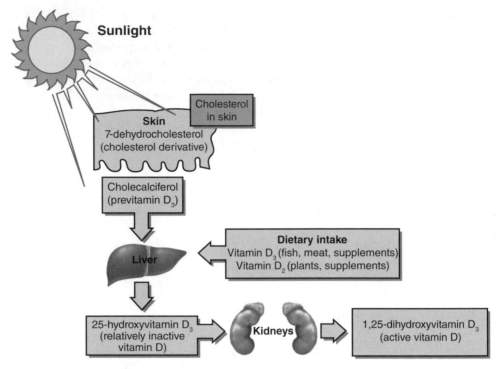

Figure 2.2 Sources of vitamin D.

A diet with an adequate intake of calcium and phosphorus but without adequate vitamin D would lead to calcium and phosphorus deficiency. The childhood disease rickets and the adult disease osteomalacia are diseases of calcium deficiency that are caused either by inadequate levels of vitamin D or the inability to convert vitamin D to the active (functional) form. Excess vitamin D intake may lead to vomiting, diarrhea, weight loss, kidney damage, high blood calcium levels, and death.

A great deal of current science suggests that vitamin D promotes growth and mineralizes bones and teeth by increasing the absorption of calcium and phosphorus. But vitamin D also has other important characteristics that may influence both health and athletic performance. Vitamin D contributes to the following:[70-74]

- Bone health (through regulation of calcium and phosphorus absorption)

- Muscle contraction (through activation of enzymes for muscle stimulation)

- Intestinal absorption (through facilitation of calcium absorption in the intestines)

- Muscle protein anabolism (through both an increase in muscle mass and a decrease in muscle breakdown; muscle increase is for Type II power muscle fibers)

- Improved immune function (through accumulation of fluid and immune cells in injured and inflamed tissues and through release of antimicrobial peptides; the outcome is reduced risk of cancer, intestinal disease, cardiovascular disease, and muscle soreness)

- Improved anti-inflammatory action (through increased production of anti-inflammatory cytokines and interleukin-4 and decreased production of inflammatory agents interleukin-6, interferon-y, and interleukin-2)

There is a long history of ultraviolet light (i.e., vitamin D) therapy for athletes.[71] In the mid-1920s, sunlamps were used by swimmers in Germany, and the effect was sufficiently positive that it was considered a form of illegal doping by some. Russian and German athletes also used ultraviolet (UV) light therapy in the 1930s and 1940s, and it significantly improved performance. In the mid-1940s in the United States, the combined effect of a fitness program plus ultraviolet irradiation produced significantly better fitness results than athletic training without the ultraviolet irradiation. The general consensus during these years was that UV irradiation had a positive impact on speed, strength, endurance, reaction time, and pain. Some have even pondered whether the greater UV irradiation of the Mexico City Olympic Games, because of the city's higher altitude, contributed to the high number of world records set there.

It is also possible that vitamin D plays a role in injury resistance. Athletes in some sports may have dramatically lower sunlight exposure because all training sessions take place inside a building. This lower UV exposure may reduce vitamin D synthesis to a point where both growth and bone density are negatively affected. Lower bone densities are known to place athletes at higher risk for developing a stress fracture, an injury that can end an athletic career.[75-77] In a survey of U.S. national-team gymnasts, the factor most closely related to bone density was sunlight exposure. Those athletes with higher densities had the greatest exposure.[78] Also, sunlight exposure was more important as a predictor of bone density in this group than vitamin D or calcium intake from food.

Table 2.13 Vitamin D Quick Guide

Alternative names	Cholecalciferol, calcitriol, calciferol
Dietary reference intake (DRI)	Adult males: 15 mcg/day (600 IU/day) Adult females: 15 mcg/day (600 IU/day)
Recommended intake for athletes	15 mcg/day (600 IU/day)
Functions	Absorption of calcium and phosphorus, healthy skin
Good food sources	Ultraviolet light exposure, fatty fish (catfish, salmon, mackerel, sardines, tuna), fish liver oil, lesser amounts in eggs and canned fish, fortified milk, and margarine
Deficiency	Rickets (children), osteomalacia (adults), increased risk of stress fractures, increased risk of osteoporosis
Toxicity (high toxicity potential)	Tolerable upper intake levels: 100 mcg/day (4,000 IU/day) for all teenagers and adults Symptoms: nausea, diarrhea, loss of muscle function, organ damage, skeletal damage

Vitamin E

Vitamin E is a generic term for several of the tocopherols with similar activity, and the unit of measure is based on the level of tocopherol with an activity equivalent to that of beta-tocopherol. Beta-tocopherol (β-tocopherol) has a lower level of activity than alpha-tocopherol (α-tocopherol), so more of it would be necessary for the same effect. The adult DRI for vitamin E is 15 milligrams per day, a level easily obtained by consuming green leafy vegetables, vegetable oils, seeds, seed oils, nuts, liver, and corn. The vitamin E content of commonly consumed vegetable oils is closely linked to the level of polyunsaturation of the oil. Interestingly, higher polyunsaturated lipid consumption results in greater vitamin E intake, and this higher level of vitamin E is needed to protect the consumed polyunsaturated lipids from oxidation. A failure to consume sufficient vegetables, nuts, or vegetable oil may place adults at risk of an inadequate intake. Any problem with the fat absorption system (i.e., bile production, pancreatic lipase production, or dietary lipoprotein metabolism) is also likely to negatively affect vitamin E status.

Vitamin E is a potent antioxidant that protects membranes from destruction by peroxides. Peroxides are formed when fats (especially polyunsaturated fats) become oxidized (rancid). These peroxides are called free radicals because they bounce around unpredictably inside cells, altering or destroying them. Since vitamin E is an antioxidant, it helps capture oxygen, thereby limiting the oxidation of fats to protect cells.

It is difficult to induce a vitamin E deficiency in humans, but when it occurs it is associated with damage to the central nervous system and red blood cell hemolysis. There is some indication that vitamin E deficiency can result in muscle breakdown in humans,[79] but there is no indication that taking supplemental doses improves performance or that athletes are at risk for deficiency. In fact, there is evidence that taking a supplemental dose of 800 IU a day for 2 months actually promotes lipid peroxidation and inflammation during endurance activity.[5] A meta-analysis of the effect of high-dose supplementation of vitamin E indicates that chronically high supplemental intakes of greater than 400 IU a day increases all-cause mortality and should, therefore, be avoided.[80]

Several studies on vitamin E and physical performance have been conducted, but none has found an improvement in either strength or endurance with vitamin E supplementation.[81-84] Studies evaluating whether vitamin E supplementation reduces exercise-induced peroxide damage have mixed results. Some show a clear reduction in peroxidative damage,[85,86] but others have found that vitamin E has no benefit.[87] It seems clear that more information on vitamin E is needed before a definitive exercise-related benefit can be claimed from taking doses of the vitamin outside normal food consumption.

Table 2.14 Vitamin E Quick Guide

Alternative names	Tocopherol, alpha-tocopherol, gamma-tocopherol
Dietary reference intake (DRI)	Adult males: 15 mg/day Adult females: 15 mg/day
Recommended intake for athletes	15 mg/day
Functions	Antioxidant protection of cell membranes
Good food sources	Polyunsaturated and monounsaturated vegetable and cereal oils and margarines (corn, soy, safflower, olive); lesser amounts in fortified cereals and eggs
Deficiency	Rare; if it occurs, possible increased risk of cancer and heart disease
Toxicity	Tolerable upper intake levels: 200 to 300 mg/day for young children (age 1-8) 600 to 1,000 mg/day for children and adults (age 9-70+)

Vitamin K

Vitamin K is found in green leafy vegetables and in small amounts in cereals, fruits, and meats. Bacteria in the intestines also produce vitamin K, so the absolute dietary requirement is not known. This vitamin is needed for the formation of prothrombin, which is required for blood to clot. Recent work suggests that vitamin K may also have importance in bone metabolism and vitamin D activity. Several studies show that vitamin K deficiency caused from inadequate dietary intake, albeit rare in human populations, results in low bone mineral density and an increase in skeletal fractures.[88] It has been found that vitamin K–associated lower bone density can be improved with vitamin K supplementation.[89] In addition, women obtaining a minimum of 110 micrograms of vitamin K are at significantly lower hip fracture risk than women who have a lower intake.[90] The Framingham Heart Study also found a relationship between higher vitamin K intakes and reduced hip fracture risk.[91]

It is possible for people who regularly take antibiotics that destroy the bacteria in the intestines to be at increased risk for vitamin K deficiency. A deficiency would cause an increase in bleeding and hemorrhages. The DRI for vitamin K is 90 micrograms per day for adult women and 120 micrograms per day for adult men. There is no established upper limit for this vitamin. Vitamin K appears to be relatively nontoxic, but high intakes of synthetic forms may cause jaundice. Supplemental doses also interfere with anticoagulant drugs. People taking Warfarin (a blood thinner) must be aware that vitamin K supplements or foods containing vitamin K may reduce the effectiveness of their medication.

Vitamin K is found in many foods (including vegetable oils and dark green leafy vegetables), and with bacterial production of the vitamin in the gut, it would seem difficult to develop a deficiency. Nevertheless, a survey has found that an important segment of Americans, particularly children and young adults, does not obtain sufficient vitamin K.[92] No studies have examined the relationship between vitamin K and athletic performance. Further, it is difficult to think of a theoretical framework in which such a relationship might exist. It seems clear that, especially for athletes involved in contact sports, adequate vitamin K is necessary to avoid excessive bruising and bleeding. However, there is no documented evidence that these athletes are at a particularly high risk for a deficiency.

Table 2.15 Vitamin K Quick Guide

Alternative names	Phylloquinone, menoquinone, antihemorrhagic vitamin
Dietary reference intake (DRI)	Adult males: 120 mcg/day Adult females: 90 mcg/day
Recommended intake for athletes	700 to 900 mcg/day
Functions	Formation of blood clots, enhancement of osteocalcin function to aid in bone strengthening
Good food sources	Phylloquinone: a variety of vegetable oils and dark green leafy vegetables (cabbage, spinach) Menoquinone: formed by the bacteria that line the gastrointestinal tract
Deficiency	Rare; if it occurs, results in hemorrhage
Toxicity	Tolerable upper intake levels not established

MINERALS

Minerals are unique in that, unlike other nutrients, they are inorganic. Nevertheless, they work in unison with other organic nutrients (vitamins and energy substrates). An obvious example of this inorganic–organic integration is the well-established relationship between the mineral calcium and vitamin D. Individually, these nutrients are essentially useless, but when available together, they work in concert to sustain bone density. Minerals have numerous functions, including the following:

- Adding to the strength and structure of the skeleton, keeping it strong and resistant to fracture.
- Maintaining the relative acidity or alkalinity of the blood and tissue. For athletes, hard physical activity tends to lower the pH level (i.e., increase the relative acidity), so having a healthy system to control acid–base balance is critical for endurance performance.
- Serving as bridges for electrical impulses that stimulate muscular movement. Since all athletic endeavors rely on efficient and effective muscular movement and coordination, this function is critically important.
- Metabolizing cells. Physical activity increases the rate at which fuel is burned. Therefore, the effective control of fuel burned at the cellular level is necessary for athletic endeavors.

All these functions are important for athletes. Athletes with low-density bones are at increased risk for stress fractures; poor acid–base balance leads to poor endurance; poor nerve and muscle function results in poor coordination; and altered cell metabolism limits a cell's ability to obtain and store energy.

The established roles of minerals in the development of optimal physical performance include involvement in glycolysis (obtaining energy from stored glucose), lipolysis (obtaining energy from fat), proteolysis (obtaining energy from protein), and the phosphagen system (obtaining energy from phosphocreatine).[93] Inorganic mineral nutrients are required in the structural composition of hard and soft body tissues. Minerals also participate in the action of enzyme systems, muscle contractions, nerve reactions, and blood clotting. These mineral nutrients, all of which must be supplied in the diet, are of two classes: major elements (macrominerals) and trace elements (microminerals).

Macrominerals

The total mineral content of the body is approximately 4 percent of body weight. Macrominerals are present in the body in relatively larger amounts than microminerals (thus the name) and include calcium, phosphorus, magnesium, sodium, chloride, and potassium. Calcium makes up approximately 1.75 percent of total body weight, phosphorus makes up approximately 1.10 percent of total body weight, and magnesium makes up approximately .04 percent of total body weight. See tables 2.16 through 2.22 for a summary of the functions, sources, and possible problems associated with macrominerals.

Calcium

Calcium is an important mineral for bone and tooth structure, blood clotting, and nerve transmission; it has a DRI of 1,000 milligrams per day for adult men and women. Deficiencies are associated with skeletal malformations (as in rickets), increased skeletal fragility (as in osteoporotic fracture and stress fractures), and blood pressure abnormalities. There are few reports of toxicity from taking high doses of calcium, but it is conceivable that a high and frequent intake of calcium supplements may alter the acidity of the stomach (making it more alkaline), thereby interfering with protein digestion. Since there is competitive absorption between bivalent minerals (calcium, zinc, iron, and magnesium) in the small intestine, it is also possible that a high amount of calcium may interfere with the absorption of other minerals if they are present in the gut at the same time. Therefore, taking high-dose calcium supplements with a meal that contains iron, for example, may result in the malabsorption of iron and eventually lead to iron-deficiency anemia.

Food sources of calcium include dairy products (milk, cheese, yogurt), dark green vegetables (collards, spinach, chard, mustard greens, broccoli, green peppers), and dried beans and peas (lentils, navy beans, soy beans, and split peas). Calcium and several other minerals (especially iron, magnesium, and zinc) are easily bound to the oxalic acid in dark green vegetables, making the minerals unavailable for absorption. Therefore, although dark green vegetables are potentially good sources of calcium and several other minerals, these foods don't make the minerals easily available to us unless they are properly prepared. Oxalate is highly water soluble, so by dipping the vegetables for a few seconds into boiling water (blanching), a good deal of the oxalate is removed, but most of the minerals remain. The vegetables can then be prepared as needed. This technique dramatically improves the delivery of calcium from vegetables and has been used by cultures that have not traditionally consumed dairy products (especially in Asia) for thousands of years. As a side benefit, vegetables that are blanched may also be more acceptable to eat. Oxalic acid has a bitter taste. Therefore, removal of oxalate has the added benefit of making the vegetables more pleasant tasting.

Numerous studies have assessed the relationships among calcium intake, physical activity, and bone density. Athletes most often take calcium supplements to reduce the risk of fracture (i.e., by improving bone density), not for the purpose of improving physical performance. Physical activity is known to enhance bone density, just as physical inactivity is known to lower bone density. However, the development and mineralization of bone are complex processes involving several factors, including growth phase (childhood and adolescence are associated with faster bone development) hormonal status (especially estrogen for women), energy adequacy, vitamin D availability, and calcium intake.

Since the early 1990s, the increased availability of an accurate bone-density measuring device called dual energy X-ray absorptiometry (DEXA) has dramatically improved the ability to measure bone density and determine fracture risk. Studies that used DEXA indicate that children and adolescents who have a calcium intake at or slightly above the RDA (up to 1,500 milligrams) have higher bone densities. Adequate calcium intake in adults may not increase bone density, but it lays the groundwork for stabilizing the bone. It seems prudent, therefore, to make certain that calcium intake is maintained at the DRI level, that adequate physical activity is maintained (not a problem for most athletes), and that the intake of vitamin D is adequate. A survey of elite gymnasts indicates that sunlight exposure is more related to bone mineral density than is calcium intake. This points to the integrated relationship between calcium and vitamin D and how critical it is to have nutrients working together to ensure optimal health.[94]

Another concern of many female athletes is amenorrhea (cessation of menses), which is strongly associated with either poor bone development in young athletes or bone

Phytochemicals

Phyto is the Greek word for plants, and phytochemicals (also known as phytonutrients) are plant-derived chemical compounds that are increasingly found to be important for health. Although phytochemicals have not been directly assessed for their impact on human athletic performance, they may be important to the athletic endeavor. Studies show that a number of phytochemicals have important nutrition effects. Dr. David Heber of the UCLA Center for Human Nutrition in Los Angeles, California, with the assistance of Susan Bowerman, originated a seven-color system to organize the major phytochemicals and their physiological impact:

- **Red (lycopene, phytoene, phytofluene, vitamin E):** Fruits and vegetables containing these phytonutrients include tomatoes, vegetable juice, and watermelon. These substances are potentially twice as effective as beta-carotene in eliminating cell-destroying free radicals.

- **Green (glucosinolates, folic acid, isothiocyanates, indole-3 carbinol):** Fruits and vegetables containing these phytonutrients include broccoli, brussels sprouts, bok choy, cauliflower, and cabbage. These substances have been associated with cancer-protective effects.

- **Green/Yellow (lutein, zeaxanthin):** Fruits and vegetables containing these substances include spinach, avocado, kale, green beans, green peppers, kiwi fruit, collard greens, and mustard greens. These substances are associated with antioxidant and anticancer effects.

- **Orange (alpha- and beta-carotene, beta-cryptoxanthin):** These substances include carrots, pumpkins, butternut squash, mangoes, apricots, and cantaloupe. They are associated with anticancer effects.

- **Orange/Yellow (vitamin C, flavonoids):** These substances include oranges, orange juice, tangerines, yellow grapefruit, peaches, nectarines, lemons, limes, papaya, and pineapple. They are potent antioxidants associated with anticancer effects.

- **Red/Purple (anthocyanins, ellagic acid, flavonoids):** These substances include grapes, cherries, red wine, strawberries, blueberries, blackberries, raspberries, cranberries, plums, prunes, and raisins. They appear to be 20 to 50 times more effective than vitamin C alone, appear to reduce blood clots, and may also have some anticancer and antiaging characteristics.

- **White/Green (allyl sulfides):** These are found in garlic, onion, and chives and appear to have anticancer and anti–heart disease characteristics.

Although there is still much to learn about the specific roles these individual substances play in human nutrition, they may be why people with higher vegetable intakes are found to be at lower risk for a variety of cancers. There is little reason to not eat more vegetables, as they are good sources of nutrients, carbohydrate, and phytochemicals, and we may find in the future that they also play an important role in improved muscle recovery, reduced muscle soreness, and better health. Eat your vegetables!

demineralization in older athletes. The causes of amenorrhea are complex and include inadequate energy intake, eating disorders, low body-fat levels, poor iron status, psychological stress, high cortisol levels, and overtraining. Put simply, elite female athletes who train hard are at risk. Anything that might lower risk, such as maintaining a good iron status and consuming enough energy, is useful for lowering the risk of developing amenorrhea. Even if an amenorrheic athlete has sufficient calcium intake, that alone would not suffice to maintain or develop healthy bones because the lower level of circulating estrogen associated with amenorrhea would inhibit normal bone development and maintenance.

Table 2.16 Calcium Quick Guide

Symbol	Ca
Dietary reference intake (DRI)	Adult males: 1,000 mg/day Adult females: 1,000 mg/day
Recommended intake for athletes	1,300 to 1,500 mg/day
Functions	Bone structure and strength, acid–base balance, nerve function, muscle contraction, enzyme activation
Good food sources	Dairy products, dark green leafy vegetables, calcium-fortified orange juice and other calcium-fortified foods, soy milk, legumes
Deficiency	Osteoporosis, rickets, poor muscle function
Toxicity	Tolerable upper intake levels: 2,500 mg/day for all age groups Symptoms: constipation, malabsorption of other bivalent minerals (iron, magnesium, and zinc), kidney stones, cardiac arrhythmia

Phosphorus

Phosphorus is present in most foods and is especially plentiful in protein-rich foods (meat, poultry, fish, and dairy products) and cereal grains. It combines with calcium (about two parts calcium for every part phosphorus) to produce healthy bones and teeth. It also plays an important role in energy metabolism, affecting carbohydrate, fat, and protein. The energy derived for muscular work comes largely from phosphorus-containing compounds called adenosine triphosphate (ATP) and phosphocreatine (PCr). As with calcium, the absorption of phosphorus is dependent on vitamin D, and the adult RDA is 700 milligrams per day.

Because phosphorus is so omnipresent in the food supply, phosphorus deficiencies are uncommon. If deficiencies occur, they are most likely to be seen in people on long-term antacids containing aluminum hydroxide.[95] This type of antacid binds with phosphorus, making it unavailable for absorption.[96] The adult upper limit for phosphorus is 4,000 milligrams per day, above which there may be interference with calcium absorption.

Phosphorus supplementation has been used for a long time to enhance physical activity. During World War I, Germany commonly provided its soldiers with high-phosphorus foods and supplements for the purpose of improving strength and endurance.[97] This large-population experience suggests that large doses of phosphorus are relatively well tolerated over time. However, there is no direct evidence that strength and endurance were actually improved with this high intake. More recent studies on the effect of phosphorus supplementation yielded mixed results. Runners, rowers, and swimmers taking 2 grams of sodium dihydrogen phosphate 1 hour before exercise all experienced performance improvements, while only half the nonsupplemented athletes showed improvements.[98] Another study found that $\dot{V}O_2$max was improved on a treadmill test after short-term phosphorus supplementation.[99] However, a study evaluating the effect of phosphate supplementation on muscular power observed no apparent benefit from taking phosphate.[100] The mixed results of these studies make it difficult to conclude that a preexercise supplement of phosphorus actually improves performance. Clearly, more well-designed studies are needed before an answer to this question can be attempted.

Table 2.17 Phosphorus Quick Guide

Symbol	P
Dietary reference intake (DRI)	Adult males: 700 mg/day Adult females: 700 mg/day
Recommended intake for athletes	1,250 to 1,500 mg/day
Functions	Bone structure and strength, acid–base balance, B-vitamin function, component of ATP
Good food sources	All high-protein foods, whole-grain products, carbonated beverages
Deficiency	Unlikely; if it occurs, results in low bone density and muscle weakness
Toxicity	Tolerable upper intake levels: 3,000 mg for young children (age 1-8) and adults over 70 4,000 mg for children and adults (age 9-70) Toxicity is unlikely, but if it occurs, results in low bone density and GI distress

Magnesium

Magnesium, a mineral present in most foods, is essential for human metabolism and for maintaining the electrical potential in nerve and muscle cells. When associated with widespread malnutrition, especially in alcoholics, a magnesium deficiency results in tremors and convulsions. Magnesium is involved in more than 300 reactions in which food is synthesized to new products, and it is a critical component in the processes that create muscular energy from carbohydrate, protein, and fat.[101] The adult DRI for magnesium ranges between 310 and 320 milligrams per day for females and 400 and 420 milligrams per day for males. The safe upper limit for magnesium is similar to the DRI but represents the intake from supplement doses only and does not include the amount obtained from food and water. Supplements are available, with different supplements containing different proportions of magnesium (see figure 2.3).

It is possible that athletes training in hot and humid environments could lose a relatively large amount of magnesium by sweating. Were this to occur, a magnesium deficiency could, given the importance of magnesium in muscle function processes, cause athletes to underachieve athletically. In one study where magnesium supplements were given to athletes, an improvement in physical performance was shown.[102] There is some limited evidence that taking magnesium supplements at the level of the DRI may positively affect endurance and strength performance in athletes with blood magnesium levels at the low end of the normal range.[103,104] In a study assessing the effect of magnesium supplements (365 milligrams per day) on well-trained marathon runners, the supplements had no impact on performance, did not improve resistance to muscle breakdown, and did not enhance muscle recovery after the race.[105] With the exception of athletes who are known to reduce total energy intake to maintain or lower body weight (wrestlers, gymnasts, figure skaters), it appears that most male athletes consume the DRI or more, and most female athletes consume at least 60 percent of the DRI.[106,107] Limited data suggest that a small magnesium deficiency could exacerbate the harmful consequences of intense physical activity.[108] A good strategy is to ensure these athletes consume foods that are good sources of magnesium (see table 2.18), and if a food strategy is not possible, to consider small periodic supplemental doses of magnesium.

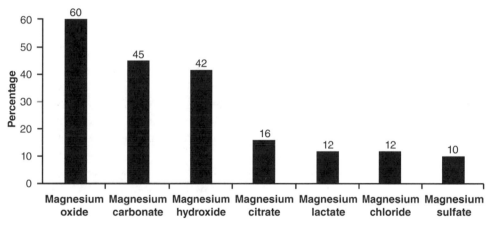

Figure 2.3 Percentage of magnesium content in oral supplements.

Source: NIH Office of Dietary Supplements, 2009, Dietary supplement fact sheet: Magnesium. Available: http://ods.od.nih.gov/factsheets/magnesium/ [August 18, 2011].

Table 2.18 Magnesium Quick Guide

Symbol	Mg
Dietary reference intake (DRI)	Adult males: 420 mg/day Adult females: 320 mg/day
Recommended intake for athletes	400 to 450 mg/day if from food sources; 350 mg/day if from supplements
Functions	Protein synthesis, glucose metabolism, bone structure, muscle contraction
Good food sources	Milk and milk products, meat, nuts, whole-grain foods, dark green leafy vegetables, fruits
Deficiency	Unlikely; if it occurs, results in muscle weakness, muscle cramps, and cardiac arrhythmia
Toxicity	Tolerable upper intake levels: 350 mg if taken as supplements Symptoms: nausea, vomiting, diarrhea

Sodium

Sodium is an essential mineral commonly referred to as salt. (Table salt is actually a combination of sodium and chloride.) It is involved in body-water balance and acid–base balance and is the major extracellular (outside the cell, including blood and fluid) mineral. Sodium is present in small quantities in most natural foods and is found in high amounts in processed, canned, cooked, and fast foods. Although most of us are capable of excreting excess sodium, some people are sodium sensitive because they lack this capacity. In these people, excess sodium retention causes edema (an excess accumulation of extracellular fluid) and contributes to high blood pressure. Sodium-sensitive persons can limit intake by concentrating food choices on natural, whole foods and avoiding high-sodium (i.e., salty) commercially prepared foods. Food labels provide information about sodium content (see table 2.20). The 2004 Institute of Medicine's recommendation for sodium intake is 1.5 grams per day, while the tolerable upper limit is 2.3 grams of sodium per day.[109]

Sodium is one of the key ingredients in sports beverages because it helps drive the desire to drink and because it helps maintain blood volume. Maintenance of blood volume is a key factor in athletic performance; it is related to the ability to deliver nutrients to cells, to the removal of metabolic by-products from cells, and to the maintenance of the sweat rate. Additional information on sodium is included in chapter 3.

Because of sweat losses, athletes are likely to require more than the 1.5 grams of sodium recommended for the general public. On hot and humid days when sweat losses of sodium are high, athletes may require more than 10 grams of sodium, a level that dramatically exceeds the upper limit of 2.3 grams per day. Therefore, the Institute of Medicine's recommendation for sodium intake is not applicable to most athletes and should not be followed. On the contrary, athletes should regularly consume salty foods and beverages when exercising or competing in hot and humid conditions. The higher athlete requirement for salt is recognized by the Institute of Medicine, which states that its recommendations for the general population are not applicable to those who sweat regularly.[110]

Table 2.19 Sodium Quick Guide

Symbol	Na
Adequate intake (AI)	Adult males: 1.5 g/day Adult females: 1.5 g/day
Recommended intake for athletes	>1.5 g/day; high sweat losses of sodium may increase requirement to >10 g/day
Functions	Water balance, nerve function, acid–base balance, muscle contraction
Good food sources	Processed and canned foods, pickles, potato chips, pretzels, soy sauce, cheese
Deficiency	Hyponatremia, with muscle cramping, nausea, vomiting, anorexia, seizures, and coma (potentially extremely dangerous)
Toxicity	Tolerable upper intake levels: 2.3 g/day (about 5.8 g of table salt); athletes may have a requirement that far exceeds the upper level Major symptom: hypertension and increased risk of cardiovascular disease and stroke

Table 2.20 Sodium on Food Labels: Understanding the Terms

Term	Definition
Sodium free	Less than 5 mg of sodium per standard serving
Very low sodium	• 35 mg of sodium or less per standard serving • If the serving weighs 30 g or less, 35 mg of sodium or less per 50 g of food • If the serving is 2 tbsp or less, 35 mg of sodium or less per 50 g of food
Low sodium	• 140 mg of sodium or less per standard serving • If the serving weighs 30 g or less, 140 mg of sodium or less per 50 g of food • If the serving is 2 tbsp or less, 140 mg of sodium or less per 50 g of food
Reduced or less sodium	A minimum of 25% lower sodium content than the food it is compared with

Chloride

Chloride is an extracellular mineral that is essential for the maintenance of fluid balance and, therefore, normal cell function. It is also an important component of gastric juices. Virtually all the chloride we consume is associated with table salt (sodium chloride), so sodium and chloride intakes parallel each other. Because chloride losses are closely linked to sodium losses, a deficiency of one is related to a deficiency of the other. Deficiencies typically occur with heavy sweating, frequent diarrhea, or frequent vomiting. Sweat losses are likely to deplete chloride and sodium to a greater degree than other minerals, including potassium and magnesium. Most people consume excessive amounts of salt (which is 60 percent chloride), so chloride intake is typically 6,000 milligrams (6 grams) or more, a level that is well above normal requirements. The DRI-estimated chloride requirement is 2.3 grams per day for both adult men and women, while the safe upper limit for chloride is 3.6 grams per day. Excess chloride and sodium may both contribute to the development of hypertension.

Table 2.21 Chloride Quick Guide

Symbol	Cl
Dietary reference intake (DRI)	Adult males: 2.3 g/day Adult females: 2.3 g/day
Recommended intake for athletes	2.3 g/day or more to match the increase in sodium intake with high sweat losses
Functions	Water balance, nerve function, parietal cell (stomach) HCl production
Good food sources	Table salt (~60% chloride and 40% sodium)
Deficiency	Associated with frequent vomiting and diarrhea, and is lost in sweat; although rare, may lead to convulsions
Toxicity	Tolerable upper intake levels: 3,500 mg/day, or the equivalent of 5,800 mg of table salt Cl intake is associated with sodium intake, both of which contribute to hypertension with excess intake.

Potassium

Potassium is the main mineral found inside cells (an intracellular electrolyte) at a concentration 30 times greater than the concentration of potassium found outside cells. It is involved in water balance, nerve impulse transmission, and muscular contractions. Dietary deficiency is rare and typically occurs only with chronic diarrhea and vomiting or laxative abuse. People taking medications for high blood pressure force the loss of sodium, and in this process potassium is also lost. These people are encouraged to replace this lost potassium through the intake of supplements or foods high in potassium (fruits, vegetables, and meats). Typical intakes of potassium range from 1,000 to 11,000 milligrams per day (1 to 11 grams per day); people consuming large amounts of fresh fruits and vegetables have the highest intakes.

There is evidence that a potassium intake of about 4.7 grams per day (4,700 milligrams per day) is useful in controlling high blood pressure.[110, 111] Adequate intake of potassium helps counteract the impact of excess sodium intake, thereby helping to control blood pressure. It also reduces the risk of decreased bone density and lowers the risk of developing kidney stones.[110] The DRI for potassium is 4.7 grams per day for both adult men and women. Although there is no established safe upper limit, potassium toxicity appears to develop with an intake of approximately 18 grams and may lead to cardiac arrest.[110, 111] People with chronic renal disease or diabetes appear to be at particular risk of death from hyperkalemia, most often resulting from high intake of salt substitutes or potassium supplements. Because of the risk of sudden cardiac arrest with an excess potassium intake, potassium supplementation is generally not recommended. It is well established that potassium is critical for heart and skeletal muscle function. However, the relatively small amount of potassium lost in sweat does not seriously affect body stores, so it does not typically have an impact on athletic performance in well-nourished athletes.[112]

Table 2.22 Potassium Quick Guide

Symbol	K
Dietary reference intake (DRI)	Adult males: 4.7 g/day Adult females: 4.7 g/day
Recommended intake for athletes	4.7 g/day or more with high levels of sweat loss
Functions	Water balance, glucose delivery to cells
Good food sources	Citrus fruits, potatoes, vegetables, milk, meat, fish, bananas
Deficiency	Hypokalemia, which is associated with anorexia, arrhythmias, and muscle cramping
Toxicity	Tolerable upper intake levels for potassium not established. Hyperkalemia, a condition that may lead to arrhythmias and altered heart function (may lead to death). Although no UL established, it appears that 18 g/day may result in cardiac arrent. Potassium supplements are generally *not* recommended for this reason.

Microminerals

Microminerals (trace elements) are present in body tissues in extremely small amounts but have critically important roles to play in human nutrition. The required intake of each micromineral is less than 100 milligrams per day, and the total body content of these minerals is less than 5 grams. They include iron, zinc, iodine, selenium, copper, manganese, and chromium. See tables 2.23 through 2.31 for a summary of the functions, sources, and possible problems associated with microminerals.

Iron

Iron is needed to form the oxygen-transporting compounds hemoglobin (in blood) and myoglobin (in muscle) and is also found in a number of other compounds involved in normal tissue function. Iron absorption is limited because there is no effective mechanism for excreting the excess once it is absorbed. To a large degree, the amount absorbed is driven by the amount of iron in storage (in ferritin and hemosiderin). The lower the iron storage level, the higher the rate of iron absorption; however, overall absorption rates rarely go above 10 to 15 percent of the iron content of consumed food. This variable absorption mechanism is aimed at maintaining a relatively constant level of iron while avoiding an excess iron uptake. Despite this variable absorption rate, people with marginal iron intakes are at risk of developing iron deficiency and, eventually, iron-deficiency anemia.

Iron-deficiency anemia is characterized by poor oxygen-carrying capacity, a condition that causes endurance problems in athletes. Iron deficiency is also associated with poor immune function, short attention span, irritability, and poor learning ability. In the United States, children experiencing fast growth, women of menstrual age, vegetarians, and pregnant women are at increased risk for developing iron-deficiency anemia. Periods of growth and pregnancy are associated with a higher requirement of iron because of a fast expansion of the blood volume, and iron is an essential component of red blood cells. Women of childbearing age have higher requirements because of the regular blood (and iron) losses associated with the menstrual period. For this reason, these women have a higher DRI for iron (18 milligrams) than do men of the same age (8 milligrams). Some people are at risk of developing iron toxicity because they are missing the mechanisms for limiting absorption. Young children in particular may be at risk for iron toxicity if they ingest supplements intended for adults. Although the iron DRI for children (~7 to 10 milligrams per day) is similar to that for male adults, many iron supplements intended for adults contain iron levels more than 300 percent of the DRI. Iron overload disease is potentially fatal.

Iron is available in a wide variety of foods, including meats, eggs, vegetables, and iron-fortified cereals. Milk and other dairy products are poor sources of iron. The most easily absorbed form of iron is heme iron, which comes from meats and other foods of animal origin. Nonheme iron, which is not as easily absorbed, is found in fruits, vegetables, and cereals. However, consuming foods high in vitamin C may enhance nonheme iron absorption. On the other hand, nonheme iron absorption may be inhibited by phytic acid (a substance associated with bran in cereal grains), antacids, and calcium phosphate. In general, red meats provide the most abundant and easily absorbable source of iron. For this reason, vegetarians are considered to be at increased risk of iron-deficiency anemia. Nevertheless, with proper planning; consumption of vegetables, iron-fortified grain products, and fruits high in iron; and sound cooking techniques that aid iron absorption, vegetarians can obtain sufficient iron. Table 2.24 lists a few ways to improve iron absorption in a vegetarian diet.

Table 2.23 Iron Quick Guide

Symbol	Fe (Fe^{2+} = ferrous iron; Fe^{3+} = ferric iron)
Dietary reference intake (DRI)	Adult males: 8 mg/day Adult females: 18 mg/day
Recommended intake for athletes	15 to 18 mg/day
Functions	Oxygen delivery (as hemoglobin and myoglobin), part of numerous oxidative enzymes, essential for aerobic metabolism
Good food sources	Meat, fish, poultry, and shellfish; lesser amounts in legumes, dark green leafy vegetables, and dried fruit; cast-iron cookware increases iron content of cooked foods
Deficiency	Fatigue, lower infection resistance, low energy metabolism (with possible hypothermia)
Toxicity	Toxic levels of tissue iron (hemochromatosis) and liver damage

Table 2.24 Maximizing Iron Intake in a Vegetarian Diet

Food type	Normal absorption	Improving absorption rate
Vegetables (all varieties)	Contain iron in the nonheme form, which has a lower rate of absorption than iron in meats	Add vitamin C to the vegetables by squeezing lemon or orange juice on them before eating.
Dark green vegetables	Contain iron but also contain oxalic acid, which reduces availability of iron for absorption	To remove the oxalic acid, blanche the vegetables by putting them in a pot of boiling water for 5 to 10 seconds. Much of the oxalate is removed, but the iron remains.
High-fiber cereals (with a high bran content)	Contain large amounts of phytic acid, which binds with iron and reduces the availability for absorption	To maximize absorption, replace bran-added cereals in the diet with whole-grain cereals.

Iron Status and Athletic Performance   Athletes have good reason to be concerned about iron status because oxygen-carrying capacity and oxidative enzyme function are critical factors in physical endurance. Iron deficiency is one of the most common nutrient deficiencies of the general public, and it appears that iron deficiency and iron-deficiency anemia have the same incidence level in athletes.[113] See table 2.25 for common causes of iron deficiency in athletes.

Dietary Intake   The dietary intake of athletes, particularly endurance athletes, typically focuses on carbohydrate foods and diminishes the intake of meats. This eating pattern is generally associated as ideal from the perspective of providing an optimal distribution of energy substrates, but it may marginalize the intake of iron. Meat clearly provides a higher concentration of iron than other foods, despite the fact that cereal grains are currently fortified with iron as a public health measure to lower the prevalence of iron-deficiency anemia. Vegetarian athletes, through their avoidance of foods that are highest in iron, are at greatest risk for deficiency.

Table 2.25 Summary of Iron-Deficiency Causes in Athletes

Low dietary intake of iron	Athletes may consume foods containing an inadequate level of iron.
Consumption of foods with low iron absorption rates	Vegetable sources of iron have lower iron concentrations and lower iron absorption rates than meats.
Increased iron losses (hematuria)	Red blood cell breakdown may occur at a faster rate because of higher intravascular compression, resulting in hemolysis. This may result in small amounts of iron (as hemoglobin and myoglobin) being lost in the urine because of a rupturing of red blood cells.
Loss of iron in sweat	Iron losses in sweat are low but may contribute to iron deficiency in athletes with marginal iron intakes.
Loss of iron from bleeding	A loss of blood, through GI losses or through abnormal menstrual losses, increases iron-deficiency risk.
Dilutional pseudoanemia (also commonly referred o as sports anemia)	Physical training results in an expansion of the blood volume, which may result in a dilution, albeit temporarily, of red blood cells.

Low Iron Absorption   Iron absorption is relatively low (rarely more than 10 percent of total dietary consumption), even in those with the greatest need. The absorption of iron is enhanced by the intake of meat and diminished by the intake of nonmeat foods. In addition, certain components of vegetables (oxalic acid) and cereals (phytic acid) bind iron and other divalent minerals and make them unavailable for absorption. Iron is competitively absorbed with other divalent minerals (most notably calcium, magnesium, and zinc), so an excessive intake of one or more of these minerals may diminish the absorption rate of iron. Given the common supplementary intake of calcium in particular, reduced iron absorption may be likely.

Increased Red Blood Cell Breakdown   A number of studies have documented higher rates of intravascular hemolysis in athletes than in nonathletes.[114] Hemolysis occurs when exertional forces cause a ballistic and premature breakdown of red blood cells (RBCs). In athletes RBCs have a life expectancy of approximately 80 days, while in nonathletes RBCs last approximately 120 days. Runners, because of frequent foot strike, and other athletes involved in concussive sports may be at increased risk of hemolysis, but hemolysis has also been documented in swimmers and dancers. The importance of foot strike on hemolysis is evident—the phrase "foot-strike hemolysis" is commonly used to describe this condition. Typically, the harder the surface the runner works out on, the greater the potential for hemolysis.[114, 115]

Loss of Iron in Sweat   The concentration of iron in sweat is low (approximately .2 milligram per liter of sweat), but the sweat loss in long-duration activities may be sufficiently high (possibly more than 2 liters of sweat per hour) that a significant amount of iron can be lost.[116] Although it appears that those athletes engaging in extremely long-duration training sessions are at risk of losing a substantial amount of iron through this route, other athletes are likely to have negligible iron losses through sweat.[117]

Loss of Iron From Blood Loss   Loss of blood is typically from menstrual losses or through the gastrointestinal tract. Of course, athletes who donate blood also lose a significant amount of iron. Blood loss through the GI tract appears to be significant and has been found in up to 85 percent of athletes engaged in intense endurance events. [118] It seems likely that nonsteroidal anti-inflammatory drugs (NSAIDs) such as aspirin and ibuprofen, frequently taken by athletes to control muscle pain, may result in a degree of GI tract irritation and blood loss.[118]

Dilutional Pseudoanemia (Sports Anemia)

Sports anemia is experienced by most athletes, typically at the beginning of an intensive training period. The initiation of intensive training is associated with an enlargement of the blood volume, which causes a dilution of the blood constituents. Because there is no reduction in blood constituents, as occurs with any form of blood loss, oxygen-carrying capacity remains at previous levels (thus the name pseudoanemia). After several weeks, the constituents of the blood (including red blood cells) have an opportunity to increase so as to normalize their concentrations. Exhaustive exercise typically results in a reduction in plasma volume, which experiences a positive recovery and expansion after rehydration in the postexercise period.[119] Harder training, particularly in endurance activities, is associated with the greatest plasma volume increase and will persist for up to 5 days after exercise cessation.[119] True iron-deficiency anemia is associated with a smaller red cell volume (i.e., lower mean cell volume, or MCV) and lower stored iron (i.e., lower ferritin), but athletic pseudoanemia is not associated with either of these biomarkers.

Iron Deficiency and Iron-Deficiency Anemia

Athletes should make every effort to avoid an iron-deficient state because oxygen-carrying capacity is of central importance for athletic endurance. Besides its obvious importance in oxygen transport, iron is also important in a large number of energy-transport enzymes and is also involved in normal nerve and behavioral function and in immune function.[120]

Iron deficiency is seen in approximately 20 percent of females of childbearing age and has a much smaller incidence (1 to 5 percent) in postmenopausal females and males.[121] Iron deficiency with anemia (i.e., low hemoglobin, low hematocrit, low MCV, low ferritin) has a lower prevalence (1 to 3 percent of the population). Athletes may have a higher prevalence of iron deficiency but not iron-deficiency anemia. Further, athletes might respond differently to the presence of frank anemia (reduction in the number and size of red blood cells) versus iron-deficiency anemia (low serum iron and low stored iron but normal red blood cells).[122] Those at highest risk for iron deficiency anemia appear to be elite female distance runners, although the condition has been reported in virtually every athlete group that has been assessed.[123,124]

Although iron-deficient athletes are known to experience a performance deficit, there appears to be no benefit in providing iron supplements to athletes who have a normal iron status.[97] Further, iron supplementation is often associated with nausea, constipation, and stomach irritation. However, in athletes with blood tests that demonstrate either an anemia or a marginal level of stored iron, iron supplementation is warranted. The usual iron replacement therapy is to provide oral ferrous sulfate, but in athletes with GI distress, ferrous gluconate can be used and appears to be better tolerated. Intermuscular injections of iron are generally not recommended because of their association with potentially serious side effects.[121]

The frequency of iron supplement intake remains a topic of ongoing debate. Some suggest the best means of reducing the chance of potential negative side effects is to take 25 to 50 milligrams every third or fourth day instead of daily doses.[125] This approach may prevent GI distress and may impart the same benefits seen with daily supplementation. Of course, taking iron supplements in the absence of iron deficiency or iron-deficiency anemia should be avoided. Besides increasing the risk of hemochromatosis (iron overload disease), which may affect 1 percent of people of northern European descent, iron supplementation may mask celiac disease and colon cancer.[126] Excess iron stores may be observed among professional road cyclists who habitually consume excessive iron supplements.[127]

Zinc

Zinc helps form a large number of enzymes, many of which function in energy metabolism and in wound healing. Inadequate dietary intake of zinc causes a variety of health problems, including stunted growth, slow wound healing, and failure of the immune system.[128] Zinc also plays an important role in the removal of carbon dioxide from cells and is part of an important antioxidant enzyme called superoxide dismutase. Excessive intake can lead to anemia, vomiting, and immune system failure. Meat, liver, eggs, and seafood are good sources of zinc. The adult DRI for zinc is 8 to 11 milligrams per day.

Zinc levels at the lower end of the normal range, or lower, have been observed in male and female endurance runners. Athletes with lower serum zinc values had lower training mileage, probably from not being able to train as hard, than those who had higher values.[129-131] Therefore, there appear to be training deficits in the small number of athletes who have poor zinc status. The effect of zinc supplementation on performance has not been extensively studied, and the level of supplementation in these studies has been extremely high (around 135 milligrams per day). Also, the athletes tested were not assessed for zinc status before the initiation of the research protocol. Nevertheless, this intake level did lead to an improvement in both muscular strength and endurance.[132] A recent study of elite athletes found an important positive relationship between normal zinc status and the athletes' ability to respond to the antioxidant mechanisms associated with intense exercise.[133] Perhaps the greatest potential problem associated with inadequate zinc is in athletes who have inadequate diets and who also use sweat loss as a means of achieving desirable weight. Athletes, usually gymnasts and wrestlers, with inadequate diets and heavy sweat losses are reported to have impaired growth and zinc deficiency.[134]

Athletes should be cautioned that chronically high zinc intakes have never been tested over time and may well have negative side effects. Toxicity and malabsorption of other nutrients are both likely with high supplemental intake.[135-137] A study assessing intake of a supplement containing zinc and magnesium (zinc magnesium aspartate) determined the supplementation did not enhance training adaptations in resistance-trained athletes.[138]

Table 2.26 Zinc Quick Guide

Symbol	Zn
Dietary reference intake (DRI)	Adult males: 11 mg/day Adult females: 8 mg/day
Recommended intake for athletes	11 to 15 mg/day
Functions	Part of numerous enzymes involved in energy metabolism, protein synthesis, immune function, sensory function, and sexual maturation
Good food sources	Meat, fish, poultry, shellfish, eggs, whole-grain foods, vegetables, nuts
Deficiency	Impaired wound healing and immune function, anorexia, failure to thrive (in children), dry skin
Toxicity	Tolerable upper intake level: 40 mg/day Symptoms: impaired immune system, slow wound healing, hypogeusia, hyposmia, high LDL:HDL cholesterol ratio, nausea

Iodine

Iodine is needed to synthesize a key hormone of the thyroid gland, thyroxine, which is involved in regulating metabolic rate, growth, and development. An iodine deficiency leads to goiter, a swelling of the thyroid gland in the front of the neck. Goiter was once common in the United States, but the use of iodized salt has eliminated the condition in this country. An excessive intake of iodine depresses thyroid activity, so taking supplemental doses of iodine is not recommended.

Table 2.27 Iodine Quick Guide

Symbol	I
Dietary reference intake (DRI)	Adult males: 150 mcg/day Adult females: 150 mcg/day
Recommended intake for athletes	120 to 150 mcg/day
Functions	Forms thyroid hormone thyroxine, which is involved in metabolism control
Good food sources	Iodized salt and seafood (depending on soil, some vegetables may also be good sources)
Deficiency	Goiter (enlarged thyroid gland with inadequate thyroxine production), with associated obesity
Toxicity	Inadequate thyroxine production

Selenium

Selenium is an important mineral antioxidant in human nutrition. Since exercise (particularly endurance exercise) is associated with an increased production of potentially damaging oxidative by-products (peroxides and free radicals) in muscle fibers, it is possible that selenium may play a role in reducing muscular oxidative stress.[139] A selenium deficiency may result in muscle weakness and increased recovery time after exhaustive exercise.[97] There is little evidence, however, that increasing the intake of supplemental selenium increases exercise performance.[140] The adult male and female DRI for selenium is 55 micrograms per day. Nutritional supplements, including sodium selenite and high-selenium yeast, are effective sources of selenium, but excessive intake may be toxic, so proper care in taking appropriate supplement levels is important. The safe upper limit is set at 400 micrograms per day for adults, with brittle hair and nails a sign of toxicity.

Table 2.28 Selenium Quick Guide

Symbol	Se
Dietary reference intake (DRI)	Adult males: 55 mcg/day Adult females: 55 mcg/day
Recommended intake for athletes	50 to 55 mcg/day
Functions	Antioxidant (part of glutathione peroxidase)
Good food sources	Meat, fish, seafood, whole-grain foods, nuts (depending on soil, some vegetables may also be good sources)
Deficiency	Unlikely; if it occurs, results in heart damage
Toxicity	Tolerable upper intake level: 400 mcg/day for adults (lower for children) Toxicity is rare; if it occurs, results in nausea, GI distress, and hair loss

Copper

Among the more important trace elements is copper, which is present in many enzymes and in copper-containing proteins found in the blood, brain, and liver. Copper is important for preventing oxidative damage to cells through the enzyme superoxide dismutase. Deficiency is associated with the failure to use iron in the formation of hemoglobin and myoglobin. The adult DRI for copper is 900 micrograms per day, and the safe upper limit for adults is set at 10,000 micrograms per day. Excess consumption may result in GI distress or liver damage. Good sources of copper include shellfish, soybean products, legumes, nuts, seeds, liver, and potatoes. As another good example of why nutrition balance is important, excessive consumption of calcium, phosphate, iron, zinc, and vitamin C all reduce copper absorption. Very few studies have been performed on the relationship between copper and athletic performance. Studies of blood copper concentrations in athletes and nonathletes have not revealed any significant differences, but the athletes have a slightly higher (3 to 4 percent) concentration of serum copper than do nonathletes.[93] In a study evaluating the copper status of swimmers during a competitive season, there was no difference in pre- and postseason copper status. In this study, the majority of swimmers were consuming adequate levels of copper (more than 1 milligram per day) from food.[141]

Table 2.29 Copper Quick Guide

Symbol	Cu
Dietary reference intake (DRI)	Adult males: 900 mcg/day Adult females: 900 mcg/day
Recommended intake for athletes	900 mcg/day
Functions	Part of iron-transport protein ceruloplasmin, oxidation reactions
Good food sources	Meat, fish, poultry, shellfish, eggs, nuts, whole-grain foods, bananas
Deficiency	Rare; if it occurs, results in anemia (inability to transport iron to red blood cells)
Toxicity	Tolerable upper intake level: 10 mg/day Toxicity is rare; if it occurs, leads to nausea and vomiting

Manganese

Manganese is a trace mineral involved in bone formation, immune function, antioxidant activity, and carbohydrate metabolism.[122] Although manganese deficiency is rare, deficiencies are associated with skeletal problems (undermineralized bone and increased risk of fracture) and poor wound healing. It appears that the greatest risk of deficiency is found in people on diets (inadequate intake) or where malabsorption occurs. Manganese is in competition with calcium, iron, and zinc for absorption, so an excess intake of these other minerals may decrease manganese absorption and lead to deficiency symptoms. Much like iron, manganese absorption is enhanced with vitamin C and meat intake. Food sources of manganese include coffee, tea, chocolate, whole grains, nuts, seeds, soybeans, dried beans (navy beans, lentils, split peas), liver, and fruits. As with several other minerals, the intake of foods high in oxalic acid (present in dark green leafy vegetables) may inhibit manganese absorption. (See the calcium section on pages 64-67 for ways of reducing the oxalic acid content of foods.) The adult DRI for manganese is 2.3 milligrams per day for men and 1.8 milligrams per day for women. The safe upper limit is set at 11 milligrams per day for both men and women, with an excess intake causing neurological symptoms. As with copper, excessive intakes of calcium, phosphorus, iron, zinc, fiber, and oxalic acid all decrease manganese absorption.

Table 2.30 Manganese Quick Guide

Symbol	Mn
Dietary reference intake (DRI)	Adult males: 2.3 mg/day Adult females: 1.8 mg/day
Recommended intake for athletes	2.0 to 2.5 mg/day
Functions	Energy metabolism, fat synthesis, bone structure
Good food sources	Whole-grain foods, legumes, green leafy vegetables, bananas
Deficiency	Poor growth and development in children
Toxicity	Tolerable upper intake level: 11 mg/day Symptoms: neurological problems, confusion, easy fatigue

Chromium

Chromium is also known as glucose tolerance factor (GTF) because of its involvement in helping cells use glucose. A deficiency is associated with poor blood glucose maintenance (either hypo- or hyperglycemia), an excessive production of insulin (hyperinsulinemia), excessive fatigue, and a craving for sweet foods. (Hypoglycemia is low blood sugar; hyperglycemia is high blood sugar). Chromium is also associated with irritability (a common condition with poor blood glucose control), weight gain, adult-onset diabetes, and increased risk of cardiovascular disease.[122] There is some evidence that frequent intense exercise, which is common for serious athletes, may increase the risk of chromium deficiency. High consumption of simple sugars (sweets) may also place people at risk for deficiency. Dietary sources of chromium include meats and whole-grain breads and cereals. Nutritional supplements, commonly in the form of chromium picolinate, are taken as a means of reducing weight or body fat, but studies on this supplement have produced mixed results. Initial studies of chromium picolinate supplementation suggest that this supplement is effective for increasing muscle mass and decreasing body fat in bodybuilders and football players.[142] However, subsequent controlled studies have failed to reach the same conclusions.[143,144] Other supplements include chromium polynicotinate, chromium chloride, and high-chromium yeast.

The adult DRI for chromium is 25 micrograms per day for females and 35 micrograms per day for males. There is no established safe upper limit, although an excess intake may result in chronic renal failure. Because chromium is not well absorbed, there is little evidence to suggest that an excessive intake will result in toxicity. However, the toxicity of chromium has not been directly tested, so athletes should be cautious about taking supplements. One study suggests that chromium picolinate has the potential to alter DNA and thus produce mutated, cancerous cells.[145] Taken together, studies of this trace mineral suggest that to maintain optimal chromium nutriture, athletes should consume foods low in sugar and a diet that contains whole grains and some meat (if not a vegetarian).

Table 2.31 Chromium Quick Guide

Symbol	Cr
Dietary reference intake (DRI)	Adult males: 35 mcg/day Adult females: 25 mcg/day
Recommended intake for athletes	30 to 35 mcg/day
Functions	Glucose tolerance (glucose–insulin control)
Good food sources	Brewer's yeast, mushrooms, whole-grain foods, nuts, legumes, cheese
Deficiency	Glucose intolerance
Toxicity	Unlikely

IMPORTANT POINTS

Vitamins

- The chronic consumption of too much of any vitamin may result in just as poor an outcome as the consumption of too little.

- Athletes who satisfy total energy requirements are also likely to satisfy vitamin requirements.

- Athletes should not shy away from eating fat, as about 20 to 25 percent of total calories from fat is needed to satisfy the need for the fat-soluble vitamins and the essential fatty acids.

- The B vitamins are associated with energy metabolism. The more energy you burn, the more B vitamins you need. However, enriched and fortified grain products contain B vitamins, so even athletes who burn a lot of energy are unlikely to have a deficiency.

- Athletes who believe they eat a poor diet and may need vitamins should consult a registered dietitian to help determine what they need and in what amounts.

Minerals

- Minerals must be consumed regularly to ensure good health. Mineral deficiencies take a long time to correct (for instance, an iron deficiency may take more than 6 months to fix), so athletes could suffer poor performance for long periods if mineral deficiencies are allowed to occur.

- Multiple studies show that athletes are most likely to be deficient in iron and calcium.

- It is typically better to spread out the intake of minerals throughout the day rather than take them in a single large dose.

- One cup of milk provides about 300 mg of calcium. With a calcium requirement of 1,000 to 1,500 milligrams per day, an athlete would have to consume 3.5 to 5 cups of milk or an equivalent amount from other foods to satisfy this daily requirement.

- Eating meat is the easiest way to obtain iron and zinc, so vegetarians may be at increased risk without careful planning to consume well-prepared dark green vegetables and enriched grains to obtain the needed amount.

- Sodium is critically important for maintaining blood volume and sweat rate. The more an athlete sweats, the more sodium is required in a sports beverage, with the normal range being 50 to 200 milligrams per cup.

Fluids and Electrolytes

Perhaps the single most important factor associated with sustaining a high level of athletic performance is maintenance of fluid balance during exercise. Despite this, most athletes experience deterioration in hydration state (with a resultant drop in blood volume) during training and competition. Studies demonstrate that, even in the presence of available fluids, athletes experience a degree of voluntary dehydration that has an inevitably negative impact on performance. Given the tremendous amount of heat that must be dissipated during exercise through sweat evaporation, athletes have no reasonable alternative for sustaining exercise performance other than to pursue strategies that can sustain the hydration state. A failure to do so will result in premature fatigue and may also lead to potentially life-threatening heatstroke. This chapter discusses the strategies related to achieving and sustaining an optimal hydration state and reviews studies that have assessed the optimal concentration of carbohydrate and electrolytes for the ideal sports beverage.

Water is the main component of blood, which delivers oxygen, nutrients, hormones, and a multitude of other substances to cells and removes metabolic by-products from cells. Water also has a protective function, cushioning the spinal cord and brain from sudden impact injury, and is a critical component of our temperature regulation mechanism. Water and its electrolyte components are involved in the control of osmotic pressure, regulating the amount of fluid inside and outside cells. See table 3.1 for a breakdown of the body's water composition.

Well-hydrated athletes are referred to as being *euhydrated* or *normohydrated*; those with below-normal body-water levels are referred to as *hypohydrated* or, if severe, *dehydrated*; and those with above-normal body-water levels are referred to as *hyperhydrated*. We have systems for the normal control of body-water levels, involving an increased retention of body water or an increased loss of body water, all mediated through a series of hormones stimulated by osmoreceptors that monitor blood osmolality and volume receptors that monitor the volume of extracellular water.

Excretion of fluids and metabolic by-products is a main function of the kidneys, which are stimulated by hormones and enzymes to adjust the volume of water and electrolytes excreted or retained.

Table 3.1 Where's the Water?

57% of an average person's total body weight is from water.
65% of total body water is intracellular.
35% of total body water is extracellular.
Well-hydrated muscles are about 75% water.
Bones are about 32% water.
Fat is essentially anhydrous, having only about 10% water content.
Blood is about 93% water.
Average males are about 60% water weight.
Average females are about 50% water weight.
Obese individuals are about 40% water weight.
Athletes are about 70% water weight.

Note: The higher the musculature and the lower the body fat, the higher the contribution of body water to total body mass.

The concentration of sodium is a primary influence on the osmolality of extracellular fluid, which is maintained within a narrow range. Because sweat is hypotonic, prolonged exercise results in a higher plasma osmolality (more water is lost than sodium). As a means of preserving body-water volume, urine production during and shortly after exercise is slightly decreased.[1,2]

If the blood has a relatively high concentration of sodium, protein, or glucose per unit volume of fluid (i.e., is hypertonic), water is drawn from cells to normalize the concentration of electrolytes. Receptors in the hypothalamus detect the fact that the blood is hypertonic through its osmoreceptors, which leads to the release of antidiuretic hormone (ADH) from the pituitary gland. ADH forces the kidneys to retain more water by producing more concentrated urine.[3] For this reason, a common test for adequate hydration status is urine color, with dark urine indicating a greater degree of underhydration than light urine. The osmoreceptors can also induce the sensation of thirst, although this sensation rarely occurs before the loss of 1.5 to 2.0 liters of water (1 liter equals approximately 1 quart; see table 3.2). Since it is nearly impossible for athletes to consume sufficient fluids during physical activity to maintain the body-water level, waiting for the thirst sensation before drinking fluids guarantees that the athlete will be exercising in a progressively worsening state of underhydration.

Table 3.2 Common Conversions

To convert Fahrenheit to Celsius, subtract 32 degrees and divide by 1.8.
To convert Celsius to Fahrenheit, multiply by 1.8 and add 32 degrees.
To convert quarts to liters, multiply quarts by .946.
To convert liters to quarts, multiply liters by 1.057.

In a state of hyperhydration, the concentrations of electrolytes, protein, and glucose are lower than normal in the blood. This condition shuts down the production of ADH so that diluted urine is produced. Fluid also tends to migrate from blood to cells to adjust for this hypotonic state.

Blood volume is affected by the concentration of sodium, the main extracellular electrolyte. A high sodium concentration is associated with an eventual enlargement of the blood volume, which results from the body's attempt to normalize the concentration of sodium per unit of fluid volume. The reverse situation, a low sodium concentration, is typically associated with an eventual reduction of the blood volume. To adjust for the natural variations in sodium intake, the hormone aldosterone is produced to retain more sodium in a low-sodium environment, and aldosterone production ceases when sodium concentrations are high so as to cause the excretion of more sodium.

Under normal circumstances, the combination of volumetric controls, osmoreceptors, antidiuretic hormone, and aldosterone maintains a relatively steady blood volume even with variations in fluid and sodium consumption. Exercise leads to an increased production of ADH and aldosterone, both of which conserve body water and sodium. This system is sufficiently effective that fluid deficiencies leading to physiological problems are rare, even in athletes. However, exercise at high intensity or of long duration (or both), particularly in a hot and humid environment, places the athlete at hydration risk because fluid loss (through sweat) may exceed the athlete's capacity to consume and absorb fluids. This can lead to a progressive reduction in blood volume, a reduced sweat rate, and other problems that negatively affect performance and health; therefore, it is important for athletes to always maintain fluid balance. See table 3.3 for the specific benefits of maintaining fluid balance.

Table 3.3 Benefits of Maintaining Fluid Balance

Maintaining fluid balance during exercise helps sustain athletic performance through the following:
Attenuation of increased heart rate
Attenuation of increased core temperature
Improvement in stroke volume
Improvement in cardiac output
Improvement in skin blood flow
Attenuation of higher plasma sodium, osmolality, and adrenaline
Reduction in net muscle glycogen usage

BALANCING FLUID LOSS AND INTAKE

Physical activity creates heat, and this heat must be dissipated for the athlete to continue performing the activity. Failure to dissipate heat will eventually lead to heatstroke and, potentially, death. One of the main mechanisms for dissipating heat is sweat production; sweat cools the body down when it evaporates off the skin. The inability to produce sufficient sweat will cause the body to overheat. Since athletes have a finite storage capacity for water, and a tremendous ability to produce sweat, fluids must be consumed during physical activity to maintain the sweat rate.

Athletes working intensely in the heat can lose 2.5 liters of sweat per hour. Sweat contains electrolytes (mainly sodium chloride but also potassium, calcium, and magnesium), with a sodium concentration that ranges from 20 to 80 millimoles per liter, depending on common sodium consumption in the diet, the sweat rate, acclimatization to the heat (better acclimatization results in lower sodium loss), and content and amount of rehydration beverages consumed.[4] See table 3.4 for concentrations of electrolytes in sweat, plasma, and intracellular water.

Table 3.4 Concentrations of Electrolytes in Sweat, Plasma, and Intracellular Water

	Sweat (mmol/L)	Plasma (mmol/L)	Intracellular water (mmol/L)
Sodium	20-80	130-155	10
Potassium	4-8	3.2-5.5	150
Calcium	0-1	2.1-2.9	0
Magnesium	<.2	.7-1.5	15
Chloride	20-60	96-110	8
Bicarbonate	0-35	23-28	10
Phosphate	.1-.2	.7-1.6	65
Sulphate	.1-2.0	.3-.9	10

Reprinted from R.J. Maughan, 1994, Fluid and electrolyte loss and replacement in exercise. In *Oxford textbook of sports medicine,* edited by M. Harries et al., pp. 82-93, by permission of Oxford University Press.

Because the electrolyte concentration of sweat is different from that of plasma and intracellular water, there are concerns that an electrolyte imbalance will develop with intense physical activity. Of greatest concern is the potential sodium imbalance that could occur. The loss of a single liter of sweat containing 50 millimoles per liter of sodium translates into a loss of nearly 3 grams of sodium chloride. Athletes who lose 2.5 liters of sweat per hour will lose almost 15 grams of sodium in 2 hours, a level that easily exceeds normal daily sodium intakes.[5]

Temperature regulation represents the balance between heat produced or received (heat-in) and heat removed (heat-out). When the body's temperature regulation system is working correctly, heat-in and heat-out are in perfect balance, and body temperature is maintained. Both internal and external factors can contribute to body heat. Radiant heat from the sun contributes to body temperature, as does the heat created from burning fuel (carbohydrate, protein, or fat). Somehow, athletes must find a way to dissipate from the body the same amount of heat that has been added to the body to maintain a constant body temperature.

The two primary systems for dissipating, or losing, heat involve (1) moving more blood to the skin to allow heat dissipation through radiation and (2) increasing the rate of sweat production. These two systems account for about 85 percent of heat removal when a person is at rest. Heat losses through conduction (the natural transmission of heat from a hotter body to the cooler air environment) and convection (heat transfer from tissue to the blood and through the skin) account for the remaining 15 percent of heat-out. During exercise, however, virtually all heat loss occurs via evaporation (sweat) (see figure 3.1).

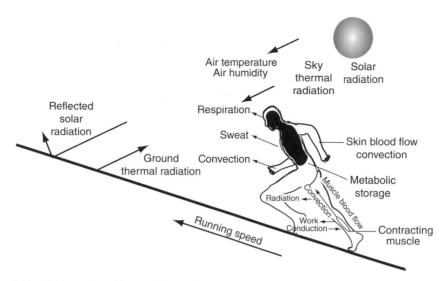

Figure 3.1 Systems for adding and removing heat in an exercising athlete.

Reprinted, by permission, from R.J. Maughan and E.R. Nadel, 2000, Temperature regulation and fluid and electrolyte balance. In *Nutrition in sport,* edited by R.J. Maughan (Oxford: Blackwell Science), 205.

Both these systems rely on maintenance of an adequate blood volume. A lower blood volume results in a reduced movement of blood to the skin, and sweat production is also reduced. Working muscles demand more blood flow to deliver nutrients and to remove the by-products of burned fuel. However, at the same time there is a need to shift blood away from the muscles and toward the skin to increase the sweat rate. With low blood volume, one or both of these systems fail, with a resultant decrease in athletic performance. In fact, the maintenance of blood volume is rightly considered by many to be the primary indicator of whether an athlete's performance can be maintained at a high rate.

Energy metabolism is only about 20 to 40 percent efficient, meaning that only 20 to 40 percent of food energy can be converted to the mechanical energy of muscular work. The remaining 60 to 80 percent of the food energy that is burned is lost as heat. However, when the rate of energy burn goes up, as happens during physical activity, the amount of heat added to the system is dramatically increased, so the heat-out systems must be "turned up." In fact, heavy exercise can produce 20 times the amount of heat produced at rest. Without an efficient means of heat removal, body temperature will rise quickly. The upper limit for human survival is about 110 degrees Fahrenheit (43.3 degrees Celsius), or only 11.4 degrees Fahrenheit (6.3 degrees Celsius) higher than normal body temperature. Body temperature has the potential to rise approximately 1 degree Fahrenheit every 5 minutes. It is conceivable, therefore, that an underhydrated athlete could be at risk for heatstroke and death less than 1 hour after the initiation of exercise.

Athletes doing very mild exercise that burns 300 kilocalories of energy during 30 minutes would use approximately 75 kilocalories for muscular work, and 225 kilocalories would be lost as heat (assuming a mechanical efficiency conversion rate of 25 percent). This excess heat must be dissipated to maintain normal body temperature. There is a loss of approximately 620 calories of heat energy for each liter of water evaporated from the skin's surface. Athletes working twice as intensely would create 450 kilocalories of excess heat that would need to be dissipated over the same 30 minutes to maintain body temperature.

It is estimated that 1 milliliter of sweat can dissipate .5 kilocalorie, so over this 30-minute period the athlete would lose approximately 900 milliliters (almost 1 liter) of sweat. In 1 hour of high-intensity activity, approximately 1.8 liters of water would be lost. On sunny and hot days when the heat of the sun is added to the heat generated from muscular work, the athlete must produce more sweat (see figure 3.2). Sweat doesn't evaporate off skin as easily when it is humid, so even more sweat must be produced. In these conditions, a person can easily lose between 1 and 2 liters of fluid (via sweat) per hour.

Well-trained athletes exercising in a hot and humid environment may lose more than 3 liters of fluid per hour. To protect athletes from placing themselves at increased heat-stress risk, the heat index was developed (see table 3.5). This index simultaneously considers environmental temperature and relative humidity to establish exercise risk.

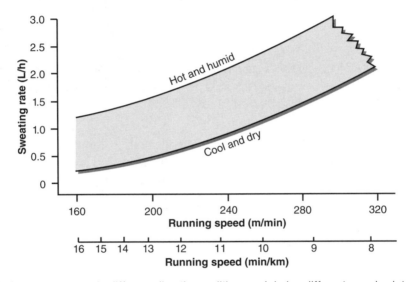

Figure 3.2 Heating rates in different climatic conditions and during different exercise intensities.

Reprinted, by permission, from M.N. Sawka and K.B. Pandolf, 1990, Effects of body water loss on physiological function and exercise performance. In *Perspectives in exercise science and sports medicine, volume 3: Fluid homeostasis during exercise*, edited by C.J. Gisolfi and D.R. Lamb (Carmel, IN: Benchmark Press), 4.

Factors Affecting Fluid Loss

Because sweat has a lower osmolality than does plasma (i.e., sweat is hypotonic), profuse sweating increases plasma osmolality. Whether or not this increased plasma osmolality affects body temperature or cooling capacity in an exercising person is, as yet, unclear, but a sufficient change in osmolality and volume does stimulate the kidneys to excrete sodium and reduce urine output by producing more concentrated urine.

Several factors affect the rate at which an athlete can produce sweat. Higher ambient temperatures result in a greater potential for sweat production. Higher humidity is also responsible for higher sweat production, but because of the difficulty in evaporating sweat into a high humidity environment (i.e., the rate of evaporation off the skin is low), the cooling potential is lower than in less humid environments. The same problem also exists with clothing that traps sweat against the skin (i.e., does not breathe). This type of clothing

Table 3.5 The Heat Index

	Environmental temperature, °F (°C)										
	70 (21)	75 (24)	80 (27)	85 (29)	90 (32)	95 (35)	100 (38)	105 (41)	110 (43)	115 (46)	120 (49)
Relative humidity	Apparent temperature, °F (°C)										
0%	64 (18)	69 (20)	73 (23)	78 (26)	83 (28)	87 (30)	91 (33)	95 (35)	99 (37)	103 (39)	107 42)
10%	65 (18)	70 (21)	75 (24)	80 (27)	85 (29)	90 (32)	95 (35)	100 (38)	105 (41)	111 (44)	116 (47)
20%	66 (19)	72 (22)	77 (25)	82 (28)	87 (30)	93 (34)	99 (37)	105 (41)	112 (44)	120 (49)	130 (54)
30%	67 (19)	73 (23)	78 (26)	84 (29)	90 (32)	96 (36)	104 (40)	113 (45)	123 (51)	135 (57)	148 (64)
40%	68 (20)	74 (23)	79 (26)	86 (30)	93 (34)	101 (38)	110 (43)	123 (51)	137 (58)	151 (66)	
50%	69 (20)	75 (24)	81 (27)	88 (31)	96 (36)	107 (42)	120 (49)	135 (57)	150 (66)		
60%	70 (21)	76 (24)	82 (28)	90 (32)	100 (38)	114 (46)	132 (56)	149 (65)			
70%	70 (21)	77 (25)	85 (29)	93 (34)	106 (41)	124 (51)	144 (62)				
80%	71 (22)	78 (26)	86 (30)	97 (36)	113 (45)	136 (58)					
90%	71 (22)	79 (26)	88 (31)	102 (39)	122 (50)						
100%	72 (22)	80 (27)	91 (33)	108 (42)							

Apparent temperature	Heat-stress risk with physical activity or prolonged exposure.
90-104 °F (32-40 °C)	Heat cramps or heat exhaustion possible.
105-129 °F (41-53 °C)	Heat cramps or heat exhaustion likely. Heat stroke possible.
130 °F and up (54 °C and up)	Heat stroke very likely.

Caution: This chart provides guidelines for assessing the potential severity of heat stress. Individual reactions to heat will vary. Heat illnesses can occur at lower temperatures than indicated on this chart. Exposure to full sunshine can increase values up to 15 °F (8 °C).

results in a reduced cooling efficiency that forces a greater sweat rate. (Sweat-soaked clothing doesn't mean an athlete is effectively controlling body temperature, it just means he is losing water.) Some new materials designed for athletes actually wick sweat away from the skin to improve evaporative efficiency. Athletes with large body surface areas may also have an enhanced sweat production capacity and, therefore, an enhanced evaporative heat loss. But these athletes may also gain more heat from the environment through radiation and convection in hot weather.[6] The conditioning or training state of an athlete makes a difference. Well-conditioned athletes have a higher sweat volume potential that results in an enhanced cooling potential. However, this higher sweat rate requires a greater during-exercise fluid consumption to avoid higher heat-stress risk.

An athlete's state of fluid balance also plays a factor. The better the hydration state, the greater the sweat potential. As athletes become progressively dehydrated, the sweat rate is reduced, and body temperature rises. This is a problem because fluid consumption during activity is rarely greater than 2 cups (480 milliliters) per hour, or only 30 to 40 percent of the amount of fluid lost in sweat, an amount that will inevitably lead to the athlete becoming dehydrated. Consider that marathoners competing in a cool temperature of 50 to 54 degrees Fahrenheit (10 to 12 degrees Celsius) lose between 1 and 5 percent of total body mass.[7] Marathoners competing in warm weather lose about 8 percent of total body mass, or between 12 and 15 percent of total body water.[8]

Factors Affecting Fluid Intake

The two main factors influencing fluid intake are thirst and taste. Thirst is a sensation of dryness in the mouth and throat related to the body's need for additional fluids. Taste is the response humans have (either good or bad) to substances in the mouth. Humans are more likely to consume more of what they like, or more of what tastes good to them. Most athletes induce voluntary dehydration because they don't drink enough despite having plenty of fluids readily available. Insufficient consumption of fluids by athletes is probably due to a lack of the thirst sensation.

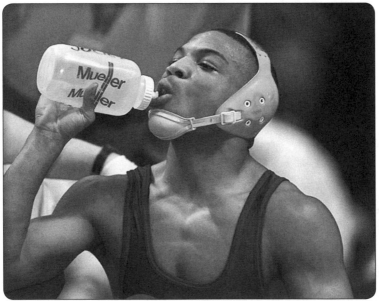

© Human Kinetics

During exercise, waiting to become thirsty before drinking may result in dehydration and reduced performance.

The onset of thirst may be the result of habit, a ritual, or the need for a warming (hot fluids) or cooling (cold fluids) effect.[9] A rise in plasma osmolality of between 2 and 3 percent is needed to produce the sensation of thirst, and sensitivity to a reduction in fluid volume is even less responsive, requiring nearly a 10 percent decrease in blood volume to stimulate thirst.[10,11] The thirst sensation, often considered delayed in athletes because it doesn't appear until an athlete has already lost 1.5 to 2.0 liters of body water, is therefore a poor indicator of fluid needs in athletes.[12] There is no hope that an athlete can return to an adequately hydrated state during exercise if fluid consumption begins at the same time the thirst sensation occurs. This apparent delay in the thirst mechanism is a primary reason for athletes to train themselves to consume fluids on a schedule, whether they feel thirsty or not.

Color, taste, odor, temperature, and texture all play important roles in determining if the beverage will be considered desirable and whether it will be consumed. It appears that athletes prefer cool beverages with a slightly sweet flavor. Heavily sweetened beverages (around a 12 percent carbohydrate solution) are not as widely tolerated during exercise as beverages with a 6 or 7 percent carbohydrate solution.[10, 13] When not exercising, however, the reverse may be true, pointing to an interesting phenomenon: Food and drink taste differently during exercise. Therefore, athletes are wise to determine the fluids they find most desirable for exercise while they are exercising.

Gastric Emptying and Fluid Delivery to Working Muscles

Several factors influence the rate at which fluids leave the stomach. Gastric emptying describes the volume of food or drink that leaves the stomach per unit of time. Food and drinks with a slower gastric emptying take longer to completely leave the stomach. This means these substances enter the small intestine more slowly, and some of the food or drink will remain in the stomach longer.

• **Carbohydrate concentration of the solution:** Sports beverages and other beverages consumed by athletes commonly contain carbohydrate. When the concentration of carbohydrate in a fluid rises above 7 percent, gastric emptying time decreases. At concentrations below 7 percent carbohydrate, gastric emptying time is not significantly affected, showing gastric emptying characteristics similar to water.[14] For this reason, the recommended carbohydrate concentration in sports beverages is below 8 percent.[15] Having said that, some ultraendurance athletes train their systems to tolerate greater concentrations because they desperately need the additional carbohydrate.

• **Type of carbohydrate in the solution:** Carbohydrates are not all the same, coming in different molecular sizes and in different molecular combinations. For instance, glucose (referred to as *dextrose* on package labels) is a monosaccharide (a single-molecule carbohydrate), sucrose is a disaccharide (two monosaccharides held together with a bond), and starch is a polysaccharide (many molecules of monosaccharides held together with bonds). The smaller the length of a carbohydrate chain, the slower the gastric emptying time. Therefore, on an isocaloric basis, pure glucose (a monosaccharide) will take longer to leave the stomach than table sugar (a disaccharide), and table sugar will take longer to leave the stomach than a simple starch (a polysaccharide).[16]

• **Amount of fluid consumed:** The amount of fluid consumed at one time has a major influence on gastric emptying time. When a large volume of fluid is consumed, gastric emptying time is initially faster, and when the volume of fluid in the stomach is reduced, gastric emptying time slows. To achieve a hydrated state before competition or practice, 14 to 22 ounces (420 to 660 milliliters) of fluid should be consumed, followed by frequent sipping on fluid to maintain fluid volume in the stomach and, therefore, a faster gastric emptying time. [16,17]

• **Temperature of the solution:** Beverage temperature only slightly affects gastric emptying time. When people are at rest, fluids at body temperature leave the stomach more quickly than either very hot or very cold fluids.[18] During exercise, however, it appears as if cool fluids leave the stomach more quickly than room-temperature or body-temperature fluids.[19] An important consideration, although not affecting gastric emptying, is that athletes may consume more cool fluids.

• **Carbonation of the solution:** Athletes commonly believe that consuming a carbonated beverage causes gastric distress and delayed gastric emptying (the first sports beverage was probably a defizzed cola), but there is little scientific evidence that this occurs. However, studies evaluating the impact of fluid carbonation on gastric emptying time have typically relied on few subjects. In general, the studies suggest that, all other things being equal (carbohydrate concentration, volume, temperature, and so on), carbonation has little impact on gastric emptying.[20,21] Nevertheless, carbonation does make athletes feel more full, thereby reducing the drive to drink. Nothing should take away the athlete's drive to drink because this can negatively affect hydration state.

• **Relative hydration state of the athlete:** Progressive dehydration and higher body temperatures associated with high-intensity activity cause a slower gastric emptying rate.[16] This is an excellent rationale for athletes to maintain hydration state during activity. Dehydration will make it almost impossible for the athlete to return to an adequately hydrated state during exercise, and if this is attempted through consumption of a large volume of fluid, it will likely lead to a sense of discomfort rather than faster rehydration.

• **Degree of mental stress:** The mental stress and anxiety associated with athletic competition are major factors in gastric emptying. Higher levels of mental stress and anxiety are associated with a reduced gastric emptying that can have a serious impact on the ability to adequately rehydrate during competition.[12, 22] The mental training techniques that can be learned from a sports psychologist to reduce stress are important for reducing the physiological effects of sports-related stress and anxiety.

• **Type of physical activity:** High-intensity activity is associated with a slower gastric emptying rate than lower-intensity activity, but the differences are minor. Additionally, the type of activity (running, swimming, cycling) does not appear to have a large influence on gastric emptying rate.[12]

ATHLETE CONDITIONING, ADAPTATION, AND AGE

The human body has wonderful adaptive mechanisms (see table 3.6), and the ability to adapt to higher or lower glucose concentrations and faster or slower rates of fluid ingestion is no exception. It seems clear that athletes can train to enhance their potential for achieving optimal hydration. Therefore, each athlete should start with general recommendations for fluid intake to maintain hydration state, then make modifications that are best suited to them.

Table 3.6 Body Adjustments During Acclimatization

Plasma volume expands to increase total blood volume.
The heart is then able to pump more blood per beat.
More blood flows to muscles and skin.
Less muscle glycogen is used as an energy source during exercise.
Sweat glands hypertrophy and produce 30% more sweat.
Salt in sweat decreases by about 60%, which helps to maintain plasma volume.
Sweating starts at a lower core temperature.
Core temperature will not rise as high or as rapidly as in unacclimatized state.
Psychological feeling of stress is reduced at a given exercise rate.

For instance, a young figure skater training in a relatively cool environment protected from direct sunlight (an indoor ice rink) is likely to satisfy hydration needs by sipping one or two mouthfuls of a sports beverage about every 15 minutes. By contrast, a distance runner on a hot and humid day should drink as much sports beverage as can be tolerated, with as high a frequency as possible. The higher sweat volume of the distance runner is also likely to result in a greater sweat sodium loss, which would need to be replenished by a higher concentration of sodium in the sports beverage than would be needed by the figure skater. Endurance sports beverages typically have sodium concentrations of approximately 150 to 200 milligrams per 240 milliliters (1 cup)—a level appropriate for this runner. Regular sports beverages typically have sodium concentrations of 50 to 100 milligrams per 240 milliliters (1 cup)—a level appropriate for the figure skater. Adjustments of this kind, modifying the concentrations of carbohydrate and sodium and the volume of fluid consumed, are a necessary part of what serious athletes must consider doing to optimize performance.

Heat tolerance is highly influenced by physical fitness: Poor physical fitness dramatically increases the risk of heat illness similarly in both men and women. However, this improved heat tolerance is partly the result of an enhanced sweat rate. Since children have fewer sweat glands and each gland produces less sweat, child athletes have a lower potential for adaptation to heat and are generally considered to have a lower heat tolerance than well-conditioned adults.[23] Poorly conditioned athletes with higher body-fat levels also have lower heat tolerance. Put simply, fat deters heat loss.

In summary, well-conditioned adult athletes with low body-fat levels must develop strategies for constantly increasing fluid intakes as their conditioning improves because sweat rates increase with better conditioning. Children and adults with higher body fat are likely to have a lower heat tolerance, making maintenance of adequate hydration even more critical.

Intestinal Absorption

As fluids leave the stomach and enter the small intestine, the water and carbohydrate that make up the solution must pass through the intestinal mucosa for take-up by blood. The main factor influencing the speed with which water and carbohydrate are absorbed is the concentration of carbohydrate in the solution that enters the intestines.[24] Slightly lower concentrations of carbohydrate and electrolytes, relative to the concentration of plasma, result in faster absorption of water than a solution that has either a much higher or much lower concentration.[25] A 6 to 7 percent carbohydrate solution appears to offer the best balance for speedy absorption. Consumption of highly concentrated carbohydrate solutions during exercise may cause a temporary shift of fluids away from muscle cells and into the intestines to dilute the solution before absorption. This would have a negative impact on both muscle function and sweat rates because it would cause, at least temporarily, a degree of plasma and tissue dehydration.

Fluid-Related Problems

Heat balance (see figure 3.3) can be described by the following equation:[26]

$$S = M \pm R \pm K \pm C - E \pm WK$$

Heat balance (S) = metabolic heat production (M), as corrected for the net heat exchange by radiation (R), conduction (K), convection (C), and evaporation (E), and as further corrected by the amount of work performed (WK).

Dehydration

Dehydration occurs when more fluids are lost than are consumed. By definition, dehydration means the amount of body water is below optimal. As little as a 2 percent drop in body water results in a measurable reduction in athletic performance. Common risks for dehydration include the following:

- Vomiting
- Diarrhea
- Inadequate fluid replacement
- Induced high sweat rates (as in saunas)
- Laxatives
- Diuretics (and substances with a diuretic effect)
- Dieting
- Febrile illness

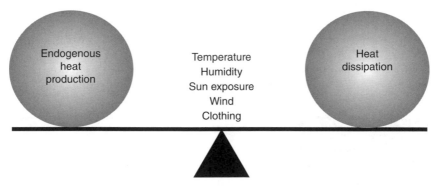

Figure 3.3   Heat balance.

Reprinted, by permission, from R.P. Sandor, 1997, "Heat illness: On-site diagnosis and cooling," *The Physician and Sportsmedicine* 25(6): 35-40.

Ideally, dehydration avoidance is the best policy. The only way to avoid dehydration is to rightly assume there is a constant output of fluids that must be dealt with by having an equally constant input of fluids. It is important for athletes to recognize the signs of dehydration. Thirst is an obvious sign, but athletes should learn to monitor urine output for volume and color. Both low urine output and dark urine color are signs of dehydration that may precede the sensation of thirst.

Some athletes dehydrate themselves to try to look better or to make a competitive weight classification, or they fail to consume fluids even when they are readily available to them (referred to as *voluntary dehydration*); other athletes become dehydrated as a result of heavy training, particularly in hot and humid environments, when adequate fluid consumption is difficult (referred to as *involuntary dehydration*). Regardless of the cause, athletes can be certain that dehydration will result in negative performance outcomes and reduced mental function.[27,28]

Heat Cramps

Heat cramps—painful spasms in the legs and abdomen—are typically the result of a fluid and electrolyte imbalance caused by severe dehydration. They are most likely to occur in people who sweat heavily and who lose a higher than normal amount of sodium and other electrolytes (including potassium, calcium, and magnesium) in the sweat (see table 3.7). For these people, drinking adequate amounts of sodium-containing beverages during exercise is particularly useful. Heat cramps appear to occur late in the day after consumption of large volumes of plain water.[29] At the first sign of involuntary muscle twitching or mild muscle cramping, athletes should consume 16 ounces (480 milliliters) of a sports drink that has been supplemented with a teaspoon of table salt.[30] This should then be followed by a steady intake of sodium-supplemented sports drinks for the remainder of the exercise session. To help meet the needs of athletes who experience frequent cramping, companies have developed products that provide a measured amount of sodium, potassium, calcium, and magnesium for adding to a given volume of sports beverage.

Heat Exhaustion

The symptoms of heat exhaustion include weakness, cold and clammy skin, a feeling of faintness, fatigue, nausea, and a weak pulse. It is also possible, when the person has severe body-water depletion, that sweating has stopped and the skin feels dry. These symptoms are associated with an inadequate blood flow to the brain, with the sufferer typically on the ground but semiconscious. Symptoms usually respond well to rapid cooling, so

Table 3.7 Indications of Cramp-Prone Athletes

History of heat cramps
Consume inadequate sodium (eat a salt-restricted diet)
Sweat profusely early in activity
Have poor hydration habits during exercise
Sweat is heavy in salt; stings eyes; tastes salty
Visible (chalky) salt on body and clothing
Not adapted to a hot and humid environment
Family history of cystic fibrosis

heat-exhaustion victims should be cooled through whatever means are available. Applying wet, ice-cold cloths to the body or placing the victim in a cold-water bath are both effective. After a return to full consciousness, the athlete can be given sips of cool fluid, but this should not be forced because it may cause nausea. There is no rational reason for a heat-exhausted athlete to try to return to physical activity on the same day. Instead, the person should spend the remainder of the day staying cool and hydrating with sodium-containing fluids, such as sports beverages. *Caution:* Under no circumstances should an athlete who has stopped sweating continue exercising because this may cause a rapid and dangerous rise in core temperature.

Heatstroke (Sunstroke)

Heatstroke is an extremely dangerous condition, typified by high body temperature (usually above 105 degrees Fahrenheit, or 40.5 degrees Celsius), hot and dry skin, and a rapid pulse. It is also possible for the athlete to be coming in and out of consciousness. The first responder should call 911 (hospitals are best equipped to deal with this life-threatening condition) and then do whatever possible to cool the athlete (fanning, cold water, sponge bath, loosening clothing, cold-water bath). Until the athlete returns to consciousness, do not give fluids. Heatstroke is caused by a combination of several factors, as shown in table 3.8.

Table 3.8 Risk Factors for Heatstroke

Increased endogenous heat load
Overexertion
Drugs (e.g., sympathomimetics, caffeine)

Increased exogenous heat load
Temperature
Sun exposure

Decreased heat dissipation
Dehydration
Lack of acclimatization
Healed burns
Rashes
Drugs (e.g., phenothiazines, antihistamines, alcohol)
Humidity
Occlusive or excessive clothing

Drugs reported to predispose to heatstroke
Amphetamines: epinephrine, ephedrine, cocaine, norepinephrine
Anticholinergics
Diuretics: furosemide, hydrochlorothiazide, bumetanide
Phenothiazines: prochlorperazine, chlorpromazine hydrochloride, promethazine hydrochloride
Butyrophenones: haloperidol
Cyclic antidepressants: amitriptyline hydrochloride, imipramine hydrochloride, nortriptyline hydrochloride, protriptyline hydrochloride
Monoamine oxidase inhibitors: phenelzine, tranylcypromine sulfate
Alcohol
Lysergic acid diethylamide (LSD)
Lithium

Other
Concurrent illness (e.g., upper respiratory infection, gastroenteritis)
Prior heatstroke

Reprinted, by permission, from R.P. Sandor, 1997, "Heat illness: On-site diagnosis and cooling," *The Physician and Sportsmedicine* 25(6): 35-40.

Hyponatremia

Exercising for long periods may cause low blood sodium (hyponatremia), a potentially fatal condition. Low blood sodium can occur if you drink excessive amounts of water, which may dilute the sodium content of your blood. The resulting edema may lead to rapid and dangerous swelling of the brain. Inadequate sodium intake also may play a role, so a failure to consume sufficient sodium when fluid and sodium losses are high can lead to hyponatremia. The word *hyponatremia* literally means low (*hypo*) sodium (Na) in the blood (*emia*); it may result from the production of a large volume of sweat (which contains both sodium and water) and the consumption of a replacement fluid that has an inadequate concentration of sodium. The sodium dilution that results leads to a reduced blood volume, which is the cause of the symptoms of hyponatremia.

The sodium concentration of sweat varies greatly between individual athletes but typically falls within the range of 2.25 to 3.4 grams of sodium per liter of sweat. (Lower sodium sweat concentrations are found in well-conditioned athletes, so they have lower hyponatremia risk.) Given the volume of sweat that can be lost during a race (may exceed well over 1 liter per hour), it is conceivable that an athlete could lose more than 40 grams of sodium over the course of a long-endurance competition. If the fluid replacement the athlete chooses has no sodium or is too low in sodium, hyponatremia can result. It has also been found that commonly consumed NSAIDs (e.g., aspirin, ibuprofen) and any substances that induce a diuretic effect may alter kidney function in a way that exacerbates hyponatremia risk during long-duration events.[31] Hyponatremia can be caused by many medications, and athletes should check with their doctors regarding the medications they use. Given the very real risks associated with hyponatremia, all reasonable steps should be taken to avoid this condition.

Hyponatremia becomes physiologically important when free water shifts from the blood to the intracellular space. Cellular edema, although well tolerated by many tissues, is not well tolerated by the brain. Therefore, the serious symptoms of hyponatremia are related mainly to cerebral edema. Hyponatremia symptoms include nausea, cramping, slurred speech, disorientation, and general confusion. If allowed to progress, athletes may experience coma and death. Put simply, hyponatremia is a potentially fatal condition that can be largely avoided if athletes consume only sodium-containing beverages with sufficient sodium concentration (between 100 and 200 milligrams of sodium per cup is desirable, with the higher concentrations for higher sweat losses) and avoid plain water during a long-duration event. Athletes experiencing any of the initial symptoms of hyponatremia, such as muscle cramping, may find that consumption of salty foods and sodium-containing sports beverages satisfactorily resolves the symptoms. However, slurred speech, disorientation, and confusion are serious symptoms that require immediate medical attention, preferably by a qualified health professional.[32] If no one is available, salt tablets can be used to recover from hyponatremia. A single salt tablet typically delivers 1 gram (1,000 milligrams) of sodium. For recovery, one or two tablets should be consumed per cup of water taken every 15 to 20 minutes, depending on the severity of hyponatremia symptoms. The total fluid consumed should return the athlete to preexercise weight but not cause the athlete to increase body weight above that point.[33] It is unlikely that salt tablets would be used in other scenarios.

There are several forms of hyponatremia, including the following:[32]

• **Hypovolemic hyponatremia:** Total body water (TBW) decreases, but total body sodium decreases to a greater extent and results in a decrease in the extracellular fluid (ECF) volume. This is likely the most common hyponatremia seen in long-endurance events. It occurs as sodium and body water lost through sweat are replaced by water or other hypotonic fluids.

- **Euvolemic hyponatremia:** TBW increases while total sodium remains normal. The ECF volume is increased minimally to moderately, but edema is not present. Euvolemic hyponatremia suggests that sodium stores are normal but there is a total body excess of free water. This occurs when athletes consume excess fluids and is one of the reasons why athletes should be cautious about not drinking a volume of fluids that would increase body weight.

- **Hypervolemic hyponatremia:** Total body sodium increases, and TBW increases to a greater extent, with higher ECF and edema present. This most likely occurs with renal failure, resulting in hypertension.

- **Redistributive hyponatremia:** Water shifts from the intracellular to the extracellular compartment, with a resultant dilution of sodium. The TBW and total body sodium are unchanged. This condition occurs with hyperglycemia.

- **Pseudohyponatremia:** The blood volume is diluted by excessive proteins or lipids. The TBW and total body sodium are unchanged. This condition is seen with hypertriglyceridemia and multiple myeloma.

Low blood sodium may also occur in athletes who habitually restrict sodium consumption in the foods and beverages they consume. In general, unless it is contraindicated because of a medical condition and the athlete is under the careful supervision of a physician, adding salt to meals and beverages is a desirable strategy for avoiding low blood electrolytes and reducing hyponatremia risk.

Signs and symptoms of low blood sodium include the following:

- Headache
- Confusion
- Nausea
- Cramping
- Bloated stomach
- Swollen fingers and ankles
- Pulmonary edema
- Seizures
- Coma

Just before the 2003 Boston Marathon, *USA Track & Field* announced fluid-replacement guidelines for long-distance runners that are designed to lower hyponatremia risk.[34] Earlier guidelines encouraged runners to drink as much as possible to "stay ahead" of their thirst, but the new guidelines advise runners to drink only as much fluid as they lose through sweat during a race. This recommendation suggests that athletes consume 100 percent of fluids lost through sweat and no more. Higher levels of consumption, particularly of plain water, could cause a drop in blood sodium concentration, leading to hyponatremia. Athletes at increased risk of hyponatremia include those who

- take NSAIDs;
- are on a low-sodium diet;
- drink water or other no-sodium beverages during exercise;
- aren't acclimatized to warm weather or are poorly trained;
- run slowly, taking longer than 4 hours to complete endurance events; and
- experience weight gain during the event (most likely due to excess fluid consumption).

The highest risk of hyponatremia appears to be in athletes who produce a large volume of sweat with a relatively high concentration of sodium and who consume large volumes of plain water (which contains no sodium).[35] Sports beverages contain approximately 20 milliequivalents (mEq) of sodium chloride (table salt), but even higher levels of sodium are recommended by a number of researchers who have assessed plasma changes during prolonged exercise in the heat.[36,37] These researchers have recommended 20 to 50 milliequivalents per liter, but it appears that most athletes with normal sweat rates and normal sweat sodium concentrations who consume commercial sports beverages and avoid consumption of plain water during endurance events are protected.[38]

If you eat during exercise, salty foods such as pretzels are a good choice. Sports drinks also are a good source of sodium, water, and carbohydrate. Dehydration during prolonged exercise is still far more common than low blood sodium. It is important, therefore, to start exercise well hydrated and to drink appropriate amounts of the right kind of fluids during exercise.[39]

HYDRATION STRATEGIES

No level of low body water is acceptable for achieving optimal athletic performance and endurance, so athletes must develop personal strategies for maintaining optimal body water while exercising. Imagine a full glass of water represents your body in a state of optimal hydration. When not exercising, it's like having a pinhole in the bottom of the glass. The water level will drop, but only at a very slow rate and at a pace that makes it easy for you to maintain an optimal hydration state. Because the water level drops so slowly, drinking an occasional glass of water or other fluid is an adequate means of maintaining hydration state. Now consider what happens when you exercise, which is equivalent to putting a pencil hole in the bottom of the glass: The rate of water loss is much faster. Within even a short period of time, the amount of water loss could be enough to affect exercise performance and endurance. Waiting to drink in this situation is not a reasonable option. If the frequency of drinking when not exercising is once every 2 hours, then the frequency of drinking during exercise should be once every 10 to 15 minutes. Water is lost so quickly during exercise that it becomes difficult, if not impossible, to replace the amount of water being lost and virtually impossible to increase body water while exercising. Waiting too long between drinks causes body water to decrease such that it cannot be adequately replaced. If you wait to drink you may be able to maintain the body's water level at its current state, but that state will be too low.

Without fluid intake, blood volume will quickly drop, sweat rates will drop, and body heat will rise quickly and dangerously, at the rate of approximately 1.8 degrees Fahrenheit (1 degree Celsius) every 5 to 7 minutes. (See table 3.9 for the effects of dehydration on aerobic performance.) Because it is so difficult to consume sufficient fluids during hard physical work, athletes should develop a fixed drinking schedule. With a loss of 1 liter of water per hour, athletes should find a way to drink 4 cups of water per hour. Athletes losing 2 liters of water per hour need to drink more than 8 cups of water per hour to replace the amount lost, but athletes rarely fully satisfy fluid needs during activity. Of course, it's difficult to know precisely how much water is being lost during activity, but a simple technique can help an athlete estimate how much is lost. One liter of water weighs approximately 2 pounds, and

Table 3.9 Effects of Dehydration on Aerobic Endurance Performance

Hypohydration of >2% loss of body weight leads to decrements in performance.
Cardiovascular function and temperature regulation are adversely affected.
Maximal aerobic performance decreases 4 to 8%, with a 3% weight loss during exercise in neutral environments.
Dehydration and GI distress are evident.
Fluid and electrolyte balance in muscle cells is disturbed.
Adverse effects of hyperthermia on mental processes contribute to central fatigue.

1 pint of water weighs approximately 1 pound. By knowing these relationships, athletes can estimate how much fluid should be consumed during physical activity by doing the following:

1. Write down what time it is just before the exercise session.
2. Write down body weight in pounds. (Preferably, this should be nude weight.)
3. Do the normal exercise, and monitor how much fluid is consumed during the exercise period.
4. Immediately after exercise, take off the sweaty clothing and towel dry. Once dry, write down body weight in pounds. (Again, this should be nude weight.)
5. Write down the current time.
6. Calculate the amount of fluid lost by subtracting ending weight from beginning weight.
7. Calculate exercise time by subtracting ending time from beginning time.
8. The amount of extra fluid that should be consumed during the activity is equivalent to 1 pint (16 ounces) of additional fluid for each pound lost, provided in 10- to 20-minute increments.

Example: If John weighs 4 pounds less after a 2-hour football practice, he should consume an additional 4 pints (8 cups) of fluid during that practice. He was already consuming 2 cups of fluid, so John's total fluid consumption should be 10 cups of fluid per 2-hour practice. In 2 hours there are 12 10-minute time increments, so John has 12 opportunities to consume 10 cups of fluid. Therefore, John should consume 6.5 ounces of fluid, or a bit more than three-quarters of a cup (10 ÷ 12 = .8), every 10 minutes or 13 ounces of fluid (about 1.5 cups) every 20 minutes.

Fluid Intake Before Exercise

It is critical for athletes to be in a state of optimal hydration before the initiation of exercise or competition. All the evidence suggests that even a minor level of underhydration (as little as 2 percent of body weight) can cause a measurable difference in endurance and performance, and the greater the underhydration, the greater the negative impact.[40,41] Furthermore, it can take 24 hours or longer to bring a dehydrated athlete back to a well-hydrated state. Therefore, waiting until just before practice or competition to bring an athlete to a well-hydrated state or simply failing to take any steps to make certain the athlete is in an optimally hydrated state will doom that athlete to having a poor practice or competition outcome.

In some sports, athletes try to achieve a particular look or try to make a specific weight. The classic body profile in rhythmic gymnastics is long, graceful lines with, essentially, no secondary sexual characteristics. It is common for rhythmic gymnasts to restrict water intake before a competition because they think it will help give them the desired look. Wrestlers have a well-established regimen for fluid restriction to achieve a particular weight class. They then have about 24 hours to rehydrate themselves before the competition. Besides the inherent health dangers (there are well-documented deaths associated with this strategy), it is unlikely that dehydrated wrestlers would be able to adequately rehydrate themselves in just 24 hours. Therefore, performance is likely to be affected.

On the other side of the continuum, some athletes try to superhydrate with fluid before exercise. This is typically a strategy of long-distance runners, whose water loss during competition is likely to be greater than their ability to replace it. The runner with the best hydration state near the end of the competition clearly has a major advantage over less hydrated competitors. When athletes constantly superhydrate they may develop a greater blood (plasma) volume, with resultant lower core temperatures and heart rates during activity, suggesting the potential for improved endurance and performance.[42,43] Consumption of large fluid volumes is also associated with frequent urination, but this may be somewhat mediated by consumption of sodium-containing fluids.[41] In addition, superhydration is associated with higher sweat rates and a lower heart rate during exercise.[44]

Glycerol (also referred to as *glycerin*) was used in the past by endurance athletes to aid superhydration because it acts as a humectant (i.e., it attracts water). See figure 3.4. Limited evidence suggests that adding glycerol at the rate of 1 gram per kilogram of body mass to preexercise fluids improves endurance performance in extremely hot and humid environments. This improvement occurs because glycerol enables retention of more of the consumed fluids.[41, 45-47] However, the World Anti-Doping Agency recently included glycerol on its banned substance list, so it should no longer be used as a hydrating agent by athletes.

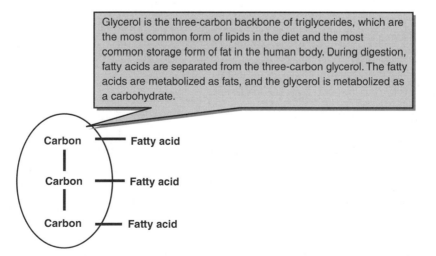

Glycerol is the three-carbon backbone of triglycerides, which are the most common form of lipids in the diet and the most common storage form of fat in the human body. During digestion, fatty acids are separated from the three-carbon glycerol. The fatty acids are metabolized as fats, and the glycerol is metabolized as a carbohydrate.

Figure 3.4 Glycerol is a simple three-carbon lipid that is metabolized like a carbohydrate.

In general, athletes should follow these hydration guidelines before exercise:

1. The sensation of thirst should not be relied on as an indicator of fluid need. Thirst should be considered an emergency sensation that occurs when the body has already lost 1.5 to 2.0 liters of water. Because the thirst sensation is likely to be delayed during exercise, waiting for thirst results in excessive water loss and a downward shift in total body water.

2. Athletes should become accustomed to consuming fluids without the thirst sensation. As a practical matter, this is made easier if athletes carry fluids with them, wherever they are and wherever they go. Fluid consumption is much more likely to occur if the fluid is readily available without the need to go looking for it, especially if the athlete doesn't feel thirsty.

3. Athletes should consume enough fluids before exercise to produce clear urine (a sign the athlete is well hydrated). Dark urine is a sign that the athlete is producing low-volume, concentrated urine that results from the need to retain as much fluid as possible—a clear sign of underhydration.

4. Approximately 1 to 1.5 hours before exercise, athletes should consume a large volume of fluid (up to half a liter) within a relatively short time to ensure adequate hydration and to improve gastric emptying. After this, athletes should sip on fluids (approximately half a cup every 10 minutes) to maintain hydration state before exercise or competition begins. Athletes should consume fluid as frequently and in as high a volume as can be tolerated to replace water losses.

5. Athletes seeking to superhydrate should not try this technique without careful monitoring. People who have compromised cardiovascular systems should never attempt superhydration. It is also something that shouldn't be tried for the first time just before a competition. As a practical matter, the safest way to superhydrate is to frequently consume fluids.

6. Athletes should avoid foods and drinks that may have a diuretic effect. For instance, caffeine and related substances commonly found in coffee, tea, chocolate, and sodas could increase the rate of urinary water excretion if consumed in large quantities. Therefore, these substances could be counterproductive in terms of optimizing hydration state before exercise.

Fluid Intake During Exercise

Athletes consuming fluids during exercise derive clear benefits, including better maintenance of exercise performance and a slowing of the exercise-induced rise in heart rate and body temperature. In addition, blood flow to the skin is improved or maintained. The degree to which the cardiovascular and heat-maintenance capacity is maintained is directly related to the degree to which dehydration can be avoided. It is clear that a failure to consume sufficient fluids during exercise is a major risk factor in the onset of heat exhaustion.[48] The best strategy for athletes to follow to avoid heat exhaustion and maintain athletic performance is to drink fluids during exercise (see figures 3.5 and 3.6).[49-51]

Most studies evaluating the interaction between hydration adequacy and athletic performance have used either plain water or sports beverages that contain, in differing degrees, carbohydrate and electrolytes (see table 3.10). The results of these studies are similar in confirming the importance of fluid consumption during exercise (see table 3.11). However, the

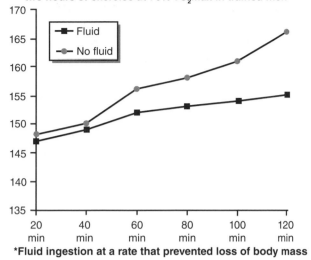

Figure 3.5 Comparison of heart rate in athletes consuming fluids and not consuming fluids during exercise.

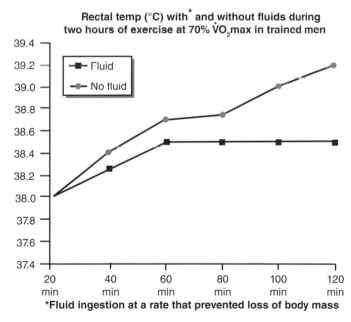

Figure 3.6 Comparison of core temperature in athletes consuming fluids and not consuming fluids during exercise.

Table 3.10 Carbohydrate and Electrolyte Content of Common Beverages

Beverage	Carbohydrate composition	Carbohydrate concentration		Sodium (mg)	Potassium (mg)
		%	Grams		
Accelerade	Sucrose, glucose, maltodextrin	7	17	127	40
All Sport	High-fructose corn syrup	9	21	55	55
Carboflex	Maltodextrin	24	55	—	—
Coca-Cola	High-fructose corn syrup, sucrose	11	26	9.2	Trace
Cytomax	Fructose corn syrup, sucrose	8	19	10	150
Diet sodas	—	—	—	Trace	Trace
Gatorade Energy Drink	Maltodextrin, glucose, fructose	23	53	133	70
Gatorade Prime	Sucrose, glucose	10.5	25	110	110
Gatorade Thirst Quencher	Sucrose, glucose, fructose	6	14	110	25
Met-Rx	Fructose, glucose	8	19	10	150
Orange juice	Fructose, sucrose	11	26	2.7	510
Powerade	High-fructose corn syrup, maltodextrin	8	19	55	30
PowerBar Endurance	Maltodextrin, dextrose, fructose	7	17	160	10
PowerBar Performance Recovery	Maltodextrin, dextrose, fructose	8.5	20	250	10
Ultima	Maltodextrin	1.7	4	8	16
Ultra Fuel	Maltodextrin, glucose, fructose	21	50	—	—
Water	—	—	—	Trace	Trace

Table 3.11 Performance Benefits of Water and Carbohydrate (Based on Performance Times)

Results:
- Performance times significantly faster with carbohydrate intake compared to no carbohydrate intake ($p>0.05$; ~6% improvement).
- Performance times significantly faster with large fluid replacement than with small fluid replacement ($p<0.05$; ~6% improvement).
- Carbohydrate intake plus large fluid replacement results in ~12% improvement compared to no carbohydrate and small fluid replacement.

Data from P.R. Below, R. Mora-Rodriguez, J. Gonzalez-Alonso, and E.F. Coyle, 1995, "Fluid and carbohydrate ingestion independently improve performance during 1 h of intense exercise," *Medicine & Science in Sports & Exercise* 27(2): 200-210.

inclusion of carbohydrate and electrolytes in the fluids affords an athlete certain advantages over plain water. Recent studies suggest that inclusion of carbohydrate in the rehydration solution improves the athlete's ability to maintain or increase work output during exercise and increases the time to exhaustion.[52-55]

Consumed carbohydrate helps athletes avoid depletion of muscle glycogen and provides fuel for muscles when muscle glycogen is low. Carbohydrate also helps maintain mental function, which is critical for maintaining endurance performance. Mental fatigue leads to muscle fatigue, even if muscles have plenty of glycogen and fluids.

Different activities result in different rates of carbohydrate utilization, but consuming carbohydrate-containing fluid consistently helps maintain athletic performance, regardless of the sport. For instance, in strenuous cycling the rate of muscle glycogen use is not affected when a carbohydrate solution is ingested;[56] in long-distance running, the rate of muscle glycogen usage is reduced when a carbohydrate-containing fluid is consumed;[57] and in stop-and-go intermittent exercise, a reduction in muscle glycogen usage is seen with the consumption of a carbohydrate-containing fluid.[58,59] In each of these scenarios, carbohydrate depletion is generally considered to be the cause of performance degradation. However, there is good evidence that consuming a carbohydrate-containing beverage may also be important for improving athletic performance in high-intensity activities where carbohydrate is not expected to be depleted because of the relatively short duration of the activity.[60-62]

These data all suggest that athletes should adjust to consuming a carbohydrate-containing fluid during exercise. However, the concentration of carbohydrate and the type of carbohydrate are important considerations. Although there are no major differences between the effects of glucose, sucrose, maltodextrins, and starch on exercise performance,[63-65] beverages containing mainly fructose may cause intestinal distress.[66,67] Maltodextrins are less sweet than sucrose and fructose, so they may be used to add carbohydrate energy to solutions without making them unpalatably sweet tasting.[40] With these exceptions aside, carbohydrate energy, regardless of whether in liquid or solid form and almost regardless of the type of carbohydrate, will aid athletic performance.[68] However, since providing carbohydrate in liquid form enables athletes to address two issues at once (energy and fluid), carbohydrate containing liquids are preferred.

The volume of carbohydrate provided during exercise is an important consideration as well; providing too much too fast may induce gastrointestinal distress and, at least temporarily, draw needed fluids away from muscle and skin to dilute this excessively concentrated solution in the gut. By contrast, providing a fluid that contains just a scant amount of carbohydrate may induce no performance benefit. Athletes should try to consume approximately 1 gram of carbohydrate per minute of exercise. This intake level can be achieved by drinking solutions that contain between 6 and 8 percent carbohydrate[69] at a volume of .6 to 1.2 liters per hour.[70,71] Some sports beverages have carbohydrate levels precisely within this range, while others have concentrations outside this range (refer to table 3.10). Concentrations above 8 percent may cause a delay in gastric emptying and do not necessarily lead to a faster or better carbohydrate metabolism during exercise.[72] Another real advantage of consuming a 6 to 8 percent carbohydrate solution is that it has a faster rate of intestinal absorption than does water alone. This means fluid status can be more efficiently maintained, and the delivery of carbohydrate to the blood and muscles is enhanced. Doctors commonly prescribe Pedialyte (sugar water) for babies with diarrhea because it induces faster water absorption than does water alone and can more quickly rehydrate the baby.

See table 3.12 for suggested fluid-replacement schedules during exercise.

Table 3.12 Opportunities for Fluid Replacement in Different Sports During Competition

Event and duration	Opportunities for fluid breaks	Fluid and carbohydrate requirements
Events lasting less than 30 min • Sprints • Jumping • Throwing • Gymnastics	Consume fluids between events but not within 15 min of event.	Not needed during the event but required between events during the course of the entire competition.
Intermediate events lasting less than 60 min • 10K run • Rowing • Aerobics class • Tennis lesson • Track cycling	Consume fluids between events. Runners should consume some fluid at least every 5 km (3.1 mi) (more often if hot and humid). All athletes in this category should bring a beverage container.	Fluid replacement is needed before, during, and after the event, and carbohydrate is needed before and after the event. However, carbohydrate will aid fluid uptake during the event, so beverages should contain carbohydrate.
Endurance events • Marathon • 80 km cycling • Olympic-distance triathlon • Tennis (5 sets)	Marathon runners should consume some fluid at least every 5 km (3.1 mi) (more often if hot and humid). Triathletes should consume fluids every 10 km (6.2 mi) during cycling and every 2 to 4 km (1.2 to 2.5 mi) during running. Tennis players should take as much time as allowable during court changes and after 3rd set to take fluids.	Fluid, electrolyte (sodium), and carbohydrate replacement are all recommended during these events. The amounts needed will vary based on environmental conditions, initial glycogen stores, and exercise intensity (e.g., difficulty of the match).
Ultraendurance events • Ironman • English Channel swim • Road cycling • Stage races such as Tour de France	Consume fluids at every opportunity, with a plan to consume fluids once every 10 min. Where fluids are not made available by race organizers (as may occur with cycling races), a fluid-consumption plan with carried fluids must be in place.	Fluid, electrolyte (sodium), and carbohydrate replacement are all recommended during these events. The amounts needed will vary based on environmental conditions, initial glycogen stores, and exercise intensity.
Team sports lasting around 90 min • Hockey • Basketball • Football • Volleyball • Baseball • Soccer	Consume fluids at breaks that naturally occur, but no less frequently than once every 15 min. Ideally, fluids should be consumed every 10 min. Naturally occurring longer breaks (halftime, between innings, between quarters) should be considered an opportunity to replenish fluids.	Fluid, electrolyte (sodium), and carbohydrate replacement are all recommended during these events. The amounts needed will vary based on environmental conditions, initial glycogen stores, and exercise intensity.

Adapted from H. O'Connor, "Practical aspects of fluid replacement," *Australian Journal of Nutrition & Dietetics* 53(4 Suppl): S27-S34. Copyright © 1996 by Wiley-Blackwell. Reproduced with permission of Blackwell Publishing Ltd.

Fluid Intake After Exercise

Athletes who have exercised intensely for an hour or longer are likely to experience some degree of underhydration. For those athletes who exercise most days (i.e., most elite athletes), postexercise fluid consumption becomes a critically important part of the exercise regimen because it helps the athlete begin each subsequent day of activity in a well-hydrated state. The important point to consider is this: It takes time to rehydrate. The less time there is to rehydrate, the lower the likelihood that the athlete will be optimally hydrated by the beginning of the next exercise session.

Athletes rarely consume fluids during exercise at a rate of more than 70 percent of sweat loss, and most athletes replace sweat losses at a rate significantly lower than this.[73,74] Therefore, most athletes require strategies to achieve adequate hydration before the next exercise session begins. Despite this clear need for fluids, athletes often remain underhydrated even when fluids are readily available to them.[75] This voluntary dehydration suggests that athletes should be placed on a fixed fluid-replacement schedule that will increase the likelihood of maintaining hydration. A way of encouraging this is to make certain that cool, good-tasting fluids are easily available to the athlete as soon as the exercise session is over.[76] Commercial sports drinks containing both carbohydrate and sodium are more effective than plain water at restoring water balance.[77] To maximize rehydration, however, it appears that a level of sodium greater than that provided in most sports drinks is desirable.[78] This added sodium can be obtained through the normal consumption of foods, many of which have added salt (sodium).[79] In general, athletes should follow these rules for fluid consumption after exercise:

1. A large volume of fluid (as much as can be tolerated, perhaps .5 liter) should be consumed immediately after exercise. This large fluid volume enlarges the stomach and increases the rate at which fluids leave the stomach and enter the small intestine to be absorbed.

2. After the initial consumption of a large fluid volume, athletes should consume approximately .25 liter of fluid every 15 minutes to achieve a fluid intake of approximately 3 liters in 3 hours. The larger the athlete and the greater the sweat loss experienced during activity, the greater the amount of fluid that must be consumed.

3. Fluids should contain both carbohydrate and sodium because both are useful in returning the athlete to a well-hydrated state. In addition, the carbohydrate content of the beverage helps return stored glycogen (energy) to muscles in preparation for the next exercise session.

4. Sports drinks typically provide 10 to 25 millimoles of electrolytes (mainly sodium) per liter of fluid. However, the optimal sodium concentration for fluid retention is approximately 50 millimoles of electrolytes per liter of fluid.[41] Since adding more sodium to fluids may make the fluid unpalatable and cause the athlete to consume less fluid, the athlete should be encouraged to consume some salted snacks (such as pretzels or saltine crackers) during the period immediately after exercise.

5. The loss in body weight that results from exercise should be the key to determining the total amount of fluid that must be replaced before the next exercise session. As a general guide, 1 pint (16 ounces) of retained fluid is equal to 1 pound of body weight. Since not all consumed fluid is retained, more fluid may need to be consumed to replace the fluid equivalent in weight loss. Athletes should weigh themselves before and after exercise in different environmental conditions as a guide for how much fluid they should consume after exercise. This requires meticulous record keeping, because hot

and humid day sweat losses will be higher than less hot and humid day sweat losses. If pre- and postexercise weight shows a weight loss, this loss is typically almost entirely from fluid losses. ***Postexercise,*** athletes should consume 1.5 pints of fluid for every pound lost during the exercise session. The rationale behind this amount is that the

Sports Gels

Sports gels are carbohydrate polymers (large molecules of many monosaccharides held together by molecular bonds). Since gastric emptying is affected by the osmolar concentration of an ingested solution (higher osmolar concentrations reduce the gastric emptying rate), consuming gels offers the possibility of delivering more carbohydrate with a lower osmolar effect.[80] This holds real promise for athletes involved in high-endurance sports (e.g., marathon, ultramarathon, triathlon, Ironman, Tour de France) where the energy requirement is far higher than could easily be provided with typical 6 to 7 percent carbohydrate sports beverages. Sports gels all deliver approximately 100 calories per gel pack and typically provide different combinations of carbohydrate polymers, such as

- maltodextrin and fructose (Gu Energy Gel; Gu Roctane; PowerBar Energy Gel; Carb-Boom! Energy Gel; and Accel Gel);
- brown rice syrup (Clif Shot); and
- maltodextrin, dextrose, and fruit juice (Hammer Gel).

These products have a wide array of sodium concentrations, ranging from a high of 200 milligrams per 240 milliliters in PowerBar Energy Gel to a low of 40 milligrams per 240 milliliters in Clif Shot. Some even contain amino acids and vitamins, although their inclusion is likely more geared toward satisfying consumer desires than providing any real performance outcomes. As you will read in chapter 4 (Ergogenic Aids), caffeine has a positive independent effect on endurance performance outcomes, and some sports gels include caffeine as well. The highest caffeine contents are found in Clif Shot Double Espresso and Carb-Boom! Double Espresso (100 milligrams), while other manufacturers and flavors have lesser concentrations.

There is evidence that mixed-carbohydrate solutions (i.e., those delivering combinations of monosaccharides) result in higher levels of carbohydrate oxidation than when an isocalorically equivalent single-carbohydrate source is used in a sports beverage.[81] It is not well understood, however, whether ingesting carbohydrate as a gel (a carbohydrate polymer) would have the same oxidative result. A recent study on well-trained cyclists suggests that carbohydrate delivery and carbohydrate oxidation are equivalent whether the delivery system is a gel or liquid drink.[82] There is also evidence that carbohydrate gel ingestion during cycling at 32 degrees Celsius (90 degrees Fahrenheit) attenuated leukocyte and neutrophil counts (measures of immune system response).[83] However, athletes must never miss an opportunity to deliver fluids to the system as well as carbohydrate, so sports gel consumption should not be considered an appropriate substitution for sports beverages. Athletes who consume them should quickly follow with a dilutional load of water to help sustain the hydration state.

athlete must replace the fluid lost during the exercise (1 pound = 1 pint; 1/2 kilogram ≈ 1 pint), but must also satisfy ongoing needs (thus, the additional 1/2 pint). These pre- and postexercise weights will also help the athlete understand how much more fluid they should try to consume ***during exercise*** on subsequent exercise days. For instance, an athlete who weighs 130 (59 kilograms) pounds before exercise and weighs 127 pounds (57.6 kilograms) after exercise should consume an additional 3 pints of fluid during the next exercise session. If the athlete consumed 2 pints of fluid during the previous exercise session, then the total fluid needs for a similar exercise session is actually 5 pints of fluid. While excess fluid consumption is rare among competitive athletes, everyone should be cautious about a level of fluid consumption that increases body weight, as this may predispose the athlete to potentially dangerous hyponatremia. Generally, athletes will find it difficult to fully satisfy sweat fluid losses; however, optimal performance is maintained when the athlete loses no more than 2 percent of body weight during an exercise session.

6. Consumption of any substance that causes a diuretic effect in an individual athlete should be avoided.

IMPORTANT POINTS

• Athletes should consume about 16 ounces of fluid approximately 1 to 1.5 hours before physical activity. After this fluid consumption, athletes should institute a sipping protocol (about half a cup every 10 to 15 minutes) with the sports beverage they will consume during the athletic endeavor. This will help ensure that exercise begins with blood sugar and blood volume at a good level.

• After the last meal and before the beginning of exercise, foods that have a long gastric emptying time (i.e., foods high in fat, protein, and fiber) should be avoided, as should unaccustomed foods and beverages.

• Thirst is an important emergency sensation indicating the body cannot tolerate a great deal more fluid loss, but athletes should not rely on thirst as the primary indicator of when to drink. When the thirst sensation first occurs, an athlete has already typically lost 1.5 to 2.0 liters of fluid.

• Before thirst sets in, athletes should drink a carbohydrate- and sodium-containing solution at fixed and well-practiced intervals. Care should be taken to not overconsume fluids during physical activity, particularly fluids devoid of sodium, as these may increase the risk of developing hyponatremia. During exercise, athletes should consume a beverage that provides about a 6 percent carbohydrate solution and a sodium concentration of between 100 and 200 milligrams per cup.

• After physical activity, athletes should consume sufficient fluids to regain a good state of hydration, as indicated by clear urine. This should be done as soon as possible after the exercise is over. As a guide, the difference in body weight before and after exercise is an indication of the amount of fluid that was not replaced during exercise. One pound of body weight is equivalent to 16 ounces of fluid. A good training program will attempt to add sufficient fluid to the training regimen so as to avoid a significant weight (i.e., body-water) loss.

Ergogenic Aids

The term *ergogenic aid* refers to any substance that can increase the capacity for bodily or mental labor, especially by eliminating fatigue symptoms. *Nutritional* ergogenic aids refer to substances that can enhance performance and are either nutrients, metabolic by-products of nutrients, food (plant) extracts, or substances commonly found in foods (e.g., caffeine and creatine) that are provided in amounts more concentrated than commonly found in the natural food supply. The nonnutritional ergogenic aids, including anabolic steroids and their analogues, continue to be used by athletes, but because they are nearly universally banned by sports organizing bodies (NCAA, IOC, USOC, and so on), they are not the focus of this chapter. Instead, this chapter focuses on the legal nutritional ergogenic aids, for which there is an increasing body of scientific information.

Companies selling ergogenic aids often target different athlete populations, with some focusing on strength and power sports while others focus on improving aerobic endurance. This chapter provides critical information on the theory behind each aid, its efficacy, and its safety (although long-term safety studies have rarely, if ever, been performed). In addition, where there may be some potential for performance enhancement by consuming an ergogenic aid, this chapter includes the best strategy for its use. Before reading this chapter, it is important that you consider this fact: The vast majority of substances advertised as having ergogenic properties do not, and those that do work would lose their ergogenic properties if the athlete consumed a regular energy and nutrient intake that satisfied need. Most importantly, the ergogenic benefit derived from a properly balanced diet is legal, far less expensive, and much more likely to be safe than any potential benefit that might be provided in bottles and pills.

In short, ergogenic aids claim to enhance performance. The nutritional ergogenic aids work by entering well-established nutritional metabolic pathways. For instance, taking extra carbohydrate to improve performance makes *carbohydrate*, by definition, a nutritional ergogenic aid. Also, taking creatine monohydrate to improve sprint performance makes creatine a nutritional ergogenic aid because creatine is a normal constituent of food, and its consumption causes creatine to enter a known metabolic pathway.[1-3] Nonnutritional ergogenic aids represent products (often of unknown origin because producers don't clearly specify what they consist of) that are neither nutrients nor other substances with nutritional properties. The best-known nonnutritional ergogenic aids are anabolic steroids.

In most cases, the performance-enhancement claims attributed to ergogenic aids exceed reality. Since many of the products are considered foods, nutrients, or nutrient-based products, there are few controls for government agencies to police these claims. The only truly credible sources of information come from published scientific works, many of which are reviewed in the website for the Office of Dietary Supplements of the National Institutes of Health (http://ods.od.nih.gov). Where improvements are seen, they are often due to a placebo effect: Consumers of a specific product *believe* it will help, so it actually helps even though there is no known biological basis for the improvement.

In other cases, improvements occur because the product provides a chemical or nutrient missing from the foods an athlete commonly consumes. For instance, bodybuilders often take protein powders or amino acid powders to aid in the enlargement of muscle mass. However, studies clearly indicate that the rate of protein usage by the body is well below the level consumed by those who take these protein powders. The body's limit for using protein to build muscle and maintain tissues is now thought to be approximately 1.5 to 2.0 grams of protein per kilogram and no more than 30 grams of protein per meal.[4,5] Nev-

ertheless, many athletes who take protein supplements often consume protein at levels that exceed 3.0 grams per kilogram per day, with single doses that provide more than 50 grams of protein. The excess protein is burned as fuel or stored as fat, but it can't be used to build more muscle. It is also known that bodybuilders frequently consume an inadequate level of energy. This energy inadequacy makes it difficult, if not impossible, for them to support their larger muscle mass.[6] Therefore, the ergogenic benefit of taking extra protein appears to be derived more from the extra *calories* provided by the protein (which helps to support existing tissue) than from its potential tissue-building effect. However, consuming protein to support caloric needs is a bad strategy, as the nitrogen that must be excreted in this process can exacerbate a negative hydration state.

Numerous ergogenic aids are available, ranging from known nutrients to supposed nutrients. Vitamin

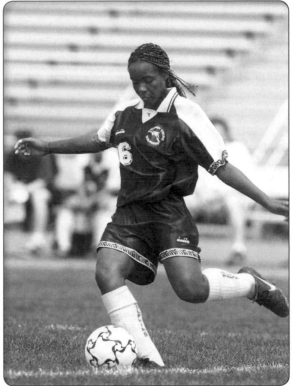

© Human Kinetics

Many athletes consume products that supposedly improve power or endurance, but few of these products provide the results promised.

Brief History of Ergogenic Aids

"The first Olympic games took place in Greece in 776 BC. From sources documenting specific training and dietary regimens for athletes in ancient times, we know that some of them ate hallucinogenic mushrooms and sesame seeds to enhance performance. Although the modern Olympic games commenced in 1896, scientific and medical interest in the diet and training of Olympic athletes did not begin until 1922. . . . In 1889, Charles Edward Brown-Séquard, a French physiologist, claimed to have reversed his own aging process by self-injecting testicular extracts. Testosterone, the primary male hormone, was first synthesized in 1935, and in the 1940s, athletes began taking anabolic steroids to increase their muscle mass. Throughout the 1950s and 1960s, amphetamines and anabolic steroids were used extensively. Concerned about that trend, the International Olympic Committee (IOC) banned their use by Olympic athletes in the early 1960s. Formal drug testing began with the 1968 Olympics. In 1988, Canadian Olympic sprinter Ben Johnson was stripped of his gold medal after testing revealed he had used an oral anabolic steroid; this was the first time a gold medallist in track and field was disqualified from the Olympics for using illegal drugs."

Reprinted from M.D. Silver, 2001, "Use of ergogenic aids by athletes," *Journal of the American Academy of Orthopaedic Surgeons* 2001; 9(1): 61-63.

B_{15}, for instance, has no official definition, varies in content by manufacturer because of no standardization of active ingredients, and is not a recognized vitamin. Many herbs sold as ergogenic aids have no known chemical content or known active ingredients. There is so much misinformation in the marketplace and in the locker room about these products that the buyer should beware. The legality of some supposed ergogenic products is also in doubt. Studies have shown that many of these products (as many as 25 percent) are laced with banned substances not listed on the label that could place an athlete at risk of failing a banned substance blood or urine test.[7] In general, athletes should avoid focusing on a magic bullet to improve performance and should take a more realistic approach by consuming a balanced intake of foods that provide sufficient energy and nutrients to support growth, activity, and tissue maintenance.

CATEGORIES OF ERGOGENIC AIDS

Ergogenic aids fall into several categories, including mechanical aids, pharmacological aids, physiological aids, nutritional aids, and psychological aids (see table 4.1). This chapter discusses pharmacological and nutritional aids. Despite widely publicized problems associated with the ingestion of many substances with ergogenic properties, athletes continue to play Russian roulette with their bodies. The side effects from taking anabolic steroids, for instance, may be irreversible and include hypertension; dysplasia resulting in tendon ruptures; liver tumors; psychosis (steroid rage); hirsutism (excessive hairiness); clitoral hypertrophy and lower voice in women; breast development, testicular atrophy, and impotence in men; and premature closure of the bone epiphyses, causing shorter stature in adolescents.[8]

Table 4.1 Categories and Examples of Ergogenic Aids
(Both Allowed and Prohibited)

Category	Examples
Mechanical aids	Free weights to develop strength; lightweight racing shoes; nasal strips to improve airflow to the lungs; running parachutes for resistance to develop strength
Pharmacological aids	Androgenic steroid hormones (and their precursors); high-dose nutrient supplements (vitamins and minerals); quasi-nutrient substances that impart a pharmacological effect (i.e., beyond the nutrition effect you would expect from a normal intake)
Physiological aids	Blood doping; sauna; massage and other forms of physiotherapy
Nutritional aids	Carbohydrate loading; sports drinks; caffeine intake and the consumption of other substances commonly available in the food supply
Psychological aids	Hypnosis; relaxation techniques; imagery techniques; motivational techniques

In addition, most ergogenic aids are taken to counter ongoing dietary shortcomings that would be cheaper, safer, and more effectively corrected with simple changes in food and fluid consumption. For instance, the amino acid delivery from protein and amino acid supplements is more than 10 times more expensive than the consumption of a small piece of chicken or meat, and the latter is known to be safe.

Of course, the legality of obtaining and consuming certain substances should also be considered. Although widely available, anabolic steroids are prescription medications that may legally be prescribed only by a doctor for a patient who presents with defined clinical symptoms. The issue of safety should not be taken lightly. Products containing combinations of caffeine and ephedrine have resulted in numerous deaths, leading to the banning of ephedra and related substances from U.S. and other markets.[9] See table 4.3 on page 124 for a summary of ergogenic aids, their potential benefits and side effects, and their legality.

Given the widespread advertisements purporting the ergogenic benefits of various substances, it is difficult for coaches and athletes to discern what works and what doesn't, what's safe and what isn't. Several points should be considered before purchasing a supplement or ergogenic aid. These include the following:[10]

- Pregnant or breastfeeding women should be cautious about taking supplements because some supplements may be dangerous to the fetus or baby.

- Certain medications and supplements can dangerously interact with each other if taken together, so people taking medications should be cautious about the supplements they take.

- Some supplements, including omega-3 fatty acids, may inhibit clotting. Athletes undergoing surgery, should be careful about what supplements they take and report consumed supplements to physicians.

- Be cautious about supplements with unfounded claims that are too good to be true. Supplements claiming cures or offering money-back guarantees are not likely to be useful.

- Choose brands labeled with NSF International, U.S. Pharmacopeia, or Consumer Lab seals. These insignia verify that the supplement actually contains the ingredients stated on the label and does not contain contaminants, potentially harmful ingredients, or banned substances not listed on the label.

- Many supplements produced outside the United States may not be regulated and may, therefore, contain potentially toxic substances.

A major problem with dietary supplements is that it is difficult to be sure of their content. Studies by Maughan (2001) demonstrate that the dietary supplements athletes take might cause them to fail a doping test because they contain nandrolone (an anabolic steroid) or other banned substances.[11] Maughan cites numerous reports of athletes failing drug tests because herbal supplements they believed to be safe and legal actually contained banned substances. Clearly, athletes should ask themselves if the risks of taking a supplement outweigh the potential benefits. They may believe they are doing nothing contrary to the rules of sports organizing committees (e.g., the IOC or USOC), but there is increasingly a zero tolerance for banned substances. If a banned substance is found in an athlete's body, the athlete will fail the test, even if the athlete didn't knowingly use the substance.

Carbohydrate as an Ergogenic Aid

Since carbohydrate is typically the limiting energy substrate in exercise (i.e., it will run out before fat or protein runs out), it is critical for an athlete to begin a bout of physical activity with enough stored carbohydrate to see him through the session; doing so will aid exercise endurance and power, regardless of the exercise modality. In high-intensity exercise, carbohydrate is the primary fuel used by the muscles. In low-intensity exercise of long duration, fat may be the primary fuel, but fat requires carbohydrate for complete oxidation.[12] In addition, the storage capacity for fat is far greater than that of carbohydrate, even in the leanest athletes. In either form of exercise, carbohydrate depletion results in a dramatically reduced exercise performance.[13,14] It is the intent of carbohydrate-loading techniques, therefore, to store the maximal amount of carbohydrate the tissues can hold. See chapter 6 for more information on carbohydrate-loading techniques.

Not all sports and activities are suitable for carbohydrate loading. Keep in mind that for every gram of stored glycogen, the body stores approximately 3 grams of water. Tissues that are packed full with glycogen and water are likely to cause some degree of muscle stiffness. In sports such as gymnastics and diving where flexibility is important, carbohydrate loading may cause difficulties. It also appears that carbohydrate loading may be less beneficial for women than for men. In a study comparing higher carbohydrate intakes in men and women, men showed both a glycogen and performance improvement, whereas women, because of a higher lipid and lower protein and carbohydrate oxidation rate than men, did not experience the same level of improvement.[15]

The type of carbohydrate does appear to make a difference. Glucose polymer products (including commercially available sports gels and polycose) and maltodextrins (which are found in numerous sports beverages) are easily digested into glucose and appear to be more effective for glycogen production than are other carbohydrates. You can find more information about sports gels, which are used primarily during events with fluids as part of a hydration regimen, in chapter 3 (see Sports Gels on page 108). However, starches from pasta, bread, rice, and other cereals are also effective at maximizing glycogen storage.[12, 16]

Different forms of carbohydrates have different rates of digestion and provide varying rates of glucose release into the blood. In a study assessing the rise of blood glucose after a high-carbohydrate meal 2.5 hours before a 90-minute bicycle ride, subjects were given a candy bar with either a high glycemic (HG) index or a low glycemic (LG) index; a no-food control was also used. Both blood glucose and insulin were higher in the LG group than in either of the other two conditions. Blood free fatty acids (FFAs) were highest in the control group, while the LG trial showed higher FFAs than did the HG trial during the ride. This study suggests that a low glycemic index food will provide more sustained energy (and thus improved endurance) during prolonged exercise.[17]

Ingesting a glucose polymer solution before exercise results in a smaller reduction in power than does a noncaloric placebo during an hour of maximal exercise. When the same amount of glucose polymer is taken in 15-minute intervals during exercise, there is no observed benefit. This suggests that glucose polymers are performance enhancing if consumed before exercise but have no ergogenic benefit if taken during exercise.[18]

How quickly an athlete can recover from exhaustive exercise by reestablishing muscle glycogen is also an important performance factor, particularly in sports where athletes compete on sequential days. Glycogen depletion may occur in 2 to 3 hours of high-intensity exercise (60 to 80 percent of $\dot{V}O_2$max) and even faster in maximum-intensity activity. Besides reducing performance, low muscle glycogen may predispose athletes to higher injury risk. In activities such as soccer and hockey, where competition frequency and exercise intensity make glycogen depletion more likely, consumption of carbohydrate during a competition or practice is a logical strategy to avoid glycogen depletion. Many athletes in these and related sports continue to miss an important ergogenic opportunity by consuming only water during an event.[19]

After exercise, it seems logical to consume a carbohydrate food (1 gram per kilogram of body weight is recommended) to reduce protein breakdown and aid in protein synthesis. Failure to consume carbohydrate after exercise results in a higher than necessary level of muscle breakdown, thereby reducing the benefit that might be derived from resistance training.[20]

Creatine Monohydrate

Creatine, a compound made from the amino acids arginine, glycine, and methionine, joins with phosphorus to make phosphocreatine (PCr). Phosphocreatine serves as a storage depot for maintaining adenosine triphosphate (ATP) levels during high-intensity activities such as sprinting, which can quickly deplete ATP (see figure 4.1). ATP is the high-energy fuel used by cells. It is believed that athletes who saturate their muscles with creatine will enhance their capacity to maintain the high-energy compound ATP and delay fatigue in high-intensity activity.[12, 21] Loading with creatine monohydrate (CrM), the supplement form of creatine, at the level of 20 grams per day for 5 to 7 days can cause muscle PCr content to increase by as much as 50 percent.

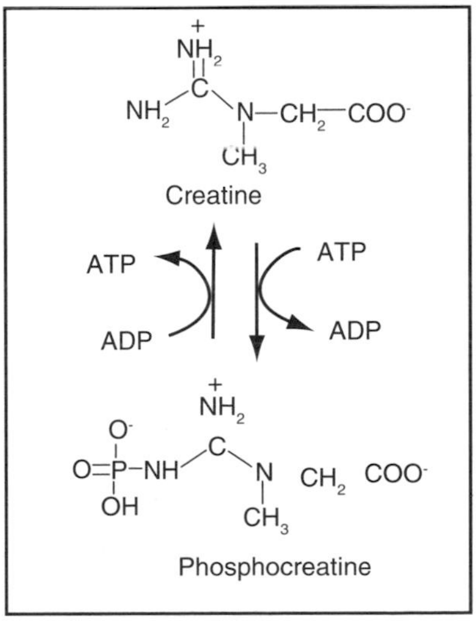

Figure 4.1 Creation of ATP from phosphocreatine.

This level of intake causes the storage of creatine to approach the theoretical upper limit of 160 millimoles per kilogram of dry muscle.[22]

Besides our cellular synthesis of creatine from three amino acids, we can also obtain creatine from meat. (*Note:* The Greek root of the word *creatine* is *creas*, which means meat.) However, normal cooking can easily reduce the preformed creatine level of foods by denaturing this simple polypeptide. Therefore, well-done meats retain relatively small preformed creatine content. To avoid the irregularities of intake from diet alone, many athletes regularly consume creatine in the form of creatine monohydrate (CrM), with evidence suggesting that CrM can cause a small but significant improvement in high-intensity sport performance.[3, 23-25] CrM may also enhance strength gains during the beginning of resistance training, a benefit that is likely to be expressed during later competitive events.[26] Limited evidence suggests an endurance performance benefit, but this is likely for the more anaerobic portions of endurance races, such as the sprint at the end of a 10K or marathon.[27,28] It also is possible that some of the benefit derived from taking creatine monohydrate may be due to the inadequate energy (caloric) intake commonly seen in athletes.[29] In a recent study on repeated jump height, a 250-calorie supplement of carbohydrate was found to be more effective at sustaining maximal jump height than was a standard creatine monohydrate supplement. In addition, the carbohydrate sustained jump height without an associated weight gain, whereas the creatine monohydrate consumption was associated with a significant increase in weight.[30,31] As previously mentioned, inadequate energy intake is one of the major problems athletes face. It is possible that athletes with an adequate energy intake would not benefit from these supplements, although this has never been adequately tested.

Athletes consuming creatine monohydrate typically dose themselves with 10 to 28 grams, divided into four doses over the day. For instance, if the goal is to take 10 grams per day, individual doses should be 2.5 grams four times daily. Smaller athletes should use smaller daily doses. There is evidence that taking daily creatine supplements causes a saturation of creatine in muscle tissue after 5 days.[32] Therefore, creatine should be consumed for no longer than 5 days, followed by about a 5-day break in supplementation. Taking creatine supplements only 5 days per month may even be sufficient to saturate muscle tissue.[3, 33] Creatine storage in muscle causes retention of water, with a concomitant increase in weight.[3]

The issue of creatine monohydrate supplementation and heat regulation has been assessed, but the study findings are inconclusive. In addition, the exercise time used in previous research was limited. Highest heat risk occurs in people who exercise longer than 60 minutes in hot and humid environments, and studies assessing whether CrM ingestion affects heat tolerance have failed to push athletes to these limits. Ideally, future CrM assessments should assess increases in muscular creatine storage after supplementation and should stress people for longer periods in hot and humid environments to determine the effect of creatine on heat stress.

The long-term safety of creatine monohydrate supplementation has never been fully tested on children, adolescents, or adults. There is also no solid evidence to suggest that creatine supplementation is unsafe for healthy adults, and there is no information on its safety if taken by children over long periods. Athletes must determine whether creatine supplementation is appropriate for them. Before an athlete tries creatine supplementation, it may be prudent to first be certain that an adequate level of energy (calories) is being consumed. If not, a simple increase in energy consumption may suffice to improve repeat high-intensity activity.

Glycerol

Glycerol (also referred to as glycerin) is a three-carbon simple lipid that is metabolized like carbohydrate. The three-carbon structure of glycerol holds dietary fatty acids together to form triglycerides. Glycerol is a powerful humectant, with a potent capacity to attract a large volume of water. A number of endurance athletes in the past have used glycerol as a means of superhydration (increasing body-water storage beyond the normal level) because of its capacity to hold water and its ability to be easily and cleanly metabolized for energy. Now the World Anti-Doping Agency (WADA) has placed glycerol on its banned substance list.

Maximizing body water may induce a level of stiffness that some athletes find uncomfortable. Indeed, athletes who consume glycerol-laced fluids before an event often complain that they feel, at least initially, stiff and sluggish. But many of these same athletes claim that the benefits of having extra water at the end of a race far outweigh the feeling of sluggishness at the beginning of the race. While other athletes are dehydrated and overheating, these athletes say they feel fresher when it counts the most.

A word of caution: Although many endurance athletes use glycerated water (i.e., water containing glycerol) to enhance their hydration state, this product has never been adequately tested for safety. Because glycerol is a normal component of the diet and is easily metabolized, it is unlikely that small amounts of glycerol, by itself, would cause any difficulty. With higher doses, headaches and blurred vision may occur.[34] Furthermore, it is unclear how much additional stress is placed on the cardiovascular system when additional water is stored in the system.

The IOC bans diuretics because of the detrimental effects of dehydration and because diuretics have been used to lower the concentration of biological markers of steroids and other banned substances in the urine. Glycerol was once classified as a diuretic, but in 1997 the U.S. Olympic Committee (USOC) removed the ban on glycerol because it was widely understood that diuresis is not likely with glycerol doses of between 1.0 and 1.5 grams per kilogram.

There is no widespread consensus on how to best consume glycerated water. The protocol established for a 155-pound (70 kg) athlete ingesting approximately 2 liters of fluid 2.5 hours before activity is as follows:[35]

- Drink 5 milliliters per kilogram of a 20 percent glycerol solution.
- Thirty minutes later: Drink 5 milliliters per kilogram of water.
- Fifteen minutes later: Drink 5 milliliters per kilogram of water.
- Fifteen minutes later: Drink 1 milliliter per kilogram of a 20 percent glycerol solution and 5 milliliters per kilogram of water.
- Thirty minutes later: Drink 5 milliliters per kilogram of water.
- Begin exercise 1 hour later.

For events lasting more than 2 hours, consuming 400 to 800 milliliters per hour of a 5 percent glycerol solution before and during the event may also be beneficial, although there is more compelling evidence that consumption of a 6 to 8 percent carbohydrate solution during competition is ergogenic. However, remember that the WADA recently placed glycerol on the banned substance list, so it should not be used by an athlete.

Bicarbonate (Sodium Bicarbonate or Bicarbonate of Soda)

Researchers have theorized that sodium bicarbonate buffers the acidity from lactic acid that is created by anaerobic metabolism. If so, this would allow for a prolonged maintenance of force or power.[36] Many activities involve mainly anaerobic metabolic processes, and it would appear that some athletes could benefit from sodium bicarbonate consumption. Study results, however, are mixed and generally indicate that well-hydrated athletes do not derive the performance benefit theorized from bicarbonate ingestion.

The sodium in the sodium bicarbonate may actually be more useful than the bicarbonate (the acid buffer). Sodium is an electrolyte that helps increase or maintain blood volume, creating a larger buffering space (i.e., more fluid) for muscles to excrete the extra acidity created by high-intensity activity. Think of sugar as the acid produced from anaerobic activity and a glass of water as the blood volume, and you can see what might happen. If the glass of water is half full and you drop a cube of sugar in it, the concentration of sugar would be higher than if you put the same amount of sugar in a full glass of water. The potential negative side effects from taking sodium bicarbonate, however—including the potential for severe gastrointestinal distress and nausea—should give athletes reason to be cautious before taking this potential ergogenic aid.

In a 1993 study of 10 collegiate varsity rowers, subjects consumed 300 milligrams of sodium bicarbonate ($NaHCO_3$) per kilogram of lean body mass 1 hour before a 2,000-meter time trial. Power, total work produced, and speed in the event were all significantly improved when compared with the consumption of a nonergogenic placebo.[37] In another study, six trained males ingested 300 milligrams of $NaHCO_3$ per kilogram of lean body mass and were assessed before, during, and after exhaustive resistance training. The $NaHCO_3$ produced no apparent improvement.[38] In an assessment of male and female runners who competed in a series of four 1,600-meter races scheduled 3 days apart, subjects ingested 400 milligrams of $NaHCO_3$ per kilogram, 500 milligrams of sodium citrate per kilogram, or a placebo (calcium carbonate) 2 hours before three of the races; one race was used as a control. The sodium bicarbonate and sodium citrate had no effect on racing time, and most of the runners complained of uncomfortable side effects. Bicarbonate loading was associated with uncomfortable side effects in the majority of athletes.[39]

Proteins and Amino Acids

Amino acids are the building blocks of proteins. Various numbers of amino acids held together in diverse sequences result in proteins with different characteristics. The protein in hair, for instance, has a particular sequence of amino acids, and the protein in muscle has another sequence of amino acids. When proteins are broken apart, the result is a pool of amino acids derived from the amino acid building blocks of the protein.

Many athletes consume protein or amino acid supplements, believing they promote muscle building. However, dietary assessments of athletes strongly suggest that any benefit of the supplement comes from helping athletes meet their caloric needs rather than independently supporting a larger muscle mass. Because this is most likely the case, most athletes would find it easier, cheaper, and safer to eat more food to obtain the needed calories than to take protein or amino acid supplements. Studies generally agree that humans use, anabolically, only about 1.5 grams of protein per kilogram of body weight.[40,41] Protein requirements can be thought of as directly related to the amount of fat-free mass a person has, plus a very small amount used to supply energy. Taken together, this amounts to a requirement range for athletes of between 1.2 and 1.7 grams per kilogram of body weight. Consuming more than this amount ensures the remaining protein will be catabolized as a source of fuel or stored as fat. Burning protein as a source of fuel is undesirable because it creates toxic nitrogenous waste (e.g., ammonia, urea) that must be excreted. This mandatory urinary excretion causes an increase in water loss and increases the chance for dehydration.

Caffeine

Caffeine, one of several methylxanthines found in coffee, tea, cola, chocolate, and a variety of other foods and beverages (see table 4.2), has been shown to help endurance-type performance in people who are unaccustomed to consuming caffeinated products.[42] Caffeine is a central nervous system stimulant and a muscle relaxant. It has recently been removed from the IOC's banned substance list. In a number of studies, caffeine ingestion significantly increased free fatty acid concentration in plasma.[43] The increased availability of FFAs enhances the ability of cells to use these fats as a fuel in endurance-type, low-intensity activities. Since humans adapt to caffeine intake, frequent and regular consumption results in a reduced dose effect. Put simply, the more you consume, the more you need to consume to achieve the same ergogenic effect. A recent review of the effect of caffeine on endurance performance has found that studies assessing the ergogenic effect of caffeine have an average improvement of about 3.2 percent (± 4.3 percent), with some studies showing an improvement of 17.3 percent.[44] The variability in benefit was likely because of subject tolerance or adaptation to caffeine, with the recommendation that the greatest performance benefit would likely occur if athletes abstained from caffeine for a minimum

Table 4.2 Caffeine Content of Common Foods, Drinks, and Medicines

Food, beverage, medicine	Serving size	Caffeine content (mg)
Coffee, brewed	250 ml	100-150
Coffee, drip	250 ml	125-175
Coffee, instant	250 ml	50-70
Coffee, espresso	250 ml	50-110
Tea, green	250 ml	25-40
Tea, black	250 ml	40-60
Cola drinks	360 ml	35-54
Energy drinks	250 ml	80-150
Chocolate, dark	50 mg	20-40
Chocolate, milk	50 mg	8-16
No-Doz	1 dose tablet	200
Anacin	1 dose tablet	64
Excedrin	1 dose tablet	130
Bufferin	1 dose tablet	0

Note: 240 ml = 8 oz; 360 ml = 12 oz

Source: USDA National Nutrient Database for Standard Reference, Version 21.

of 7 days before competition. Overconsumption of caffeine is associated with irritability, insomnia, diarrhea, and anxiety. In addition, a large volume of caffeine intake may induce a diuresis that could exacerbate the state of dehydration.

Many studies have assessed caffeine at doses ranging from 3 to 6 milligrams per kilogram, taken about 1 hour before physical activity. More recent studies use doses of 1 to 2 milligrams per kilogram provided during the last portion of endurance exercise.[45] In practical terms, this would be equivalent to providing a 50-kilogram (110-pound) athlete with one brewed cup of coffee's worth of caffeine in the last one or two hydration stations of a marathon. Caffeine consumed at doses of between 3 and 9 milligrams per kilogram or a total of approximately 250 milligrams appears to aid performance in long-endurance activity and may also improve performance in more intense short-duration exercise.[46] It remains unclear as to why caffeine has this apparent ergogenic benefit, although it was originally hypothesized that it may stimulate the sympathetic nervous system and enhance utilization of fatty acids, thereby sparing limited glycogen stores.[47,48] This is referred to as the Randle effect but has not been supported in studies.[49] As a central nervous system stimulant, caffeine may stimulate the brain into a lower level of fatigue to allow a continuation of performance at a higher level.

Although the ergogenic benefit of caffeine on endurance performance is increasingly supported by studies, limited data suggest that caffeine would induce an ergogenic benefit in high-intensity activities. Several studies have found no caffeine benefit in sprint cycling performance, but one study did show a caffeine benefit with intermittent cycling (2-minute sprints followed by 4 to 5 minutes of rest).[50,51] Contrary to popular belief, caffeine, when taken in normally consumed amounts, does not have a diuretic effect.[52] It is possible that caffeine is mistakenly thought to have a diuretic effect because it is so often consumed in liquids, which may themselves (even without the caffeine) induce diuresis.

Now that the IOC no longer bans caffeine, athletes have started using it more regularly, particularly at the end of endurance competitions when caffeine can wake up an athlete at a point in the race when muscular and mental fatigue are evident. Except for the dependence problem it creates with regular use (discontinuation produces irritability, headache, and mood shifts), it is a relatively safe substance to consume.[53]

Carnitine (Typically L-Carnitine)

L-carnitine is a common name for beta-hydroxy butyrate, a quaternary amine that was first discovered in muscles in the early 1900s. It is mainly involved in transporting long-chain fatty acids that reside inside cells into the mitochondria of the cells, where they are metabolized. Carnitine increases blood flow by improving fatty acid oxidation in the artery walls, and it detoxifies ammonia, a by-product of protein breakdown that is associated with early fatigue.[54] We synthesize carnitine from the amino acids lysine and methionine, and it is found in abundant quantities in all meats and dairy products, so a deficiency is unlikely. If a deficiency occurs, it is most likely in vegetarians who avoid consumption of dairy products. With an adequate intake of meats or dairy products, there is little reason to take this relatively expensive supplement. Although never tested, it is possible that pure vegans might benefit from L-carnitine supplementation if they perform high-intensity exercise.

Carnitine is thought to spare muscle glycogen breakdown and decrease lactic acid production, but studies generally show no benefit in low-intensity endurance activities.[55] Some studies, however, have demonstrated a benefit in high-intensity activities when L-carnitine is consumed either just before the activity or for several days. The typical dose is between 1 and 2 grams per day, but the safety of L-carnitine supplementation has not been adequately tested. The type of carnitine taken is also important. There are reports that DL-carnitine supplementation (a less expensive form of carnitine) may cause muscle weakness.[56] Therefore, if an athlete insists on taking this supplement, only the L-carnitine form should be considered.

Omega-3 Fatty Acids

Omega-3 fatty acids are available as over-the-counter supplements, but they can also be easily obtained through regular consumption of cold-water fish such as salmon, herring, and sardines. These fatty acids may be useful for reducing muscle soreness, and they may have several other benefits, including the following:[43]

- Improved delivery of oxygen and nutrients to muscles and other tissues. Omega-3 fatty acids reduce red blood cell "stickiness," thereby improving the flow of red blood cells to tissues. (*Note:* Excess consumption of omega-3 fatty acids may inhibit normal blood clotting, resulting in excess bleeding should an injury occur.)
- Improved aerobic metabolism due to better delivery of oxygen.
- Higher release of somatotropin (growth hormone) in response to normal stimuli (exercise, sleep, hunger). This may have an anabolic effect and may improve muscular recovery.
- Reduced inflammation of tissues resulting from muscular fatigue and overexertion, allowing for faster recovery.

Despite these potential benefits, results from the scientific literature do not indicate an endurance performance benefit is derived from omega-3 fatty acid supplementation.[57,58] However, there may be differences in the response to omega-3 fatty acids between trained and untrained athletes.[58] A study of well-trained soccer players found no performance benefit from taking omega-3 fatty acids. However, a study of untrained men found a lower level of perceived pain associated with delayed-onset muscle soreness in those who took omega-3 fatty acid supplements.[59]

Medium-Chain Triglycerides

Medium-chain triglycerides (MCTs) are found in coconut oil and palm kernel oil, which are among the most saturated fatty acids in human nutrition. MCTs have carbon lengths of 6 to 12 carbon atoms, while the majority of the triglycerides consumed have considerably longer carbon chains. This difference, plus their water solubility, allows these particular fats to be absorbed and metabolized differently. The liver readily takes them up, where they can be rapidly oxidized for cellular energy.[60] In addition, MCT oils do not require L-carnitine to deliver energy to cell mitochondria for metabolism (other fats require L-carnitine).[61] These oils offer several potential benefits for athletes:[62-64]

- Provide a quick source of energy
- Help mobilize body-fat stores for energy
- Increase the metabolic rate
- Spare lean body mass (muscle)

Widely available in drugstores and health food stores, MCT oils have a long history of safety. They have been used for many years as a source of energy for those on enteral (tube) feedings. Studies assessing the impact of MCTs on performance, however, have not found a benefit even though there is an apparent increase in serum free fatty acid concentration as a result of ingestion.[62-64]

Ginseng

Ginseng has been used for centuries in Asian cultures to reduce fatigue. In a limited number of studies, components of ginseng have been shown to spare glycogen usage and increase the oxidation of fatty acids.[65] Exercised animals that have been injected with a ginseng extract have shown reduced fatigue.[65] However, human studies evaluating various doses of ginseng root for periods of up to 2 months have shown no clear ergogenic benefit. There is only limited evidence that providing a supplement of ginseng extract may improve endurance performance by increasing oxygen delivery to the muscles. Ginseng ingested at either 8 or 16 milligrams per kilogram of body weight for 7 days did not improve either submaximal or maximal cycling performance.[66]

Quercetin

Quercetin is a food-derived flavonoid polyphenol that may possess ergogenic properties. In particular, there is limited evidence that quercetin may prevent the excessive accumulation of reactive oxygen species (ROS), may positively affect the central nervous system, and may also increase mitochondrial content in muscle cells (mitochondria are the energy-metabolizing factories in cells). It is a naturally occurring substance found in olives, olive oil, apples, onions, tea, and red wine. The postconsumption tissue level of quercetin reaches its peak in 1 to 3 hours and maintains this higher level for 6 to 12 hours.[67] The quercetin blood plasma level seems unaffected by gender, age, or fitness level, with evidence that quercetin supplementation increases blood plasma levels in all groups.[68] A higher blood plasma volume may be useful in sustaining delivery of blood and its components to working muscle and to sweat glands, helping to make athletes more resistant to the effects of underhydration. Both the food intake and supplement effects on plasma quercetin suggest that quercetin-containing foods and, perhaps, supplements may need to be consumed regularly to sustain quercetin levels. The food source with the highest known level of quercetin is capers (180 milligrams of quercetin per 100 grams of intake), which represents a level well below the amount needed to provide the desired antioxidant benefit.[69-72] Regular intake of quercetin-containing foods would appear necessary, therefore, to obtain a benefit.

Intense exercise increases the likelihood of several metabolic events, including the following:

- Increased lactic acid accumulation, contributing to exercise fatigue and delayed-onset muscle soreness (DOMS)
- Significantly decreased blood glucose and muscle glycogen, contributing to exercise fatigue and the need to reduce exercise intensity
- Increased oxidative stress, as measured through the production of reactive oxygen species (ROS) in a variety of tissue cells, altering cell structure and function
- Increased free radical production (related to oxidative stress), possibly modifying cellular structure and function in a way that increases cancer risk

Resveratrol

Resveratrol has been described in the popular literature as a substance that can make you look like a trained athlete without the training.[75] A study assessing mice found that an ordinary laboratory mouse can run 1 kilometer on a treadmill before reaching exhaustion. The mice that were given resveratrol, however, were capable of running twice the distance and were able to do so with a reduced heart rate similar to that seen in aerobically trained athletes.[76] In other laboratory experiments involving mice and rats, resveratrol showed anticancer and anti-inflammatory properties.[77,78] It has also been found to lower blood sugar and have a number of other positive cardiovascular effects. Although promising for rodents, these results have not yet been seen in human studies.

Resveratrol is present in the skin of red grapes and is, therefore, a component of red wine. The act of converting grape juice to wine appears to nearly double the resveratrol content.[79] It can be synthesized or derived from Japanese knotweed, which is commonly available as a nutritional supplement.[80,81] Resveratrol exists in several foods, including cocoa powder and peanuts.

The anti-inflammatory activity of resveratrol is of particular interest to athletes, and there is some evidence that its anti-inflammatory potential is more effective than aspirin and ibuprofen.[82] One animal study found that injections of resveratrol may effectively decrease tissue inflammation and reduce the cartilage destruction associated with arthritis.[83]

Resveratrol may have clear health-enhancing properties, but the limited assessment of resveratrol on human populations restricts the possibility of making a recommendation. Athletes should watch for the inevitable human performance studies that will be carried out to determine if this naturally occurring food component has true ergogenic properties.

Quercetin is an antioxidant that may potentially buffer the excessive accumulation of ROS and, therefore, free radical production. In doing so, normal cell metabolism is enhanced to enable continuation of intense physical activity. Some studies suggest that, when compared with nonsupplemented groups, quercetin improves power, peak power output, speed, and endurance.[68, 69, 70] Despite these studies supporting the potential benefit of quercetin supplementation, the scientific findings on the usefulness of quercetin are not consistent. A number of recent studies have also found that quercetin supplementation does not aid exercise performance and may even be detrimental to performance.[73,74] One of these studies found that race finish times were not different between the quercetin supplement and nonsupplement groups, and markers of oxidative stress and antioxidant activity were also not different. Of 39 competitors who finished an endurance race, the majority of finishers (21) were from the nonquercetin supplement group.

Taken together, these studies suggest that quercetin may hold some future promise for athletes, but the method of delivery (food versus supplement), the optimal amount to consume, and the best time for its consumption are yet to be definitively determined. Given the potential negative effects of supplementation, it is suggested that athletes regularly consume foods (typically fresh fruits and vegetables and olives or olive oil) that are good sources of the polyphenol antioxidants and forgo taking high-dose supplements of quercetin.

ERGOGENIC CHOICES

An almost never-ending array of products advertise their performance-enhancing properties. For the most part, however, there is little evidence that well-nourished athletes derive any of the advertised benefits from the consumption of these products. (On the other hand, those manufacturing and selling the products derive a great deal of benefit.) Athletes should carefully consider the adequacy of their own diets before attempting to use ergogenic aids. These products are expensive, few of them have ever been adequately tested for safety, their contents are often unknown, and the actual amount of the active ingredient is uncertain. Furthermore, the chance that these supplements may be laced with banned substances is real. See table 4.3 for a summary of the most common ergogenic aids and their effects.

Table 4.3 Summary of Substances Commonly Used by Athletes as Ergogenic Aids

Substance/Strategy	Potential action	Research findings	Side effects	Legality
Alcohol	Lowers anxiety	No benefit	Significantly negative	Banned in shooting events
Amino acids: arginine, ornithine, lysine	Stimulate growth hormone; enhance muscle development	No benefit	None known	Legal
Amphetamines	Lower fatigue and appetite	Mixed results; some positive	Significantly dangerous	Illegal
Anabolic steroids	Increase lean mass, exercise motivation, and strength	Clear benefit	Significantly dangerous	Illegal
Androstenediol	Increase lean mass, exercise motivation, and strength	Limited studies	Unknown	Banned by IOC
Androstenedione	Increase lean mass, exercise motivation, and strength	No benefit	Significantly negative	Banned by IOC, NCAA
Antioxidants	Enhance muscle recovery; reduce muscle breakdown	Mixed results; no clear benefit	Mild	Legal
Aspartates	Increase use of free fatty acids, thereby sparing muscle glycogen	Mixed results	Mild	Legal
Aspirin	Decreases pain associated with muscle fatigue and muscle breakdown	No benefit	Mild; potential for GI bleeding with large doses	Legal
Bee pollen	Increases strength and endurance	No benefit	Potential for allergic reaction	Legal

Substance/Strategy	Potential action	Research findings	Side effects	Legality
Beta-blockers	Lower anxiety; Improve fine motor control; reduce aerobic capacity	Mixed Benefit	Significantly negative	Banned by IOC
Blood doping	Increases aerobic capacity	Clear benefit	Significantly dangerous (increases blood viscosity)	Illegal
Boron	Increases endogenous steroid production	No benefit	Mild	Legal
Branched-chain amino acids (BCAAs)	Reduce central nervous system fatigue	Mixed results	Mild	Legal
Caffeine	Increases muscle contractility; improves aerobic endurance; improves fat metabolism	Clear benefit	Mild	Legal
Calcium	Increases muscle contractility; improves glycogen metabolism	No benefit	Mild	Legal
Carbohydrates	Improve performance; lower fatigue	Clear benefit	Mild	Legal
Carnitine	Increases fat metabolism	No benefit	None	Legal
Choline	Improves endurance	Mixed results	None	Legal
Chromium	Increases lean mass	No benefit unless preexisting deficiency	Safe up to 400 mcg/day; dangerous above this level	Legal
Chrysin	Increases endogenous steroid production	No benefit	None	Legal
Cocaine	Stimulates CNS; delays fatigue	Mixed results	Significantly negative; dangerous	Illegal
Coenzyme Q-10 (ubiquinone)	Delays fatigue; antioxidant	No benefit	None	Legal
Coenzyme Q-12	Improves aerobic capacity; speeds muscle repair	No benefit	None	Legal
Creatine	Improves repeated high-intensity activity endurance	Benefit, but no safety data available	None in short term; unknown in long term	Legal

(continued)

Table 4.3 *(continued)*

Substance/Strategy	Potential action	Research findings	Side effects	Legality
Dehydroepiandosterone (DHEA)	Improves endogenous steroid production	No benefit in healthy athletes	Potentially dangerous	Banned by IOC and other groups
Diuretics	Lower body mass to lower resistance	Limited benefit	Potentially dangerous	Banned by IOC
Ephedrine and related substances	Stimulate CNS; delay fatigue; encourage weight loss	No benefit	Potentially dangerous	Banned by IOC and other organizations; illegal to sell in USA and several other countries
Ephedrine plus caffeine	Increases energy; stimulates weight loss	Some benefit	Potentially dangerous; fatal at higher doses	Banned by IOC and other organizations; illegal to sell in USA and several other countries
Erythropoietin (EPO)	Increases aerobic capacity	Clear benefit	Significantly negative; dangerous	Illegal
Fluids	Increase endurance	Clear benefit	Some danger of hyponatremia	Legal
Folic acid	Increases aerobic capacity	No benefit	None	Legal
Gamma-Hydroxybutyric Acid (GHB)	Stimulates growth hormone release and muscle growth	No clear benefit	Significantly negative (dose related); abuse potential	Illegal
Ginseng	Increases endurance; improves muscle recovery	No clear benefit	Mild; abuse syndrome reported	Legal
Glucosamine	Serves as NSAID alternative; enhances muscle recovery	Limited benefit	None	Legal
Glutamine	Boosts immunity and growth hormone levels	May boost immunity	None	Legal
Glycerol	Improves hydration and endurance	Some benefit	Mild	Legal
Beta-Hydroxy beta-methybutyric acid (HMB)	Decreases muscle breakdown; enhances recovery	Limited studies; some strength benefits	None	Legal
Human growth hormone	Has anabolic effect on muscle growth; increases fat metabolism	Limited benefit	Significantly negative; dangerous	Illegal

Substance/Strategy	Potential action	Research findings	Side effects	Legality
Inosine	Enhances energy production; improves aerobic capacity	No benefit	Mild	Legal
Iron	Increases aerobic capacity	No benefit unless preexisting deficiency	Mild; toxic at high doses	Legal
Leucine	Decreases muscle breakdown; spares muscle glycogen stores	Limited studies; no benefit	None	Legal
Ma huang (herbal ephedrine)	Stimulates CNS; delays fatigue; promotes weight loss	No benefit	Potentially dangerous	Banned by IOC and other organizations
Magnesium	Enhances muscle growth	No benefit unless preexisting deficiency	Mild at high doses	Legal
Niacin	Increases energy and endurance	No benefit unless preexisting deficiency	Mild at high doses; extremely high chronic doses associated with hepatitis	Legal
Oxygen	Increases aerobic capacity; improves recovery	No benefit	Mild	Legal
Phosphates	Increase ATP production, energy, and muscle endurance	Mixed results	Mild at high doses	Legal
Phytosterols	Stimulate release of endogenous steroids and growth hormone	No benefit	Little data; allergic reaction possible	Legal
Protein	Optimizes muscular growth and repair	Slightly increased need for protein with increased activity	None	Legal
Pyruvate	Increases lean body mass	No benefit	None	Legal
D-ribose	Increases cellular ATP and muscle power	No human research	None known	Legal

(continued)

Table 4.3 *(continued)*

Substance/Strategy	Potential action	Research findings	Side effects	Legality
Selenium	Enhances antioxidant functions	Limited studies; no benefit	Mild at high doses	Legal
Sodium bicarbonate	Buffers lactic acid production; delays fatigue	Some benefit	Mild; dangerous at high doses	Legal
Tryptophan	Decreases pain perception; increases endurance	Mixed results; no benefit in trained athletes	Mild; potentially dangerous	Legal
Vanadyl sulfate	Increases glycogen synthesis; enhances muscle recovery	No benefit	Mild	Legal
Vitamin B_1 (thiamin)	Enhances energy production; increases aerobic capacity; improves concentration	No benefit unless preexisting deficiency	None	Legal
Vitamin B_2 (riboflavin)	Increases aerobic endurance	No benefit unless preexisting deficiency	None	Legal
Vitamin B_6 (pyridoxine)	Enhances muscle growth; decreases anxiety	No benefit unless preexisting deficiency	None	Legal
Vitamin B_{12} (cyanocobalamin)	Enhances muscle growth	No benefit unless preexisting deficiency	None	Legal
Vitamin B_{15} (dimethylglycine)	Increases muscle energy production	No benefit; may make things worse	None proven, but concerns raised	Legal
Vitamin C	Acts as antioxidant; increases aerobic capacity and energy production	No benefit unless preexisting deficiency	Mild at high doses	Legal
Vitamin E	Acts as antioxidant; improves aerobic capacity	Some positive findings	Mild	Legal
Yohimbine	Increases endogenous steroid production	No benefit	Mild	Legal
Zinc	Enhances muscle growth; increases aerobic capacity	No benefit unless preexisting deficiency	Mild	Legal

Reprinted, by permission, from D.M. Ahrendt, 2001, "Ergogenic aids: Counseling the athlete," *American Family Physician* 63(5): 913-922.

Athletes choosing to use an ergogenic aid should proceed cautiously. Speak with an appropriately credentialed health professional (e.g., a doctor, dietitian, or pharmacist) to obtain as much information on the product as possible, and determine if there is a simple dietary fix that would make the supplement unnecessary. When any supplement is consumed for the first time, carefully observe whether gastrointestinal distress or nausea occur, and document your sense of well-being after taking it. Most ergogenic aids are powerful chemicals that are easily handled if taken in the small amounts that naturally appear in the foods we eat. However, when they are taken in the large doses often prescribed to achieve an ergogenic benefit, the impact on your body may be entirely different and unexpected.

Of all the ergogenic aids mentioned in this chapter, it is very clear that carbohydrate holds the greatest promise for improving both endurance and power performance. Before trying anything else, athletes should consider a regular consumption of carbohydrate with plenty of fluids. This is, perhaps, the single most important thing an athlete can do to ensure both an adequate total energy intake and an appropriate consumption of the energy substrate most easily depleted.

Some athletes use ergogenic strategies, such as blood doping, taking erythropoietin (EPO), and consuming anabolic steroids or human growth hormone, that are widely banned by sports organizing committees and the IOC. Because of the widespread use of anabolic steroids and other banned or illegal ergogenic aids, the World Anti-Doping Agency (WADA) was established in 1999 in an attempt to avoid giving athletes who use these substances an unfair competitive advantage. Since the origination of WADA, most national and international sports governing bodies, including the United States Olympic Committee (USOC) and the National Collegiate Athletic Association (NCAA), have signed onto the WADA code, which is intended to do the following:[84]

- Protect athletes' fundamental right to participate in doping-free sport and thus promote health, fairness, and equality for athletes worldwide
- Ensure harmonized, coordinated, and effective antidoping programs at the international and national levels with regard to detection, deterrence, and prevention of doping

For a comprehensive and up-to-date list of widely restricted and banned ergogenic aids, along with prohibited methods for achieving performance enhancement, visit the following website: www.wada-ama.org/en.

It should be clear to the reader that this book fully supports the WADA mission, and this chapter's discussion of how ergogenic aids function to improve performance is not an endorsement to take these substances. Indeed, healthy athletes who consistently match nutrient and energy intakes with requirements are rarely in need of other ergogenic substances to support the athletic endeavor.

IMPORTANT POINTS

- Claims made about ergogenic aids that are hard to believe and that have little or no scientific support are not likely to be true, even if a famous athlete claims he won a gold medal because he used an ergogenic substance. The athlete is most likely well known because he did everything else right: a good training program, a good coach, and a solid nutrition program.

- Most products sold as ergogenic aids have not been tested to determine whether or not they are safe. Athletes may be jeopardizing long-term health and performance for a hypothetical short-term gain.

- Recent studies show that about 25 percent of the ergogenic aids targeting athletes contain banned substances that are not listed on the labels. Athletes are at risk for sanctions if these substances are consumed, whether intentionally or not. Athletes should check with their sport's national governing body (e.g., U.S. Track and Field, U.S. Figure Skating) to obtain lists of supplements and ergogenic aids that have been determined to be safe, effective, and free of banned substances.

- Athletes who consume ergogenic aids should look for products that have the USP (United States Pharmacopeia) symbol on the label. This symbol indicates the products have passed tests that ensure content and purity.

- Many ergogenic aids work because they fulfill a dietary weakness, which most often occurs with an inadequate energy intake. Consuming enough energy at the right time and in the right amount is a cheaper, safer, and more effective strategy for optimizing performance.

- There is no ergogenic aid that can make up for a proper fluid intake, a solid nutrition intake, an appropriate training regimen, and sufficient rest.

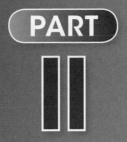

PART II

Nutrition Aspects of Optimal Performance

GI Function and Energy Delivery

Athletes need more energy nutrients, more fluids, more vitamins, and more minerals than nonathletes need, and all these essential substances must pass through the gastrointestinal (GI) tract to be digested and absorbed for delivery to organs and muscles. It is critically important, therefore, that athletes be familiar with numerous issues relating to the delivery of nutrients and fluids through the gastrointestinal tract. Understanding the issue of gastric emptying will enable athletes to adopt the best strategies for delivering the greatest amount of energy, fluids, and electrolytes without inducing nausea or vomiting. Understanding the digestion and absorption process for nutrients and fluids helps athletes develop optimal timing strategies for delivering needed nutrients and fluids to working muscles while maintaining blood volume, both of which are critical issues for performance. The best food-consumption strategies, based on GI tract function, have the combined benefit of enhancing performance while minimizing the potentially damaging effects of poorly timed and constituted meals. For athletes who require iron supplements, calcium supplements, or both, understanding GI tract processing of these minerals will help athletes plan the best strategy for incorporating them into their dietary intake.

This chapter presents issues to consider when delivering the nutrients and fluids that athletes highly require. The goal for athletes should be to deliver the most needed nutrients while lowering the risk of gastrointestinal distress, particularly when training and during competition. The information is presented in a way that helps readers understand GI function in exercise and nonexercise conditions so they'll acquire the tools to make the best eating and drinking decisions in a variety of situations.

GASTROINTESTINAL (GI) TRACT

Food is the carrier of nutrients, and it is the responsibility of the GI tract to break down (i.e., digest) food into its nutrient components (vitamins, minerals, energy) and bring these nutrients into the blood and lymph for delivery to cells via absorption and transport. Humans are amazingly efficient at digesting and absorbing

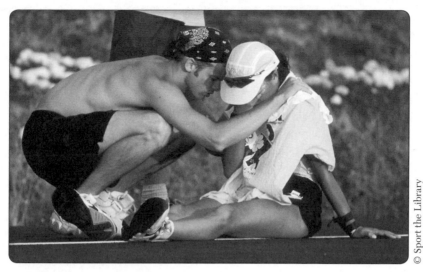

GI problems may contribute to dehydration, which could result in serious health risks for the athlete.

nutrients and transporting the absorbed nutrients to body tissue—a process that begins when you place food in your mouth and continues through the stomach and intestines. As it travels through the GI tract, food is mechanically ripped apart, attacked by chemicals to aid in the release of nutrients, exposed to radical changes in acidity, and compacted for removal of what is left.

Mouth and Esophagus

Mouth and esophagus health is important for athletes because problems with either inevitably lead to food intake restrictions that limit nutrient consumption and, ultimately, result in malnutrition. Given the predisposition of athletes to consume a relatively high level of simple carbohydrates in snacks and sports beverages, which have a high cariogenic (i.e., cavity-causing) potential, frequent visits to a dentist to ensure healthy teeth and gums are advised. In addition, the intense abdominal forces inherent in many sporting activities (e.g., weightlifting) may predispose athletes to hiatal hernias that lead to esophagitis. An acutely irritated esophagus is painful, makes swallowing difficult, and inevitably leads to food restrictions.

Placing food in your mouth initiates a series of events that begins the digestive process. Chewing breaks apart food so it can be mixed more completely with digestive enzymes, and salivary amylase begins the digestion of carbohydrates (mainly the conversion of cooked starch to dextrins and maltose). The secretion of saliva and amylase occurs from the thought, sight, smell, and taste of food. All the food placed in the mouth is covered with saliva, which contains the glycoprotein mucin. With its excellent lubricating properties, mucin helps foods slide into the stomach through the esophagus without irritation. The pH of the mouth is approximately neutral (between 6.0 and 7.0; see table 5.1), and the pH remains neutral in the esophagus.

The feel and taste of foods and drinks in the mouth have much to do with whether they are acceptable to an athlete. These food and drink properties, commonly referred to as their organoleptic properties, may be altered during exercise, which is an important consideration for the athlete. Therefore, taste testing a sports beverage while sitting on a couch and watching television is not an appropriate strategy for determining how palatable this sports beverage will be during exercise. Put simply, foods and drinks taste and feel differently while you're exercising than while you're not.

Table 5.1 The pH Ranges in the GI Tract

Location	pH
Mouth	6.0-7.0 (neutral)
Esophagus	6.9-7.1 (neutral)
Stomach	2.0-2.5 (very acidic)
Small intestine	6.9-7.1 (neutral)
Large intestine	6.9-7.1 (neutral)

Note: pH of 1 = battery acid.

If you're a cyclist wishing to try a carbohydrate gel for your next race, try it after you've been cycling for a while or you could be in for a big surprise during the event. In summary, always try a food, whether it's a sports beverage or snack, during the activity for which its use is intended.

Stomach

Food passes from the esophagus to the stomach, where additional digestive processes take place. A rapid shift in pH occurs from ~6.0 to 7.0 to between 2.0 and 2.5 when food enters the stomach. This highly acidic stomach environment (similar in pH to battery acid) initiates a series of events that promotes protein digestion while continuing the mixing action that was initiated in the mouth. Specialized cells in the stomach also produce intrinsic factor, which is important for the absorption of vitamin B_{12}. Vitamin B_{12} is necessary for the production of new red blood cells, and a persistent failure to adequately absorb vitamin B_{12} eventually results in a condition called pernicious anemia.

Risk factors for an acute irritation of the stomach, referred to as gastritis, include excessive use of nonsteroidal anti-inflammatory drugs (NSAIDs), excessive consumption of alcoholic beverages, and increasing age. The common cause of gastritis in athletes would most likely be regular NSAID use, which may irritate the stomach lining. NSAIDs come in prescription (e.g., Naprosyn) and over-the-counter (e.g., aspirin or ibuprofen) forms. These common pain relievers reduce a protective substance in your stomach called prostaglandin. When taken infrequently and short term, NSAIDs usually don't cause many stomach problems, especially if taken with antacids or food. However, regular use may result in gastritis and, eventually, in stomach ulcers as well. Other factors could be associated with gastritis in athletes:

- Stress
- Overtraining
- Alcohol abuse
- Bacterial infection from *Helicobacter pylori* (*H. pylori*). This common bacterium is the cause of the majority of all stomach ulcers.
- Cocaine use

Gastric emptying refers to the speed at which food and drink leave the stomach. High-fat, high-protein meals take longer to digest and require more processing time in the stomach. Therefore, precompetition or pretraining meals should be consumed with gastric emptying time in mind. With the goal of exercising with no solid food in the stomach, higher-protein and higher-fat meals should be finished a minimum of 2.5 hours before physical activity, while low-fiber, starchy carbohydrate meals should be finished a minimum of 1.5 hours before physical activity. The size of the meals also influences when they should be consumed. Smaller meals are more easily tolerated closer to physical activity. Exercising with food in the stomach may lead to nausea and vomiting. Furthermore, the sensation of fullness may inhibit adequate fluid consumption, which could lead to dehydration and heat stress. Cyclists may better tolerate solid foods in the stomach while exercising because of less bouncing motion, but in general, all athletes should be wary of eating meals too close to the time of exercise.

The following known factors affect gastric emptying:[1,2]

- Ingested volume (higher volumes result in faster gastric emptying, but there is more to empty)
- Energy concentration (higher concentrations result in slower gastric emptying)
- Type of carbohydrate (glucose results in slower gastric emptying than other mono- and disaccharides)
- Osmolality (the concentration of particles per unit volume of fluid) (the higher the sugar content of a beverage, the higher the osmolality of the beverage; higher osmolar solutions result in slower gastric emptying)
- pH (deviations from neutral pH slow gastric emptying)
- Exercise intensity (higher intensities result in slower gastric emptying)
- Stress (severe psychological stress slows gastric emptying)

See chapter 3 for additional information on gastric emptying and related issues.

Small Intestine

The small intestine has three distinct compartments: the duodenum (closest to the stomach), jejunum (middle), and ileum (closest to the large intestine). The liquid mass of consumed food formed by the stomach is passed into the small intestine for additional digestive processing and for absorption into the blood and lymph. The pyloric valve separates the stomach from the small intestine. The small portion of the small intestine closest to the pyloric valve is the primary absorption site for the divalent minerals iron, calcium, magnesium, and zinc—all of which are important to athletes. (*Note:* The term *divalent* is used here to refer to minerals with a similar chemical structure and to indicate that these minerals share the same absorption site.)

These divalent minerals are competitively absorbed because the site of absorption is relatively small. Therefore, an excessively high intake of one divalent mineral may occupy the entire absorption site and make the absorption of other divalent minerals difficult. The principle of nutrient balance is critical (i.e., more than enough is not better than just enough). For instance, female athletes are often appropriately concerned about iron status, but a frequent high-dose intake of iron may lower the absorption of calcium, magnesium, and zinc to create a series of other nutrition problems. Put simply, the strategy for divalent mineral intake is crucial for optimizing nutrition health and, because these minerals are so closely tied to muscle function and bone health, athletic performance.

A short distance from the proximal duodenum where divalent minerals are absorbed, the bile duct and pancreatic duct enter the small intestine (pancreatic duct and bile duct meet to form a single duct—the common bile duct). The pancreas is stimulated by secretin, which travels up the pancreatic duct to cause the release of pancreatic juice into the duodenum. Because of its large volume (between 20 and 27 ounces daily, or about three-quarters of a liter) and highly alkaline pH of ~8.0, pancreatic juice neutralizes the acidity of the food mass that has left the stomach. The pancreas also releases several digestive enzymes, including

- pancreatic amylase to digest starch into dextrins and maltose;
- pancreatic proteases to digest larger proteins into smaller proteins or polypeptides; and
- pancreatic lipase to digest fats into monoglycerides, individual fatty acids, and glycerol.

Of course, the pancreas also produces powerful hormones (insulin by the beta cells and glucagon by the alpha cells) for controlling blood sugar. (Both insulin and glucagon are discussed fully in following chapters.)

The liver manufactures bile, which is stored in the gallbladder until it is required. Cholecystokinin, which is produced in the small intestine, travels up the bile duct to stimulate the gallbladder to release its stored bile into the small intestine. Bile is a powerful emulsifying agent (unique chemicals that are water soluble on one end and fat soluble on the other) that helps in the digestion of fats. The fat-soluble end attaches itself to fat droplets, and the water-soluble end surrounds the fat droplet. This allows the fat to mix (and stay mixed) in a water-based environment. The daily bile volume is between 17 and 37 ounces (500 and 1,100 ml), helping to explain our efficiency at digesting and absorbing fats. Bile has an interesting feature in that it is 50 percent cholesterol. Higher intakes of fat stimulate a higher production of bile, which is absorbed with the fats it has emulsified. This higher bile production–absorption cycle increases circulating cholesterol, even if the intake of dietary cholesterol is zero. Therefore, dietary fat intake is more of a culprit in high circulating cholesterol levels than dietary cholesterol intake.

The mucosal (border) cells of the small intestine (mainly in the duodenum) produce enzymes that break down disaccharides into their component monosaccharides. Specifically, these disaccharidases do the following:

- Sucrase breaks down sucrose to glucose and fructose.
- Maltase breaks down maltose to two molecules of glucose.
- Lactase breaks down lactose to glucose and galactose.

These seemingly minor digestive enzymes are important for athletes to consider, particularly as they relate to the composition of sports beverages. For instance, a sports beverage deriving 100 percent of its energy from pure glucose (the ultimate energy source for cells) would induce delayed gastric emptying and, once absorbed, would produce a sudden, high, and relatively short-lived rise in blood sugar (glucose). On the other hand, an isocaloric sports beverage containing a combination of sucrose and glucose would have some inherent advantages in maintaining blood sugar for a longer period of time. The lower concentration of glucose in the beverage would not significantly delay gastric emptying, so there would be a more rapid infusion of glucose into the blood without achieving such a high peak. The sucrose would be digested into its component glucose and fructose, a process that takes some time. The glucose from this breakdown would follow the glucose already absorbed, and the fructose would be converted to glucose in the liver (still more time required) before infusion into the blood. The end result is a lower glucose peak but a much more sustained infusion of glucose into the blood, helping the athlete feel energized for a longer time.

Nutrients are absorbed mainly in the duodenum and jejunum, but some absorption also takes place in the ileum and the large intestine:

- Minerals are mainly absorbed in the proximal duodenum.
- Monosaccharides and water-soluble vitamins are mainly absorbed in the jejunum.
- Fat-soluble vitamins, amino acids, fats, vitamin B_{12}, and bile salts are absorbed mainly in the ileum. Vitamin B_{12} requires intrinsic factor, which is produced by the parietal cells of the stomach, for absorption in the ileum. A failure to produce intrinsic factor will cause vitamin B_{12} deficiency disease (pernicious anemia), regardless of the amount of B_{12} consumed.

The interior surface of the small intestine is composed of microvilli that dramatically enlarge its absorptive surface, accounting for an extraordinary efficiency in absorbing consumed energy substrates: 98 percent of all digestible carbohydrate is absorbed; 95 percent of all fat is absorbed; and 92 percent of all protein is absorbed.

Large Intestine

The large intestine is made of six parts, including the cecum, ascending (right) colon, transverse colon, descending (left) colon, sigmoid colon, and rectum. The small intestine connects to the large intestine at the cecum, which is actually the beginning part of the ascending colon. A small projection attached to the cecum, called the appendix, serves no well-understood function. However, the appendix is predisposed to becoming infected, a condition referred to as appendicitis. The main function of the large intestine is to reabsorb water from the stool and eliminate the remaining relatively dry waste. Food and drink consumption and intestinal secretions result in approximately 5 gallons (19 L) of fluid being placed in the large intestine daily. A failure to adequately reabsorb this fluid would result in dehydration. The following factors keep a GI tract healthy:

- Adequate dietary fiber, both viscous (soluble) and nonviscous (insoluble)
- Optimal bacterial flora
- Adequate fluids
- Regular movement; physical activity
- Balanced diet with adequate folate
- Reduced intake of simple sugars
- Avoidance of bacterial contamination
- Avoidance of antibiotics (disrupt microflora) (*Note:* Antibiotics may be needed to resolve infections, so they should be taken until finished if prescribed. However, afterward it is important to return the gut microflora to a normal state, perhaps by taking macrobiotics or by consuming live-culture yogurt.)

The large intestine is populated by bacteria, many of which are essential for human nutrition. Some of these bacteria manufacture vitamin K (an important substance for blood clotting). The bacterial flora is also important for normal large intestine function by creating gas that aids peristalsis and by aiding in the digestion of certain materials. Certain consumed foods may create a healthy bacterial flora, which can help overwhelm "bad" bacteria that try to populate the gut. For instance, live-culture yogurt often contains *Lactobacillus bulgaricus* and *Streptococcus thermophilus*, which convert pasteurized milk to yogurt during fermentation. In addition, some yogurts contain *Lactobacillus acidophilus* and *Bifidobacterium bifidum*. The amount of intestinal bacteria varies depending on diet and use of antibiotics but can make up more than half the weight of fecal material. An infection with "bad" bacteria creates an irritation that causes an increase in mucus production and a failure to reabsorb water from stool, leading to diarrhea. Of course, the use of antibiotics disturbs the bacterial flora in the gut and often leads to abnormal gut function until the healthy bacteria return.

Common problems of the large intestine include constipation, diarrhea, diverticulosis or diverticulitis, and colon cancer. Constipation, diverticular disease, and colon cancer risks are increased with low fiber intakes; there is also evidence suggesting that poor vitamin D status is associated with colon cancer.[3] Currently, Americans consume approximately half of the 20 to 35 grams of dietary fiber recommended to reduce disease risk and maintain healthy gut function. To obtain the recommended level of fiber, athletes would need to consume at least five servings of fresh fruits and vegetables and three servings of whole-grain products daily as well as legumes occasionally. Because of the gas and bloating caused by higher fiber intakes, athletes could experience performance difficulties unless the fiber intake is timed correctly so it does not interfere with training or competition. The issue of food timing is comprehensively discussed later in this book.

FACTORS INFLUENCING FOOD CONSUMPTION

Several factors may influence food consumption and, therefore, total nutrient intake. These factors range from appetite stimulation or loss, which may result from conditions as varied as temporary depression to consumption of certain drugs; micronutrient deficiency or toxicity, which may alter appetite through the impact it has on taste sensitivity; dieting, which purposefully lowers total food consumption with the hope of achieving a desirable weight loss or body profile; and overtraining, which is considered to be a major problem for many athletes.

Appetite Loss A loss of appetite (anorexia), regardless of the cause, interferes with food consumption and may result in malnutrition if it continues for an extended period. Appetite may be affected by both nutrition and nonnutrition factors. A death in the family, for instance, often leads to some reduction in appetite, while a zinc deficiency is associated with appetite loss. Inadequate consumption of carbohydrate, as is possible on excessively high-protein, high-fat, low-carbohydrate diets, may result in some degree of ketosis, which is associated with nausea and a loss of appetite. Consumption of certain drugs is also known to result in an altered taste perception or an appetite loss, both of which may result in lower energy and nutrient consumption.

Even something as seemingly minor as a small toothache can reduce food intake or, at the very least, reduce the variety of foods consumed so as to create a below-optimal nutrient and energy intake. Dental caries, cold sores, sensitive gums, and swollen tongues all have the potential to limit food intake and, therefore, restrict nutrient and fuel exposure to needy tissues. Regular visits to a dentist will resolve the majority of these problems. A B-vitamin deficiency, particularly of riboflavin (B_2) and pyridoxine (B_6), may also lead to mouth and tongue problems that inhibit food intake.

A loss of appetite lasting more than several days may be a sign of a more serious problem, including cancer, tuberculosis, hypothyroidism, heart disease, lung disease, and liver disease, so it should not go unattended for long. See table 5.2 for a list of possible causes of loss of appetite and altered taste perception.

Micronutrient Deficiency or Toxicity   Micronutrients also play a role in appetite, creating a problem that is difficult to address. A deficiency of any single vitamin, such as thiamin, may result in poor appetite. However, because this deficiency creates poor appetite, it becomes increasingly difficult to increase food intake to reverse the deficiency. Often a single nutrient deficiency will lead to multiple nutrient deficiencies because of the appetite-mediated lower intake of food. Toxicity resulting from the excess intake of nutrients may also lower appetite.

Table 5.2   Possible Causes of Loss of Appetite and Altered Taste Perception

Loss of appetite	Altered taste perception
Anorexia nervosa	Amphetamines
Cancer (colon, ovarian, stomach, leukemia, and pancreatic)	Ampicillin
Chronic kidney failure	Benzocaine
Chronic liver disease	Clofibrate
Cirrhosis of the liver	Griseofulvin
Congestive heart failure	Lidocaine
Diabetes mellitus	
Emotional upset, nervousness, loneliness, boredom, tension, anxiety, loss, and depression	
HIV/AIDS	
Hypothyroidism	
Infections (any febrile disease, including influenza)	
Medications and street drugs:	
• Amphetamines	
• Amphojel	
• Antibiotics	
• Azulfidine	
• Chemotherapy drugs	
• Cocaine	
• Codeine (or acetaminophen with codeine)	
• Colchicine	
• Cough and cold medications	
• Digitalis	
• Demerol	
• Heroin	
• Morphine	
• Sympathomimetics, including ephedrine	
• Tamoxifen	
Pregnancy (first trimester)	

Sources: (1) *New York Times* Health Section, October 30, 2010. (2) L.K. Mahan and S. Escott-Stump, 2000, *Krause's food, nutrition, & diet therapy*, 10th ed. (Philadelphia: W.B. Saunders), 401.

For instance, an established symptom of excess vitamin A intake is nausea, which directly affects appetite. See table 5.3 for a list of vitamins and minerals that may create a loss of appetite from either an excessive or deficient intake.

Dieting Popular diets are, by design, *meant* to restrict the intake of foods. Some diets achieve this by eliminating whole food groups, while others encourage the intake of some energy substrates (typically protein and fat) while discouraging the intake of other substrates (typically carbohydrate). Regardless of the diet plan, most diets involve a massive reduction in calories that ultimately results in a loss of lean mass, a lowering of the strength-to-weight ratio, and a reduction in performance. Sudden and large reductions in caloric intake result in a lowering of fat-free mass (i.e., lean mass), which results in a lowering of metabolic rate. This condition forces people to constantly eat less to adapt to the frequent ratcheting down of metabolic rate. At some point, low-calorie diets become low-nutrient diets, with all of the potential dangers associated with a chronically inadequate nutrient intake.

Overtraining Overtraining can lead to a cascade of problems including sleep loss, increased illness frequency, and appetite loss. The major point to remember is this: Anything that interferes with food intake is likely to have a major impact on nutrition status and energy intake, both of which will diminish athletic performance and will likely place the athlete at increased disease risk. Athletes who experience sleepless nights, constant fatigue, frequent illness, appetite loss, weight loss, and large mood swings are likely overtraining.

Table 5.3 Vitamins That Can Affect Appetite

Vitamin	Inadequate intake	Excessive intake
Thiamin (vitamin B_1)	Poor appetite; mental depression	
Riboflavin (vitamin B_2)	Tongue sores; mouth sores	
Niacin (vitamin B_3)	Poor appetite; weakness	Nausea; liver damage
Pyridoxine, Pyridoxal, Pyridoxamine (Vitamin B_6)	Tongue sores	
Pantothenic acid	Poor appetite; nausea (extremely rare deficiency)	
Choline		Nausea; GI distress
Ascorbic Acid (Vitamin C)	Bleeding gums	
Copper		Nausea (extremely rare toxicity)
Zinc	Poor appetite; altered sense of taste; reduced sense of taste	

FACTORS INFLUENCING DIGESTION AND ABSORPTION OF NUTRIENTS

Any number of factors may result in maldigestion or malabsorption, either of which will diminish nutrient delivery to needy cells. It is important to consider that a problem early in the GI tract (i.e., the mouth or esophagus) is likely to create a cascade of problems later in the GI tract. For instance, the pain associated with esophagitis (an irritation in the esophagus from frequent vomiting, frequent alcohol consumption, or gastric reflux) may inhibit normal eating and drinking patterns to the point of changing normal bowel habits, thereby causing constipation, colonic irritation, and of course, dehydration. Other inhibitors of digestion and absorption are food sensitivities and allergies, intestinal inflammation from Crohn's disease, and drug interactions. Celiac disease is now generally considered the most common food-intolerance GI disorder.

Food Sensitivity and Allergic Response   Food sensitivities are the result of a toxic response to a component chemical in the food, due to either an allergic response involving the immune system or a food intolerance involving, most typically, a missing enzyme. The common symptoms of food allergies include vomiting, diarrhea, hives and other skin rashes, runny nose, and bleeding stools. There are well over 100 foods that people can have allergic reactions to, but milk, wheat, shellfish, eggs, strawberries, and peanuts are among the most common. The offending allergic substance is commonly a protein that the person's system cannot properly process. For instance, the cow's milk protein casein is the offending substance in milk allergies, and the protein gluten is the common offending substance in wheat allergies.

Celiac Disease   Celiac disease is an intestinal intolerance of the protein gluten (found in wheat, barley, rye, and oats). It is associated with dermatitis herpetiformis, which occurs in 70 to 80 percent of people with gluten-induced GI tract damage.[4] This form of dermatitis produces an extremely itchy rash of small sandpaper-like bumps and blisters and tends to persist until the offending substance (in this case gluten) is removed from the diet.

Celiac disease has a strong genetic association, so relatives of someone who has celiac disease may also develop the condition.[4,5] Uncontrolled celiac disease results in intestinal damage, with associated malabsorption, and causes diarrhea, steatorrhea (fat malabsorption), iron-deficiency anemia, other vitamin deficiencies, and eventually weight loss.[5] Malabsorption-related weight loss and a profoundly uncomfortable sense of well-being can further diminish the desire to eat, resulting in what appears to be a full-fledged eating disorder. A person may be asymptomatic for years before these symptoms occur, or some signs, such as milk intolerance or iron deficiency, may be present without any of the other signs. According to the National Institutes of Health (2008), digestive symptoms are more common in infants and children than in adults, but they may occur in all age groups (see table 5.4).

The more we learn about GI disorders, the greater the problem appears to become. The prevalence of celiac disease was estimated at 1 in 100,000 people, but current studies suggest it is actually 1 in 133 people.[4] It is uncertain whether the medical profession is sufficiently aware of the high prevalence of this disorder to consider it as a possible cause when an athlete presents with vague symptoms. A prime example is runner Amy Yoder Begley, who for more than 2 years could not run 30 minutes without having to use the bathroom.[6] Doctors investigating her condition wrongly diagnosed ovarian cysts, irritable bowel syndrome, thyroid issues, and even depression. She was eventually found to have celiac disease, which finally allowed her to correct her problem and train to the point where she became an Olympian, running the 10,000 meters for the United States in Beijing. There are other examples of athletes who were ultimately found to have celiac disease, but only after long histories of GI difficulties and inappropriate cures.[7,8]

Athletes with malabsorption, frequent diarrhea, iron deficiency, or any of the other symptoms of GI dysfunction associated with celiac disease should consider the possibility

Table 5.4 Celiac Disease Symptoms in Infants, Young Children, and Adults

Infants and young children	Adults (left-column symptoms possible)
Abdominal bloating and pain	Iron-deficiency anemia (no apparent cause)
Chronic diarrhea	Fatigue
Vomiting	Bone or joint pain
Constipation	Arthritis
Pale, foul-smelling, or fatty stool	Bone loss or osteoporosis
Weight loss	Depression or anxiety
	Tingling and numbness in hands and feet
	Seizures
	Missed menstrual periods
	Canker sores inside mouth
	Dermatitis herpetiformis (itchy skin rash)
Common and shared symptoms	
Intermittent diarrhea	
Abdominal pain	
Bloating	

Sources: (1) NIH National Digestive Diseases Information Clearinghouse. Available: http://digestive.niddk.nih.gov/ddiseases/pubs/celiac/ [August 18, 2011]. (2) Mayo Clinic. Available: www.mayoclinic.com/health/celiac-disease/DS00319/ [August 18, 2011].

that they do not tolerate gluten. It is quite possible that at least a proportion of those people who report feeling so much better on the Atkins diet (a high-protein, low-carbohydrate diet that restricts bread intake) improve because of the elimination of gluten rather than any of the other purported benefits of the Atkins regimen. For those wishing a firm diagnosis of celiac disease, clinically accepted tests are available, often involving a small bowel biopsy, to confirm the presence of the disease.

For those diagnosed with celiac disease, the solution is total gluten avoidance. That means avoiding bagels; bread; breakfast cereals that contain wheat, barley, rye, malt or malted products; crackers; pasta; most sports bars; and pizza. Eating is made even more complex by the fact that gluten is found in foods you would never expect. French fries, which should be a safe food in celiac disease, are often coated in a fine spray of wheat to make them more crispy; going to an Asian rice-based restaurant sounds like the perfect solution for the gluten avoider, until you realize the rice is coated in soy sauce, which is wheat based; a French chef in Paris making a sauce might use corn starch as a thickener, but a chef in the United States will almost surely use wheat flour instead; and those energy bars runners swear by to fill the energy gap nearly always have enough wheat in them to make life difficult for a person with celiac disease. Foods labeled *gluten free* must contain less than 20 parts per million of gluten (about two tiny bread crumbs in a large plate of food), and it is difficult to meet that standard if gluten-free foods are processed on equipment that also processes wheat, barley, and rye. Foods labeled *wheat free*, therefore, are not necessarily gluten free.

According to the NIH (2008), wheat products containing gluten are even found in vitamins, medicines, and lip balms.

Persons with celiac disease who remove gluten-containing products from the diet are initially distressed at having this limitation in food consumption, but the improvement in bowel function with gluten restriction often allows them to comfortably consume other foods that may previously have caused GI distress. Virtually all celiac patients feel so much better with the restriction of gluten-containing products that they are self-motivated to continue with a gluten-free diet.[4] In addition, many gluten-free bread products on the market, typically made of rice or corn, are excellent substitutes for wheat and rye breads. There are numerous online resources on gluten-free foods and recipes for readers who wish additional information. See table 5.5 for a list of common foods that are high in gluten and foods that have no gluten.

Table 5.5 Sample of Gluten-Containing and Gluten-Free Foods

Gluten-containing foods	Gluten-free foods
Wheat (wholemeal, whole-wheat, and wheatmeal flour; wheat bran; spelt)	Amaranth
Barley	Arrowroot
Rye (rye flour)	Buckwheat
Bulgur	Corn and maize
Durham	White potatoes and potato flour
Farina	Sweet potatoes
Graham flour	Rice, rice bran, rice flour
Kamut	Tapioca
Matzo meal	Soya, soya bran, soya flour, soya products
Semolina	Hominy grits
Triticale	Polenta
All foods made from these grains, including barley-based drinks, malted drinks, and beer; pasta, noodles, pastry, pies, wafers, and cakes (unless specifically labeled gluten free)	Quinoa
	Eggs, milk, cream, butter, cheese, curd cheese
	All fruits and vegetables
Sauces, dressing, and soups that contain wheat and, therefore, gluten	Fresh meats, fish, and poultry (not breaded or marinated)
Oat cereals that contain wheat	Beans (except certain brands of baked beans and beans with a gluten-containing sauce)
Breaded food products, such as fried chicken	Tea, coffee
Imitation meats or seafood and processed luncheon meats	Cocoa
	Most alcoholic drinks
	Jam, marmalade
	Sugar, honey
	Salt, pepper, vinegar, herbs, and spices

Note: Wheat products are often used as fillers or thickeners in foods the consumer may not realize have been processed. The habitual reading of labels is an important means of eliminating foods that contain the grains listed in the first column (or their derivatives) to be certain of consuming a gluten-free diet.

Lactose Intolerance   Depending on ethnicity, the prevalence of lactose intolerance ranges from 5 percent to more than 50 percent. Most young children produce the enzyme lactase, which digests the milk sugar lactose (found in all mammalian milk) into its component parts (glucose and galactose).[9] Lactase production may decrease, however, in some people after the age of 3, and it is this decrease in the production of lactase that limits a person's ability to tolerate the sugar lactose. Adults of northern European descent appear to have the lowest prevalence of lactose intolerance (between 5 and 17 percent of the population), while populations from South America, South Africa, and Asia have much higher prevalence rates of more than 50 percent.[10]

When lactose is not digested because of the inadequate production of lactase in the small intestine, it enters into the large intestine as an intact disaccharide, which in some people results in abdominal pain, bloating, gas, and diarrhea within a relatively short time after consumption of the lactose-containing food. The gas and bloating are likely caused by an increase in the processing of lactose by gut bacteria. These symptoms may be easily confused with other GI problems, so people with lactose intolerance may not properly attribute the problem to milk consumption. When lactose intolerance is properly diagnosed, typically with a lactose hydrogen breath test, there should be a severe reduction or elimination of lactose-containing foods to eliminate the symptoms. Every person has an individual lactose-tolerance threshold, above which symptoms will occur. All dairy products contain lactose, but the highest lactose contents are found in fluid milk, condensed milk, and dried skimmed milk.

Crohn's Disease   Crohn's disease is a regional inflammation of the ileum but may affect the entire small or large intestine. It is associated with abdominal pain and frequent diarrhea, with bowel obstruction being a serious problem for the Crohn's patient.[11] This form of irritable bowel syndrome (IBD) causes a thickening of the intestinal wall that reduces the internal transit diameter of the affected portion of the intestines. This reduced interior intestinal diameter is responsible for the bowel obstruction. Crohn's disease equally affects men and women and appears to run in families, although about only 20 percent of Crohn's patients have a relative with the disease. The disease has no known cause, but it is theorized that an immune system reaction against a bacteria or virus causes the inflammation. It appears clear that, unlike some intestinal disorders, Crohn's disease is not related to stress. For an athlete, Crohn's can have a debilitating effect on the capability to absorb sufficient nutrients, and the associated diarrhea affects fluid and electrolyte balance.

The ileum (the main intestinal area affected by Crohn's disease) is the site of vitamin B_{12} absorption. A failed absorption of vitamin B_{12} will eventually lead to megaloblastic hypochromic anemia, which negatively affects oxygen-carrying capacity. Athletes who have been diagnosed with Crohn's disease are most commonly treated with an anti-inflammatory drug (commonly containing mesalamine; sulfasalazine is the most common of these drugs), along with treatments that aim to correct the nutrition deficiencies and relieve the pain and diarrhea.[12] Treatment with fluids and electrolytes is common for patients suffering from frequent diarrhea. Some drugs also reduce the immune response so as to reduce the cause of the inflammation. An irritated GI tract may require that no solid foods be consumed to allow for a reduction in the inflammation and to reduce the chance for a bowel obstruction. Liquid full-nourishment meals are often consumed during these periods.

No foods appear to universally increase the GI inflammation of Crohn's disease, but doctors often ask patients to limit the intake of foods that are not well tolerated in large portions of the population or foods that are known irritants (e.g., milk, alcohol, spicy foods).[13] In the presence of a vitamin B_{12} deficiency, consumption of oral supplements or foods high in vitamin B_{12} (foods of animal origin) does not resolve the deficiency because, regardless of the amount consumed, the absorption of vitamin B_{12} is sufficiently corrupted that the vitamin will not enter the blood. Periodic injections of vitamin B_{12}, which bypass the GI tract, are typically needed to correct the deficiency.

Drugs   Certain drugs can have an effect on the digestion and absorption of nutrients. Antibiotics destroy the intestinal microflora (bacteria) that assist in digestive and absorptive processes and that are involved in creating certain nutrients, such as vitamin B_{12}. The commonly prescribed antibiotic neomycin, for instance, causes a malabsorption of fat, protein, sodium, potassium, and calcium.[14] Because of the competitive absorption of divalent minerals (calcium, iron, magnesium, and zinc), a high intake of calcium-containing antacids could, for instance, take up most of the absorption site and interfere with the absorption of the other minerals.[15] As previously mentioned, the nonsteroidal anti-inflammatory drugs (NSAIDs) commonly taken by athletes to resolve the bumps, bruises, aches, and pains of athletic endeavors may create a GI irritation that results in blood loss and an iron-deficiency anemia.[16] These are but a few examples of how drugs can result in an altered fuel intake and utilization. Athletes should be fully aware that virtually every drug taken, including over-the-counter drugs, is likely to have a digestive, absorptive, or metabolic impact that could be a detriment to performance. Athletes should therefore consult with an appropriate health care professional rather that pursue self-diagnosis and self-prescription.

FACTORS INFLUENCING ENERGY METABOLISM

Nutrients that are consumed, digested, and absorbed must still be delivered to the correct tissues for metabolic purposes. A number of factors may inhibit the normal metabolism of nutrients, including nutrient–nutrient interactions, drug–nutrient interactions, and excess alcohol consumption. Of these, regular alcohol consumption is likely to present the greatest difficulties for athletes.

Alcohol   Alcohol is absorbed in the stomach and small intestine. Although it is a nutrient that provides 7 calories per gram, it must also be considered an antinutrient because of the way it inhibits the normal metabolism of vitamins and, therefore, the main energy substrates (carbohydrate, protein, and fat) if consumed in excess. Most important, alcohol should not be mistaken for an essential nutrient, which it is not. It is a toxic substance that humans have a limited capacity to detoxify, and in the process, alcohol leaves other toxic substances in its wake.

A regular high intake of alcohol increases disease risk, including cancers of the liver, mouth, throat, and esophagus (these latter three cancers are even more likely if combined with smoking) as well as cirrhosis of the liver (a condition where increasing portions of the liver become fibrotic and are no longer able to function). In addition, alcohol can be an irritant to all segments of the GI tract and, as a result, can cause the malabsorption of nutrients. To make matters worse, alcohol increases the urinary excretion of calcium and magnesium. Magnesium is a cofactor in enzymes transferring phosphate groups, so it is a needed ingredient in energy metabolism. Regular alcohol intake lowers the resorption of magnesium (increasing urinary losses) and also increases magnesium excretion in sweat. The result is an increase in muscle cramps, weakness, and cardiac arrhythmias. Athletes cannot afford creating a magnesium deficiency associated with regular alcohol consumption.[17]

Because liver function is impaired, alcohol may also interfere with the normal metabolism and storage of nutrients. Further, alcohol increases nutrient requirements so as to repair the damage it creates and to counteract the malabsorption it produces. Chronic alcohol abuse may weaken the heart; alter brain and nerve function; increase blood lipids (particularly triglycerides); result in a fatty, cirrhotic liver that malfunctions; and cause pancreatitis (which can have a major impact on blood glucose control and digestive processes.) Besides the increased risk of athletic injury induced by alcohol consumption, there is also evidence that more than one drink per day can have a clear effect on performance by negatively affecting reaction time, coordination, and energy metabolism.[18]

Alcohol dehydrogenase, a liver enzyme, is made by the liver to dehydrogenate the active form of vitamin A (retinol, an alcohol). However, with alcohol (ethanol) consumption, the limited production of alcohol dehydrogenase is shunted to dehydrogenate ethanol, thereby leaving the potentially toxic form of vitamin A in the alcohol form. The result is an adverse interaction between alcohol and vitamin A that can result in liver toxicity and increased cancer risk.[19]

The risk of alcohol-related health effects is real in athletes. Although elite athletes consume alcohol half as often as age-equivalent nonathletes, many athletes (particularly those in team sports) still consume far more alcohol than would support good health, good nutrition, and optimal athletic performance.[20] Nonelite adolescent athlete groups are more likely to engage in problem drinking than their nonathlete counterparts.[21] Male athletes appear more likely than female athletes to consume alcohol daily.[22] See table 5.6 for a list of the major effects of alcohol on athletic performance.

Nutrients   Nutrient intake and availability clearly affect energy metabolism. Even a deficiency in one nutrient can corrupt the normal metabolic pathways for energy utilization and therefore affect athletic performance. Given the potential hazards of inadequate intake, maldigestion, malabsorption, and altered metabolic processes from drug or alcohol ingestion, it is a credit to the human system that most people are able to supply nutrients to

Table 5.6   Effects of Alcohol on Human Performance

Effect	Consequence
Increased risk of hypoglycemia	In prolonged exercise, hypoglycemia is more likely because alcohol suppresses liver gluconeogenesis
Increased heat loss	Hypoglycemia results in impairment of temperature regulation, particularly in cold environments
Reduced performance in middle- and long-distance running	As alcohol intake increases, performance deficits are seen in middle- and long-distance events
Reduced vertical jump height and sprint performance	A 6% reduction in vertical jump height and a 10% reduction in 80 m sprint performance
Adverse effect on concentration	Central nervous system effect
Adverse effect on visual perception	Central nervous system effect
Adverse effect on reaction time	Central nervous system effect
Adverse effect on coordination	Central nervous system effect
Increased risk of dehydration	Alcohol has a diuretic effect
Poor postexercise glycogen recovery	Alcohol impairs carbohydrate status of the liver and may also impair muscle glycogen storage
Poor postexercise recovery	Alcohol impairs the repair of injured tissues

Adapted from L.M. Burke and R.J. Maughan, 2000, Alcohol in sport. In *Nutrition in sport*, edited by R.J. Maughan (Oxford: Blackwell Science), 405-414.

the tissues that need them at the time they're required. However, any chronic insult from poor intake, heavy alcohol abuse, or untreated illness will eventually have a negative effect on performance, a fact that athletes and their coaches should constantly bear in mind.

Physical activity increases the need for fuel and for the metabolic processes that are involved in its utilization. Anything that either limits the provision of adequate calories to support the cellular requirement or alters the cells' capacity to properly metabolize the provided fuel will have a negative impact on performance. Some factors are within athletes' control, including adequate food consumption, careful consumption of drugs and supplements, and avoidance of regular alcohol consumption; other factors are not within athletes' control, including disease states that may alter food intake or food absorption. This book is filled with information on how to best provide the fuels needed for successfully pursuing athletic endeavors. For those conditions that are not within the direct control of the athlete (e.g., celiac and Crohn's disease and other GI tract disorders), an increasing number of medical solutions are available; athletes should not hesitate to seek medical advice that can ameliorate the impact these conditions have on health and performance. Ultimately, if the fuel doesn't make it to a cell that has the capacity to burn it, athletic endeavors cannot be successfully pursued.

GI CONCERNS FOR ATHLETES

Gastrointestinal (GI) problems are considered so common by many athletes that they have become a natural part of the athletic experience. Many athletes have even accepted the symptoms of GI distress (pain, diarrhea, gas, vomiting, bloating) as an inherent and normal part of training and competition, having suffered for so long they can't imagine life without these problems. Of course, GI distress that results in these symptoms is anything but normal and natural, and left untreated, some GI problems may cascade into disease states that can seriously compromise a runner's health.

There are many GI concerns for athletes. Frequent fluctuations in hydration state can cause digestion and absorption difficulties that require a constant vigilance to make sure fluid consumption is adequate. The stress associated with competition and overtraining is also a concern; GI dysfunction (e.g., nausea, gastritis, colitis) is a common outcome with persistent stress and a lack of adequate rest. Once stress-related GI problems occur, nutrient intake drops. This gives rise to numerous other nutrient-deficiency disorders that can be adequately dealt with only when the athlete returns to a more stress-free and rested state.

Runner's diarrhea is well recognized in endurance runners but may affect athletes in other sports as well.[23-25] As part of this same syndrome, a significant proportion (20 percent) of marathon runners report blood in their stools after the completion of a marathon.[26] There are likely several causes for runner's diarrhea, including[27]

- an irritated colon from electrolyte imbalance,
- a change in bowel transit speed from greater stimulation of pancreatic hormones,
- a travel-associated change in bacterial exposure, and
- excess consumption of vitamin or mineral preparations.

Athletes may be able to alleviate GI distress through consumption of better beverages; an improvement in the content and timing of foods and fluid relative to exercise or competition; and targeted, conservative supplement consumption.

Sports Beverages

A common source of GI distress is sports beverages. There are three common scenarios: (1) The athlete fails to adequately adapt to the beverage; (2) the beverage has an excessively high osmolarity (i.e., the concentration of electrolytes, sugar, or protein is too high); and (3) the athlete has an intolerance or sensitivity to a specific carbohydrate source in the beverage.

Poor Beverage Adaptation Humans are highly adaptable to nutrition regimens, but athletes often fail to train in a way that fully mimics competition, making adaptation to the competition routine impossible. There is every reason to believe that adapting to a drinking strategy (both qualitatively and quantitatively) is extremely important in helping athletes determine the adaptation limits. For instance, runners often go on beverage-free training runs every day but then appear at a competition venue with beverages they intend to drink every 3 miles (5 km). Without practicing consumption of a known beverage at the expected volume per unit of time, these athletes have not adapted to a given strategy and have no idea of their tolerance limits. The inevitable result will be over- or underconsumption of a beverage, with dehydration, hyponatremia, or diarrhea the likely outcome.

Beverage Osmolarity The concentration of electrolytes and energy substrates (typically only carbohydrate, with some beverages also containing protein) affects the osmotic pressure created by the beverage. The higher the osmolar concentration, the greater the delay in gastric emptying, which increases the chance of GI distress. Most sports beverage companies are acutely aware of this issue and create beverages that most athletes find tolerable; the delay in gastric emptying after consuming these beverages is not severe enough to cause excess fluid buildup in the stomach when large volumes must be consumed to match sweat rates.

When the sodium concentration of a beverage goes up, the carbohydrate concentration must be adjusted downward to sustain an acceptable osmolar concentration. In general, most athletes find a 6 to 7 percent carbohydrate solution with 50 to 150 milligrams of sodium per 240 milliliters acceptable, and this is the typical range of carbohydrate and sodium found in most sports beverages. There are notable exceptions to this, as some beverages have extremely low sodium (less than 20 milligrams per 240 milliliters), and endurance beverages may have sodium concentrations of 200 milligrams per 240 milliliters in an attempt to sustain blood volume when runners are covering marathon distances or higher. Some athletes use protein-containing sports beverages, but protein causes an additional delay in gastric emptying and, therefore, may increase the chance for GI distress when large volumes are consumed, as in very hot and humid environments. Assuming that each athlete will fall under the typical tolerance limits is a mistake, since athletes are individuals who have large differences in their capacity to tolerate a given osmolar solution delivered at a given volume per unit of time. Therefore, the only sure way to know if a specific beverage will result in no GI distress is to consume it at the predicted rate in training sessions that closely emulate the competition's environmental conditions.

A note of caution about swilling beverages (i.e., keeping a solution in the mouth without swallowing): A research project has assessed the effects of swilling a cooling menthol-containing solution and found that it can help reduce heat stress.[28] This should not be interpreted by athletes that swilling a carbohydrate and electrolyte solution is also effective and, therefore, could be a strategy for avoiding some GI distress. There is no evidence that swilling a carbohydrate and electrolyte sports beverage is an effective means of maintaining hydration state and avoiding heat stress.

Sensitivity to the Carbohydrate Source Sports beverages that deliver multiple carbohydrate sources (e.g., sucrose plus glucose) are generally better tolerated than those that deliver one carbohydrate source. Imagine a room of 100 people who must quickly leave out of a single door. Now imagine the same room of 100 people who must quickly leave out of three doors; three doors will result in a three times faster exit. Each carbohydrate monosaccharide (single sugar) has a different receptor (i.e., exit door) for passing through the intestinal wall and into the blood. Providing the same caloric load, therefore, with different carbohydrate sources enhances absorption and reduces the chance that carbohydrate will stay in the intestines long enough to cause a fluid inflow that results in diarrhea.

Another problem is that some people have very few receptors or enzymes for certain sugars, resulting in diarrhea and bloating if these sugars are consumed. Lactose (milk sugar) is a well-known problem in about 10 percent of the population, and many athletes complain of diarrhea and bloating from consuming fructose-only beverages. An important distinction should be made here, however, since people commonly associate high-fructose corn syrup (HFCS)—a common ingredient in many sports beverages—with pure fructose. The HFCS used in sports beverages is indistinguishable from table sugar (sucrose), as the concentration of glucose and fructose is nearly identical. Beverages that contain high concentrations of free fructose (not HFCS) are the ones associated with a high frequency of GI distress because most runners don't have sufficient receptors to properly deal with it, and they experience the expected result: diarrhea and bloating.

Content and Timing of Foods and Fluids

The discussion of optimal fluids and foods for enhancing exercise and reducing the risk of GI distress often focuses on issues related to the content and quantity of foods and fluids consumed but rarely adequately focuses on optimal timing of their intake. Both are equally important in reducing the risk of GI distress and optimizing the performance-related benefit of the foods and fluids.

Before Exercise   In the period immediately before training or competition, nutritionally balanced meals are not needed and may even be counterproductive. The goal for athletes in the preexercise period is to make certain that blood sugar is maintained, that hydration state is optimal, and that the stomach is empty. To do this, the focus should be on starchy, low-fiber carbohydrate foods and fluids for the last meal before exercise, followed by a sports beverage sipping protocol that maintains blood glucose and volume up to the beginning of the training or competition. Eating the final meal too soon may cause blood sugar to become low just before the exercise period, and eating the final meal too close to the activity may leave food in the stomach.

During Exercise   Perhaps the most common error during physical activity is to delay drinking fluids until the sensation of thirst manifests itself. Besides the fact that drinking at this point is not likely to adequately hydrate working muscles during the activity (see chapter 3), the natural response to thirst is to drink a large volume of fluid at one time. Because the thirst sensation suggests the athlete is already dehydrated, gastric emptying will be delayed, which will make the athlete feel nauseated. In general, care should be taken to never allow thirst to occur during exercise so that consumed fluids will rapidly leave the stomach and be delivered quickly to needy muscles. Additionally, no solid foods or high-concentration carbohydrate beverages (e.g., beverages with a carbohydrate concentration that exceeds 8 percent) should be consumed during physical activity unless the athlete knows these foods and beverages do not cause GI distress.

After Exercise   The greater the degree of dehydration, the greater the fluid requirement. However, since dehydration causes a delay in gastric emptying, dehydrated athletes should be

GI Recommendations for Athletes

If gastrointestinal symptoms are cramping your style, start with the simplest adjustments to your routine before moving on to more complicated and possibly unnecessary or harmful interventions.

Evaluate whether overtraining, stress, and inadequate rest are contributing to your GI symptoms. Is your training helping you improve, or are you getting more and more tired? Are you constantly nursing injuries? Are you sleeping enough or sleeping a lot and still feel fatigued? Any of these signs of overtraining can send your autonomic nervous system into overdrive, affecting normal GI function.

• **Cultivate predictable bowels.** Don't let practices or competitive events disrupt your normal bowel habits. Get up and eat breakfast early enough to ensure a complete bowel movement before start time. An adequate breakfast will not only give you the required energy for your physical effort but also stimulate bowel function, allowing the bowels to evacuate before leaving home. Try adding a hot beverage.

• **Maintain a continuous optimal hydration state.** Dehydration, overhydration, and improper choice of hydration beverages can contribute to GI distress. Noticeable GI distress can result from a fluid loss of 2 percent of body weight. Just taking the time to predict and adequately replace event sweat losses will minimize the chances of cramping and diarrhea during an event. However, hydration requires constant vigilance, even outside of training hours. Consider your hydration plan to be as important as your training and food plans.

Diligently consume sports beverages with 6 to 7 percent carbohydrate during practice and competitions. These beverages are specifically formulated to increase the speed of fluid absorption from the intestines to working muscles, leaving less unabsorbed liquid in the intestines to contribute to loose stools or diarrhea. Avoid fructose-only sports beverages. Higher-carbohydrate beverages, such as juice or sodas, can shift fluid absorption away from working muscles and leave greater amounts of fluid in the intestines, causing diarrhea. Athletes in some activities, including those of relatively short duration or conducted in temperature-controlled environments, are not likely to require as much sports beverage as athletes involved in longer-duration activities in hot environments. Any sporting activity, however, will speed the rate at which blood sugar is lowered, with the effect of causing mental fatigue and related muscular fatigue. Therefore, while sports beverage intake is likely to be useful for all athletic endeavors, individual athletes should follow strategies to ensure optimal consumption patterns that avoid inadequate and excess intakes. Pre- and postactivity body weights are a good way to adjust fluid intakes to meet individual needs.

• **Practice the preexercise meal.** The last food you put in your stomach before exercise can trigger upper gastrointestinal symptoms, such as nausea, cramping, esophageal reflux, chest pain, and vomiting. Gastric emptying and intestinal motility increase with exercise, creating a mechanical source of GI symptoms. But the timing, volume, nutrient density, consistency, and temperature of your preexercise meal can also affect gastric emptying. Liquid emptying from the stomach is increased with light exercise, and solid-food emptying is delayed with vigorous exercise. Dietary fat and fiber also delay gastric emptying. Develop a list of high-carbohydrate, low-fat, low-fiber foods that are tried and proven as your pre-event meal.

• **Save high-fiber foods for after practice.** Fiber intake is crucial for healthy digestion, but fiber can also be a source of GI distress. In general, food sources of insoluble fiber, such as wheat and corn bran, flax seeds, nuts, and fruit and vegetable peels are more likely to contribute to diarrhea. Eat high-fiber cereals after practice. If mild to moderate diarrhea and loose stools are a problem, increasing total daily soluble fiber intake can help relieve symptoms. Soluble fiber will soak up a significant amount of water, making stools firmer and slower to pass through the digestive tract. Beans, oats, barley, fruits, and vegetables contain soluble fiber. Fiber supplements should be used with caution and preferably with professional advice. Be aware that many commercial food products not previously considered high-fiber food sources, such as yogurt, now have added fiber, which may or may not be desirable. Soluble fiber overload can produce another negative GI symptom—gas and bloating.

• **Discontinue any dietary and herbal supplements**. If symptoms disappear, first consider whether it is necessary to reintroduce the offending supplements into your nutrition plan. If necessary, decrease the amount of supplement in the gut at one time by taking smaller, more frequent dosages.

• **Try lactose-free dairy products.** The digestive enzyme lactase breaks down lactose—a naturally occurring sugar in dairy products. Humans produce limited amounts of lactase, and production also tends to decrease with age, illness, and stress. The total amount of milk products consumed in one day may put you over the limit of your lactase capacity and cause diarrhea. Or that large latte ingested 45 minutes before your run may be the cause. Lactose-free milk and yogurt are readily available and can serve as dairy substitutes. If you find some symptom relief with a lactose-free diet, you may want to ask your physician for a lactose breath test to determine that lactose is indeed your offending substance.

• **Don't try too many remedies at once.** When making dietary changes, more is not necessarily better. Any major changes to your dietary intake can adversely affect your gut. Make one change at a time, and give your system several days or even weeks to adjust before making more changes. For example, do not add a high-fiber cereal, a fiber-enriched yogurt, and a fiber supplement at the same time. Also, probiotics, marketed as a remedy for constipation, increase stool bulk and are very common additions to many commercially available food products. Delay adding new substances until you have your symptoms under control, and tolerance to new foods can be individually evaluated.

• **Talk to your physician about whether testing for celiac disease is appropriate**. Undertaking a diet that prohibits all wheat-, rye-, and barley-based foods is not an easy task, especially since it eliminates favorite high-carbohydrate foods, such as pasta and breads. In addition, starting the diet without complete testing will make a proper diagnosis difficult.

wary of taking in large volumes of fluid at one time. Instead, athletes should continually sip on fluids until they feel the dehydration resolving itself. For athletes involved in sequential day practices or competition, the immediate postexercise period is an opportunity to replenish depleted glycogen stores, to reduce exercise-associated muscle soreness, and to return to a well-hydrated state. The enzyme glycogen synthetase is highest when glycogen stores are most depleted. This enzyme converts glucose to glycogen, so consuming high-carbohydrate foods, as tolerated, immediately after exercise is a desirable practice. This practice is inhibited by the relative degree of dehydration experienced by the athlete. The greater the degree of dehydration, the smaller the amount of food tolerated (because of delayed gastric emptying). Ideally, therefore, the postexercise period should be high in fluids that can help rehydrate the athlete. Consumption of chocolate milk or similar beverages after exercise satisfies multiple needs: fluid and sodium for rehydration, sugar for glycogen replenishment, and protein for reducing postexercise muscle soreness.

Medications, Herbal Remedies, and Supplements

A common reaction to GI distress is to increase the intake of vitamins, minerals, and other "cures" in the hope they will somehow alleviate the problem. It is possible, however, that high intakes of vitamins, minerals, antibiotics, and NSAIDs may exacerbate rather than lower the GI distress an athlete is trying to resolve.[29] Many common vitamin and mineral supplements can wreak havoc on the GI tract. The supplements commonly associated with lower gastrointestinal symptoms are high-dose vitamin C, magnesium, and iron. The high doses of common over-the-counter vitamin and mineral preparations are sufficiently con-centrated in micronutrients that a residual of unabsorbed nutrients will inevitably remain in the GI tract, causing irritation and associated fluid inflow that can contribute to diarrhea. NSAIDs are known to be associated with GI bleeding, which may be the cause of bleeding diarrhea in runners.

IMPORTANT POINTS

• The greater the volume of food and fluids that must be consumed, the greater the number of meals the athlete should consume. Simply increasing the amount of food con-sumed at each meal creates problems.

• The timing of food intake is important. No solid food should be consumed within 1.5 hours of physical activity (longer if the food is high in protein or fat); between the last meal and exercise, athletes should sip on sports beverages to maintain blood sugar and avoid hunger. During activity, a sports beverage containing sodium and carbohydrate will help maintain blood volume and blood sugar. Athletes should avoid foods with a high level of fiber immediately before and during physical activity. After activity, athletes should consume foods and fluids to restore muscle glycogen and hydration state.

• Certain factors can delay gastric emptying, which could result in GI upset. These include beverages with a carbohydrate concentration of 8 percent or more, beverages that contain a high level of free fructose, high exercise intensity, and high psychological stress.

• GI distress is a common problem in athletes, resulting in pain, diarrhea, gas, vomiting, and bloating. Although common, these problems should not be considered insignificant. Athletes should consult a physician to determine the cause. Athletes with GI distress should consider the consumed beverage, sensitivity to the carbohydrate source, celiac disease, food allergies, and food sensitivities as possible causes.

Nutrient and Fluid Timing

The traditional view of energy and nutrient delivery is to provide recommendations in units of 24 hours. Although these general guidelines may be useful for some people, they are not particularly useful for athletes wishing to optimize fuel and fluid delivery to enhance performance. Put simply, the dynamics of energy and fluid *intake* should match the dynamics of energy and fluid *usage*. Any delivery system that deviates widely from this principle diminishes the usefulness of fuel and fluid recommendations in helping athletes train and perform at their best. The body does not work in 24-, 48-, or 72-hour units. We have an endocrine system and a central nervous system that is constantly making microadjustments in biological values (blood glucose, insulin, and so on) to optimize system function. Assessing nutrient and fluid intake in a way that ignores these dynamic microadjustments only ignores important within-day adjustments that could make an important difference in performance and body composition. Studies have shown that matching intake and expenditure dynamics helps athletes maintain lean mass, reduce body-fat levels, improve sense of well-being, and enhance athletic performance.

Exercise has two major effects on the requirement for nutrients. It results in an increase in the rate of energy usage and, because of the greater heat production associated with higher levels of energy metabolism, an increase in the rate of water lost as sweat. Athletes must increase energy substrate and fluid consumption to meet this additional nutrition burden, yet nutrition surveys suggest that athletes don't eat enough and don't drink enough.[1-3] Moreover, it appears that energy consumption is not well timed, which negatively affects both body composition and performance.[4-6]

The outcome of this widespread athletic malnutrition is all too well understood: an excessive reliance on supplements and ergogenic aids to overcome the deficits created by inadequate energy and fluid consumption. Athletes will likely achieve better results by paying attention to food and drink intake than by following any other course of action. Focusing on food and drink is a less expensive, more dependable, and safer strategy for improving athletic performance than relying on supplements and ergogenic aids, which may have indefinite content and unpredictable quality.

This chapter provides a critical summary of studies that have looked at within-day energy balance and eating frequency and the underlying physiological and nutrition principles that show the importance of reducing the magnitude of energy surpluses and deficits during the day. In addition, the chapter provides practical strategies for how athletes involved in morning and afternoon, afternoon and evening, or one-time daily training regimens can sustain an optimal within-day energy and fluid balance.

INTAKE FOR PERFORMANCE ENHANCEMENT

Much of the discussion on energy intake focuses on the optimal distribution of the energy substrates: carbohydrate, protein, and fat. Despite the popular recommendations for high-protein, low-carbohydrate diets, there is no question that focusing on a diet high in complex carbohydrates, moderate in high-quality protein, and relatively low in fat is performance enhancing. But this discussion has little meaning in the face of energy intake inadequacy. Put simply, it doesn't matter if high-octane fuel is put in the system if there isn't enough fuel to get you where you want to go. Weight and lean-mass stability are the best indicators that energy intake matches need. A failure to consume sufficient energy leads to either a reduction in weight or a reduction in lean mass (or both) as the body tries to compensate for this energy deficit. For most athletes, a lower relative lean mass and higher relative fat mass is not desirable and is a physiological marker associated with decreased performance, even if weight is lowered. Knowing how weight has changed (more or less fat; more or less muscle) is critically important in knowing if the food intake strategy has been successful. Weight alone simply fails to give you that critical information.

In what must be considered a terribly unwise reaction to this relatively higher fat mass, athletes commonly reduce energy intake still further to reduce the excess fat. The impact of this constant ratcheting down of energy intake is weight loss with a greater loss of lean mass than fat mass, with fat constituting an ever-higher proportion of body weight.[7,8] If caloric intake is inadequate, the body reduces the metabolic mass (i.e., the muscle mass) to make a downward adjustment in the metabolic rate and the need for calories.

It is possible that this cycle of lowering energy intake to adapt to a constantly rising relative fat mass is predictive of the eating disorders seen too often in athletes where appearance plays a factor in a sport's subjective scoring.[9] To emphasize this point, it should be noted that at death, persons with

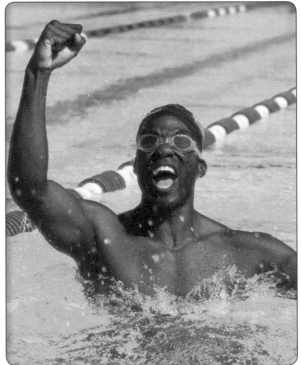

© Human Kinetics

Energy intake should dynamically match energy expenditure to optimize performance.

anorexia nervosa show a terrible loss of weight and a terrible loss of lean mass (the weight of the heart is typically 50 percent of normal) but have a relatively high body-fat percentage. Severely deficient caloric intakes, therefore, lead to a greater wasting away of lean mass than of fat mass.[10] The concept that a significant reduction in calories (i.e., dieting) results in an improved body profile and body composition simply does not stand up to scrutiny. Although a short-term lowering of body weight may be temporarily associated with enhanced performance, the long-term effect of such low-calorie diets is to lower the intake of needed nutrients (a problem that can manifest itself in disease frequency and increased risk for low bone density); to lower the muscle mass (as an adjustment to the inadequate caloric intake);

Nutrient Timing and the Immune System

The immune system protects people from environmentally present infectious substances, including bacteria and viruses, and from the inevitable exposure to toxic substances in the air we breathe and the water we drink. There is good evidence that intense training and exhaustive competition cause immunosuppression in athletes and greatly increase the risk of infectious disease of the upper respiratory tract.[11,12] There is also increasing evidence that delayed eating, excess or inadequate intake of certain nutrients, inadequate carbohydrate consumption, and mistimed intake of protein may all play a role in degrading the athlete's immune system.[13] The combination of heavy training and poor nutrition habits certainly lowers athletic performance, but it also creates a higher risk of illness frequency and even, perhaps, a higher risk of developing certain cancers.[14] To complicate matters, many athletes purposefully consume diets that have an imbalance in protein or carbohydrate intake, and they often emphasize the intake of certain vitamins and minerals at the expense of others. Athletes commonly take nutrient supplements, but they are helpful only when a deficiency is present and the supplements consumed specifically target the at-risk nutrient.

Glucose and the amino acid glutamine are the only fuels used by the immune system. A rapid decline in blood glucose results in a decrease in immune function by lowering macrophage and lymphocyte function.[15] Therefore, appropriately timed intake of carbohydrate-containing beverages and foods to avoid hypoglycemia during physical activity is useful both from a performance and immune function standpoint.[16] Chronically undersupplying energy, as so often happens with athletes, has also been shown to compromise immune cell activity.[17] A successful strategy for avoiding both episodic and chronic low energy intake is to time meals in a way that dynamically matches requirement. Doing so necessarily results in timed food intake opportunities of six or more per day. Even a subtle delay in food consumption after activity may negatively affect the immune system. For instance, ingestion of a carbohydrate and protein solution immediately after, rather than 1 hour after, prolonged strenuous exercise prevented degradation of the immune system.[18] Combining exercise with fasting makes matters even worse, compromising both the immune and antioxidant systems and predisposing the athlete to disease.[19] Taken together, these data strongly suggest that consuming sufficient total energy, with carbohydrate and protein intake that is timed in a way to avoid hypoglycemia, and avoiding inadequate micronutrient deficiencies are critical for maintaining immune system health.[20]

and to regain the weight, which is made up of less lean tissue and more fat. To make matters worse, the lowering of lean mass makes eating normally without weight gain more difficult.

A microeconomic view of the energy-balance issue may shed some light on how athletes should eat to achieve an optimal body composition that enhances performance. A study of four groups of national-level female athletes (rhythmic gymnasts, artistic gymnasts, middle-distance runners, and long-distance runners) found that those who deviated most widely from perfect energy balance during the day had the highest body-fat levels, regardless of whether the energy deviations represented surpluses or deficits (see figure 6.1).[5] In fact, the rhythmic gymnasts, who as a group had the most pronounced energy deficits (nearly 800 kilocalories), had the highest body-fat percentages of all the groups assessed, while middle-distance runners had the best within-day energy balance and the lowest body-fat percentages.

This strongly suggests that the common eating pattern of athletes, which is typified by infrequent meals with a heavy emphasis on a large end-of-day meal, is not useful for meeting athletic goals because it is guaranteed to create large energy deficits during the day. Although this energy deficit may be made up for at the end of the day to put an athlete in an energy-balanced state, this eating pattern is typified by weight stability but higher than desirable body-fat levels. The reason for the higher body-fat level becomes clear when you consider how blood sugar fluxes (after a meal, it rises, levels off, and drops over a period of 3 hours). With delayed eating, blood sugar drops and the amino acid alanine is recruited from muscle tissue to be converted to glucose by the liver. Although this stabilizes blood sugar, it does so at the cost of the muscle mass. In addition, both low blood sugar and large meals are associated with hyperinsulinemia, which encourages the manufacture of fat. So, delayed eating followed by an excessively large meal, which is typical of the athletic eating paradigm, is an ideal way to lower muscle mass and increase fat mass . . . not what athletes want to do. Frequent eating reduces the size of within-day energy deficits and surpluses and helps stabilize blood sugar.

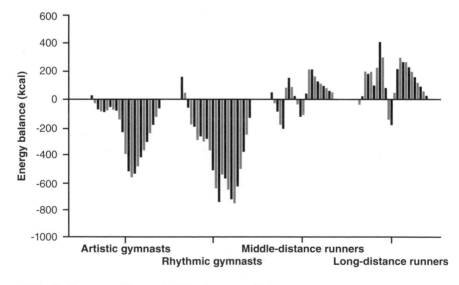

Figure 6.1 Body composition and within-day energy balance.

Reprinted, by permission, from R.C. Deutz, D. Benardot, D. Martin, and M. Cody, 2000, "Relationship between energy deficits and body composition in elite female gymnasts and runners," *Medicine & Science in Sports & Exercise* 32(3): 659-668.

Many athletes concerned about weight have learned to cope with the feeling of low blood sugar by consuming a diet product (diet colas are popular). Although these diet products do nothing to resolve the very real physiological need for energy to maintain an adequate blood sugar, they do provide a central nervous system stimulant (usually caffeine) that masks the sensation of hunger. However, since this strategy maintains the low blood sugar level, the outcome will inevitably be less muscle and more fat. It is clear from these studies that the only appropriate strategy for weight loss is a subtle energy deficit that results in only a slight deviation from a within-day energy-balanced state.

Benefits of Analyzing Energy Balance

It has recently been suggested that there is a benefit to analyzing energy balance and nutrient intake at smaller time intervals because it better addresses physiologic need in real time.[21,22] The thermic effect of food may be higher or lower depending on the frequency and regularity of nutrition delivery.[23] In essence, the body's response to energy intake is not a caloric calculation made each day at midnight but rather is dynamic, occurs in real time, and is highly changeable.

The act of eating more frequently, in and of itself, appears to play a role in the thermic effect of food (the number of calories burned as a result of eating; a higher burn rate is considered good because it is associated with lower body fat). The thermic effect of food is higher in subjects eating at regular, short intervals when compared with subjects eating at irregular, longer intervals.[23] Humans and other animals more efficiently process 1,000 kilocalories delivered in one meal than the same caloric amount delivered in four meals. This has been demonstrated in mongrel dogs fed either small or large meals at varying frequency.[24] After each meal, respiratory quotients and $\dot{V}O_2$peak were observed, and the amount of energy expended after eating was twice as large when meal frequency was increased, suggesting that small and frequent feedings are more energy costly and, therefore, more conducive to a lean body composition. Many studies assessing eating frequency have come to the same conclusion: The more frequent the eating pattern, the lower the body fat and the higher the muscle mass.[25-27] In addition, frequent eating patterns provide a simple, workable strategy for increasing energy intake while simultaneously reducing GI discomfort associated with larger meals.[25]

A study assessing the impact of meal frequency on body composition and weight in boxers found that, even with isocaloric intakes (both groups had the same caloric intake for 2 weeks), the group consuming two meals each day experienced a significant reduction in lean body mass, whereas the group consuming six meals each day did not.[6] In another study of wrestlers, athletes who recorded cyclic weight changes, typified by long periods of very low caloric intakes, had lower metabolic rates, suggestive of a loss of lean body mass.[28]

These studies suggest that large within-day energy deficits clearly cause muscle catabolism, which can be avoided by supplying energy in smaller but more frequent meals. This finding is consistent with a recent study of 60 male and female collegiate athletes that assessed the impact of adding a 250-calorie snack or a noncaloric placebo between each major meal and after dinner (i.e., between breakfast and lunch, between lunch and dinner, and after dinner, for 750 calories provided as snacks each day). After 2 weeks of this protocol, the group consuming the caloric snack experienced a significant reduction in body fat, a significant rise in lean body mass, a significant improvement in anaerobic power and anaerobic endurance, no change in weight, and no change in total caloric intake.[29] Weight stayed the same because energy intake did not change (an important principle of energy thermodynamics), a result that presents an interesting point. When snacks were provided with no instructions regarding the other meals, the athletes spontaneously reduced the size of the other meals to compensate for the snacks. A failure to do so would have increased total caloric intake and resulted in a weight gain.

The snacks were removed 2 weeks into the study. The athletes were remeasured 4 weeks later; they had assumed their old eating patterns and returned to baseline values for body fat and muscle mass. The findings of this study make it clear that an athlete's eating pattern will default to her usual practice (e.g., two or three meals a day, with the largest meal at the end of the day) unless a new pattern becomes the accepted standard. Indeed, studies have found that the environment (e.g., whom the athletes tend to eat with; food availability) plays a major role in eating patterns.[30] Getting athletes to eat more frequently on their own, in opposition to the environmental norm, is extremely difficult.

Animal studies have also found benefits to increasing meal frequency so that large within-day energy deficits and surpluses can be avoided. A study using dogs found that providing a set amount of calories in small but frequent meals rather than large infrequent meals significantly reduces the insulin response to food, even in dogs fed a high-carbohydrate meal. In addition to this clear benefit, more meals result in higher thermogenesis (faster energy metabolic rate) and better fat utilization.[31] What does this mean for athletes? A high insulin response to food translates into high fat production, so having a reduced insulin response means less fat production. Having a faster metabolic rate makes it easier for athletes to eat without getting fat because more calories are being burned per unit of time. These factors, plus a more efficient fat utilization, all translate into eating more, taking in more nutrients, maintaining muscle mass, and lowering body-fat percentage. A failure to eat frequently, causing a mini-starvation state during the day, has just the opposite effect on metabolic rate. The resulting lower metabolic rate is associated with a higher fat mass and more difficulty eating normally without gaining fat.[32-34]

The benefits of eating frequently enough to reduce the magnitude of within-day energy deficits and surpluses go beyond body composition, weight, and performance. There is also evidence that people with frequent eating patterns have lower serum lipid levels, a risk factor in cardiovascular disease.[26] A study assessing the impact of food restriction during the period of the Ramadan fast found that insulin production was increased, as was the production of leptin (a hormone produced by fat cells), both of which are associated with a greater fat-mass production.[35]

Assessing energy intake and expenditure dynamically (i.e., in real time) may have other advantages. A recent study by a graduate student of nutrition determined that the traditional modality of assessing energy balance in units of 24 hours would have missed entirely the most significant factor associated with amenorrhea in active women: the number of hours during the day spent in an energy deficit versus the number of hours spend during the day in an energy surplus. Even in cases of energy balance, more time spent in an energy deficit during a day was significantly more associated with amenorrhea.[36]

What are athletes to do? Never get hungry. This is not easy with a typical three-meal-a-day eating pattern, which provides for a refueling stop every 5 to 6 hours, and the typical athlete eating patterns that heavily backload intake make it even more difficult. Since blood sugar is known to rise and fall in 3-hour units, it makes sense to have planned snacks. If an athlete is weight stable, the best way to initiate this process is to eat a bit less at breakfast, eat the remainder at midmorning, and do the same for lunch and dinner. Total caloric intake will remain the same, but the athlete will avoid sharp energy deficits and surpluses during the day. Besides the improved nutrient intake and better body composition associated with this type of eating pattern, athletes can also expect improved mental acuity and enhanced athletic performance. See chapters 16 through 18 for diet plans that provide examples, at different caloric intakes, of how to avoid large within-day energy surpluses or deficits.

Considerations for Fluid Intake

Studies have demonstrated that athletes experience a degree of voluntary dehydration, even in the presence of available fluids, that lowers blood volume and negatively affects performance.[3] Given the tremendous amount of heat that must be dissipated during exercise through sweat evaporation, athletes must pursue strategies that will sustain the hydration state. Failure to do so will result in poor performance and may also lead to heat illness.

Temperature regulation represents the balance between heat produced or received (heat-in) and heat removed (heat-out). When the body's temperature regulation system is working correctly, heat-in and heat-out are in perfect balance, and body temperature is maintained.[37] The two primary systems for dissipating, or losing, heat while at rest are (1) moving more blood to the skin to allow heat dissipation through radiation and (2) increasing the rate of sweat production. These two systems account for about 85 percent of the heat lost when a person is at rest, but during exercise virtually all heat loss occurs from the evaporation of sweat.

Working muscles demand more blood flow to deliver nutrients and to remove the metabolic by-products of burned fuel, but at the same time there is a need to shift blood away from the muscles and toward the skin to increase the sweat rate. With low blood volume, one or both of these systems fail, with a resultant decrease in athletic performance.

Heavy exercise can produce heat that is 20 times greater than the heat produced at rest. Without an efficient means of removing this excess heat, body temperature will rise quickly. The upper limit for human survival is about 110 degrees Fahrenheit (43.3 degrees Celsius), or only 11.4 degrees Fahrenheit (or 6.3 degrees Celsius) higher than normal body temperature. With the potential for body temperature to rise at the rate of about 1 degree Fahrenheit every 5 minutes, it is conceivable that underhydrated athletes could be at heatstroke risk only 57 minutes after the initiation of exercise.[38]

An athlete who is working hard for 30 minutes can create 450 kilocalories of excess heat that need to be dissipated to maintain body temperature. Since 1 milliliter of sweat can dissipate approximately .5 calorie, athletes would lose about 900 milliliters (almost 1 liter) of sweat. In 1 hour of high-intensity activity, approximately 1.8 liters of water would be lost. On sunny and hot days when the heat of the sun is added to the heat produced from muscular work, athletes would need to produce even more sweat to remove more heat. Sweat doesn't evaporate off the skin as easily when it is humid, so even more sweat must be produced in hot and humid weather. Well-trained athletes exercising in a hot and humid environment may lose more than 3 liters of fluid per hour.[39]

No level of low body water is acceptable for achieving optimal athletic performance and endurance, so athletes should have a strategy for maintaining optimal body water during exercise. The problem is that athletes often rely on thirst as the marker of when to drink. Since the thirst sensation occurs only after a loss of 1 to 2 liters of body water, thirst is an inappropriate indicator of when to drink.[40] Instead, an athlete should strategize on how to never get thirsty. Ideally, this strategy should involve helping athletes determine how much fluid is lost during typical bouts of physical activity and developing a fixed fluid-consumption schedule from that information (typically 3 to 8 ounces every 10 to 15 minutes of a sodium-containing 6 to 7 percent carbohydrate solution). See the section Hydration Strategies in chapter 3 for more specific recommendations.

Considerations for Energy Intake

The question most frequently asked by athletes is what to eat before competition. Although this is important, it is of relatively small importance when compared with how the athlete should eat most of the time. It is impossible to properly prepare for a competition by consuming some pancakes several hours before the feet are placed in the starting blocks. It takes a consistent and long-term effort in conditioning and good nutrition. There is no way an athlete with iron deficiency can magically cure the condition by consuming some red meat the day before an event. It may take 6 months on a proper diet to reach a state of normal iron status. Therefore, the first and most important step in preparing for competition is to consistently eat enough energy and nutrients to support the body's energy and nutrient requirements. Failure to do so will inevitably lead to a poor competition outcome, no matter what the athlete does just before the competition.

In addition to consuming enough energy and nutrients, it's equally important to eat foods when the body can benefit the most from them. The timing of meals is also important to make certain the muscles have enough energy and nutrients to grow and get stronger during training sessions rather than get burned for energy because the athlete hasn't eaten enough. Put simply, it's important to get enough and get it on time. This isn't easy to accomplish because athletes have terribly hectic schedules, and it takes strategic thinking and good scheduling to ensure food is consumed when it's needed. Although careful meal planning may not seem as important as having a well-developed training plan, both should be considered equally important. They should also be thought of collectively to make certain the training plan can be properly supported with the foods that are consumed.

If the general food intake is supportive of the training plan, what should an athlete do differently on the days leading up to a competition? The sequence of events for the seven days before a competition should meet three major goals:

1. **The athlete should gradually become rested.** This may be a problem for many athletes and coaches because athletes (either with or without the encouragement of the coach) often increase the training schedule during the week leading up to a competition. Overtraining is a big problem and may increase the risks of getting sick or getting injured. It certainly doesn't help an athlete do his best at the upcoming competition.

2. **The athlete should gradually build up muscle glycogen (energy) stores.** The main purpose of gradually reducing the intensity and duration of training sessions before the competition is to be sure the athlete can begin the competition with full muscle glycogen stores. The storage capacity for glycogen is relatively small, and athletes are heavily reliant on stored glycogen for muscular work (it's the limiting fuel for muscular work, regardless of the type of exercise the athlete is doing). Therefore, it's important to eat plenty of carbohydrate and reduce work so glycogen stores are full going into the competition.

3. **The athlete should become well hydrated.** When athletes work hard it is difficult (if not impossible) to maintain an optimal hydration state. It takes time to return lost body water, and athletes should give themselves the opportunity to do so by reducing the training intensity and duration and by drinking plenty of fluids. An additional benefit of becoming well hydrated is that glycogen storage is enhanced. The gradual tapering of training during the 7 days before competition makes it easier for the athlete to start the competition in a well-hydrated and optimally energized state.

Of course, many sports don't provide athletes the luxury of tapering activity on a 7-day cycle. Basketball and hockey players play several games each week during the season, and baseball players play nearly every day. Although their schedules don't permit 7-day activity tapering, the principles behind tapered activity, glycogen storage, and optimal hydration should be remembered and, when possible, adhered to. For athletes with daily schedules that eliminate the possibility of tapering, consumption of high-carbohydrate diets and maintenance of optimal hydration become even more important components of athletic performance. Athletes with these schedules should develop eating and drinking plans that are as solid as their training and competition plans.

All too often athletes prepare for a big competition by increasing their training regimen as the competition draws nearer. This is a big mistake. Coaches working in high-skill sports, such as figure skating and gymnastics, may ask their athletes to perform multiple runthroughs of their routines the day before competition just to be sure they can do them. The message this sends to an athlete (i.e., "I don't believe you're ready, and we're going to keep practicing until you get it right") is counterproductive. There is nothing more confidence building for athletes than entering the competition well rested and knowing the coach is secure in their ability to do a good job. This is true whether an athlete is a professional or a tee ball player in Little League baseball.

Carbohydrate Ingestion Before Exercise

A high-carbohydrate meal that is completed approximately 90 minutes before physical activity has been shown to improve endurance performance. After this preexercise meal, athletes should consume carbohydrate right up to the beginning of the training session or competition to avoid low blood glucose. Two strategies can be followed:

1. Ingest a carbohydrate-containing sports beverage using a sipping strategy, where approximately 2 to 4 ounces (60 to 120 ml) of beverage is consumed every 10 to 15 minutes.

2. Snack on low-fiber, starchy foods (such as saltine crackers) every 15 minutes, washed down with ample quantities of water.

Athletes should avoid eating patterns that could stimulate a reactive hypoglycemia, which is caused by ingestion of large quantities of foods with a high glycemic index, but should also avoid the hypoglycemia that could occur from consuming no carbohydrate or from delayed eating. Snacking and sipping procedures appear to be well tolerated and help maintain blood glucose.

Carbohydrate Maintenance During Exercise

Avoiding low blood glucose and avoiding depletion of muscle glycogen stores are both critical for maintaining exercise performance. Consumption of carbohydrate-containing beverages (e.g., sports beverages) and food during exercise delays fatigue and improves performance, even if the consumption occurs late in the exercise session. This strategy delays fatigue through the following mechanisms:

1. Maintains blood glucose, which preserves liver glycogen

2. Maintains branched-chain amino acid (BCAA) levels, which prevents central fatigue by maintaining the ratio of tryptophan and BCAAs

3. Inhibits the production of cortisol, which is catabolic to muscle tissue

4. Reduces the usage of muscle glycogen by providing a constant source of glucose from the blood to working muscle cells

During exercise, carbohydrate is best obtained through a 6 to 7 percent carbohydrate solution, with 4 to 8 ounces (120 to 240 ml) taken every 10 to 20 minutes (the amount to consume depends on sweat rate; see chapter 3). A number of carbohydrate solutions are available to athletes, each with a different concentration and composition of carbohydrate. Issues of gastrointestinal distress and osmolarity should be considered. Of equal 6 percent concentrations of glucose, fructose, or sucrose, the fructose has been shown to cause more gastrointestinal distress. Therefore, athletes should carefully check their tolerance of fructose-only beverages before consuming them in critical situations. (Most sports beverages contain multiple carbohydrate types.)

Few sports beverages are milk based or use lactose as a predominant form of carbohydrate because of the relatively common problem of lactose intolerance. This condition, caused by an inadequate production of the enzyme lactase, results in diarrhea, gas, and abdominal pain. Given the possibility of lactose intolerance in some athletes, it is prudent for athletes to avoid lactose-containing products immediately before and during physical activity.[41]

Glucose polymers have the advantage of being able to deliver more carbohydrate in a lower osmolar solution. Osmolality is determined by the number of particles in a solution, not the size of the particles. Therefore, you can deliver more carbohydrate with a lower osmolality when polymers (strands of attached glucose) are used instead of individual glucose molecules.

Isocaloric beverages typically contain simple sugars, but glucose polymers may improve gastric emptying and enhance absorption. Athletes involved in extremely high-intensity activity for a long duration may need a high volume of carbohydrate calories during physical activity, and glucose polymers may provide a good solution for these athletes.

Carbohydrate Replenishment After Exercise

Glycogen and fluids are usually, to a degree, depleted after exercise, and protein requirements are also higher to aid in muscle recovery. The protein and fluid issues are discussed in other sections of this book. The carbohydrate and glycogen issues are presented here.

One of the main postexercise goals is to replenish glycogen to prepare the athlete for the next bout of exercise. As glycogen becomes depleted, the enzyme glycogen synthetase becomes elevated in the blood. Providing glucose or sucrose (but not fructose) while glycogen synthetase is elevated efficiently replaces muscle glycogen stores.[42] Glycogen synthetase reaches its peak at the point of greatest glycogen depletion, which is immediately after exercise. Therefore, athletes should consume carbohydrate as soon as physical activity ends. Ideally, the carbohydrate consumed for the first 2 hours after exercise should be high glycemic, followed by medium-glycemic carbohydrate for another 2 hours and finally medium- to high-glycemic carbohydrate for the remainder of the day. Athletes should plan on consuming 200 to 400 kilocalories from carbohydrate (50 to 100 grams) immediately after physical activity, followed by sufficient carbohydrate to fulfill the guidelines presented in table 1.7 (Carbohydrate Requirement for Athletes, page 18).

CARBOHYDRATE LOADING

Consumption of carbohydrate before exercise improves carbohydrate stores and reduces the chance for premature fatigue, regardless of whether the sport is high endurance and low intensity, intermittent (as in many team sports), or high intensity and low endurance.[43-48]

Carbohydrate loading is a strategy commonly followed by many athletes before an endurance competition to increase muscle glycogen storage. The general technique is to gradually increase carbohydrate and fluid intake each day, beginning the week before competition, while exercise is tapered downward.[49] This reasonable, safe strategy maximizes glycogen storage. (Glycogen storage requires extra fluid in a 3:1 ratio of water to glycogen.) See figure 6.2 for a comparison of the techniques commonly followed to maximize glycogen storage.

An older strategy for carbohydrate loading involved depleting carbohydrates by exercising intensely while consuming low-carbohydrate foods.[50] This was followed by the technique described in the previous paragraph. This older carbohydrate-loading technique is dangerous (depletion of glycogen stores may cause a sudden and dangerous drop in blood pressure), and there is no evidence that it better optimizes glycogen stores.

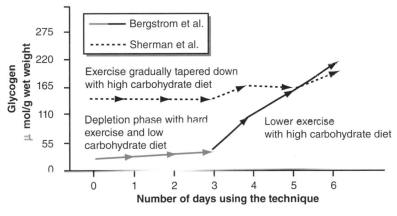

Figure 6.2 Comparison of the Bergstrom et al. (1967) and Sherman et al. (1983) glycogen-loading techniques. (Note: The Bergstrom et al. depletion phase is potentially dangerous and is not recommended.)

Seven-Day Taper

The following tables provide an example of how the principles for maximizing carbohydrate storage can be put to work. They illustrate what and how athletes might eat if they typically train twice daily. You'll notice the food is spread out over six smaller meals rather than two or three larger ones. You'll also notice that the caloric level of the meals does not emphasize dinner at the end of the day. Although dinner is important, training takes place before dinner, so ample energy must be available when the athlete needs it the most. Breakfast comes before the morning workout; when an athlete wakes up, blood sugar is marginal and the liver is virtually depleted of energy, so maintaining blood sugar is virtually impossible. Eating some food before the morning workout ensures that the muscles will benefit from the training and makes the athlete feel better. Nobody feels good with low blood sugar.

As indicated by the tables, foods should be consumed long enough before the training session so an athlete feels no discomfort from training because there is food in the stomach. In addition, the meal plan always includes some carbohydrate immediately after a workout. This helps ensure an effective replenishment of the glycogen that was used up during the training. Waiting too long after training to eat can diminish the efficiency of muscle glycogen replacement. Tables 6.1 through 6.6 provide a unique view into both the volume and timing of food and drink that must be consumed to sustain a reasonably good energy balance (i.e., ± 400 calories) throughout the day. The goal is to never allow so much energy into the body at a single time that a hyperinsulinemic response is likely, followed by an inevitable high fat storage. It is also important to never have so little energy that the catabolic hormone cortisol is increased, followed by the inevitable loss of lean tissue. Put simply, both the volume and timing of intake must match the volume and timing of energy expenditure to enhance the athletic endeavor.

Seven Days Before Competition

One week before competition is the time for a complete, total, and exhaustive workout. The athlete should practice all skills completely and repetitively, focusing on her weakest area. If a basketball player has trouble making foul shots during the game, then she should spend a good deal of time shooting from the foul line after all the other practice regimens have been followed. She should get a sense of what it's like to feel a bit tired, just like in a game. In other words, 7 days before the competition is not a time for being timid about the workout. Give your body a sufficiently good workout so you know you've really gone through the paces. See table 6.1, page 166 for a sample schedule for competition minus 7 days.

During this workout, all the protocols discussed earlier in this book should be followed. It's important to drink plenty of carbohydrate-containing fluids during the workout (see chapter 3). It's also important to follow the workout with plenty of carbohydrate. Consuming at least 400 calories from carbohydrate (100 grams) immediately after the training regimen is desirable, followed by at least 800 calories (200 grams) during the next several hours. This is your first attempt at getting your muscles to replace the glycogen that has been lost during the workout.

Six Days Before Competition

Six days before competition represents the first day of tapered exercise plus maintenance of a high-carbohydrate intake with plenty of fluids. Since activity is reduced, total energy intake should also be trimmed to match needs. Activity can be decreased by reducing total time spent in training or by reducing the intensity of the training activities. For instance, a weightlifter could do fewer repetitions or could do the same number of repetitions with less weight. Regardless of the technique followed, competition minus 6 days should provide a training schedule that is not as exhaustive as competition minus 7 days. See table 6.2, page 168.

Five Days Before Competition

On the second day of reduced exercise intensity and duration, a consistent high carbohydrate and fluid intake is still maintained. Again, total energy intake should be reduced to match needs. This day, competition minus 5 days, is characterized by activity that is discernibly less than the athlete is accustomed to doing. See table 6.3, page 170.

Four Days Before Competition

Four days before the event is a good time for making your final strategic plans for the competition. Your training regimen should focus on key elements of the special skills you have, with an emphasis on practicing skills in a way that keeps you from becoming exhausted. As with the previous days, you should maintain a high carbohydrate and fluid intake to support your needs.

This is also a good time to eat a little extra protein, up to 1.7 grams per kilogram per day to make certain all your tissue-repair needs are covered and to support the manufacture of creatine. For a 190-pound (86 kg) athlete, 1.7 grams of protein per kilogram of body weight amounts to 146.2 grams of protein, which is well within the reach of most diets. Even if your protein requirement is at the lower end of the recommended range of 1.2 to 1.7 g/kg, providing a little extra protein may provides some assurance that protein intake is not a limiting factor in performance.

Three Days Before Competition

Similar to 4 days before competition, 3 days before competition places a continued emphasis on low- to moderate-intensity exercise, a high carbohydrate intake, and a low fat intake, along with a maintained emphasis (up to 1.7 grams per kilogram on protein. Other activities during the day should also be reduced, with more time made available for both physical and psychological relaxation. The athlete should absolutely avoid becoming overheated or exhausted from any activity. Use table 6.4, page 172 as a sample exercise and eating schedule for competition minus 4 days and competition minus 3 days.

Two Days Before Competition

Two days before an event is an excellent time to get more rest, and a good way to achieve this goal is to eliminate the morning training schedule. The afternoon training should be reduced to no more than 1.5 hours, with a moderate to low intensity. The focus should be on reviewing skills and reinforcing the mental strategy it will take to compete effectively. Of course, carbohydrate and fluid intake should remain high. See table 6.5, page 174.

One Day Before Competition

The day before competition should be characterized by plenty of rest (both physical and mental) and relaxation. Athletes and coaches should refrain from running through multiple full routines, a full-speed run, or a full "game intensity" practice. Walking parts of the course, getting familiar with the competition venue, or watching video of your opponents are OK activities but only if you know they won't make you anxious and unable to relax. Sport psychologists indicate it's probably better to watch video of your own successful competitions than to watch video of what your opponent might do. By the day before competition, you should have been briefed about who you're competing against and what strategy to follow.

This is almost your last chance to make certain your glycogen stores are at peak values, and you should maintain a steady fluid intake to ensure optimal hydration going into the next day's activities (see table 6.6, page 176). The carbohydrate foods you consume should be high in starch and relatively low in fiber. Pasta, bread, rice, and fruits (without seeds or skins) are excellent choices. Vegetables and legumes tend to have lots of fiber but may produce gas (causing you to become uncomfortable and bloated). Vegetables in the cabbage family (cabbage, brussels sprouts, kohlrabi) are particularly notorious for their gas-creating capabilities.

Table 6.1   Sample Exercise and Eating Schedule for Competition Minus 7 Days

Energy-balance graph

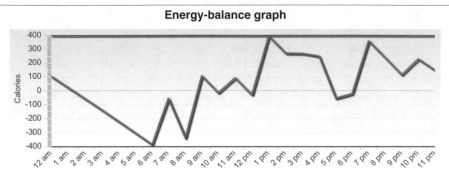

Hours anabolic (calories > 0) = 13; hours catabolic (calories < 0) = 11; anabolic:catabolic ratio = 1.18

Energy Substrate Distribution

Total calories: 3,186   **Carbohydrate %:** 68   **Protein %:** 18   **Fat %:** 14

Hour	Activity	Food	Amount	Calories
7-8 a.m.	Normal daily activity. Wake-up and breakfast.	Orange juice	16 oz (480 ml)	223
		Sports beverage	12 oz (360 ml)	95
		Multigrain bread, toasted	2 slices	138
8-9 a.m.	Vigorous run.	Sports beverage	16 oz (480 ml)	127
9-10 a.m.	Light stretching and other cool-down activities.	Egg, hard boiled, chopped	2/3 cup	139
		Multigrain bread, toasted	3 slices	207
		Orange	1 large	86
		Cereal, whole-grain (Total)	3/4 cup	100
		1% milk	8 oz (240 ml)	102
10-11 a.m.	Relaxed activities.	Water	As desired	0
11 a.m.-12 p.m.	Normal household or workplace activities; important to consume a high-carbohydrate snack midday.	Yogurt, fruited, low fat	1/2 cup	121
		Banana	1 medium	109
12-2 p.m.	Normal household or workplace activities. Lunch.	Chicken breast, baked, no skin	4 oz	196
		Tomatoes, cherry	1 cup	27
		Potato, baked	1 large	277
		Sour cream	2 tbsp	46
		Water	16 oz	0
2-5 p.m.	Casual household or desk activities.	Granola bar, hard, almond	1 bar	119
		Grapes, red, fresh	1 cup	104
5-6 p.m.	Moderate-intensity run.	Sports beverage	8 oz (240 ml)	62

Hour	Activity	Food	Amount	Calories
6-7 p.m.	Light cool-down activities.	Chocolate milk	8 oz (240 ml)	195
7-8 p.m.	Casual, sitting. Dinner.	Spaghetti, enriched, cooked with salt	1 cup	220
		Marinara sauce	1/2 cup	111
		Beef steak, round, lean	3 oz (90 g)	138
		Squash	2 cups	36
		Water	16 oz	0
8-10 p.m.	Casual, sitting.	Water	As desired	0
10-11 p.m.	Evening snack. Snack ensures normal liver glycogen.	Popcorn, air popped	4 cups	124
		Apple juice	8 oz (240 ml)	114
11 p.m.	Sleep			

Meal totals for selected nutrients

Total kcal	3,186	Iron (mg)	34	Vit C (mg)	383	Vit B_{12} (mcg)	7.96
Carbohydrate (g)	551	Calcium (mg)	1,428	Vit B_1 (mg)	3.08	Folic acid (DFE)	933
Protein (g)	147	Zinc (mg)	19	Vit B_2 (mg)	4.99	Vit A (RAE)	1,041
Fat (g)	52	Magnesium (mg)	658	Niacin (mg)	51.5	Vit D (IU)	221
Sodium (mg)	3,017	Potassium (mg)	7,165	Vit B_6 (mg)	5.5	Vit E (mg)	8

Note: The food intake in this example meets the needs of a 190 lb (86 kg) athlete with a twice-per-day exercise schedule. Athletes with different weights should adjust food intake amounts. This represents a full-bore workout day, with subsequent diet intake examples reducing both energy expenditure and energy intake to reduce glycogen utilization but to also achieve energy balance. Athletes weighing more or less than this would consume proportionately more or less food, while maintaining the same frequency of intake.

Source: Energy balance and nutrient intake values were derived using NutriTiming®. The energy balance graph is copyrighted by NutriTiming LLC and is used with permission.

Table 6.2 Sample Exercise and Eating Schedule for Competition Minus 6 Days

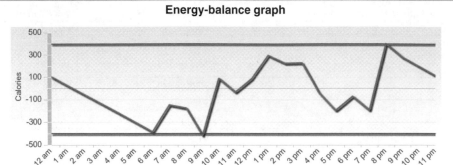

Energy-balance graph

Hours anabolic (calories > 0) = 11; hours catabolic (calories < 0) = 13; anabolic:catabolic ratio = 0.85

Energy Substrate Distribution

Total calories: 3,221   **Carbohydrate %:** 70   **Protein %:** 14   **Fat %:** 16

Hour	Activity	Food	Amount	Calories
7-8 a.m.	Small breakfast to ensure normal blood sugar during morning exercise.	Multigrain bread, toasted	2 slices	161
		Cranberry juice	8 oz (240 ml)	137
		Sports drink	8 oz (240 ml)	62
8-9 a.m.	Initiate sipping protocol with sports beverage to prepare for run. Stretch to prepare for morning run.	Sports drink	16 oz (480 ml)	125
9-10 a.m.	Moderate-intensity run for 60 min; carry sports drink in drink belt and consume every 10 to 15 min.	Sports drink	16 oz (480 ml)	125
10-11 a.m.	Postrun stretch followed by hearty breakfast; focus on carbohydrate to replenish muscle and liver glycogen; consume fluids liberally.	Eggs, poached	2 large eggs	142
		English muffin, mixed grain	1 muffin	155
		Jam	1 tbsp	56
		Blueberries	1 cup	84
		Cereal, bran flakes	1 cup	120
		Milk, 1% fat	8 oz (240 ml)	102
		Water	16 oz	0
11 a.m.-12 p.m.	Normal daily activities.	Water	As desired	0
12-1 p.m.	Normal daily activities. Snack.	Yogurt, fruited, low fat	1 cup	243
1-2 p.m.	Lunch.	Spaghetti, enriched, cooked with salt	1 cup	220
		Marinara sauce	1/2 cup	111
		Water	8-16 oz	0
2-3 p.m.	Light stretching for afternoon workout.	Sports drink	8 oz (240 ml)	62
3-4 p.m.	Very low-intensity warm-up for 30 min.	Sports drink	24 oz (720 ml)	187
4-5 p.m.	Moderate-intensity skills practice at comfortable pace.	Sports drink	8 oz (240 ml)	62
5-6 p.m.	Continued comfortable pace for an additional 30 min.	Sports drink	8 oz (240 ml)	62

Hour	Activity	Food	Amount	Calories
6-7 p.m.	Cool-down and stretching.	Banana	1 medium	109
		Mozzarella, part-skim	1 oz (30 g)	71
		Rye crackers	3	110
		Water	24 oz	0
7-8 p.m.	Total relaxation for remainder of evening.	Water	As desired	0
8-9 p.m.	Dinner	T-bone steak, broiled	4 oz (120 g)	324
		Potato, baked	1 medium	160
		Broccoli, steamed	1 large stalk	98
		Rice pudding	4 oz (125 g)	133
		Water	As desired	0
9-10 p.m.	Relax	Water	As desired	0
10 p.m.	Sleep			

Meal totals for selected nutrients

Total kcal	3,221	Iron (mg)	30	Vit C (mg)	347	Vitamin B_{12} (mcg)	8.16
Carbohydrate (g)	578	Calcium (mg)	1,424	Vit B_1 (mg)	2.40	Folic acid (DFE)	987
Protein (g)	113	Zinc (mg)	19	Vit B_2 (mg)	3.48	Vit A (RAE)	925
Fat (g)	58	Magnesium (mg)	513	Niacin (mg)	35.45	Vit D (IU)	211
Sodium (mg)	4,263	Potassium (mg)	5,405	Vit B_6 (mg)	4.35	Vit E (mg)	11

Note: The food intake in this example meets the needs of a 190 lb (86 kg) athlete with a twice-per-day exercise schedule. Athletes with different weights should adjust food intake amounts. This represents a full-bore workout day, with subsequent diet intake examples reducing both energy expenditure and energy intake to reduce glycogen utilization but to also achieve energy balance. Athletes weighing more or less than this would consume proportionately more or less food, while maintaining the same frequency of intake.

Source: Energy balance and nutrient intake values were derived using NutriTiming®. The energy balance graph is copyrighted by NutriTiming LLC and is used with permission.

Table 6.3 Sample Exercise and Eating Schedule for Competition Minus 5 Days

Energy-balance graph

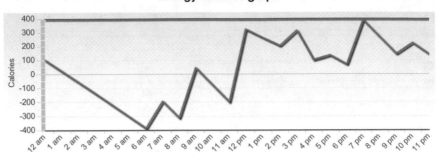

Hours anabolic (calories > 0) = 15; hours catabolic (calories < 0) = 9; anabolic:catabolic ratio = 1.67

Energy Substrate Distribution

Total calories: 2,948   **Carbohydrate %:** 73   **Protein %:** 15   **Fat %:** 12

Hour	Activity	Food	Amount	Calories
7-8 a.m.	Important to immediately consume carbohydrate and fluids upon waking up.	Italian bread	2 large slices	163
		Grape juice	8 oz (240 ml)	152
8-9 a.m.	More carbohydrate and fluids to ensure normal liver glycogen hydration; begin moderate-intensity exercise about 8:30 a.m.	Sports drink	16 oz (480 ml)	125
9-10 a.m.	Immediately after exercise, eat breakfast from 9:40-10:00 a.m.; focus on carbohydrate, good-quality protein, and fluids.	Egg, poached	1 large	71
		Multigrain bread, toasted	2 slices	138
		Orange	1 cup sections	81
		Oatmeal	1/3 cup	102
		Milk, 1% fat	6 oz (180 ml)	76
		Cranberry juice	8 oz (240 ml)	116
10 a.m.-12 p.m.	Shower and dress.	Water	As desired	0
12-1 p.m.	Lunch.	Italian bread	2 large slices	163
		Spaghetti	1.5 cup	330
		Marinara sauce	1/2 cup	111
		Cheese, parmesan	2 tbsp	42
		Water	As desired	0
1-4 p.m.	Relax; sip on sports beverage and have snack to maintain normal blood sugar and liver glycogen in preparation for afternoon exercise.	Sports drink	16 oz (480 ml)	125
		Apple juice	8 oz (240 ml)	114
		Granola bar, hard	1 bar	119
4-5 p.m.	Low-intensity nonexhaustive skills training for 45 min.	Sports drink	8 oz (240 ml)	62
5-6 p.m.	Fluid and carbohydrate replenishment.	Bagel, cinnamon-raisin	1 small	156
		Water	As desired	0
6-7 p.m.	Snack.	Kiwi fruit, fresh	1	56

Hour	Activity	Food	Amount	Calories
7-8 p.m.	Dinner. Focus on good-quality protein, carbohydrate, and fluids.	Chicken breast, baked, no skin	3 oz (90 g)	147
		Brown rice	1 cup	216
		Broccoli raab, cooked	1 cup	80
		Water	8-16 oz	0
8-9 p.m.	Relax. Consume water as needed.	Water	As needed	0
10-11 p.m.	Evening snack. Consume carbohydrate to ensure normal liver glycogen through entire sleep.	Popcorn, air popped	3 cups	93
		Orange juice	8 oz (240 ml)	110
11 p.m.	Sleep			

Meal totals for selected nutrients

Total kcal	2,948	Iron (mg)	22	Vit C (mg)	567	Vitamin B_{12} (mcg)	1.86
Carbohydrate (g)	542	Calcium (mg)	1,113	Vit B_1 (mg)	3.06	Folic acid (DFE)	962
Protein (g)	109	Zinc (mg)	12	Vit B_2 (mg)	2.40	Vit A (RAE)	851
Fat (g)	40	Magnesium (mg)	558	Niacin (mg)	42.24	Vit D (IU)	111
Sodium (mg)	3,091	Potassium (mg)	4,507	Vit B_6 (mg)	2.91	Vit E (mg)	16

Note: The food intake in this example meets the needs of a 190 lb (86 kg) athlete with a twice-per-day exercise schedule. Athletes with different weights should adjust food intake amounts. This represents a full-bore workout day, with subsequent diet intake examples reducing both energy expenditure and energy intake to reduce glycogen utilization but to also achieve energy balance. Athletes weighing more or less than this would consume proportionately more or less food, while maintaining the same frequency of intake.

Source: Energy balance and nutrient intake values were derived using NutriTiming®. The energy balance graph is copyrighted by NutriTiming LLC and is used with permission.

Table 6.4 Sample Exercise and Eating Schedule for Competition Minus 4 Days and Minus 3 Days

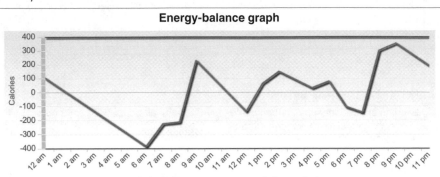

Energy-balance graph

Hours anabolic (calories > 0) = 13; hours catabolic (calories < 0) = 11; anabolic:catabolic ratio = 1.18

Energy Substrate Distribution

Total calories: 2,921   **Carbohydrate %:** 69   **Protein %:** 16   **Fat %:** 15

Hour	Activity	Food	Amount	Calories
7-8 a.m.	Stretch and warm up for 30 min.	Egg bagel, toasted	1 small	192
		Grape juice	8 oz (240 ml)	152
8-9 a.m.	Consume cereal at 8:00. Exercise at light intensity from 8:30-9:00; consume a sports beverage during the exercise.	Shredded wheat	1/2 cup	92
		Sports drink	16 oz (480 ml)	125
9-10 a.m.	Continue exercise until 9:30, then breakfast immediately after exercise; focus on good-quality protein, carbohydrate, and plenty of fluids.	Grapefruit juice	4 oz (120 ml)	51
		Eggs, scrambled	1/2 cup	184
		Multigrain bread, toasted	2 slices	138
		Strawberries	2 cups	97
		Cereal, whole grain	3/4 cup	100
		Milk, 1% fat	6 oz	76
		Water	As desired	0
10 a.m.-1 p.m.	Shower and dress; relaxed activity (reading, walking, desk work).	Water	As desired	0
1-2 p.m.	Relaxed lunch.	Tomatoes, cherry	1 cup	27
		Romaine lettuce	1 cup	8
		Grilled chicken, chopped	3 oz (90 g)	147
		Caesar dressing, low cal	2 tbsp	33
		Egg noodles, cooked with salt	1/2 cup	110
		Water	8-16 oz.	0
2-3 p.m.	Relaxed activity; snack.	Grapes, red	2 cups	208
3-5 p.m.	Exercise preparation; afternoon workout.	Sports drink	16 oz (480 ml)	126
5-6 p.m.	High-carbohydrate snack and sports drink early in hour to prepare for exercise.	Banana	1 medium	109
		Sports drink	8 oz (240 ml)	62
6-7 p.m.	45-min skills training exercise; light intensity only.	Sports drink	8 oz (240 ml)	62
7-8 p.m.	Shower and dress.	Crackers, saltines	5	81

Hour	Activity	Food	Amount	Calories
8-9 p.m.	Dinner.	Steak, broiled, lean	4 oz (120 g)	225
		Potato, baked	1 medium	145
		Green snap peas, boiled	1 cup	44
		Pudding, chocolate	4 oz (125 g)	153
		Water	As desired	0
9-10 p.m.	Evening snack high in carbohydrate and fluids.	Cherries	1/2 cup	43
		Strawberries	1 cup	49
		Blueberries	1 cup	84
10 p.m.	Sleep			

Meal totals for selected nutrients								
Total kcal	2,921	Iron (mg)	40	Vit C (mg)	565	Vitamin B_{12} (mcg)	11.54
Carbohydrate (g)	518	Calcium (mg)	1,735	Vit B_1 (mg)	3.80	Folic acid (DFE)	1,376
Protein (g)	117	Zinc (mg)	30	Vit B_2 (mg)	4.38	Vit A (RAE)	795
Fat (g)	51	Magnesium (mg)	485	Niacin (mg)	56.93	Vit D (IU)	171
Sodium (mg)	2,993	Potassium (mg)	5,584	Vit B_6 (mg)	6.08	Vit E (mg)	21

Note: The food intake in this example meets the needs of a 190 lb (86 kg) athlete with a twice-per-day exercise schedule. Athletes with different weights should adjust food intake amounts. This represents a full-bore workout day, with subsequent diet intake examples reducing both energy expenditure and energy intake to reduce glycogen utilization but to also achieve energy balance. Athletes weighing more or less than this would consume proportionately more or less food, while maintaining the same frequency of intake.

Source: Energy balance and nutrient intake values were derived using NutriTiming®. The energy balance graph is copyrighted by NutriTiming LLC and is used with permission.

Table 6.5 Sample Exercise and Eating Schedule for Competition Minus 2 Days

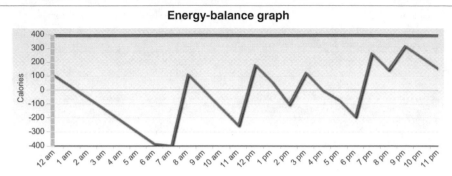

Energy-balance graph

Hours anabolic (calories > 0) = 12; hours catabolic (calories < 0) = 12; anabolic:catabolic ratio = 1.00

Energy Substrate Distribution

Total calories: 2,630   **Carbohydrate %:** 65   **Protein %:** 19   **Fat %:** 17

Hour	Activity	Food	Amount	Calories
6-7 a.m.	No morning workout today, only rest and relaxation.			
7-8 a.m.	Snack, shower, and dress. Important to ensure blood sugar maintained in normal range.	Orange juice	8 oz (240 ml)	110
8-9 a.m.	Relaxed breakfast.	Eggs, poached	2 large	142
		Multigrain bread, toasted	2 slices	138
		Jam	1 tbsp	56
		Cereal, whole grain	3/4 cup	100
		Milk, 1% fat	6 oz (180 ml)	76
		Cantaloupe melon	1 cup cubes or balls	60
		Sports drink	8 oz (240 ml)	62
9 a.m.-12 p.m.	Relax.	Water	As desired	0
12-2 p.m.	Lunch.	Baked turkey, light meat	3 oz (90 g)	134
		Rye bread	2 slices	165
		Mayonnaise, light	1 tbsp	49
		Grapes, red	1 cup	104
		Pretzels, hard, salted	1 oz (31 g)	106
		Water	As desired	0
2-4 p.m.	Practice skills, without exhaustion; keep workout light while sipping on a sports beverage (30 min is sufficient for workout).	Sports drink	8 oz (240 ml)	62
4-5 p.m.	Postexercise carbohydrate replenishment.	Banana	medium	109
		Yogurt, fruited, low fat	1 cup	243
		Water	As desired	0
5-8 p.m.	Snack and relax.	Strawberries	1 cup	49
		Water	As desired	0

Hour	Activity		Food	Amount	Calories
8-9 p.m.	Dinner.		Salmon, baked	4 oz (120 g)	262
			Rice, white	1 cup	205
			Green peas, boiled	3/4 cup	101
9-10 p.m.	Snack.		Pineapple, fresh	2 cups	164
			Rice pudding	4 oz (125 g)	133
			Water	As desired	0
10 p.m.	Sleep.				

Meal totals for selected nutrients									
Total kcal	2,630	Iron (mg)	35	Vit C (mg)	532	Vitamin B_{12} (mcg)	12.90
Carbohydrate (g)	435	Calcium (mg)	2,005	Vit B_1 (mg)	3.73	Folic acid (DFE)	1,464
Protein (g)	124	Zinc (mg)	27	Vit B_2 (mg)	4.23	Vit A (RAE)	1,003
Fat (g)	50	Magnesium (mg)	553	Niacin (mg)	54.76	Vit D (IU)	168
Sodium (mg)	3,176	Potassium (mg)	4,908	Vit B_6 (mg)	5.53	Vit E (mg)	17

Note: The food intake in this example meets the needs of a 190 lb (86 kg) athlete with a twice-per-day exercise schedule. Athletes with different weights should adjust food intake amounts. This represents a full-bore workout day, with subsequent diet intake examples reducing both energy expenditure and energy intake to reduce glycogen utilization but to also achieve energy balance. Athletes weighing more or less than this would consume proportionately more or less food, while maintaining the same frequency of intake.

Source: Energy balance and nutrient intake values were derived using NutriTiming®. The energy balance graph is copyrighted by NutriTiming LLC and is used with permission.

Table 6.6 Sample Exercise and Eating Schedule for Competition Minus 1 Day

Energy-balance graph

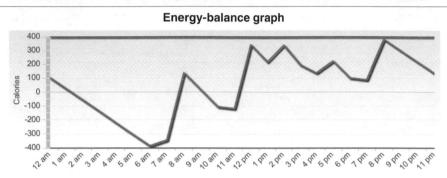

Hours anabolic (calories > 0) = 14; hours catabolic (calories < 0) = 10; anabolic:catabolic ratio = 1.4

Energy Substrate Distribution

Total caloric: 2,562   **Carbohydrate %:** 67   **Protein %:** 19   **Fat %:** 14

Hour	Activity	Food	Amount	Calories
7-8 a.m.	No workout today; orange juice important for sustaining normal blood sugar immediately after waking. Shower and dress.	Orange juice	12 oz (360 ml)	164
8-9 a.m.	Breakfast.	Oatmeal	1 cup	159
		Multigrain bread, toasted	2 slices	138
		Jam	1 tbsp	56
		Blueberries	1 cup	84
		Walnuts	1/2 oz	93
		Milk, 1%	6 oz (180 ml)	76
9-11 a.m.	Relax.	Water	As desired	0
11 a.m.-12 p.m.	Snack.	Banana	1 medium	109
12-1 p.m.	Lunch.	Lean roast beef	3 oz (90 g)	157
		French bread	2 slices	185
		Swiss cheese	1 oz (30 g)	51
		Carrots, baby	1 cup	84
		Pretzels, hard, salted	1 oz (31 g)	106
		Water	As desired	0
1-2 p.m.	Relax.	Water	As desired	0
2-3 p.m.	Snack.	Yogurt, fruited, low fat	1 cup	243
3-5 p.m.	Extremely relaxed walk around neighborhood, sipping on sports beverage every 10 to 15 min.	Sports drink	8 oz (240 ml)	62
5-6 p.m.	Relax, hydration, and carbohydrate snack.	Grapes, red	2 cups	208
		Water	As desired	0

Hour	Activity	Food	Amount	Calories
6-7 p.m.	Relax.	Water	As desired	0
7-8 p.m.	Snack.	Banana	1 medium	109
8-9 p.m.	Dinner.	Potato, baked, no skin	1 medium	145
		Chicken breast, baked	4 oz (120 g)	196
		Zucchini squash	1 cup	51
		Sour cream	1 tbsp	23
		Water	As desired	0
9-10 p.m.	Relaxed activities.	Water	As desired	0
10 p.m.	Sleep.			

Meal totals for selected nutrients

Total kcal	2,562	Iron (mg)	31	Vit C (mg)	305	Vitamin B_{12} (mcg)	4.11
Carbohydrate (g)	441	Calcium (mg)	1,382	Vit B_1 (mg)	2.61	Folic acid (DFE)	743
Protein (g)	127	Zinc (mg)	17	Vit B_2 (mg)	2.84	Vit A (RAE)	2,369
Fat (g)	41	Magnesium (mg)	541	Niacin (mg)	42.54	Vit D (IU)	94
Sodium (mg)	1,946	Potassium (mg)	6,414	Vit B_6 (mg)	5.24	Vit E (mg)	4

Note: The food intake in this example meets the needs of a 190 lb (86 kg) athlete with a twice-per-day exercise schedule. Athletes with different weights should adjust food intake amounts. This represents a full-bore workout day, with subsequent diet intake examples reducing both energy expenditure and energy intake to reduce glycogen utilization but to also achieve energy balance. Athletes weighing more or less than this would consume proportionately more or less food, while maintaining the same frequency of intake.

Source: Energy balance and nutrient intake values were derived using NutriTiming®. The energy balance graph is copyrighted by NutriTiming LLC and is used with permission.

Competition Day

It is particularly important that athletes avoid doing anything they are unaccustomed to doing, or eating anything they are unaccustomed to eating, on the day of an event. Athletes should have a checklist prepared of what is needed and where it is. Competition day is not the time for running around the house screaming, "Where did I put my running shoes!" Leave nothing to chance, and have a backup plan for everything that might go awry (e.g., transportation).

Eating and drinking appropriately on competition day is important, so make certain you have the right foods and drinks immediately available (don't leave it to chance). Take charge of knowing what you need, and take charge of getting it. Imagine drinking sports beverage X during practice all year, then getting up the morning of the competition to discover that your spouse couldn't find sports beverage X at the store, so he bought sports beverage Y instead. Avoid being put in any situation that will cause you stress on competition day.

Early-Morning Competition If the competition is early in the morning, you should get out of bed 2 to 3 hours beforehand. If you have difficulty getting up early in the morning, practice it for several days before the competition. Give yourself enough time to eat some carbohydrate, drink some fluids, and get to the competition. Finish eating at least 1.5 hours before the start of your competition (assuming you are eating mainly starchy carbohydrate foods). Different athletes process foods differently, so knowing the best time differential between eating and the competition is important. Some athletes feel best when they finish eating 2 hours before competition, while others feel best finishing 3 hours before an event. Find out what works best for you, making whatever minor adjustments are needed if you eat with a team. After eating, maintain a sipping protocol on sports beverages for the entire time leading up to the competition. An athlete should not be placed in a position of feeling rushed. When that happens, the food inevitably gets the short end of what should be done, and the athlete suffers, either through poor endurance or GI distress, during the entire competition.

Late-Morning or Early-Afternoon Competition   People often feel tired and hungry in the late morning and early afternoon because the food they ate for breakfast has stopped providing energy by this time. Therefore, it's important for athletes to eat something every 2.5 to 3.5 hours. For an 11:00 a.m. competition, wake up and have breakfast at 6:30 a.m., and eat again at 9:00 a.m. After the 9:00 a.m. meal, initiate your constant fluid-sipping protocol until competition time. For an early-afternoon competition (at 1:00 p.m.), have your last meal at 10:30 a.m., then begin your fluid-sipping protocol. Going into competition hungry is a sure formula for failure.

Midafternoon or Early-Evening Competition   It's difficult to compete in the midafternoon or early evening, especially if it's an outdoor sport and it's hot. Athletes typically go off schedule with a midafternoon competition. The best thing to do is spend the morning eating and drinking as usual (breakfast, midmorning snack, lunch) and then begin the countdown to the competition by having some starchy carbohydrate foods (e.g., a banana, toast, or crackers) and some fluids about 1.5 to 2 hours before the competition starts. The fluid-sipping protocol should then be initiated until competition time. The excitement of the competition can make athletes forget they're hungry. Therefore, it's a good idea to develop a well-rehearsed eating, snacking, and drinking schedule—and stick to it.

Late-Evening Competition   The late evening is also a difficult time to compete; the body wants to sleep, but the competition is keeping it awake. Therefore, sleeping late and eating something every 2.5 to 3 hours will help keep your energy level up until it's time to compete. Keep checking your hydration state (urine should basically be clear). Remember that a successful late-evening competition is sweet and will help you get a good and restful night's sleep.

SEVEN DAY WRAP-UP

The main idea behind getting ready for competition is to set your body up so it has a full tank of both carbohydrate (as glycogen) and fluid. The muscles and psyche should be well rested, and the athlete should be getting clear messages of confidence from the coach. Getting sufficient rest before competition can't be overemphasized. When athletes are involved in sports that require frequent competition, sufficient rest is critical. Anything that keeps you from getting a good night's sleep and being well rested will cause performance difficulties. The keys to good preparation for competition include the following:

1. Get plenty of rest.
2. Begin tapering physical activity 6 or 7 days before competition.

3. Eat enough carbohydrate to maximize glycogen stores.

4. Drink sufficient fluids to maximize fluid stores.

5. Eat frequently, approximately once every 3 hours, to maintain blood glucose and muscle glycogen levels and to feel good.

6. Consume enough energy before activity to ensure there's enough fuel in the system to support the activity and to avoid burning muscle as a fuel.

7. Practice the eating and drinking schedule of your competition day in advance so you know what makes you feel good.

8. Don't do anything on competition day that you haven't practiced doing beforehand.

9. Be ready with everything you'll need (sports beverages, snacks, and so on) long before the competition day arrives.

Both hunger and thirst are emergency sensations marking the onset of performance-reducing problems. As such, they should be avoided through a planned eating and drinking timetable that is integral to an athlete's training schedule and lifestyle. Perhaps no other two factors have the potential for making such an enormous positive impact on health and performance. Put simply, athletes interested in performing up to their conditioned abilities and skill levels should never get hungry and never get thirsty.

IMPORTANT POINTS

• Infrequent eating intervals increase the likelihood that blood glucose will drop, with a resultant increase in the body's creation of glucose to sustain mental function. The amino acid alanine, derived from the breakdown of muscle, is a major substance used to create glucose when blood glucose drops.

• Consuming too much energy in a single meal encourages excess insulin production and excess fat storage. If someone has fewer eating opportunities to deliver the required energy, then they are obligated to eat more at each meal than someone with the same energy requirement but with more eating opportunities.

• Infrequent eating patterns are associated with the loss of lean mass and a higher body-fat percentage. The greater the body fat, the greater the insulin produced, guaranteeing an even larger fat mass.

• Restrained eating triggers hunger, which is associated with stress hormone (cortisol) production, making the loss of lean mass and bone mass more likely.

• An inadequate consumption of fluid, particularly during physical activity, results in dehydration, causing early exercise fatigue and poor performance.

• Physical activity is heat producing, and this heat must be dissipated via sweat production. A failure to remove this excess heat because of poor hydration will lead to heat stress.

• Eating small, frequent meals that dynamically match energy utilization and a liberal intake of fluids with these meals before, during, and after exercise help athletes maintain both energy and fluid balance.

Oxygen Transportation and Utilization

It is difficult to imagine how an athlete could be successful without fully functional mechanisms for pulling in enough oxygen, transporting oxygen through the blood to working cells, using the delivered oxygen efficiently by having sufficient oxidative enzymes in mitochondria, efficiently excreting oxygen by-products (carbon dioxide), and dealing with the side effects of excess oxygen exposure through adequate antioxidant intake. Every one of these functions has an important nutrition component, with iron playing the critical role for oxygen delivery and carbon dioxide removal; vitamins B_{12} and folic acid playing a role in red blood cell formation; and the antioxidant nutrients beta-carotene, vitamin C, vitamin E, and selenium protecting cells from oxidation reactions. Strenuous physical activity, in and of itself, may increase the rate of energy utilization 20 to 100 times above the energy expended in a resting state, and the nutrient–oxygen relationship is a critical factor in ensuring this can continue to happen.[1] This chapter reviews the nutrient relationship in the utilization of oxygen as well as the critical relationship between oxygen, nutrition, and human performance.

OXYGEN UPTAKE

Air is breathed in through the nostrils and mouth before entering the left and right bronchi of the lungs. Gas exchange in the lungs occurs in the 150 million alveoli humans have in each bronchi. The average adult male can inhale approximately 4 liters (close to 4 quarts) of air with each breath, from which the oxygen is diffused into the alveoli, passes into the blood through capillaries, and enters the hemoglobin in red blood cells. At the same time, carbon dioxide in the blood passes to the alveoli and is exhaled. The oxygen content of air is approximately 21 percent, and the oxygen content of expired air is approximately 15 percent, indicating that only a proportion of the oxygen in air is captured by the lungs. The typical water content of air is .5 percent, while the water content of expired air is approximately 6 percent, which clearly explains why rapid respiration is a major route of water loss in athletes.

The rate of cellular respiration increases with exercise intensity, with vigorous high-intensity exercise causing a 25-fold increase in the demand for oxygen in working muscles. This increase in oxygen requirement is satisfied by an increase in the rate and depth of breathing. However, it is the rising rate of carbon dioxide, rather than the higher demand for oxygen, that triggers the increased breathing rate. A higher carbon dioxide level causes the medulla to stimulate the motor nerves controlling the intercostal and diaphragm muscles to increase their activity. Diseases that affect the lungs, such as pneumonia, asthma, emphysema, bronchitis, chronic obstructive pulmonary disease, and lung cancer, compromise a person's ability to obtain sufficient oxygen and excrete sufficient carbon dioxide.

Exercise-Induced Asthma

Exercise-induced asthma (EIA) compromises an athlete's ability to inspire oxygen. The prevalence of EIA in athletes ranges from a low of 12 percent in basketball players to a high of 55 percent in cross-country skiers.[2,3] Athletes involved in cold-weather or cold-environment sports appear to have a higher prevalence of EIA, and it may occur in people who do not suffer from chronic asthma, with symptoms (including coughing, wheezing, tight chest, shortness of breath, and early fatigue) beginning within 5 to 20 minutes after the initiation of exercise.[4] Symptoms are most obvious immediately after stopping exercise and usually dissipate within an hour. The underlying cause of asthma-related chronic lung inflammation is unknown, but there does appear to be a genetic component (i.e., a family history), and some people are born with a predisposition to develop the condition. A trigger is required to cause asthma, and in EIA the trigger appears to be a large volume of cold and dry air moved into the lungs; mouth breathing during exercise in cold and dry environments may also play a factor. Because of this, sports requiring continuous activity with faster breathing (i.e., endurance sports), especially in cold weather, are most likely to induce EIA. The chlorine in pools may also trigger EIA.[5]

Oxygen Delivery and Cellular Utilization

Several elements, vitamins, and protein carriers are involved, as a primary function, in the delivery and cellular utilization of oxygen. These elements work in unison to capture oxygen from the environment, transport oxygen through the blood to cells for metabolic actions, and remove the by-products (including carbon dioxide) of the oxygen-related metabolic activities.

Iron Iron is a critical element in the delivery of oxygen to working tissues. It is part of red blood cell hemoglobin, muscle myoglobin, and enzymes involved in electron transfer for energy metabolism. The body uses a priority-based system for iron, with hemoglobin at the top of the priority system. If stores of iron become sufficiently low to cause hemoglobin to drop, iron in myoglobin and iron-containing enzymes are scavenged to maintain red blood cell hemoglobin. Because of this, it is possible for an athlete to experience a reduction in performance even if hemoglobin and hematocrit (the two most common measures of iron status) appear to be in the normal range. It is important, therefore, that ferritin (stored iron) also be measured as a normal component of a blood test intended to screen for iron status (see table 7.1).

Table 7.1 Terms Related to Iron Status

Ferritin	Ferritin is an iron-storage protein found in the liver, spleen, and bone marrow, with only a small amount in the blood. The amount in the blood is thought to be proportionate to the amount stored in the liver, spleen, and bone marrow, so a blood ferritin test is an indicator of the amount of stored iron. The lower the ferritin level, even within the normal range, the more likely a patient is iron deficient. Athletes should include a ferritin measure with all blood tests intended to assess iron deficiency or iron-deficiency anemia. Normal ferritin values: • Adult males: 20 to 300 ng/ml • Adult females: 20 to 120 ng/ml **Note:** ng/ml = nanograms per milliliter
Hematocrit	Hematocrit is the proportion of whole blood that is composed of red blood cells; it is often referred to as the number of red blood cells per unit of blood. Normal hematocrit values: • Adult males: 42 to 52% • Adult females: 36 to 48%
Hemochromatosis	Hemochromatosis is an iron-overload disease caused by uninhibited iron absorption. It can result in liver damage if the iron concentration is not lowered.
Hemoglobin	Hemoglobin is the iron-containing, oxygen-carrying protein in red blood cells.
Hemosiderosis	Hemosiderosis is a disease condition that results from excess iron in the body, often from blood transfusions. It is often seen in persons with thalassemia.
Serum iron	Serum iron represents the total amount of iron in the blood serum. Normal serum iron values: • Adult males: 75 to 175 mcg/dl • Adult females: 65 to 165 mcg/dl
Total iron binding capacity (TIBC)	The TIBC test measures the amount of iron the blood could carry if transferrin were fully saturated with iron molecules. Since transferrin is produced by the liver, the TIBC can be used to monitor liver function and protein-status nutrition.
Transferrin	The transferrin test is a direct measurement of the protein transferrin (also called siderophilin) in the blood. The saturation level of transferrin can be calculated by dividing the serum iron level by TIBC. Normal transferrin values: • Adult males: 200 to 400 mg/dl • Adult females: 200 to 400 mg/dl Normal transferrin saturation values are between 30 and 40%.

A typical iron-deficiency anemia is microcytic (small cell) and hypochromic (red blood cells are light in color). It is characterized by an inadequate number of red blood cells and existing cells that are smaller than normal due to low hemoglobin levels.

Transferrin   Transferrin is a blood protein that carries iron through the blood to the bone marrow, spleen, and liver for either the storage of iron as ferritin or the manufacture of new red blood cells. It is a protein with a relatively short half-life that can be a marker for recent protein status, and it is used for this purpose. Low blood transferrin may be an indicator of protein or calorie malnutrition, resulting in inadequate synthesis of transferrin by the liver, or it can result from excess protein loss through the kidneys (proteinuria). A systemic infection or cancer can also lower the blood transferrin level. A high blood transferrin is a marker of iron deficiency. If an athlete has a low blood transferrin level, the production of hemoglobin can be impaired and can lead to anemia, even if there is ample iron in the body.

Ceruloplasmin   Ceruloplasmin is a copper-containing protein involved in transporting iron from transferrin to hemoglobin in the formation of new red blood cells, or in removing iron from old red blood cells for inclusion in new ones. A copper deficiency results in low ceruloplasmin and can lead to anemia that appears similar to iron-deficiency (microcytic, hypochromic) anemia, possibly leading to a misdiagnosis. A ceruloplasmin deficiency may result in iron accumulation in the pancreas, liver, and brain, resulting in neurological disorders.

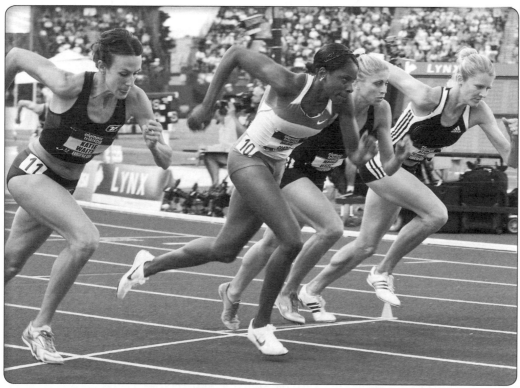

© Human Kinetics

Nutrient deficiencies can inhibit oxygen delivery to cells, which will impair an athlete's performance.

Vitamin B$_{12}$ Vitamin B$_{12}$ is a cobalt-containing vitamin that is also referred to as cobalamin. Two of its primary functions are the formation of red blood cells and the preservation of a healthy nervous system. The absence of vitamin B$_{12}$ when red blood cells are being formed results in cells that have a weak membrane. These cells, called megaloblasts, are fragile and live approximately half as long as a normal red blood cell (60 days versus 120 days). The shortened life of these cells requires a constantly faster production of red cells to maintain normal oxygen-carrying capacity. However, this fast level of red cell production cannot be maintained, eventually resulting in anemia. The anemia resulting from vitamin B$_{12}$ deficiency is referred to as pernicious anemia because it develops slowly over several years. Pernicious anemia is a megaloblastic, hypochromic anemia, meaning the red blood cells are large and misshapen and are low in color (the hemoglobin is spread out over a larger cell area, diluting the color). Besides the reduced oxygen-carrying capacity from the anemia, pernicious anemia is associated with neurological symptoms and nerve degeneration. Although only a small amount of vitamin B$_{12}$ is needed to avoid anemia (the amount in one egg is likely to be sufficient for more than a month), vegetarian athletes are considered at risk of deficiency because it is derived almost exclusively from meat sources.

Folic Acid   Folic acid, vitamin B$_{12}$, and vitamin C are all involved in protein metabolism. In conjunction with vitamin B$_{12}$, folate is needed for the production of red blood cells. Folate is also involved in nerve tissue development, and in females with good folate status, it is known to nearly eliminate the risk of neural tube defects in newborns. The anemia associated with inadequate folate is similar to that produced by a deficiency of vitamin B$_{12}$ (megaloblastic, hypochromic anemia), and the reduced oxygen-carrying capacity that results is equally severe. However, although vitamin B$_{12}$ is obtained primarily from animal sources, folic acid is best obtained from fresh fruits, fresh vegetables, and legumes.

The Oxygen-Nutrient Performance Relationship

There is no question that physical activity can alter blood-iron status and that blood-iron status can also alter physical activity performance. One study assessing 747 athletes and 104 untrained controls found that endurance athletes had lower hemoglobin and hematocrit levels than either power- or mixed-trained athletes, suggesting the difference may be due to dilutional pseudoanemia and, perhaps, a greater degree of foot-strike hemolysis.[6]

Athletes with higher exercise durations and workloads also appear to store less iron (ferritin). These findings imply that athletes are indeed at higher risk of compromised iron status than are nonathletes, and higher exercise durations within the athlete pool create even greater iron-status risk. Endurance athletes who put in large numbers of training hours (and miles) are therefore at highest risk of poor iron status even though they rely most on aerobic metabolic processes to achieve their endurance.

Restrictive intakes, as are common among athletes involved in weight-classification or aesthetic sports, almost always supply inadequate levels of vitamins and minerals. There is real risk, therefore, that a significant proportion of the athlete population has less than optimal oxygen-utilization capacity—a fact that surely inhibits optimal performance. Iron deficiency, even without anemia, reduces muscle work potential, and iron-deficiency anemia makes matters worse because of a further reduction in oxygen-carrying capacity.

Iron-deficiency anemia is likely to be more prevalent among athletes (particularly female athletes) than among nonathlete groups.[7] The effects include reduced athletic performance and impaired immune function. Young female athletes should consider either consuming more iron-rich foods (particularly red meats) or taking iron supplements under the supervision of a doctor.

Iron deficiency occurs in athletes for many reasons, including inadequate intake, hemolysis, and menstrual blood loss in females.[8] However, the most common iron problem in athletes is caused not by blood loss but by an enlargement of the blood volume without a concomitant increase in the constituents of the blood, including red blood cells. This is likely to occur when athletes add more intensity to an existing exercise program or when they are at the beginning of a training season. Because the blood volume increases at a faster rate than the red blood cells, it appears as if these athletes have anemia. Since this condition is transient (eventually the concentration of red cells becomes normal), it is referred to as a dilutional pseudoanemia (also known as sports anemia or athletic anemia; see figure 7.1). Repeated foot strike associated with running causes red blood cells to break down and is referred to as foot-strike hemolysis. Red cells circulating in capillaries through the bottom of the feet are crushed by the foot strike. The faster the rate of red blood cell breakdown from foot-strike hemolysis, the more difficult it is for athletes to maintain a normal concentration of red blood cells because their bodies can't make the red blood cells fast enough, resulting in anemia.

The underconsumption of other nutrients may also affect oxygen utilization. Magnesium deficiency increases oxygen requirements needed to perform submaximal exercise, thereby reducing endurance performance.[9] Folate and vitamin B_{12} deficiencies result in megaloblastic anemia, a condition that results in malformed red blood cells with a reduced life expectancy.

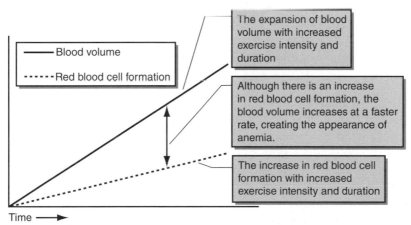

Note: The differential in blood volume and red cell concentration becomes noticeable after 3 to 5 days of an increase in exercise duration or intensity. After a period of time, blood volume ceases to increase and red cell production catches up, removing the appearance of anemia.

Figure 7.1   Dilutional pseudoanemia (also called *sports anemia*).

This reduced functional duration makes it difficult for athletes to constantly manufacture red cells, which are also being destroyed through foot-strike hemolysis. The result is fewer cells that can carry oxygen and remove carbon dioxide, a sure formula for poor athletic performance. Data from past studies indicate a higher prevalence of hematuria (i.e., blood in the urine) in athletes, with multiple causes that include the following:[10]

- Foot-strike hemolysis—the break-down of red blood cells from the sudden compression of capillaries caused by foot strike and other concussive movements.
- Renal ischemia—poor blood flow to the kidneys, likely a result of dehydration-related low blood volume.
- Hypoxic kidney damage—damage caused by poor oxygen delivery to the kidneys, possibly resulting from iron deficiency anemia or renal ischemia.
- Release of a hemolyzing factor—increased breakdown of red blood cells from any of a number of factors, including bacteria, parasites, sickle-cell disease, and, in athletes, an acidification of the blood pH.
- Bladder or kidney trauma that may be caused by hits in concussive sports such as football or boxing or in other physical activity.
- Nonsteroidal anti-inflammatory drug (NSAIDs) intake may cause subtle transient changes in kidney function, allowing blood to be released into the urine.
- Dehydration—reduced blood flow to the kidneys as a result of dehydration is causally related to both hypoxic kidney damage and renal ischemia, described earlier in this list.
- Increased circulation rate—higher blood velocity, as caused by faster heart rates and higher cardiac stroke volumes increase red blood cell breakdown.
- Myoglobinuria release (referred to as *rhabdomyolysis*)—exercise may result in muscle breakdown and the release of the iron-containing myoglobin molecule, which is released by the kidneys into urine. Excess myoglobin release from a high level of muscle breakdown is associated with renal obstruction and dysfunction.
- Peroxidation of red blood cells, which occurs when the lipid membrane of red blood cells become oxidized, resulting in the breakdown of the cell and removal of the cell via the kidneys.

A chronic loss of red blood cells in the urine, a condition brought on by frequent high-intensity and long-duration practice sessions, would contribute to anemia, a problem that reduces competitiveness in any athlete. Athletes should be careful, therefore, to take in sufficient nutrients (particularly iron) to replace what is lost. Luckily, the erythropoietic process (production of new red blood cells) appears to be remarkably resilient in the face of exercise stress; it is capable of producing a large and adequate number of red blood cells provided a sufficient nutrient base (in particular iron, folate, and vitamin B_{12}) is available.[11] Some athletes try to enhance erythropoiesis by taking erythropoietin (EPO), but this blood-doping technique is illegal and has the potential for increasing blood viscosity, with subsequent thrombosis and potentially fatal results.[12]

OXIDATIVE STRESS

Oxidative stress refers to the creation of an increased volume of reactive oxygen species (ROS) because of an inadequate presence of antioxidants.[13] Also referred to as peroxides and free radicals, ROS cause damage to cells because their radical movement inside cells destroys them, producing "clinkers" (dead cells). The body inhibits ROS production through antioxidant vitamins and minerals (see table 7.2). The minerals work to regulate enzyme activity so as to diminish ROS production, while vitamins accept ROS to remove them from the cellular environment, thereby limiting their potential hazards. Early studies of vitamin E, a fat-soluble antioxidant vitamin found mainly in vegetable oils, initially showed promise in reducing ROS. However, there has been a recent concern that vitamin E supplementation, by itself, may place the pool of antioxidants out of balance, thereby diminishing the overall defenses humans have to prevent ROS. A proposed strategy to prevent this imbalance is to regularly consume a cocktail of antioxidants from foods rather than a single antioxidant vitamin supplement. In doing so, the sensitive balance between the antioxidants can remain intact while there is an increase in antioxidant presence to provide an improved defense against ROS.

Table 7.2 Antioxidant Nutrients

| Nutrient | Daily recommended intake (age 19 to 30) | | Functions |
	Male	Female	
Vitamin C	90 mg/day	75 mg/day	Vitamin C scavenges reactive oxidants in leukocytes and in lung and gastric mucosa, and it reduces lipid peroxidation in cells.
Vitamin E	15 mg/day	15 mg/day	Vitamin E mainly prevents the peroxidation of lipids.
Selenium	55 mcg/day	55 mcg/day	Selenium functions through selenoproteins, which form oxidant defense enzymes. The DRI is based on the amount needed to synthesize selenoprotein glutathione peroxidase.
Beta-carotene	(900 mcg/day)	(700 mcg/day)	12 mcg of beta-carotene can form 1 mcg of retinol (vitamin A). The human nutrient requirement is for vitamin A, not beta-carotene. However, there is no question that beta-carotene is more than just a precursor to the production of vitamin A. Besides being an important biomarker for the intake of fresh fruits and vegetables, it has important antioxidant properties.

Nutrient imbalances can also cause difficulties with immune function. Excess vitamin E can negatively affect the immune system, but inadequate levels of this vitamin, iron, selenium, zinc, calcium, and magnesium can also create immune problems.[14] All this information points to the importance of maintaining a balance of all the nutrients rather than pushing one or two with the hope of inducing a desirable biochemical effect.

Oxidative metabolic processes are constantly working, even during events that are primarily anaerobic. The anaerobic athlete who just completed a 10-second high-intensity sprint has something in common with a gymnast who just completed a 90-second floor routine: the need to breathe a large volume of air (oxygen) to recharge the fuels they will need for the next bout of high-intensity exercise. Iron is a primary element for transporting oxygen to working tissues and carbon dioxide away from working tissues—it is a critical nutrient for athletes. Nevertheless, iron is the most common nutrient deficiency, and athletes may be at even greater risk for iron deficiency than the general public because of the hemolysis and hematuria commonly experienced. Other nutrients are also important to ensure a healthy red blood cell production (vitamin B_{12} and folate) and to ensure all the oxygen brought into the system will not be damaging (the antioxidant nutrients beta-carotene, selenium, vitamin C, and vitamin E).

Oxygen is sufficiently important for athletic performance that athletes of all sizes, sports, and ages should regularly check their iron status via a blood test that measures hemoglobin, hematocrit, and ferritin. Only with the information from such a test will athletes know if they should alter food intake or consume iron or other supplements to ensure that oxygen will not be a negative factor in performance.

IMPORTANT POINTS

• Iron is critically important for oxygen delivery, but iron deficiency is the most prevalent of the nutrition deficiencies. Women of childbearing age and vegans are at highest risk of developing iron deficiency.

• Normal athletic activities can increase iron-deficiency anemia risk from a faster destruction of red blood cells or an increased loss of red blood cells via the urine and sweat. As a result, athletes should get periodically tested to determine if they are anemic. Athletes whose tests indicate a deficiency should seek the advice and supervision of a physician for the best route of corrective action. This typically involves assessment of hemoglobin, hematocrit, and ferritin. Importantly, the cause of the deficiency (e.g., inadequate intake, poor absorption, increased losses) should be determined.

• Vitamins B_{12} and folate are important in the formation of red blood cells, deficiencies of which can result in anemia and lower oxygen delivery.

• Studies have shown that athletes may be under higher oxidative stress than nonathletes, suggesting it is important to consume adequate amounts of the antioxidant vitamins and minerals. However, athletes should be cautious of overconsuming these antioxidant nutrients because an excess intake may inhibit normal antioxidant processes.

Strategies for Anti-Inflammation and Muscular Health

Experienced by virtually all athletes, muscle soreness is associated with a lower range of motion and reduced muscular strength and therefore has a negative impact on performance.[1,2] Athletes feel an indistinct aching muscular pain, and the affected muscle feels stiff and tender, but mainly only when the muscle is used. Because muscle soreness reaches its peak about 24 to 48 hours after exercise, it is commonly referred to as delayed-onset muscle soreness, or DOMS. Typically, DOMS has a duration of 2 to 4 days and is considered a minor muscle strain injury that may be associated with microtears of the affected muscle.[3-5] The related pain is thought to be most associated with eccentric muscular motion, which has the effect of stretching the muscle with contraction.[6] (Imagine how sore your thigh muscles can become after running downhill for a long distance.) This lengthening muscle action is more likely to result in muscle damage and the associated muscle inflammation and pain. DOMS is also more likely to occur with unfamiliar activity, so athletes who frequently do familiar eccentric activities will adapt and reduce the likelihood and severity of DOMS. The resultant muscle damage creates more production of reactive oxygen species (ROS) and poor use of the high-energy compound adenosine triphosphate (ATP), the latter of which is the likely cause of DOMS-associated muscle weakness.[7,8]

DIETARY INTAKE AND DOMS

There is limited evidence that certain nutrients or nutritional supplements affect DOMS. The nutrients and supplements that have been assessed include L-carnitine, antioxidants (vitamin C and vitamin E, individually and in combination), flavonoids, branched-chain amino acids, protein, omega-3 fatty acids, and vitamin D. Fish oil, which is high in the omega-3 fatty acids eicosapentaenoic acid (EPA) and docosahexaenoic acid (DHA), has been found to reduce the joint inflammation of rheumatoid arthritis, and some studies were performed on the theory that these oils may also buffer the inflammatory response of intense exercise.[9, 10] A review of the literature confirms two things: (1) The studies are scant, and (2) where evidence exists for an association with DOMS, the evidence is weak (see table 8.1).

In addition, although some studies (not many) have assessed food intakes with the tested supplements that deliver these nutrients, they have not assessed how the nutrient delivery (i.e., all at once or spread out evenly in smaller units during the day, or before or after exercise) may affect DOMS.

Table 8.1 Summary of Findings on Nutrient Associations With Muscle Soreness

Variable	Evidence for effect*	Nutrient
Cytoskeleton disruption	None	
MRI-assessed tissue disruption	Weak	L-carnitine (2 g/day)
Muscle force	Weak	Vitamin C (ascorbic acid) (500 mg/day) + vitamin E (tocopherol) (1,200 IU/day)
Interleukin 6 (IL-6) C-reactive protein (CRP)	Weak	Mixed tocopherols, DHA, flavonoids (combination)
Delayed onset muscle soreness (DOMS)	Weak	Vitamin C (1-3 g/day)
	Weak	Vitamin E (400 IU/day) (in combination with vitamin C)
	Weak	Branched chain amino acids (BCAAs) (5 g/day)—women only
	Weak	L-carnitine (2 g/day)
Creatine kinase (CK) Lactate dehydrogenase (LDH)	Weak	Vitamin E (400-1,200 IU/day)
	Weak	Vitamin C (1-3 g/day)
	Weak	Beta-hydroxy beta-methylbutyric acid (HMB) (1.5-3 g/day)
	Weak	L-carnitine (2 g/day)
Girth	None	
Range of motion (ROM)	None	
3-Methylhistidine (3-MH)	Weak	Beta-hydroxy beta-methylbutyric acid (HMB) (1.5-3 g/day)

*Strength of evidence is based on outcome as well as the number of studies demonstrating a benefit. If there is evidence for an effect in 1 or 2 studies for a given variable, the effect is listed as weak. If there is evidence for an effect in 3 to 5 studies for a given variable, the effect is listed as moderate. If there is evidence for an effect in more than 5 studies for a given variable, the effect is listed as strong.

Adapted, by permission, from R.J. Bloomer, 2007, "The role of nutritional supplements in the prevention and treatment of resistance exercise-induced skeletal muscle injury," *Sports Medicine* 37(6): 519-532.

Omega-3 Fatty Acids

Omega-3 fatty acids may reduce DOMS because they work both as antioxidant and anti-inflammatory agents. Other supplements, such as vitamins E and C, function as potent antioxidants but have no specific anti-inflammatory action. Omega-3 fatty acids may reduce inflammation by competing with arachidonic acid for eicosanoid generation, which stimulates a greater production of anti-inflammatory agents. The proposed effect of omega-3 fatty acids is that they become part of cellular membranes and alter the release of these inflammatory agents, including 2-series prostaglandins, thromboxanes, and prostacyclins. It is possible, therefore, that this anti-inflammatory effect could contribute to a reduction in DOMS.

A study evaluated 27 male subjects (mean age 33.4 years), who were assessed for perceived pain after omega-3 fatty acid supplementation and eccentric exercise.[11] Subjects consumed a fish oil capsule containing 324 milligrams of eicosapentaenoic acid (EPA) and 216 milligrams of docosahexaenoic acid (DHA) once per day for 30 days preexercise and for two days postexercise. The subjects also consumed a supplement containing 100 IU of d-alpha-tocopherol acetate (i.e., vitamin E) in addition to the omega-3 capsule, but the administration frequency of the vitamin E was not described. The group taking the omega-3 fatty acids had significantly better (i.e., lower) pain scores 48 hours after eccentric exercise but not at 24 hours postexercise. Thigh circumference was used as a marker of inflammation (higher circumference is associated with inflammation-associated swelling) and was significantly smaller in the omega-3 group at both 24 hours and 48 hours after eccentric exercise. It is possible that the addition of vitamin E (a potent antioxidant) could have contributed to the DOMS reduction by reducing ROS, but the effect of vitamin E is inconclusive.

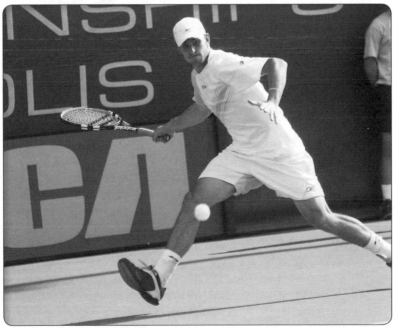

© Human Kinetics

Eating foods high in omega-3 fatty acids may reduce DOMS, but nothing is likely to trump food conditioning.

Another study assessing the effect of omega-3 fatty acids on DOMS was performed on 10 untrained males (average age 22.7 years) and 6 untrained females (average age 24.5 years).[1] Subjects were organized into three supplement groups: (1) a fish oil group (fish oil is an excellent source of omega-3 fatty acids), (2) an isoflavone group receiving a combination of soy isolate and a *non*-omega-3-rich fat blend, and (3) a placebo group receiving the non-omega-3-rich fat blend plus wheat flour. All groups were supplemented 30 days before and during the week of the exercise intervention. The subjects also received 100 IU of vitamin E to help lower fat oxidation. After 30 days of supplementation, the subjects performed eccentric exercise to induce muscle soreness, which was measured 2, 4, and 7 days after the eccentric exercise. There was a significant increase in serum EPA and DHA in the omega-3 fatty acid (i.e., fish oil) group, but there were no significant differences in DOMS level between any of the groups.

A study assessing the effect of fish oil and isoflavones on DOMS found significant increases in pain and arm circumference in all groups, regardless of fish oil and isoflavone consumption.[10] This study randomly selected 22 subjects into 3 different groups: fish oil supplement, isoflavone supplement, or placebo. All groups received the intervention substance plus 100 IU of vitamin E (to reduce the possibility of lipid peroxidation) for 30 days prior to the eccentric exercise. The authors concluded that the intervention substances had no effect on reducing DOMS.

The bottom line: These studies suggest there may be a minor reduction in DOMS, given the right mix of the following variables:

- Specific types of activity (eccentric)
- Specific nutrient mix (omega-3 fatty acids plus vitamin E)
- Gender (muscle damage is similar between genders, yet the inflammatory response is not as great in women compared to men.[12])
- Period of time supplement is provided (needs to be long enough before the eccentric activity)

Given these results, it seems prudent to suggest that athletes regularly consume foods that are good sources of omega-3 fatty acids and vitamin E, but that supplementation of these substances is not likely to reduce exercise-associated pain. These foods include fresh vegetables, fish, and flax.

Vitamin D

The eicosapentaenoic acid (EPA) and docosahexaenoic acid (DHA) used to supplement subjects with omega-3 fatty acids are mainly from cold-water fatty fish. These same fish are also excellent sources of vitamin D, making it possible that vitamin D or the combination of vitamin D with EPA and DHA is at least partially responsible for any soreness reduction attributed to omega-3 fatty acids. It is also possible that vitamin D alone is the nutrition factor associated with DOMS. In a study of native Australians with chronic muscle pain and vitamin D deficiency,[13] eight age- and gender-matched pairs were selected, with one person from each pair complaining of muscle pain and the other without muscle pain. Using blood tests to determine the presence of vitamin D deficiency, it was found that *all* the subjects who had lower serum vitamin D were the ones experiencing muscle pain, while none of the subjects with normal serum vitamin D values were experiencing pain.

Decreased muscular strength may also be associated with vitamin D deficiency. Another study assessed 976 elderly subjects who were diagnosed with vitamin D deficiency, insufficiency, or normal vitamin D status.[14] Using two sessions with a handgrip dynamometer, the study found that vitamin D status was significantly associated with handgrip scores (the higher the score, the better the vitamin D status). Since both decreased muscular strength and increased muscle soreness are features of DOMS, it is conceivable that vitamin D status could either ameliorate or magnify DOMS. The bottom line: Athletes who do much of their sport indoors (e.g., gymnasts, figure skaters, basketball players), thereby inhibiting the formation of vitamin D from sunlight exposure, should seriously consider having a serum vitamin D test to determine vitamin D status. Vitamin D supplementation would seem like a prudent strategy to reduce DOMS, but only for those athletes who have low serum vitamin D.

Vitamin E

At least two studies assessing omega-3 fatty acid supplementation and DOMS used products that also contained tocopherols (vitamin E).[10,11] The studies concluded that the vitamin E impact on DOMS was either inconclusive or not important. However, since vitamin E is a potent antioxidant, it has the potential to inhibit oxygen-mediated cellular damage that results from exercise-induced muscle damage. One study examined the antioxidant effects of vitamin E and also tested its anti-inflammatory impact. Male college students were organized into a vitamin E supplement and placebo group, with the vitamin E group taking 800 IU of d-alpha-tocopherol acetate once per day for 14 days preexercise and 7 days postexercise.[15] Those taking vitamin E supplements reported significantly lower muscle soreness scores than the placebo group 2, 4, and 7 days after the eccentric exercise regimen. The vitamin E group also had significantly lower oxidative damage than the placebo group on days 4 and 7. Despite these findings, there was no evidence that consuming the supplemental vitamin E resulted in less inflammation. The bottom line: Athletes should be wary of taking supplemental vitamin E because it could blunt the body's normal protective antioxidant mechanisms (see the information on vitamin E in chapter 2). However, if athletes fail to satisfactorily consume foods that contain vitamin E (mainly vegetable oils and fresh vegetables), an occasional mild supplemental intake may reduce DOMS severity.

Vitamin C

The effect of vitamin C on DOMS remains unclear. In a study examining vitamin C supplementation on 18 untrained men (mean age 23 years), the subjects were organized into a vitamin C supplementation group (3 grams L-ascorbate) and a placebo group.[16] The supplementation period was 2 weeks before and 4 days after the eccentric exercise intervention. The pain scores of the supplemented group were significantly lower 24 hours after the eccentric exercise than the scores reported by the placebo group. To ensure the total vitamin C intake was understood, this study used a dietary recall to make certain diet did not create an unknown intake of either vitamin C or vitamin E (antioxidants that work together). Another study assessed 24 untrained male and female subjects who were divided evenly into placebo and supplemented groups, with the supplemented group receiving 3 grams of vitamin C per day for 3 days before the eccentric exercise intervention and 5 days afterward.[17] There were no differences found between the supplemented group and the placebo group on muscle soreness. The bottom line: It appears from these studies that the length of time taking a supplement is an important factor in its potential effectiveness. However, it must be understood that 3 grams (i.e., 3,000 milligrams) of vitamin C is a huge dose that is more than 300 times the dietary reference intake. There should be a clear understanding of the potential hazards of regularly taking such a large dose (e.g., higher kidney stone risk; decreased cellular sensitivity to the vitamin) before an athlete tries to reduce DOMS through such a protocol.

Branched-Chain Amino Acids

Branched-chain amino acids (BCAAs) are essential amino acids (i.e., they must be consumed in the diet because we are incapable of synthesizing them) that can be oxidized in skeletal muscle. This oxidation is promoted by exercise, giving rationale to supplementing the diet with BCAAs to replace those lost. Without adequate replacement of BCAAs before and after exercise, exercise-induced muscle damage may occur and muscle-protein synthesis may be inhibited.[18] A study assessed BCAA supplementation and its effect on DOMS using 30 untrained men and women, aged 21 to 24. Fifteen minutes before the eccentric exercise protocol, subjects consumed a solution containing 5 grams of BCAAs, 1 gram of green tea, and 1.2 grams of sugar substitute.[19] (The green tea and sugar substitute were used to mask the taste of the BCAAs.) The female subjects recorded soreness scores that were significantly lower after consuming the BCAAs at 24, 48, and 72 hours. The male subjects, however, did not experience a benefit, perhaps because the amount of BCAAs provided was fixed rather than standardized by weight. The bottom line: It appears the one-size-fits-all paradigm does not work with BCAAs and that the dosage may need to be linked to body mass. That said, it also appears that even a small amount of BCAAs (5 grams = 20 calories) is sufficient to produce a benefit for females, so 10 grams may be a sufficiently high dose for males. This could easily be provided by a high-quality supplement, such as whey protein isolate, added to a carbohydrate beverage before and after activity.

Protein Intake

Exercise often results in muscle damage, particularly if it is unfamiliar eccentric exercise. The muscle damage is associated with muscle protein breakdown and depletion of muscle glycogen stores. These outcomes suggest that exercisers have an increased need for dietary protein, particularly at the beginning of a new training program that may include a large amount of strength training.[20] However, since the maximal rate of protein utilization appears to be about 1.5 grams per kilogram of body weight (an amount about double the reference intake for nonathletes), only a subtle change in diet would be needed to achieve this level of intake. In fact, most people (athletes and nonathletes alike) already consume protein at a level at or above the recommendation for athletes. A study of collegiate female athletes assessed the effects of whey and casein protein consumption and found that a resistance training program with pre- and postexercise protein supplementation is able to induce positive changes in both performance and body composition.[21] Chocolate milk is a useful beverage for recovering more quickly from exercise, perhaps because it has a combination of carbohydrate and high-quality protein that enables faster cellular return to normalcy.[22,23] The bottom line: Even a small amount of well-targeted and high-quality protein can make a difference in reducing muscle soreness and improving performance. In general, the protein studies suggest it is far better to sustain the amino acid pool through frequent delivery of small amounts of protein (about 30 grams per meal) than through large single supplemental doses.

Fluid Intake

Dehydration has for many years been associated with higher muscle soreness. In a study examining the effect of dehydration on DOMS in 10 untrained men (mean age 21 years), subjects were organized into a well-hydrated and dehydrated group before physical activity. DOMS was present in both groups, but the muscle soreness in the dehydrated group was significantly (44 percent) higher than in the well-hydrated group.[1] The bottom line: There are many reasons to try to stay well hydrated, and muscle soreness is one of them. Remember that *the solution to pollution is dilution.* Having a larger fluid pool allows the metabolic by-products produced during exercise to be diluted and, therefore, have a lower impact on working muscles.

Studies suggest differences in the amount and frequency of alcohol consumption among different sports teams and between male and female athletes, but heavy alcohol consumption is common, particularly at social events, regardless of sport or gender.[24,25] Although alcohol is a potential source of energy (7 calories per gram), it also behaves as an antinutrient by inhibiting the conversion of B vitamins to their active coenzymes, which are involved in the derivation of energy from carbohydrate, protein, and fat. Studies have found that alcohol consumption, depending on frequency and volume, may have an impact on the cardiovascular system, energy metabolism, muscle damage and recovery, thermoregulatory mechanisms, and neuromuscular function, all of which may affect performance.[26,27] At relatively high doses, alcohol affects the central nervous system, resulting in reduced motor skill functions, lower cognitive function, and behavioral changes, all of which impede the athletic endeavor. To make matters worse, these effects may be long lasting, having a measurable effect for hours or days after alcohol intoxication.

Alcohol appears most likely to affect sports performance through alterations in glycogen metabolism and storage and through changes in hydration and thermoregulatory function. The resynthesis of glycogen stores in the liver and muscle is dramatically inhibited by alcohol consumption; it takes up to twice as long to replace glycogen stores in athletes who have consumed alcohol compared with athletes who have not.[28] Alcohol is a potent diuretic that can seriously compromise hydration state. Drinks containing 4 percent alcohol tend to also significantly delay the recovery process by promoting an increase in urinary fluid loss.[29] Dehydration and poor glycogen storage are both associated with inflammation and muscle function. Therefore, the performance-compromising effects associated with alcohol consumption should be considered by all athletes who wish to perform optimally.

IMPORTANT POINTS

Our current state of understanding of the impact of nutrients on muscle soreness can be summarized by five points:[30]

• There is limited evidence for an effect with vitamin C taken alone and also in conjunction with vitamin E. There is also limited evidence for flavonoids when taken with tocopherols and docosahexaenoate and for HMB in untrained people.

• Nutritional supplements are not useful for eliminating muscle injury, but they *may* be useful in reducing certain signs and symptoms of muscle injury, including pain.

• If nutritional supplements are used, it seems they must be consumed for days or weeks before the exercise stress for them to have any hope of effectiveness. However, the optimal pretreatment period is unknown and may be different for each nutrient.

• The optimal dosage of nutrients to reduce muscle injury and soreness is unknown because different doses have not been assessed. In addition, few studies have evaluated food consumption to determine if food delivery of a nutrient may have skewed total nutrient intake, further complicating our understanding of what constitutes the optimal nutrient delivery dosage.

• The reduction in muscle injury and associated soreness that *may* occur with targeted nutrient intake appears to be most appropriately generalized to non-resistance-trained persons. Resistance-trained persons already have adapted to the activity most associated with DOMS and are, therefore, already more DOMS resistant.

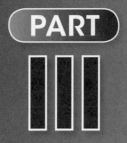

PART

III

Factors Affecting Nutrition Needs

Travel

Whether traveling for pleasure or competition, serious athletes should try to maintain a regular training and eating regimen. Regardless of where in the world athletes find themselves, it is important that they follow certain key principles that will help them adapt more quickly to their new environments, reduce the nutrition stresses associated with eating in a nonfamiliar setting, and adjust their circadian rhythms to the local time zone. Only a few scientific studies have addressed this issue, but there are many well-tested practical strategies that athletes can follow to avoid the performance problems associated with jet lag, food intolerance, consumption of unsafe diarrhea-causing foods, and dehydration. This chapter focuses on useful strategies for reducing the potentially negative impact of travel on performance.

Serious athletes inevitably find themselves competing away from home, often in locations with unfamiliar foods. Regardless of the distance traveled, planning ahead is essential to ensure the final performance matches the athlete's trained capabilities. Sadly, few athletes and their coaches take the necessary steps to minimize the negative physical and psychological impact of traveling long distances. Perhaps it is because many athletes and coaches believe that home advantage consists of nonmodifiable factors, and the impact of travel is relatively unimportant compared with site familiarity and officials' bias.[1] Others believe, however, that part of the home advantage includes the impact of travel, particularly if the team or individual athletes must cross multiple time zones without sufficient time to adapt.[2]

Creating a plan that ensures the availability of the right kinds of foods and fluids at the right time is critical when competing at home, and it is no less critical when competing away from home. Perhaps the biggest mistake athletes can make when traveling to a competition is to assume that what they need to eat and drink will be there waiting for them. No such assumption should be made. If an athlete doesn't take care of his own training and eating plan, no one else will either. Of course, an inadequate knowledge of nutrition makes it impossible for athletes to make the correct dietary choices, particularly if presented with new foods in a new environment. There is no single perfect food that will guarantee an optimal athletic performance, but athletes must know the basic elements of the best foods and fluids to consume.

Both food and adaptation are important considerations. It takes time for an athlete's circadian rhythms to adapt to a new location, so adequate time at the new location is required for these adaptive changes to take place. The desynchronization of an athlete's normal rhythms results in malaise, loss of appetite, fatigue, and disturbed sleep, all of which can affect performance.[3] The severity of these effects depends, to a large degree, on the number of time zones crossed, the direction of the flight, the age of the athlete, and the steps taken by the athlete before travel to minimize the disruption in normal rhythm.[1,4] Even a relatively brief air travel that crosses only two time zones can negatively affect team performance.[5] This clearly suggests that, when possible, athletes should arrive at the competition early enough for their circadian rhythms to return to normal before the competition begins.[6] Each athlete has a different capacity to adapt to a new location. Therefore, to the greatest degree possible, the adaptive strategy should be individualized.[7] Studies assessing the impact of jet lag on members of the U.S. women's soccer team traveling to Taiwan, North American students traveling to Western Europe, and European students traveling to North America found that mood state, anaerobic power and capacity, and dynamic strength were all negatively affected. It took 3 or 4 days to eliminate the impact of travel on these performance measures.[8]

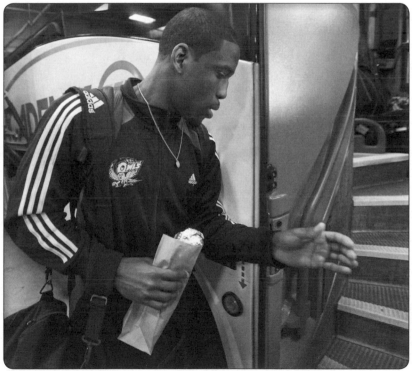

© Associated Press

Careful planning for having the right foods and beverages available during travel is critical when competing away from home.

Some athletes consider massage or chiropractic adjustment a critical component of a speedy adaptation. However, there is limited evidence that this approach is truly useful. One study of Finnish junior elite athletes investigated whether the impact of jet lag could be reduced with chiropractic adjustment after a trip. Looking at sleep patterns and mood score (via the Profile of Mood States instrument), it was found that the chiropractic care had no impact on the effects of jet lag.[9]

Acclimatization is particularly important for athletes traveling to locations that are hotter and more humid than where training normally occurs. Physiological adjustments to heat take 7 to 14 days, and without adequate heat adaptation, performance will clearly be affected.[1] Planning ahead to ensure optimal access to the right foods and fluids and to allow for sufficient adaptation time is the key to success.

Travel must also be considered a time of increased disease risk. The traveling athlete may be exposed to unfamiliar pathogens (i.e., those for which the body has yet to develop protective systems); and the lack of sleep, increased mental stress, and increased fatigue associated with travel may increase the chance of infection. Strategizing for how to rest and eat properly before, during, and immediately after a trip is a critical component of staying healthy and reducing the risk that a disease state compromises athletic performance.[10] Maintaining personal hygiene and washing the hands frequently can reduce the risk of infection—these habits should become a regular component of the traveling athlete's strategy for keeping healthy.[11]

GENERAL GUIDELINES FOR EATING ON THE ROAD

Most guidelines require advance planning. Just as an athlete must pack her uniform, she should also give thought to where, when, and how the right foods and beverages can be obtained to satisfy needs. The worst thing that can happen to an athlete while traveling is to become hungry or thirsty and not have anything quickly available to eat or drink. Make sure this doesn't happen by trying to follow these general tips for eating on the road:[12]

• Bring your own snacks. Fresh fruits, fruit juices, crackers, low-fat rice and pasta salads, and low-fat energy bars are nutritious and easy to carry (see table 9.1).

• Watch out for hidden fats. Creamy soups, bread-type flaky pastries, mayonnaise-based salad dressings, and sauces in sandwiches add unnecessary fat to food. However, good alternatives are available. Consuming clear, broth-based soups instead of creamy soups may provide all the nutrients with considerably less fat. Using lemon juice–based salad dressing rather than mayonnaise-type dressing lowers the fat and makes it possible to eat more salad.

• Consume grilled, baked, boiled, and broiled foods rather than fried or sauteed foods. You must ask for it the way you want it. Make no assumptions about how food will be prepared by the way it is described on the menu. When possible, request lower-fat dairy products and lower-fat salad dressings.

• Order a la carte to get exactly what you want. Full dinners often don't fit the way a serious athlete should be eating. For instance, the grilled fish may be exactly what you want, but the full dinner may come with mashed potatoes that are soaked in gravy, broccoli that is covered with cheese sauce, and a piece of apple pie with ice cream. The serious athlete would be better off with broiled fish, a plain baked potato, broccoli with lemon juice, and fresh fruit for dessert.

Table 9.1 Good Snacks for Athletes to Take With Them When Traveling

Food	Approximate energy substrate distribution[1]		
	% carbohydrate	% protein	% fat
Bagel	76	14	10
Breadsticks	76	13	11
Breakfast cereal, unsweetened (such as Cheerios)	70	15	15
Cheese[2]	7	37	56
Cookies (such as oatmeal)	65	4	31
Crackers (such as saltines or graham crackers)	66	8	26
Cut-up vegetables (such as carrots and celery)	94	4	2
Dried fruit (such as apricots)	93	6	11
Energy bar, breakfast bar, granola bar	91	4	5
Fresh fruit (such as apples, oranges, and grapes)	75	10	15
Fruit juice (such as apple, grape, and orange)	99	0	1
Pretzels	78	10	12
Sports beverages	100	0	0
Trail mix (including nuts, dried fruit, and M&Ms)	43	11	46
Yogurt with fruit[2]	75	17	8

[1]Energy substrate distribution varies with brand name and type.

[2]May require refrigeration.

• If you travel by air, tell the travel agent you'd like to eat vegetarian. There's a greater chance you'll receive foods that are higher in carbohydrates and lower in fat. However, you need to give fair warning of your special dietary requirements, so make certain to notify the airline at least 24 hours in advance of the flight.

• If you travel by air, bring something to drink on the plane with you. There may be a significant delay between the time you take off and when you receive your first drink. Air travel is one of the most dehydrating experiences a person can have. Because of this, passengers often contract sore throats and other upper respiratory illnesses. As a preventive measure, keep sipping on fluids during the flight to keep your mouth and throat moist. Drink bottled water or sports beverages.

- Good choices to bring on the plane include any foods that are relatively high in complex carbohydrates, have a lean source of protein, and are relatively low in fats (fried foods are not good choices). Examples include salad with broiled chicken strips (request oil and vinegar or lemon juice instead of dressing); baked potato stuffed with vegetables (go easy on the melted cheese, or request a lower-fat cheese); and taco salad with corn tacos, beans, rice, broiled chicken strips, and tomato salsa (avoid fried taco bowls).

- If you're changing time zones, get on the local schedule as soon as possible. Have dinner when the local population is eating rather than at the time you eat at home. You'll still have difficulty getting your eating pattern on track because traveling and changing time zones are tiring and disorienting. To make certain you're completely ready to compete, try to arrive at the competition site early.

MINIMIZING JET LAG

Jet lag results in temporary disturbance of circadian rhythms, which last until the person has fully adapted to the local time zone. The most commonly experienced symptoms include poor concentration, irritability, depression, fatigue, inability to sleep, disorientation, poor appetite, and GI problems. Leaving enough time to adjust to long-distance travel is important. It has been found that 3 days are needed to resynchronize psychomotor performance rhythms after a westward flight from Germany to the United States, but 8 days are required for the reverse (easterly) direction.[13] Even the most seasoned travelers suffer from jet lag, and most of them don't have to run, jump, hit, kick, flip, or swim when they reach their destinations. Jet lag can impart a feeling of illness, will lower appetite, and can disturb normal sleep.[14] Jet lag comes in two forms: (1) travel involving small but consecutive trips, causing multiple small shifts in usual eating patterns; and (2) travel involving one large trip that crosses multiple time zones, causing a major change in eating and sleeping behaviors. Athletes should never delay eating when the sensation of hunger occurs, so snacks should always be quickly available to fill the gap in time until a regular meal can be obtained. The following recommendations may help alleviate the effects of jet lag:[3]

1. **For small consecutive time-zone changes (called phase shifts):**
   - Eat meals at regular local times after arriving at the new destination. This will help you get on the local schedule quickly and aid your adjustment to the new time zone.
   - Drink plenty of liquids. Plane cabins are notoriously dry, and dehydration is the cause of many complaints, including headaches and mild constipation.
   - Alternate light meals with heavy meals before the flights. The stress of travel may increase protein requirements slightly, so eat a high-protein breakfast and a low-protein, high-carbohydrate dinner after the phase shift.
   - Avoid caffeine until the end of the flight. Large volumes of caffeine-containing beverages can have a diuretic effect that can increase water loss in an environment that is already dehydrating. Consume fluids that will help you maintain hydration state (water, sports beverages, fruit juices).

- Avoid alcohol during and after the flight. Besides the negative metabolic alterations that alcohol causes, it is also a diuretic that can increase water loss. There is *no* reason why serious athletes should drink alcoholic beverages at any time.

- Engage in social activity or exercise after the flight. This will help you get on the local schedule more quickly and will aid in reducing the stress associated with travel.

2. For a large phase shift:

- Arrive at your destination at least 1 day early for each time zone crossed. For flights crossing more than six time zones, a minimum of 4 days and preferably 1 week should be allowed to return to a normal circadian rhythm and a feeling of well-being. Cost and scheduling limitations may keep athletes from arriving as early as needed, so getting on the local schedule as quickly as possible, but with as much rest as possible, is important.

- Exercise and get involved in social activities on your arrival in the new location. It helps to become familiar with your new environment right away. The exercise and social activities will reduce the stress of travel and will help you get on the local schedule more easily.

- Maintain regular sleeping and eating times on arrival to your new destination. The sooner you can eat and sleep on the schedule of your new destination, the more quickly your body will feel as if it can perform well. Eating and sleeping regularly and on schedule are keys to doing well when you travel.

- Continue to eat and drink frequently before, during, and after travel. Creating a snacking schedule at your new location may be difficult because you may not know where to buy good high-carbohydrate snacks. However, maintaining a frequent eating and drinking schedule (eating something about every 3 hours) is an important strategy for helping you adjust to your new environment. Bring some snacks with you to get started, and then find a good source of snacks once you arrive. However, always avoid alcohol.

- If you have a dietary restriction, such as gluten-containing foods, have a card made in the language of the country where you are traveling. In this example, the card could say, "I cannot eat any food that contains wheat or wheat flour, or other foods that contain gluten, including . . ." Give this card to your server when eating out so there is no question about what you can eat.

- Have more protein than usual. The stress associated with travel may slightly increase your protein requirement, so make a conscious effort to consume a little more protein each day. For instance, consuming a higher-protein breakfast (add a boiled egg to your normal intake) could be useful in ensuring that your protein requirement is met. However, the focus of your intake should continue to be carbohydrate.

Several aids help athletes cope with jet lag and adapt more quickly to their new environment. These include the following:

- **Compression hose:** A significant number (about 10 percent) of air travelers develop deep vein thrombosis (DVT, a form of blood clots and a sign of poor vascular circulation). Travelers wearing compression hose are less likely to develop DVT.[15] If you choose to obtain compression hose, make certain they have graduated compression, with the greatest compression at the ankle and a lower level of compression going up the calf. The effect of mild compression slightly constricts blood flow, thereby increasing blood flow velocity (i.e., the same volume traveling through narrower "tubes"), with two effects: (1) It keeps blood fluids in circulation instead of causing edema (fluid pooling around the tissues, outside the blood), and (2) it limits the possibility of clot formation. *Caution:* Compression hose should not be excessively tight and should not be confused with support hose, which exert the same level of pressure throughout the entire length of the stocking.

- **Melatonin:** A review of 10 research trials suggests that, if taken in the right amount and at the right time, melatonin is remarkably effective at reducing jet lag when flights are crossing multiple time zones.[16] Nine of these studies determined that when melatonin is taken at a time that closely approximates the target bedtime at the destination (between 10 p.m. and midnight at the target location), there was a lessening of jet lag when flights crossed more than 4 time zones. Daily doses of melatonin between .5 milligram and 5 milligrams appeared to be similarly effective, except that people fall asleep faster with the larger dosage. There is no apparent benefit of doses that exceed 5 milligrams. The benefit is likely to be greater the more time zones are crossed, but it appears less effective for flights going west (delayed sleep time) than for flights going east (earlier sleep time). Reports suggest that melatonin is contraindicated for those with epilepsy or taking Warfarin.

- **Caffeine:** A study assessing slow-release caffeine (SRC) determined it was effective at combating daytime sleepiness after an eastbound flight crossing 7 time zones.[17] In this double-blind, randomized, placebo-controlled study, subjects were provided with 300 milligrams of SRC for each of 5 days after the flight, with a positive effect on jet lag symptoms.

- **Timing and composition of meals:** Although there is limited study in this area, it does appear that certain foods influence circadian rhythm adjustments.[18] A relatively high-carbohydrate and low-protein meal may enhance brain exposure to tryptophan and, through its conversion to serotonin, enhance sleep. This should occur, therefore, in conjunction with melatonin intake. By contrast, a relatively higher-protein and lower-carbohydrate meal may expose the brain to more tyrosine that, through conversion to adrenaline, may enhance alertness. This should occur, therefore, once the athlete has arrived at the location if he remains sleepy and fatigued. Some caution here: Athletes should be careful to not consume such a low level of carbohydrate that glycogen storage and blood sugar are compromised, as this would have a profoundly negative impact on performance, regardless of the sport.

TRAVEL LOCATION

When traveling to most places in the United States, Canada, and Western Europe, there's a high likelihood familiar foods will be available. Breakfast cereals, for instance, can be found in virtually every grocery store, and there is bread everywhere you go. The preparation of many of the foods is different, however. If you're accustomed to having a cup of coffee in the morning, you may be surprised (perhaps even shocked!) at the variety of ways different cultures treat the coffee bean.

All this information indicates that athletes should do whatever they can to sustain dietary and sleep habits because it is impossible to know what the outcome will be if there is a sudden change in usual lifestyle practices and procedures. A particularly useful gadget to have with you is an in-cup electric water heater that has the appropriate power adapters for the country. These little heaters allow consumption of familiar soups, and athletes can brew familiar-tasting coffee. For a traveling athlete, this is one of the best inventions ever.

Some countries have reputations for unsafe water or food supplies. If there is any doubt whatsoever about the safety of the food or water supply, call your nearest consular office or your travel agency. Employees should be able to provide you with the information you need. Pick up a good travel book for the location you're heading to. A good book will describe the foods that will be available and will tell you about the water supply.

When traveling abroad, take the following items with you even if you think the food and water supply is safe and familiar (you can adjust the quantities depending on your length of stay):

- Power-cord adapters and converters to fit the power supply of the country you're traveling to
- An in-cup electric heater
- A water-filter pump
- A box of saltine crackers
- Powdered sports beverage packets to make 20 quarts (20 L) of beverage
- Two quarts (2 L) of bottled water
- A medium-size box of raisins (or other favored dried fruit)
- Five individually packaged low-fat granola bars
- Two nonfat powdered milk packets
- One small box of your favorite cereal

Water Supply It doesn't matter where the travel destination is, athletes will, for one reason or another, need water. Different water supplies can cause gastrointestinal (GI) difficulties, even if the water supply is perfectly safe. Different and unaccustomed levels of bromide or fluoride in the water may, for instance, cause severe gut pain. Of course, drinking bottled water or bottled sports drinks is a good solution if these are available. However, if bottled drinks are not easily available, you need a way to deal with the situation. It is virtually impossible to travel with a significant number of bottled drinks, but athletes should travel with powdered packages of sports beverages and a water filter to purify the water. The best water filters are those capable of removing microscopic parasites and bacteria—check your local camping goods store. These water filters are also at the top of the list of excellent inventions for the traveling athlete. They don't take up much space and work extremely efficiently, giving you the peace of mind you need so you can deal with other more pressing matters.

Eating Locations Travel inevitably keeps athletes from eating when and where they'd like, so plan ahead for what you might select before you enter an eating establishment. Seeing the dizzying array of foods and menu items can easily influence your order if you're not already committed to your selection. Airports are filled with fast-food restaurants that typically offer high-fat and high-sugar foods. These are not easy places to make the right selections. In general, athletes should stick with foods that aren't fried. However, if you don't have a choice, minimize the fried (fatty) food and maximize the carbohydrate. For instance, instead of a double-patty hamburger, it would be better to order two regular hamburgers because you get twice the bread (carbohydrate).

Try to find pasta, baked potatoes, bread, vegetables, and salads in restaurants. It might be necessary to request a substitution (e.g., a baked potato instead of French fries), but don't be afraid to ask. Restaurants in airports or ports may be less likely to want to satisfy your special needs because they know they'll probably never see you (or your business) again. Nevertheless, it's important that athletes always ask for exactly what they want. Even when ordering baked potatoes, ask for everything on the side rather than on the potato. See table 9.2 for key words to look for when viewing a menu.

The key to successful travel is advance planning. Make no assumptions about the availability of foods or drinks that will satisfy your needs. Bring some items with you when traveling to be certain you have some key foods and drinks that will keep you happy and nourished. Don't try new foods until after the athletic event, and then only on the recommendation of your local hosts. Experimenting on your own can be dangerous. Find out as much as you can about where you're going by visiting a bookstore or library, or do some research on the Internet. Your travel agent and nearby consular office are also excellent sources of information. Give yourself plenty of time to get acclimatized to the location you're traveling to. It takes about 1 day for each time zone you cross, so for a trip from New York to Paris, you should arrive at least 6 days before the event. If that's not possible, do whatever you can to reduce stress by getting plenty of rest, relaxing with friends, and getting on the local schedule as soon as possible.

Table 9.2 Selecting Items Through a Careful Review of the Menu

Cuisine	Foods to avoid	Foods to seek
General	Fried, crispy, breaded, scampi style, creamed, buttery, au gratin, gravy	Marinara, steamed, boiled, broiled, tomato sauce, in its own juice, poached, charbroiled
Mexican	Deep-fried shells, fried flour tortillas, refried beans, corn chips, sour cream, guacamole	Low-fat refried beans, chicken or lean beef and bean burritos, baked soft corn tortillas, salsa, rice, baked flour tortillas
Italian	Cream sauces, high-fat dressings, rich desserts	Pasta with marinara sauce, cheese or vegetable pizza, salad with dressing on the side, low-fat Italian ice, low-fat frozen yogurt
Chinese	Deep-fried egg rolls, deep-fried wontons, sweet and sour pork, tempura	Stir-fried and steamed dishes, chicken and vegetables with rice, clear broth soups
Burger places	High-fat dressings in salad bars, mayonnaise, French fries, milk shakes	Low-fat dressings in salad bars, baked potatoes, grilled items
Cafes	Prebuttered items, excessive coffee intake	Pancakes, toast, bagels, waffles, fruit, fruit juices, whole-grain cereals, breads, muffins

Adapted, by permission, from E.R. Burke and J.R. Berning, 1996, *Training nutrition: The diet and nutrition guide for peak performance* (Carmel, IN: I.L. Cooper), 134.

IMPORTANT POINTS

- Athletes should travel to a new location early enough to allow time to adjust. Eating at the same times the local population eats and sleeping at the times the local population sleeps will help you adjust more quickly. Exercising lightly may also help.

- Wearing compression hose with light compression while traveling long distances helps keep blood fluids circulating and avoids edema, which will help you feel better on arrival and adapt more quickly to the new environment.

- Traveling with some familiar foods is a good idea, particularly if the competition takes you to an unfamiliar country and culture. These key staples can give you some time to find local foods you can eat.

- If you have a dietary restriction of any kind, have a card made in the language of the country where you are traveling. The card should clearly spell out in the local language the foods that you cannot eat. Give this card to the server when eating out so there is no question about what you can eat. (Google Translate can help you do this yourself, with more than 55 languages that can be translated.)

- Drink plenty of fluids while traveling. Sipping on fluids constantly will help you avoid the dry throat that increases the risk of getting an upper respiratory illness.

- Avoid alcohol consumption, as alcohol is a diuretic that can make you dehydrated and may also contribute to GI upset.

- Caffeine consumption at the new location may help you adjust more quickly, but excessive intake of caffeine-containing beverages may have a diuretic effect that contributes to dehydration.

High Altitude

Performing physical work at high altitude presents enormous challenges, whether a person climbed to get there or was taken there via helicopter as a member of a search crew. High altitudes are likely to be cold, often to the extreme; the oxygen concentration of the air is lower, and the terrain is sufficiently harsh that the human system is under constant strain to do physical work. Moving quickly from lower to higher altitude, as often occurs when athletes train at high altitude to enhance oxygen-carrying capacity, may result in headache and nausea, both of which can negatively influence food and fluid consumption. The lower oxygen level of high-altitude air results in early fatigue, and the difficulty of eating and drinking normally may lead to enough tissue loss that cold tolerance is decreased. Maintaining body-fluid balance in extreme cold is just as difficult as maintaining fluid balance in hot and humid environments, with both increased urinary flow and voluntary dehydration contributing to higher risk of dehydration. Simply finding a way to keep drinking fluids from freezing presents a challenge, and cooking takes much longer at higher altitudes than at lower altitudes, necessitating more cooking fuel to be carried. The challenges of performing physical work at high altitude are daunting, but good nutrition strategies can help people attain their goals in this unfriendly environment, whether it's a 3-day 14,400-foot (4,400 m) climb up Mount Rainier or a week-long trek up the 19,300-foot (5,900 m) Mount Kilimanjaro. This chapter reviews the physiological and nutrition stresses the human body experiences when working at high altitude and presents recommendations for successfully dealing with this environment.

The live high, train low (LHTL) training paradigm has been with us for more than 20 years and has surpassed the popularity of the earlier live high, train high paradigm, which presented far too many difficulties and training limitations. In fact, training at high altitude results in reduced speeds, reduced power output, and reduced oxygen flux, none of which provide any advantage to training. By contrast, LHTL improves performance in athletes of all abilities.[1] The purpose of the LHTL training regimen is to create a tissue adaptation that improves oxygen-carrying capacity, which results in better endurance through improved fat metabolism and lower carbohydrate metabolism. To optimally benefit from this LHTL strategy, athletes are required to live at an elevation of 2,000 to 2,500 meters (6,600 to 8,200 feet) for a minimum of 4 weeks.[2]

The best strategy for avoiding any of the high-altitude illness (HAI) syndromes is to allow sufficient time for acclimatization. The commonly suggested acclimatization protocol is to have a graded ascent of no more than 600 meters (2,000 feet) per day to the ultimate altitude, with a rest day every 600 to 1,200 meters (2,000 to 4,000 feet).[3]

HIGH-ALTITUDE EXERCISE

A series of physiological adjustments can help athletes acclimatize to low-oxygen (i.e., hypoxic) environments. These include the following:[4]

- An increase in ventilation, termed the hypoxic ventilatory response (from 14 breaths per minute to 20-plus breaths per minute compared with the same activity at sea level)
- A catecholamine-mediated increase in heart rate
- A catecholamine-mediated increase in cardiac output
- Eventual pulmonary, hematologic, and tissue adaptations that occur over several days provided the increase in altitude is gradual (rapid ascents that provide inadequate adaptation time are associated with high risk of high-altitude sickness)

The oxygen concentration is lower at higher altitudes, requiring that athletes undergo a degree of adaptation before training regimens and performance can approach sea-level expectations, particularly for aerobic (predominantly endurance) activities. Even for anaerobic events, a degree of adaptation is necessary to adjust to the lower oxygen concentration of high altitude to avoid altitude illness that can impede training. Because the concentration of oxygen is lower at progressively higher altitudes, a stepwise progression to higher and higher altitudes makes sense to allow for an efficient and illness-free adaptive response.

Athletes training at higher altitudes can expect a faster respiration and faster heart rate, which are adaptations to the lower oxygen being pulled into the lungs with each breath. Although the athlete may adapt to this lower-oxygen environment with alterations in cardiac output, breathing frequency, and oxygen diffusion from the blood to the cell, raising the number of red blood cells is the most efficient

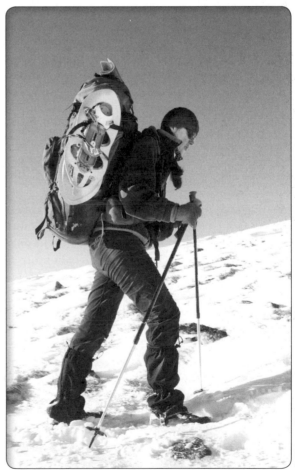

© Human Kinetics

High-altitude and cold environments create unique hydration challenges that must be planned for.

way of improving oxygen delivery and, therefore, sport performance.[5] Although there are several illegal means of doing this, including blood doping or EPO injections, there are perfectly legal nutritional means by ensuring an adequate intake of calories, iron, folic acid, and vitamin B_{12}. A healthy diet may satisfy most of these requirements, but care should be taken that iron in particular be consumed at the level of approximately 18 milligrams per day. This may be more difficult than it seems because athletes often complain of a loss of appetite at high altitude. (See table 10.1 for a definition of what constitutes high altitude.)

Table 10.1 Common Definitions of Altitude

High altitude	1,500 to 2,500 m (5,000 to 8,200 ft)
Very high altitude	2,500 to 5,500 m (8,200 to 18,000 ft)
Extreme altitude	Above 5,500 m (above 18,000 ft)

Cold environments cause heat loss through both convection and conduction, although humans do have systems that help maintain core body temperature and increase heat production.[6] This process of thermoregulation helps ensure survivability when exposed to cold temperatures. With cold exposure, the body attempts to lower the amount of heat loss through peripheral vasoconstriction. However, the reduced blood flow to the skin and extremities predisposes people to frostbite, particularly of the fingers and toes. To counteract this risk, the body initiates a process referred to as cold-induced vasodilation (CIVD) after approximately 10 minutes of cold exposure. The pulsing of peripheral vasoconstriction and vasodilation results in the preservation of core temperature, but at the cost of fluctuating temperatures of the skin and peripheral tissues.[6]

Humans mainly produce heat when muscles work. Of the calories used by working muscles, approximately 30 to 40 percent actually results in muscular movement, while 60 to 70 percent is lost as heat. Put simply, as warm-blooded animals we are more efficient at creating heat than creating movement. We can also produce heat by shivering, which is an involuntary central nervous system–induced mechanism that is invoked by a 3 to 4 degree drop in body temperature.[7,8] The increase in muscle contraction from shivering results in a 2.5-fold increase in total energy expenditure, most of which is the result of increased carbohydrate oxidation.[9] Cold stress also increases muscle glycogen utilization as a result of increased plasma catecholamines.[10]

Therefore, consumption of sufficient amounts of carbohydrate is important when exercising in an environment where cold stress and shivering occur.[11] Older people who have experienced some degree of muscle loss fare less well in cold environments, mainly because their lower level of muscle mass reduces their capacity to produce heat, whether from work or shivering.[12] However, older age would not automatically increase hypothermic risk if a program of regular exercise were instituted to maintain the lean mass.

Cold-weather exposure creates a significant dehydration risk. Soldiers in cold environments commonly lose up to 8 percent of body weight from dehydration.[13] There are several reasons for this dehydration, including difficulty obtaining adequate amounts of potable water, high levels of water loss (particularly if excess clothing is worn or heavy equipment is being carried), respiratory water loss, and cold-induced diuresis (CID).

The lower-oxygen environment of high altitudes may pose serious health risks to athletes who fail to properly and gradually acclimatize to higher altitudes. These health risks, generically referred to as high-altitude illness, or HAI (see table 10.2), include three syndromes:

- **Acute mountain sickness (AMS)**: The most common but least serious of the HAI syndromes; includes nausea, vomiting, loss of appetite, dizziness, weakness, and sleeping difficulty.
- **High-altitude cerebral edema (HACE)**: Associated with a change in mental status and loss of coordination.
- **High-altitude pulmonary edema (HAPE):** Associated with dyspnea, cough, weakness, and chest tightness or congestion.

Many experienced skiers and mountain climbers are aware of the potential for nausea, confusion, and easy fatigue with high-altitude work. It takes time to adapt to this relatively hypoxic environment, mainly by improving the capacity to deliver oxygen to working tissues. High-altitude exposure increases oxidative stress, a fact that may alter nutrient requirements in favor of more antioxidant intake.[14] It is estimated that most humans are 80 percent acclimatized after 10 days at altitude and approximately 95 percent acclimatized by 45 days at altitude.[15] People can expect certain normal changes when going to a higher altitude. These include faster breathing, increased shortness of breath, higher urination frequency, and altered sleep patterns. The lower barometric pressure of high altitude lowers the oxygen concentration of every breath, forcing a more frequent breathing pattern in an attempt to pull in the same level of oxygen. However, it is impossible to take in the same level of oxygen at high altitude when compared with sea level, no matter how fast the breathing pattern. For this reason, physical work will always be more difficult, and fatigue will occur more quickly at high altitude. A failure to properly acclimatize to the altitude may result in additional symptoms:[16]

- Headaches
- Vomiting
- Anorexia (loss of appetite)
- Malaise
- Nausea

Factors that can increase the risk of developing altitude sickness include the following:

- A fast rate of ascent
- High-fat, high-protein, low-carbohydrate diets
- A long stay at altitude
- A high level of exertion
- A higher altitude

Table 10.2 Signs and Symptoms of High-Altitude Illness (HAI)

	Diagnosis (Lake Louise Consensus Criteria)[1]	Treatment	Prevention
AMS	Presence of headache and one of the following symptoms: • Gastrointestinal issue (anorexia, nausea, or vomiting) • Fatigue or weakness • Dizziness or light-headedness • Difficulty sleeping	Mild symptoms: • Halt ascent, rest, acclimatize • Descend >500 m (1,600 ft) • Acetazolamide 125-250 mg by mouth twice daily Moderate to severe symptoms: • Descend >500 m (1,600 ft) • Low-flow oxygen, 1-2 L/min • Portable hyperbaric chamber • Acetazolamide 125-250 mg by mouth twice daily • Dexamethasone 4 mg (by mouth or intramuscular injection) every 6 hr • Use combination of approaches until symptoms resolve	• Slow ascent (max 600 m/day) (2,000 ft/day) • Sleep at lower altitude • Avoid overexertion • Avoid direct transport to elevations >2,750 m (9,000 ft) • Acetazolamide 125-250 mg by mouth twice daily, starting 1 day before ascent and continuing for 2 days at altitude • Dexamethasone 2 mg every 6 hr or 4 mg every 12 hr
HACE	Presence of a change in mental status or ataxia in a person with AMS *or* Presence of a change in both mental status and ataxia in a person without AMS	• Immediately descend >1,000 m (3,300 ft) • Oxygen (2-4 L/min) to maintain SaO_2 >90% • Dexamethasone 8 mg (by mouth, intramuscular injection, or intravenous) initial dose then 4 mg every 6 hr • Portable hyperbaric chamber (if descent delayed)	• Slow ascent (max 600 m/day) (2,000 ft/day) • Sleep at lower altitude • Avoid overexertion • Avoid direct transport to elevations >2,750 m (9,000 ft) • Acetazolamide 125-250 mg by mouth twice daily, starting 1 day before ascent and continuing 2 days at altitude • Dexamethasone 2 mg every 6 hr or 4 mg every 12 hr
HAPE	At least two symptoms and two signs from the following: Symptoms: • Dyspnea at rest • Cough • Weakness or decreased exercise performance • Chest tightness or congestion • Signs: • Crackles or wheezing in at least one lung field • Central cyanosis • Tachypnea • Tachycardia	• Oxygen (4-6 L/min until improved, then 2-4 L/min) to maintain SaO_2 >90% • Descend 500-1,000 m (1,600-3,300 ft) or more • Portable hyperbaric chamber (2-4 psi continuously) if descent delayed • Consider nifedipine (20-30 mg sustained release every 12 hr) • Consider salmeterol 125 mcg twice daily • Consider expiratory positive airway pressure mask • Dexamethasone (if HACE develops)	• Slow ascent (max 600 m/day) (2,000 ft/day) • Sleep at lower altitude • Avoid overexertion In HAPE-susceptible persons: • Consider nifedipine (20-30 mg sustained release every 12 hr) • Consider salmeterol 125 mcg twice daily, starting 1 day before ascent and for 2 days at maximum altitude • Consider tadalafil (10 mg twice daily) or sildenafil (50 mg every 8 hr)

[1]In the setting of acute exposure to altitude environment.

Reprinted, by permission, from R. Derby and K. deWeber, 2010, "The athlete and high altitude," *Current Sports Medicine Reports* 9(2): 79-85.

Acute mountain sickness (AMS), which commonly occurs at altitudes exceeding 6,600 feet (2,000 m), produces the following symptoms:[17,18]

- Nausea
- Dyspnea on exertion and at rest
- Poor sleep
- Ataxia
- Headache
- Altered mental status
- Lassitude
- Fluid retention (higher antidiuretic hormone production)
- Cough

An assessment of athletes competing in the Primal Quest Expedition Adventure Race in Colorado found that 4.5 percent had altitude illness at the start of the race; 14.1 percent had altitude illness during the race that required medical treatment (of which 13.3 percent was AMS; .8 percent was pulmonary edema); and 14.3 percent withdrew from the race because of altitude-related illness.[19] This race begins at an altitude higher than 9,500 feet (2,900 m) and rises to an altitude of more than 13,500 feet (4,100 m). Illness occurring at high altitude should be treated by descent to a lower altitude and by administering oxygen, if available. People with worsening symptoms should never delay descent because worsening symptoms may evolve to high-altitude cerebral edema (HACE) or high-altitude pulmonary edema (HAPE), both of which are life threatening.[20] Capillary leakage in the brain or lungs is the cause of this edema. Symptoms of HACE, which can progress rapidly and result in death within a matter of a few hours, include the following:[21]

- Gait ataxia (walks like someone intoxicated)
- Confusion
- Psychiatric changes of varying degree
- Disturbances of consciousness that may progress to deep coma

The cause of HAPE (fluid in the lungs) is not well understood, but it rarely occurs at altitudes below 8,000 feet (2,400 m). A failure to treat HAPE immediately, typically by immediate descent, may result in death. Symptoms of HAPE result from a lower oxygen–carbon dioxide exchange and include the following:[22]

- Extreme fatigue
- Gurgling or rattling breaths
- Breathlessness at rest
- Chest tightness, fullness, or congestion
- Cough, possibly with pink sputum
- Blue or gray lips or fingernails

Ultimately, to prevent HAI, athletes must learn that high-altitude training programs cannot mimic training programs at lower attitudes. Training adaptations include slowing down if premature hyperventilation occurs at any point during a competition or training; synchronizing limb movements with the new breathing patterns; allowing ample recovery time after sprints; and reducing the total volume of training.[23]

Obese persons are more likely to suffer from acute mountain sickness (AMS) than are nonobese persons.[24] However, people with periodic altitude exposures appear to adapt and reduce the symptoms of AMS.[25] Other strategies, including magnesium supplementation and Ginkgo biloba supplementation, have been tried for reducing AMS, but these have not been found successful.[26,27]

The combined impact of AMS symptoms is a severe appetite depression with a concomitant reduction in foods and fluids. The high caloric requirements and fluid consumption difficulties of cold weather, combined with the anorexia of high altitude, create the two most serious problems of work at high altitude: maintenance of weight and fluid balance.

Even those who are part of well-organized mountain-climbing expeditions and regularly exposed to high altitude typically fail to consume sufficient calories, which leads to a loss of body weight. An assessment of people taking part in a Himalayan trek found that body weight was significantly reduced by the end of the trek, and energy intake was significantly lower at high altitude than at low altitude.[27] Food intakes are usually 10 to 50 percent lower at high altitude, depending on the speed of the ascent. This appears to be true even when people are not exposed to severe cold (as in a hypobaric chamber).[28] Only when there is a conscious effort to consume more food, often with forced eating, do people at higher altitude have energy intakes that approach physiological needs.[29]

The level of sweat loss in extremely cold environments can equal that of hot and humid environments. It has been estimated that moderate to heavy exercise in typically insulated winter clothing will result in a sweat loss of nearly 2 liters per hour.[13] Therefore, the principle strategy for ensuring adequate hydration is to have enough fluids readily available so they can be consumed frequently and in appropriate quantities. There are real problems, however, in making enough fluids available and ready to drink in cold, high-altitude environments. Fluids can freeze unless there are means of keeping them fluid. This is not an easy task in environments that are often well below freezing temperatures. In addition, fluids are heavy to transport in sufficient quantity to meet needs. One option is to acquire fluids from the local environment by melting and purifying ice and snow, but this option is extremely costly in heating fuel. It could take more than 6 hours and a half-gallon (2 L) of gas to melt enough ice and snow to support the fluid needs of a single person.[13]

MEETING ENERGY AND NUTRIENT NEEDS

Energy expenditures of humans climbing Mount Everest average 2.5 to 3 times higher than at sea level.[30] It is easy to understand why weight loss from reduced energy intake is a common outcome of exercise in cold or high-altitude environments.[31] Athletes performing in these environments should make a conscious effort to eat at frequent intervals. They should focus on carbohydrate foods because these foods take less oxygen to metabolize than do fat or protein foods, help replace glycogen stores, and have a protein-sparing effect. In addition, inadequate carbohydrate consumption will eventually result in low blood sugar, which leads to mental confusion and disorientation. Some reports indicate that mountaineers show a preference for carbohydrate and an aversion to fat.[32] However, this finding is not consistent; other studies indicate that athletes at high altitude do not shift their food selections away from high-fat items and toward high-carbohydrate foods.[33] The same report indicates that high-altitude environments blunt the sense of taste, which may contribute to inadequate energy intake. This inadequate energy intake leads to a weight loss (including muscle weight) that negatively affects strength, endurance, and the capacity to produce heat. The goal should therefore be to consume an adequate volume of food to provide sufficient calories rather than place undo importance on the distribution of energy substrates.

Athletes should have foods available to them that they will eat in large quantities and that make them feel good after they are consumed. To make matters even more difficult, the time to cook a meal doubles for each 5,000-foot (1,500 m) climb in elevation. Prepackaged high-carbohydrate snacks and foods are a good alternative for most meals, with cooked meals reserved for those times when athletes have available water and time. Good quick-access foods include lower fat, whole-grain energy or granola bars, and there are now a number of higher-protein bars that would provide some variety to what is consumed.

The intake of vitamins and minerals should be considered before exposure to either cold or high altitude. Iron status in particular should be excellent before attempting a high-altitude trek because oxygen-carrying capacity is stretched to its limit in this environment. Taking iron supplements while on the climb is not likely to be of much benefit because it takes months to improve a poor iron status. Oxidative stress may be higher in hot and cold environments, so consumption of foods that contain antioxidants or periodic consumption of a multivitamin and multimineral supplement should be considered.[34] A study of oxidative stress in humans at high altitude found that those receiving an antioxidant mixture had lower breath pentane (a marker of oxidative stress) compared with those receiving single-antioxidant supplements. Consuming a variety of antioxidants, such as ascorbic acid, beta-carotene, selenium, and vitamin E (as would be present in a broad-spectrum supplement), is therefore likely a better strategy than focusing on a single antioxidant.[35]

MEETING FLUID NEEDS

Consuming sufficient fluids in cold and high-altitude environments presents unique challenges, all of which must be overcome to ensure an adequate hydration state. These factors include providing adequate availability of drinking fluids, avoiding the freezing of drinking fluids, and overcoming voluntary dehydration. High-altitude athletes may be motivated to drink beverages that contain both alcohol (they believe it may help warm them . . . it does not) and caffeine (shown to improve endurance activity). However, the combination of alcohol and caffeine is unhealthy.

Providing Adequate Availability of Drinking Fluids   Fluids are heavy and not easy to transport in the best of circumstances. In cold weather and treacherous high-altitude terrains, fluid availability becomes an even greater issue. Using a CamelBak or similar hydration pack requires much less energy than accessing fluid from another type of container. Also, sipping water sometimes relieves any nausea. The basic strategy is for each person to ensure availability of a minimum of 2 liters of fluids and preferably 4 liters of fluids per day. The 2 liters is truly a minimum because hard physical work in a cold, high-altitude environment may result in 2 liters of water loss per hour. The base-camp strategy of moving large amounts of food, water, and other living essentials to the highest possible altitude with the use of helicopters, automobiles, or animal packs is a logical strategy. Climbing to a higher altitude could then proceed from the base camp, with climbers carrying sufficient food and fluid for the amount of time away from the base camp. Using melted snow or ice as the source of fluids is not a reasonable planning option; melting snow and ice at high altitude takes a great deal of time and adds significant weight in fuel, pots, and stoves. In addition, it is possible that the available ice and snow is impure and not fit for consumption. Giardia lamblia, a diarrhea-causing intestinal parasite, is present in high-altitude regions.[36] Of course, in emergency situations any available fluids should be consumed, but the risk of infection is present if purification devices are not used.

Avoiding the Freezing of Drinking Fluids   Climbers should carry drinking fluids close to the body to keep them from freezing and should even consider keeping fluids with them inside their sleeping bags while sleeping. The alternative (frozen fluid) is simply too difficult to deal with. A unique strategy for keeping fluids from freezing is to add glycerol (see chapter 4), which may improve fluid retention, adds calories to fluids, and reduces the freezing point.[13] The last characteristic of glycerol is rarely considered, but for the athlete working in a cold environment, it is extremely important. The added calories are also an important benefit of glycerol because both cold-weather and high-altitude work commonly induce a hypocaloric state. Glycerol, however, also carries certain risks as a plasma enlarger, so it should only be used with care. In addition, glycerol was recently placed on the banned substance list by the World Anti-Doping Agency, so it should not be consumed by any athlete competing in a sanctioned event.

Overcoming Voluntary Dehydration   When left to their own devices, athletes typically consume less fluid while exercising than is needed to sustain an optimal hydration state. This condition, termed voluntary dehydration, may be an even greater problem when athletes exercise in the cold than when they exercise in the heat. The basis for this remains unclear, but two theories, one physiological and one practical, have been suggested as the possible cause:[13] (1) There is a possibility that cold skin or lower core body temperature modifies the thirst sensation, and (2) the voluntary restriction of fluids seems to occur most often late in the day, an act that blunts the necessity for an athlete to leave a warm tent to urinate in a cold and unfriendly environment during the night. The only reasonable solution to avoid voluntary dehydration is for athletes to place themselves on a fixed drinking schedule, whether or not the sensation of thirst exists.[37] Having small sips of fluids at regular intervals also eliminates the need to consume a large volume of fluid at one time, which may stimulate the need to urinate.

Alcoholic Energy Drinks Should Be Banned

WASHINGTON (AP) — A New York senator says federal regulators are expected to move to ban caffeinated alcoholic drinks as soon as this week. Democratic Sen. Charles Schumer, who has pushed the Obama administration to ban the beverages, said Tuesday that the Food and Drug Administration is expected to find that caffeine is an unsafe food additive to alcoholic drinks, essentially banning them. The Federal Trade Commission will then issue letters to caffeinated alcoholic beverage manufacturers warning that marketing them could be illegal. College students have been hospitalized after drinking the beverages, including the popular Four Loko, and they have been banned in four states.

Source: The Associated Press, 12:15pm EST, Nov 11, 2010

IMPORTANT POINTS

• High-altitude illnesses includes acute mountain sickness (AMS), high-altitude cerebral edema (HACE), and high-altitude pulmonary edema (HAPE). Symptoms range from nausea and dizziness to more serious loss of coordination and chest congestion.

• It takes time to adapt to high-altitude environments, so athletes should not try full-intensity training until they have fully adapted.

• People who are out of shape are more likely to suffer from AMS, but failure to provide sufficient time to adapt to a high-altitude environment can cause difficulties in even well-conditioned athletes.

• Athletes in high-altitude, low-oxygen environments will not adapt well if they are iron deficient, and simply taking iron supplements will not have an immediately discernible positive effect. It takes many weeks to return an iron-deficient athlete to a normal state.

• Fluid consumption is critically important in high-altitude environments, where dehydration may not seem as obvious as when training in hotter and more humid environments.

• High-altitude environments are also often cold environments, which cause an increase in total energy (particularly carbohydrate) expenditure. Therefore, sufficient energy and carbohydrate intake is important. Consumption of adequate calories, iron, vitamin B_{12}, and folic acid will help athletes adjust better to a high-altitude environment, but the intake of these nutrients should be well established before high-altitude training.

• Alcohol consumption in high-altitude environments causes difficulty and is unhealthy, particularly if combined with caffeine. Beverages providing both caffeine and alcohol should be avoided.

Gender and Age

There are specific gender and age-related nutrition recommendations that will help athletes perform at their conditioned best. Female athletes have a unique set of stressors that should be considered to sustain health and optimize performance. The female athlete triad (eating disorder, menstrual dysfunction, and low bone density) should be addressed with strategies that, as much as possible, prevent its development. Child athletes and older athletes are on opposite ends of the developmental scale, a fact that alters nutrition requirements and risks. Children have fewer sweat glands that produce less sweat per gland than those of adults; children are also susceptible to voluntary dehydration.[1] These factors place them at increased risk of overheating unless established programs are in place when children are involved in sporting activities.

In addition, the nutrition requirements of growth are compounded by a large volume of physical activity. Unless there is careful planning, it is nearly impossible to satisfactorily fulfill the combined needs of exercise and growth in children and adolescents. It must also not be assumed that physical activity alone is preventive for later obesity. In fact, a failure to satisfy the energy requirements in real time may be predictive of later obesity.[2] A simple truth is that a failure to adequately satisfy energy needs causes a logical adaptation that makes fat weight more likely to increase. The body's reaction to an inadequate energy intake is to lower the tissue that *needs* calories (i.e., lean mass) to adjust to the inadequate energy exposure, increasing the risk of later obesity. Heat illness, impaired growth and development, menstrual dysfunction, eating disorders, and higher injury risk are all potential outcomes of inadequate nutrient and energy intakes in athletes.[3]

Older athletes have a different set of concerns, particularly as they relate to increased heat-stress risk, age-related changes in body composition, and the increased rate of recovery from strenuous athletic endeavors. There are, however, certain nutrition truths that apply to all groups regardless of age or gender. A failure to provide sufficient energy at the right time will result in a loss of metabolic mass, an increase in fat mass, a reduction in athletic performance, and a failure to quickly recover from intense activity.

FEMALE ATHLETES

A quick review of the dietary reference intakes (DRIs) demonstrates clearly that females have different nutrient requirements than males. Many of the requirement differences are based on body size (males being larger than females) and differences in body composition (males have a higher metabolic mass), but some are due to clear physiological differences, as is the case with iron (females require twice as much) because of the blood-iron loss associated with normal menses.

Energy intakes, for all athletes, are based on total weight, weight of the metabolic mass, and duration and intensity of exercise. Surveys of female athletes commonly report an underconsumption of energy, leading many to conclude that female athletes are at an elevated risk of developing eating disorders regardless of the type of sport they are participating in.[4] In addition, the literature is filled with reports of the impact intense exercise has on the female reproductive system, with amenorrhea or oligomenorrhea a common outcome. These reports suggest that increasing energy intake to offset the high energy demand may be sufficient to reverse the menstrual dysfunction and halt the associated reduction in bone mass.[5] The reduction in bone mass caused by menstrual dysfunction is clinically relevant for female athletes because it places them at current increased risk for stress fractures and later increased risk for osteoporosis. Amenorrhea is associated with lower circulating estrogen, which is an inhibitor of osteoclasts, the cells that break down bone. As a result, amenorrheic and oligomenorrheic athletes are at high risk for developing low bone density. In one study of 46 female athletes (31 with multiple stress fractures and 15 without stress fractures), nearly half of all athletes with stress fractures had menstrual irregularities, with a particularly high prevalence observed in endurance runners with high weekly training mileage.[6] Although consuming sufficient calories and calcium will not correct the biomechanical factors associated with stress fractures, often associated with a high longitudinal foot arch and leg-length inequality, it will substantially reduce risk if this strategy helps females return to normal menstrual function.[7] See table 11.1 for stress fracture risks.

The energy substrate distribution is of interest to female athletes. Studies indicate that females have a higher lipid, lower glycogen (carbohydrate), and lower protein utilization than do male athletes during endurance exercise.[8] Because glycogen storage is limited, the lower rate of glycogen utilization gives female athletes what appears to be a clear advantage over men in long-duration, lower-intensity athletic events.[9] This also gives rise to the following question: Should female endurance athletes have a different energy substrate consumption pattern than male endurance athletes given the difference in the pattern of substrate utilization? No solid evidence indicates there should be a difference in intake, and the nature of endurance and ultraendurance events still makes carbohydrate storage (glycogen) the limiting substrate in performance. Whether an endurance athlete is male or female, when glycogen is depleted the athletic performance will drop (or stop). A series of studies assessing the carbohydrate consumption pattern of female athletes involved in different sports indicated a wide range of intakes (see table 11.2). Few of the assessed female athlete groups meet the recommended carbohydrate intake of 5 to 7 grams per kilogram per day for general training and 7 to 10 grams per kilogram per day for endurance athletes.[10]

The general (nonathlete) recommendation for protein consumption in adults is .8 gram per kilogram per day. The athlete recommendation is approximately double this and ranges

Table 11.1 Risks for Developing Stress Fractures

Risk factor	Nutritionally related?
Genetics	Possibly (if related to food allergies or intolerances)
Female gender	No
White ethnicity	No
Low body weight	Possibly (if not related to genetic predisposition)
Lack of weight-bearing exercise	No
Intrinsic and extrinsic mechanical factors	No
Amenorrhea	Yes
Oligomenorrhea	Yes
Inadequate calcium intake	Yes
Inadequate caloric intake	Yes
Disordered eating	Yes

Adapted from A. Nattiv and T.D. Armsey Jr., 1997, "Stress injury to bone in the female athlete," *Clinics in Sports Medicine* 16(2): 197-224.

Table 11.2 Carbohydrate Consumption Patterns in Female Athletes

Study	Amount CHO (g/kg/day)	Sport
Gabel et al., 1995a	18	Ultraendurance cycling (14 to 16 hr per day)
Peters & Goetzsche, 1997b	4	Ultraendurance
Steen et al., 1995c	4.9	Heavyweight collegiate rowing
Walberg-Rankin, 1995d	3.2 to 5.4	Anaerobic sports (gymnastics, bodybuilding)
Walberg-Rankin, 1995e	4.4 to 6.2	Aerobic sports (running, cycling, triathlon)

between 1.2 and 1.7 grams per kilogram per day, depending on the degree to which the athlete is involved in endurance activity.[11] This recommended level is likely to be greater than actual needs, provided adequate total energy consumption is obtained. It should be noted that no specific protein requirement data are available for female athletes, so these values are derived from mixed-athlete or male studies. Until female-specific protein requirement data are determined, female athletes should try to consume a protein level within the currently established range.

Fat consumption is targeted by female athletes wishing to lower body weight, as indicated in a study showing amenorrheic athletes have a fat intake that is 6 percent lower than eumenorrheic athletes.[12] To obtain a sufficient energy intake, fat consumption should not be eliminated from the diet. Given the high energy needs of athletes, plus the fact that female athletes have an excellent system for catabolizing fat for energy, fat intakes should range in the area of 20 to 25 percent of total energy intake.

Female athletes appear to have less than adequate vitamin B_6 intake, assessed either in absolute values or in ratio to protein consumption.[13,14] With the exception of this vitamin, female athletes who are not on energy-restrictive food intakes appear to obtain adequate vitamins to sustain health and physical activity.

There is no question that calcium and iron intakes are of concern in the diets of female athletes. Adequate calcium consumption is necessary to develop and maintain high-density bones that are resistant to fracture, and iron is necessary for oxygen delivery to working cells. For athletes concerned about dairy product consumption, calcium-fortified orange juice is an excellent alternative and, per equal volume, has the same calcium concentration as fluid milk. Ensuring an adequate calcium intake is within easy reach of every athlete, but it should be understood that calcium intake by itself does not guarantee good bones. Calcium, vitamin D, estrogen, and physical stress are all needed for bone development.

Surveys have found low storage iron (ferritin) in female runners, and other studies have found that female athletes with anemia can improve aerobic performance through a program of iron supplementation.[15,16] Unnecessarily taking iron or other supplements in the absence of iron deficiency is not desirable. Given the very real risks that iron depletion poses, female athletes should regularly (at least yearly) have iron status assessed, with the inclusion of ferritin in the assessment protocol.

General Recommendations for Female Athletes

1. Female athletes should be made fully aware of the negative consequences associated with menstrual dysfunction and the role energy inadequacy plays in its development.[17] Put simply, female athletes should consume sufficient energy to, at the very least, eliminate the risk that menstrual dysfunction results from inadequate energy consumption.

2. A preparticipation physical examination should be a standard feature for all athletes involved in all sports. For female athletes, the screening should include an assessment for the presence of the female athlete triad and any of its sequelae.[18]

3. Calcium and iron intakes and status should be assessed and, if inadequate, corrected through a program of altered food intake (preferred) or through a doctor-supervised supplementation program. A reasonable means of assessing calcium status is to periodically assess bone density (once every 3 years if no osteopenia or osteoporosis; more often if bone disease is present). In addition, a dietary intake analysis will determine if consumed foods are providing sufficient calcium. Iron status should be assessed yearly, with special attention paid to stored iron (ferritin). In the event of iron deficiency, a supervised program of iron supplementation with follow-up blood tests should be immediately implemented.

Female athletes are at higher risk than male athletes for eating disorders, inadequate bone density, and inadequate iron consumption. They also have the unique risk of dysmenorrhea. Most of these difficulties can be controlled with the intake of a nutritionally balanced diet that delivers an adequate caloric load. To achieve this, female athletes should understand that an underconsumption of calories, while lowering weight, is likely to have a greater catabolic impact on lean mass than on fat mass. This altered body composition, by forcing the athlete to consume a still lower food intake to achieve a desired body profile, will place the athlete at greater future risk of malnutrition and associated diseases.

YOUNG ATHLETES

The energy and nutrient requirements for growth and development are so high that it is difficult to imagine how growing children involved in regular intense physical activity can possibly meet their nutrition needs unless extraordinary measures are taken.[19] An inadequate energy supply may result in a failure to achieve the genetically prescribed growth potential, and insufficient nutrients may result in poor development of organ systems. For instance, a poor calcium uptake during the adolescent growth spurt will result in less than optimal bone density, which has a lifetime of health implications. Careful attention to the provision of an adequate energy and nutrient intake is the essential construct for ensuring that youth sports result in healthy outcomes. In particular, athletes who achieve elite status at a young age, as is typical of female gymnasts, may fail to obtain sufficient nutrients at a time when growth and sports-related training and performance stresses are at their highest. These athletes should be frequently assessed to ensure they remain in a healthy state and have a normal growth velocity.

The adolescent growth spurt in girls begins around the age of 10 or 11 and reaches its peak by age 12; girls typically stop growing by age 15 or 16. The adolescent growth spurt in boys begins about 2 years later at age 12 or 13 and reaches a peak by age 14; boys typically stop growing by the age of 19. It is common for girls and boys to grow approximately 11.8 inches (30 cm) between ages 5 and 10; but boys have a greater than 3.9 inch (10 cm) per year growth during the adolescent growth spurt, and adolescent girls have a greater than 3.5 inch (9 cm) growth per year during the adolescent growth spurt. It is estimated that 25 percent of the total bone mass is acquired during the adolescent years.[20] See table 11.3 for typical ages of the child development periods.

Although the stimulation imposed on the skeleton through physical activity is important for bone development, adequate calcium, protein, and energy intakes are also critical during this period. See table 11.4 for a summary of height and weight values of children and adolescents.

Adolescence is the time when girls achieve menarche. Less than 10 percent of girls in the United States start to menstruate before 11 years, and 90 percent of all girls in the United States are menstruating by 13.75 years of age, with a median age of 12.43 years.[20] Athletic females typically begin menstruating 1 to

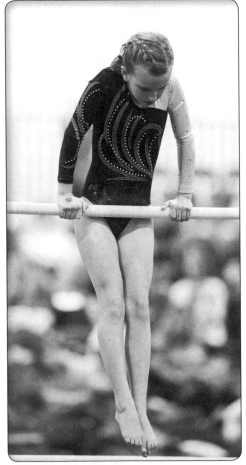

© Human Kinetics

It is critical that adolescent girls, particularly those who achieve elite athletic status at a young age, obtain adequate nutrient intake to ensure optimal bone density.

Table 11.3 Child Development Periods

Stages	Definition	Approximate age of onset (y)
Adrenarche	The period of time just before puberty when there is an increase in adrenal gland activity	7
Gonadarche	The time of the earliest gonadal changes of puberty. In girls, the ovaries grow and the production of estradiol increases; in boys, the testes grow and testosterone increases.	8
Thelarche	In girls, the time when breast development begins at the beginning of puberty	11
Pubarche	The time when pubic hair first appears	12
Menarche (females)	The time of the first menstrual period	12.5
Spermarche (males)	The time marked by the beginning of sperm development	13.4

Table 11.4 Normal Height and Weight Values of Male and Female Children and Adolescents

Age	Height, females		Height, males		Weight, females		Weight, males	
	(in)	(cm)	(in)	(cm)	(lb)	(kg)	(lb)	(kg)
1	27-31	68.6-78.7	28-32	71.1-81.3	15-20	6.8-9.1	17-21	7.7-9.5
2	31.5-36	80-91.4	32-37	81.3-94	22-32	10-14.5	24-34	10.9-15.4
3	34.5-40	87.6-101.6	35.5-40.5	90.2-128.3	26-38	11.8-17.2	26-38	11.8-17.2
4	37-42.5	94-108	37.5-43	95.3-109.2	28-44	12.7-20	30-44	13.6-20
6	42-49	106.7-124.5	42-49	106.7-124.5	36-60	16.3-27.2	36-60	16.3-27.2
8	47-54	119.4-137.2	47-54	119.4-137.2	44-80	20-36.3	46-78	20.9-35.4
10	50-59	127-149.9	50.5-59	128.3-149.9	54-106	24.5-48.1	54-102	24.5-46.3
12	55-64	139.7-162.6	54-63.5	137.2-161.3	68-136	30.8-61.7	66-130	29.9-59
14	59-67.5	149.9-171.5	59-69.5	149.9-176.5	84-160	38.1-72.6	84-160	38.1-72.6
16	60-68	152.4-172.7	63-73	160-185.4	94-172	42.6-78	104-186	47.2-84.4
18	60-68.5	152.4-174	65-74	165.1-188	100-178	45.4-80.7	116-202	52.6-91.6

Source: Centers for Disease Control and Prevention, National Center for Health Statistics, 2000, CDC growth charts: United States. [Online]. Available: www.cdc.gov/growthcharts [October 13, 2011].

2 years later.[21] The blood loss experienced approximately every 4 weeks by girls who are having menstrual periods is an important nutrition consideration. The iron loss in conjunction with the periodic bleeding may predispose adolescent girls to iron deficiency or iron-deficiency anemia that, if allowed to occur, would have a significant impact on endurance capacity. Although all adolescent girls should be cognizant of the importance of obtaining an adequate iron intake, athletic girls must make a particular effort to obtain enough of this mineral. The DRI for iron is 15 milligrams per day for girls between the ages of 14

and 18. This represents nearly a 100 percent increase over the iron requirement for girls between the ages of 9 and 13, when the DRI for iron is 8 milligrams per day. Obtaining 15 milligrams of iron per day is not easy, even if the athlete is a red-meat eater. For non-meat-eating athletes, regularly obtaining 15 milligrams of iron daily becomes nearly impossible without iron supplementation.[22] If adequate iron consumption from food (see table 11.5) is not possible, the risk of iron deficiency, reduced performance, and impaired immune function associated with inadequate iron intake should motivate athletes to seek a well-tolerated strategy for consuming enough iron.[23]

Consumption of sufficient energy is critically important for ensuring normal growth and development and supporting physical activity. It appears that substrate distribution is less important for young athletes than it is for adults. The general adult recommendation for the distribution of substrates is 60 percent from carbohydrate, 15 percent from protein, and 25 percent from fat, but the energy utilization pattern of children may allow for a greater proportion of calories from fat. Studies have found that children use more fat and less carbohydrate than adults during endurance activities and more intense activities.[24,25] Because fat is a more concentrated source of energy, a slightly higher fat intake may make it easier to satisfy the high caloric requirements of these young athletes.

Adolescent females, including adolescent female athletes, often diet to control the change in body morphology and weight associated with growth. Dieting may increase the risk of eating disorders, particularly among adolescent female athletes involved in sports where appearance and size matter (e.g., diving and gymnastics), and it may also alter production of major hormones (see table 11.6). Adrenarche, which may occur prematurely in children who are overweight, is typically associated with development of pubic hair, a change of sweat composition that results in adult body odor, a higher oiliness of the skin and hair, and some mild acne. In most boys these changes match closely with the beginning of puberty. In girls the adrenal androgenic hormones produce most of the early signs of puberty (body odor, skin oiliness, acne). Early onset of premature puberty in females may result in hirsutism (increase in body hair) or menstrual irregularities due to anovulation, the latter of which is referred to as polycystic ovary syndrome (POS). POS is also associated with overweight.

Compared with athletes in team sports, athletes in appearance sports are at greater risk of having inadequate intakes of energy, protein, and some micronutrients including calcium and

Table 11.5 Iron Content of Selected Foods

Food	Iron (mg)
Apple (medium, raw)	.2
Beef steak (3 oz; 90 g)	2.7
Bread, white (2 slices)	1.4
Broccoli (1 cup)	1.1
Burrito, bean	2.7
Chicken breast (3 oz; 90 g)	1.8
Chicken filet sandwich	2.7
Cola (12 oz; 360 ml)	.4
French fries (from 1 medium size potato)	1.8
Grapes (1 cup fresh grapes)	.5
Grilled cheese sandwich	1.6
Hamburger (1/4 pounder; 120 g) with bun	4.5
Hot dog with bun	2.3
Milk (8 oz; 240 ml)	—
Orange juice (8 oz; 240 ml)	.4
Peanut butter (1 tbsp)	.4
Pizza, cheese (1 large slice)	.9
Rice (1 cup)	1.9
Taco with beef	1.5

Table 11.6 Major Hormones in Childhood

Kisspeptin and Neurokinin B	Hypothalamic neuronal hormones that switch on the release of GnRH at the start of puberty.
GnRH (gonadotropin-releasing hormone)	Hypothalamus hormone that stimulates gonadotrope cells of the anterior pituitary.
LH (luteinizing hormone)	Secreted by gonadotrope cells of the anterior pituitary gland. The main targets are the Leydig cells of the testes and the theca cells of the ovaries. LH levels increase about 25 X with the onset of puberty, compared with the 2.5-X increase of FSH.
FSH (follicle-stimulating hormone)	Secreted by gonadotrope cells of the anterior pituitary. The main target cells are ovarian follicles and the sertoli cells and spermatogenic tissue of the testes.
IGF-1 (insulin-like growth factor 1)	Rises during puberty in response to rising growth hormone. Likely main mediator of pubertal growth spurt.
Testosterone	Steroid hormone produced mainly by the testes and also by the theca cells of the ovaries and the adrenal cortex. The primary androgen.
Estradiol	Steroid hormone produced from testosterone. Principal estrogen and acts on estrogen receptors. Mainly produced by ovarian granulose cells, but also derived from testicular and adrenal testosterone.
Adrenal androgens (AAs)	Steroids produced by the adrenal cortex in both sexes. Major AAs are dehydroepiandrosterone, androstenedione (which are precursors of testosterone), and dehydroepiandrosterone sulfate (which is present in large amounts in the blood). Contribute to androgenic events of early puberty in girls.
Leptin	Protein hormone produced by adipose tissue. Primary target is the hypothalamus. The leptin level gives the brain a rough indicator of adipose mass for purposes of regulation of appetite and energy metabolism.

iron. These are not minor issues; an inadequate calcium intake could predispose a young athlete to stress fractures and later osteoporosis, and an iron deficiency leads to poor endurance. Studies have confirmed that energy and nutrient intakes of male and female adolescent athletes, despite being better than that of nonathletes, are below recommended levels, which increases disease and injury risk and diminishes athletic performance potential.[3]

Typical school schedules that mandate a breakfast before school, a moderate lunch at midday, and a dinner that often follows sports practice create an environment that guarantees an energy imbalance. Athletic children should eat at frequent intervals to increase their total energy and nutrient exposure, to guarantee that sufficient energy is provided when it is most needed, and to reduce the chance of energy deficits that can encourage the loss of lean mass and the relative increase in fat mass.

The risk of athletes developing musculoskeletal injuries during periods of fast growth is high. This is not to say that physical activity is bad for children. On the contrary, the right amount and intensity of physical activity stimulates musculoskeletal development. However, excess physical activity that does not allow for sufficient rest and nutrient intake can result in overuse injuries, including tendinitis, Osgood-Schlatter disease, and stress fractures.[21] The timing of nutrient intake is critical for several human systems, including the skeleton. Young athletes expose themselves to a lifetime of problems by failing to provide energy or nutrients sufficient to match the combined requirements of growth and physical activity. Even inadequate sunlight exposure due to training indoors can result in low vitamin D status and compromised bone development.[26] In addition, secondary amenorrhea often occurs during periods of intense physical activity. To avoid overworking specific muscle groups or skeletal areas, it has been suggested that young children participate in a variety of sports and specialize in a specific sport only after puberty. Those who follow this strategy perform better, have lower injury risk, and continue in the sport longer than those who specialize in a single sport early.[27]

Hydration issues remain a concern for young athletes because, compared with adults, they have lower sweat rates, produce more heat per unit of body weight, experience a faster rise in core body temperature, are predisposed to voluntary dehydration, and do not acclimatize as quickly to warm environments.[28] These factors dramatically increase a young athlete's risk of developing heat injury. As a result, coaches and parents should become fully aware of the mental and physical signs of dehydration and heat injuries and should pay careful attention to the ambient temperature and humidity and take appropriate measures for reducing risk. The fact that young athletes are predisposed to voluntary dehydration (i.e., they consume insufficient fluids to maintain hydration state even when they are available) should persuade adults to encourage drinking and observe drinking patterns. It is also useful to have beverages available that young athletes are more likely to consume.[29] These include beverages that have a sweet taste and include small amounts of salt to help sustain blood volume and sweat rates.

General Recommendations for Young Athletes

1. Energy intake level should be sufficient to support normal growth and development plus the added energy requirement of physical activity. As a general guide, young athletes should track normally on charts that measure height for age, weight for age, and weight for height (often used by pediatricians). A flattening of the growth percentile is a sign of inadequate energy intake.

No Logic in School Eating Patterns

When children are in elementary school in the US, they are often provided with a midmorning and midafternoon snack of milk and a cookie, with lunch between the snacks. This is a desirable and needed strategy. However, when children move up to junior high school, just at the time they are hitting their adolescent growth spurt and in need of a huge amount of nutrients and energy, the snacks are removed. This makes no sense whatsoever. Junior high school teachers often complain that this is the most difficult school age to deal with but do nothing to ensure a stable blood sugar, a strategy that could have a major beneficial effect on behavior and nutrition status. Maintaining a snack in elementary, junior high, and high schools would help satisfy energy needs and, as an aside, do much to control undesirable behavior. It's not fun to be around people who are hypoglycemic.

2. To estimate the energy requirement of physical activity in young athletes, it is important to remember that children use more energy per unit of body weight to do the same activity as adults. Add 20 to 25 percent to the adult energy expenditure values for children 8 to 10 years old; add 10 to 15 percent for children 11 to 14 years old.[29]

3. The distribution of energy substrates is important, but parents and coaches should understand that total energy intake adequacy is more important than the amount of carbohydrate or fat in the diet. Slightly liberalizing the fat intake from 25 to 30 percent of total calories will make it easier for young athletes to obtain the calories they need. Protein intake is important but need not rise above 15 percent of total calories or 1.5 grams per kilogram of body weight provided total energy intake adequacy is satisfied.

4. Young athletes tend to underconsume fluids, predisposing them to dehydration and increasing the risk of heat illness. Supervising adults should encourage physically active youth to take regular drinks, even when fluids are readily available. This may require fixed time-schedule drinking patterns that involve stoppage of play every 10 to 20 minutes, depending on the ambient heat and humidity.

5. Young female athletes are at risk for primary and secondary amenorrhea, both of which may be caused by excess physical activity, inadequate energy intake, and other factors. If a young female has a delayed menarche beyond age 14, she should be assessed by a pediatrician to make certain there is no underlying medical condition. In addition, the adequacy of nutrient and energy intake should be carefully assessed.

6. Young athletes should not diet because delayed eating and severe low-calorie intakes are counterproductive to achieving ideal body weight and body composition and negatively affect growth and development. The eating strategy should allow for frequent eating, with an opportunity to consume food approximately every 3 hours.

7. It is difficult for young female athletes to obtain sufficient iron, and surveys suggest that calcium intake is also marginal. Therefore, the parents of young athletes should consult with the family doctor to determine if iron or calcium supplements are warranted.

Young athletes have an extraordinary nutrition burden because they must satisfy the combined nutrition needs of growth plus the needs of physical activity. Young athletes should receive a minimum of six eating opportunities to ensure that nutrition needs can be met. Fluid consumption should be planned to lower dehydration risk. In addition, pediatricians should be satisfied that young athletes are maintaining normal and expected growth patterns at annual preparticipation physical examinations. Adolescent female athletes should be assessed for primary or secondary amenorrhea, with steps taken to resolve the amenorrhea as quickly as possible.

OLDER ATHLETES

There are far too many examples of older athletes performing well to suggest there is a definite time to put away the athletic shoes. The World Masters Athletics association lists many athletes who are still competing above 60 years of age in virtually every athletic discipline including steeplechase, pole vault, marathon, and the 10,000-meter run. The world-record holder for the men's outdoor 100 meters in the 100-year-old group is Hidekichi Miyazaki of Japan, with a time of 29.83 seconds, and Ron Taylor from Great Britain holds the record for 60-year-olds, an impressive 11.70 seconds. Older female athletes also excel. In 1994

Yekaterina Podkopayeva (Russia) won the world indoor 1,500 meters at the age of 42 with a time of 3:59:78. In the 80-year-old group for women, Nina Naumenko from Russia has the world record time of 58:24:70 in the outdoor 10,000 meters. Clearly, being older does not make stopping exercise mandatory. Nevertheless, the aging process does bring with it certain undeniable changes that should be addressed to ensure that exercise remains a healthful activity. Of particular concern are the age-related changes in body composition and the impact this has on resting energy expenditure; the lowered capacity to quickly recover from intensive or long bouts of exercise; a gradually diminishing bone mass; subtle changes in GI tract function that could influence nutrient absorption; and the possibility of a progressively lower heat tolerance.[30,31]

The increased risk of heat stress in older athletes should be seriously considered because the result of heat exhaustion and heatstroke is often death. During periods of high heat and humidity, those most likely to become seriously ill or die are the elderly. Although the elderly population should not be confused with the older athlete population, even if they are in the same age group, there may be an age-related drop in the capacity to dissipate heat regardless of fitness level[32] (see table 11.7).

Table 11.7 Factors That Change With Age That Could Affect Heat Tolerance, Regardless of Chronological Age

1. Lower aerobic capacity and associated variables

2. Sedentary lifestyle

3. Lower lean body mass; higher relative fat mass

4. Chronic hypohydration from lower fluid intake or higher fluid excretion by the kidneys, or both

5. Higher prevalence of chronic diseases, including hypertension, diabetes, and heart disease

6. Higher use of medications, including diuretics, adrenergic blockers, vasodilators, and anticholinergics

Adapted, by permission, from W.L. Kenney, 1993, "The older athlete: Exercise in hot environments," *GSSI Sports Science Exchange* #44 6(3). [Online]. Available: www.gssiweb.com/Article_Detail.aspx?articleid=17 [June 27, 2011].

An important factor in sweat production and cooling capacity is the ability to increase blood flow to the skin. Blood flow to the skin in older, fit athletes is lower than in younger athletes.[33,34] In addition, the lower blood flow associated with increasing age appears to be independent of hydration state. It also appears that, although sweat-gland recruitment is similar to that of younger athletes, older athletes produce less sweat per gland.[35] There is a wide genetically based variability in sweat production, but these studies suggest that older athletes should be vigilant about following a regular fluid-consumption schedule while exercising to optimize their capacity to produce sweat. Older athletes and their exercise partners should be cognizant of the symptoms of heat exhaustion and heatstroke. They should also be aware that most heat exhaustion occurs before heat acclimatization. Therefore, normal exercise intensities and durations should be reduced for the first few days in a new environment until the athlete has adapted.

Bone density becomes progressively lower with age, and females experience a faster drop in bone density after menopause when they lose the bone-protective action of estrogen. This is one of the primary reasons it is so important to achieve a high bone density by young adulthood so that, even with a progressive loss of density later on, there will be sufficient density to prevent reaching the fracture threshold in older age. The rate of change in bone density can be altered through an adequate intake of calcium, periodic and regular exposure to the sun for vitamin D, and regular stress on the skeleton through weight-bearing exercise. In addition, women may choose to take, through the advice of their doctors, estrogen replacement therapy (ERT). ERT may be particularly useful when there is a family history of osteoporosis or a woman has been diagnosed with low bone density. Certain cortisone-based drugs taken for the control of pain or osteoarthritis appear to be catabolic to bone, so regular use of these drugs would place the older athlete at increased risk of low bone density. The fact that older athletes continually stress the skeleton through regular physical activity is a major protective factor in keeping bone density elevated.

It would be expected that older athletes experience some degree of progressive GI dysfunction and changes in nutrient requirements, although no athlete-specific studies confirm that this, indeed, occurs. The typical effects of age on the GI tract include reduced motility; decreased absorption of dietary calcium, vitamin B_6, and vitamin B_{12}; and greater requirement for fluid and fiber to counteract reduced GI motility. The absorption of iron and zinc may also be a concern.[36] Energy expenditure decreases approximately 10 calories each year for men and 7 calories each year for women after the age of 20. However, fit people who maintain their lean body (muscle) mass are typically able to sustain energy metabolism. It is unclear, therefore, how or if the typical reduction in energy metabolism affects older athletes.

Changes in immune function should also be considered, but regular long-term exercise appears to attenuate the changes in the immune system that are typically associated with aging.[37] Vitamin and mineral supplementation is common among older athletes, often in an attempt to boost the immune system. There is little evidence that this is a useful strategy, but if the supplements target nutrients that aren't well absorbed, they may be warranted. Rather than guess, however, older athletes should consult with their doctors to determine the best strategy for delivering needed nutrients. In some cases, as in the case of vitamin B_{12}, a periodic injection may be the only strategy that reduces the risk of pernicious anemia. Taking oral supplements of vitamin B_{12} simply does not work. Good protein status is an important component of a stable immune function, but there is no evidence that protein intake should in any way be increased beyond the normal values established for athletes (between 1.2 and 1.7 grams per kilogram per day). On the contrary, aging often brings with it a reduction in kidney function, so reducing the amount of nitrogenous waste by lowering protein intake may be warranted. A good strategy would be to consume less protein but of higher quality to reduce the amount of nitrogenous waste produced.

General Recommendations for Older Athletes

1. Older athletes should take steps to reduce the risk of dehydration. Developing a fixed drinking schedule and being aware of the signs of heat stress are important because older athletes are likely to have lower sweat rates than younger athletes involved in the same activity.

2. GI function may require additional vitamin and mineral intake, perhaps through supplements. Older athletes should regularly consult with doctors to determine the biological need for specific supplements and take them only in reasonable prescribed doses. Vitamins and minerals of particular concern are calcium, iron, zinc, vitamin B_6, and vitamin B_{12}.

3. Reduced gut motility requires a slight increase in fiber consumption, but this should always take place in conjunction with additional fluid intake. Focusing on fresh fruits and vegetables as well as whole-grain products is an excellent means of obtaining additional fiber, plus these foods provide needed carbohydrate energy.

4. Frequent illness may be a sign that immune function is depressed. There is no perfect weapon for combating a reduction in immune function, but exercising reasonably, eating well, and resting well are useful strategies. Older athletes with infrequent eating patterns should consult with their doctors.

5. It takes longer for older athletes to adapt to new environments, so reducing exercise intensity and frequency for several days after travel is a logical and useful step to prevent overheating and illness.

Older athletes can expect some slowing of the metabolic rate, which makes it more difficult to sustain a desirable body composition and weight without making the appropriate reduction in energy consumption. At the same time, nutrient requirements mandate the consumption of a diet with a high nutrient density (i.e., a higher nutrient-to-calorie ratio). The avoidance of overtraining is important for injury reduction and sustaining immune function. This is particularly important because healing time for both injury and disease is longer with increasing age. Finally, adequate fluid intake is critically important to prevent dehydration and to sustain gut motility because the frequency of urination associated with advanced age may inhibit fluid consumption.

IMPORTANT POINTS

- Menstrual dysfunction is prevalent in female athletes and has associated problems that could affect short and long-term health. Inadequate energy intake is significantly associated with amenorrhea in female athletes, regardless of body-fat level.

- Women of childbearing age are at higher risk for iron-deficiency anemia, which compromises both health and physical performance. Female athletes should be tested annually to determine functional and stored iron status (hemoglobin, hematocrit, ferritin).

- Women with irregular menses should have a bone-density test (typically via dual-energy X-ray absorptiometry) to determine risk of osteopenia, osteoporosis, and fracture. If low bone density is present, a strategy for improving density should be discussed with a physician.

- Young athletes have extremely high energy requirements to support the combined needs of growth and physical activity. Planning is necessary to ensure they receive the needed energy and nutrients. Besides its impact on athletic performance, poor nourishment places children at a higher risk for current and future diseases.

- The body system for dissipating heat is not as well developed in children, so they should be carefully monitored for heat stress, particularly in hot and humid environments.

- Lower energy metabolism and altered GI function are normal changes in older adults and must be taken into account in older adults involved in sport.

- Because older adults take longer to adapt to unfamiliar environmental conditions, they should not exercise too intensely or frequently when first arriving in a different time zone with a different altitude, heat, or humidity.

Body Composition and Weight

The strength-to-weight ratio is a critical factor in overcoming resistance (drag) associated with sport, and in many skill sports the marker of success is related to the athlete's appearance (e.g., figure skating, diving, gymnastics). To improve the strength-to-weight ratio or the body profile, athletes typically resort to what amounts to a weight-loss strategy by increasing activity, reducing energy intake, or doing both. Although they may temporarily lower weight, this strategy results in an undesirable change in body composition that negatively affects the strength-to-weight ratio. Under ideal circumstances, athletes should incorporate strategies that improve appearance, overcome sport-specific resistance, and also enhance the capacity to sustain power output during practice and competition. Traditions in sport are hard to change, however, and these traditions often create unnecessary difficulties for athletes.

Ultimately, athletes themselves must understand the basic science behind how to achieve a desirable body weight without losing muscle and power and without increasing body-fat percentage in the process. Athletes and their coaches must also understand the very clear risks associated with the cyclic weight-loss patterns often experienced by athletes before, during, and after the competitive season. These risks include changes in the hormonal milieu that are associated with higher risk of skeletal problems, including higher stress fracture risk, and modifications in metabolic rate (adaptive thermogenesis) that make it more difficult for an athlete to sustain a desired weight and body composition without a constant ratcheting down of food intake—a strategy that leads to nutrient deficiency and disease. At the very least, poorly achieved weight loss nearly always reduces muscle mass and increases fat mass, making it more difficult for the athlete to achieve top performance.

This chapter helps athletes and their coaches understand weight-loss and body-composition issues so they can apply the appropriate strategies to achieve the optimal strength-to-weight ratio for their sports. In addition, the chapter provides an up-to-date review of the methods commonly used for assessing body composition, with the aim of helping athletes better understand what the values derived from these methods really mean. Finally, this chapter discusses eating disorders and how they can develop from the cyclic weight-control strategies so often followed by athletes.

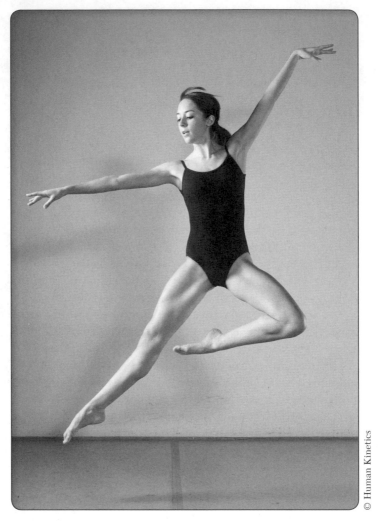

© Human Kinetics

Athletes in appearance sports are at higher risk of pursuing unhealthy means of weight loss.

WEIGHT LOSS AND BODY COMPOSITION

The body is made up of different components (water, muscle, fat, bone, nerve tissue, tendons, and so on), and each has a different density. For instance, muscle has a higher density than fat, so one pound of muscle takes up less space than one pound of fat. Athletes are often asked to lose weight, when they really should maintain muscle and lose fat. Weight, therefore is the wrong metric. Imagine an athlete who was asked to lose 4 pounds (2 kg). After his or her efforts, the athlete was assessed and found to have lost 4 pounds of fat and gained 4 pounds of muscle. Weight would be the same, but the strength-to-weight ratio would be better and the athlete would look smaller. As a result, performance would likely improve. However, if only weight was measured, this athlete would have been deemed a failure for not complying with the weight-loss mandate.

From a functional standpoint, tissues are grouped together into those that are mainly fat (fat mass), which is mainly anhydrous (has very little water associated with it), and those that have little fat (fat-free mass), which is hydrous (has a great deal of water associated with it). Fat-free mass is mainly water and protein but also includes small levels of minerals and stored carbohydrate (glycogen). The main constituents of fat-free mass include skeletal muscle, the heart, the skeleton, and other organs. Although total body weight is approximately 60 percent water, the water content of the fat-free mass is 70 percent. This can be compared with the water content of the fat mass, which is below 10 percent.[1] Fat-free mass is commonly referred to as lean mass, although this is viewed by many to be an inaccurate description because of the amount of water it contains. Athletes typically have a higher fat-free mass and a lower fat mass than do nonathletes. Sophisticated and widely accessible techniques, some of which include bone mass assessment, are now available for estimating body composition. The typical and usual body-composition techniques, however, try to estimate the fat mass and everything else (i.e., the fat-free mass).

Fat mass has two components: essential fat and storage fat. The essential fat is a necessary and required component of the brain, nerves, bone marrow, heart tissue, and cell walls that we cannot live without. Approximately 12 to 15 percent of total body weight in adult females is essential fat, the majority of which is associated with reproductive function and includes the additional fat associated with breast tissue. Because males do not have this reproductive function, male essential-fat levels are lower. Storage fat, on the other hand, is an energy reserve that builds up in adipose tissue underneath the skin (subcutaneous fat) and around the organs (interabdominal fat). There is also fat in muscle cells (particularly in Type I slow-twitch endurance muscle fibers) that serves as a ready energy reserve for aerobic metabolism. Healthy men and women have a storage-fat level that contributes approximately 11 to 15 percent to total body weight. Combining the essential-fat and storage-fat components, normal body-fat percentage for healthy, relatively lean males is about 15 percent (3 percent essential; 12 percent storage). Normal body-fat percentage for healthy, relatively lean females is about 26 percent (15 percent essential; 11 percent storage).[2]

Each technique for predicting body composition uses different assessment strategies that produce slightly different values. Therefore, each technique may use different normal standards that are specific to the method of analysis. For this reason, it is important that body-composition values derived using different assessment techniques not be used as an indication the athlete has changed. For instance, the body-composition values from dual-energy X-ray absorptiometry (DEXA) may produce higher body-fat values in the same person, taken at approximately the same time, as body-fat values derived from bioelectrical impedance analysis (BIA). It would be misleading, therefore, to use DEXA as a baseline value and BIA 4 weeks later, because the perceived change in body fat may be due more to the technique used than any actual change in body fat that has occurred.

Women with extremely low body-fat percentages may be at risk of developing reproductive system difficulties, commonly manifested as irregular menstrual periods (see table 12.1 for common terms associated with the menstrual cycle). Oligomenorrhea and amenorrhea are associated with increased fracture risk and low estrogen production, which increases the risk of osteoporosis (a bone disease associated with low bone density). There is some evidence that a body fat percentage of 17 to 22 percent is needed to maintain a normal menstrual cycle in most women.[3] There is also evidence that physiological and psychological stress is a trigger for disrupting the reproductive system.[4]

Table 12.1 Common Terms Related to the Menstrual Cycle

Term	Definition
Amenorrhea	Absence of the menstrual period for 6 months or absence of the menstrual cycle for 3 cycles
Primary amenorrhea	Considered present in a woman 18 years of age and older who has never had a period (delayed menses)
Secondary amenorrhea	Considered present in a woman who has experienced menses in the past but is not currently experiencing periods over a span of time (several months or even years)
Dysmenorrhea	Painful and irregular menstrual periods
Eumenorrhea	Normal menstrual frequency; no abnormalities of flow, timing, or pain
Oligomenorrhea	Infrequent menstrual frequency; fewer than 8 periods a year or periods at intervals greater than 35 days
Background	The hypothalamus (an organ in the brain) detects a lowered amount of estrogen and progesterone in the bloodstream during a period and secretes gonadotropin-releasing hormone (GnRH), which stimulates the pituitary gland to secrete follicle-stimulating hormone (FSH), which stimulates the ovaries to make estrogen to build up tissue in the uterus and to mature an egg within a follicle that holds it until ovulation, and luteinizing hormone (LH), which stimulates the release of that egg (ovulation). After ovulation, the remaining emptied follicle makes progesterone, which matures the built-up tissue in the uterus in preparation for implantation (pregnancy). Without implantation, the hormone levels fall, and the built-up uterine lining cannot hold together. The sloughing away of the uterine lining is referred to as the menstrual period.

A closer look, however, at both the body-fat and stress hypotheses for irregular menstrual function shows that these may not be correct. There is strong evidence that energy (calorie) availability, not body fatness or stress, is the primary regulator of female reproductive function. Women falling below an energy intake level of 30 calories per kilogram of fat-free mass per day are at significantly higher risk of menstrual dysfunction.[5,6] In addition, these data strongly suggest that women consuming 45 calories per kilogram of fat-free mass per day are resistant to developing menstrual dysfunction regardless of body-fat level or physical stress. Given the large number of normally menstruating athletic females who are lean (i.e., who have low body-fat levels), the energy availability hypothesis is more logical.

Women who develop an excessively low body-fat percentage or total body mass typically exercise excessively for the amount of energy they consume, or they have an eating disorder. The female athlete triad, a condition prevalent in many female athletes, includes the interrelated presence of an eating disorder, amenorrhea, and low bone density (either osteopenia or osteoporosis). See figure 12.1 for an illustration of the female athlete triad.

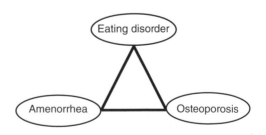

Figure 12.1 The female athlete triad.

WEIGHT

The measurement of weight (pounds) or mass (kilograms) by itself does not discriminate between fat mass and fat-free mass, so it is not a measure of body composition. Therefore, the statement "My weight is increasing, so I must be getting fat" is common but not necessarily correct. It is possible for an athlete to increase fat-free mass (i.e., muscle) without increasing fat mass. The result would be an increase in weight but not an increase in fat weight. It is also possible for an athlete to maintain weight but experience changes in fat mass or fat-free mass. This could be either desirable or undesirable depending on which element is increasing. All athletes, regardless of sport, find it desirable to achieve a high strength-to-weight ratio, which is associated with a relative increase in the ratio of fat-free mass to fat mass. This can be achieved by maintaining the fat-free mass while fat mass is decreased (lower total weight); increasing the fat-free mass while fat mass is maintained (higher total weight); increasing the fat-free mass while fat mass is decreased (lower total weight); or increasing the fat-free mass more than the increasing fat mass (higher total weight). As you can see, monitoring a change in weight alone is an inadequate means of understanding what really matters: The components of weight change. Although tracking weight is one indicator of an athlete's energy balance, it does nothing to explain whether the components of the weight are changing in a desirable direction. It is for this reason that body-composition evaluation should be a standard component of the athlete assessment protocol, with minimal reliance on weight alone.

Measures for Determining Desirable Weight

There are several common means of predicting ideal body weight. Ideally, these formulas could be used for beginning athletes as a starting goal, but since athletes typically have more lean mass per unit of height, it is likely they would exceed these ideal weight values.

Body Mass Index

Body mass index (BMI) is a useful tool for categorizing the weight of populations. However, it is not likely to be useful for individual athletes because athletes typically have more muscle per height than do nonathletes, which increases the weight-to-height ratio. BMI considers weight in relation to height using one of the following formulas:

BMI = weight in kilograms divided by height in meters squared

$$BMI = kg/m^2$$

or

BMI = weight in pounds divided by height in inches squared multiplied by 703

$$BMI = ([lb/in^2] \times 703)$$

Table 12.2 provides BMI values and their corresponding classifications.

Table 12.2 BMI Classification

Classification	BMI value
Underweight	<18.5
Normal	18.5-24.9
Overweight	25.0- 29.9
Obese	≥30

Weight and Body-Composition Issues

There is no question that total body weight is an important issue for athletes because it influences how easily they can perform their skills. A study assessing the relationship between body composition and fundamental movement skills among children and adolescents found that unhealthy weight gain reduced movement skill.[2] However, monitoring weight by itself may provide athletes with a misleading picture of what is good or bad about their body composition. In a number of sports, athletes will increase the time or intensity of a training regimen to improve performance, but then they inappropriately use changes in weight as a marker of success or failure. Imagine a football player who comes to training camp at a weight much higher than the coach is accustomed to seeing in this player. It may well be that the football player worked hard during the off-season to increase muscle mass, and the increase in weight is a result of more muscle. Wouldn't the coach be wrong in telling that player he has to lose weight? Gymnasts often reach their competitive peak during adolescence, a time when fast growth is the normal biological expectation. Despite this, gymnasts and other athletes are often weighed weekly or more often to make certain they are maintaining their weight. Shouldn't all the training they're doing increase their muscle mass and therefore their weight? Shouldn't they be growing and thus increasing their weight? These are examples of how weight is often used arbitrarily, incorrectly and, often, punitively. Tracking the constituents of weight makes much more sense and provides valuable information on the nature of body changes that are occurring. See table 12.3 for weight management strategies for athletes.

The principle of energy thermodynamics is always with us. Consumption of more calories than the body burns leads to a weight gain; consumption of fewer calories than the body burns leads to a weight loss; and consumption of exactly the same number of calories that the body burns leads to weight stability. But making a change in body weight is not as straightforward as the principle of energy thermodynamics may make it seem.

The most common belief is that low-calorie dieting is an effective but unpleasant means of weight and fat loss. It seems logical that a 25 percent reduction in energy intake will lead to a 25 percent reduction in weight. The reality, however, is that energy expenditure after weight loss is less than would be expected by the amount of weight that was lost.[7, 8,9] This means the adjustment in energy expenditure resulting from inadequate intake is greater than the mathematical expectation and leads to a return to the original weight, even with a lower energy intake. In simple terms this means that the less you eat, the less you can eat to maintain weight. A close look at the reason for this lower metabolic rate is clear. With an inadequate caloric intake, the body catabolizes the metabolic (lean) mass to lower the need for energy so survival is assured. This is a perfectly reasonable adaptation.

Table 12.3 Weight Management Strategies for Athletes

Setting and monitoring goals	• Set realistic weight and body-composition goals. Ask the athlete:
	  • What is the maximum weight you would find acceptable?
	  • What was the lowest weight you maintained without constant dieting?
	  • How did you derive your goal weight?
	  • At what weight and body composition do you perform best?
	• Focus less on the scale and more on healthful habits such as stress management and making good food choices.
	• Monitor progress by measuring changes in exercise performance and energy level, the prevention of injuries, normal menstrual function, and general overall well-being.
	• Help athletes develop lifestyle changes that maintain a healthful weight for themselves—not for their sport, for their coach, for their friends, for their parents, or to prove a point.

Suggestions for food intake	• Low energy intake will not sustain athletic training. Instead, decreases in energy intake of 10 to 20% of normal intake will lead to weight loss without the athlete feeling deprived or overly hungry. Strategies such as substituting lower-fat foods for whole-fat foods, reducing intake of energy-dense snacks, maintaining portion awareness, and doing activities other than eating when not hungry can be useful. • If appropriate, athletes can reduce fat intake but need to know that a lower-fat diet will not guarantee weight loss unless a negative energy balance (reduced energy intake and increased energy expenditure) is achieved. Fat intake should not be decreased below 15% of total energy intake because some fat is essential for good health. • Emphasize increased intake of whole grains and cereals and legumes. • Five or more daily servings of fruits and vegetables provide nutrients and fiber. • Dieting athletes should not skimp on protein and need to maintain adequate calcium intakes. Accordingly, consuming low-fat dairy products and lean meats, fish, and poultry is suggested. • A variety of fluids—especially water—should be consumed throughout the day, including before, during, and after exercise. Dehydration as a means of reaching a body-weight goal is contraindicated.
Other weight management strategies	• Advise athletes against skipping meals (especially breakfast) and allowing themselves to become overly hungry. They should be prepared for times when they might get hungry, including keeping nutritious snacks available for those times. • Athletes should not deprive themselves of favorite foods or set unrealistic dietary rules or guidelines. Instead, dietary goals should be flexible and achievable. Athletes should remember that foods can fit into healthful lifestyle. Developing lists of "good" and "bad" foods is discouraged. • Help athletes identify their own dietary weaknesses and plan strategies for dealing with them. • Remind athletes they are making lifelong dietary changes to sustain a healthful weight and optimal nutrition status rather than going on a short-term diet.

Figure 3. Weight management strategies for athletes. (Adapted from: Manore MM. Chronic dieting in active women: What are the health consequences? *Women's Health Issues.* 1996;6:332-341. Copyright 1996, with permission from Elsevier.)

Reprinted from *Journal of the American Dietetic Association* 109(3), American Dietetic Association, Dietitians of Canada, and the American College of Sports Medicine, "Position paper: Nutrition and athletic performance," 509-527, copyright 2009, with permission from Elsevier. Adapted from *Women's Health Issues* 6, M.M. Manore, "Chronic dieting in active women: What are the health consequences?," 332-341, copyright 1995, with permission from Elsevier.

Logic also suggests that a 25 percent increase in energy intake will lead to a 25 percent increase in weight. In fact, although weight gain does occur, it doesn't appear to increase as much as the increase in energy intake suggests it should, but it's close. When people are purposefully overfed to gain weight, the amount of weight gain is proportionate to the amount of overfeeding. [10-15] These studies strongly suggest that we have homeostatic mechanisms during periods of energy deficit that help us maintain our weight. This may be a "survival of the species" mechanism that helps humans survive periods of famine. We also appear capable of storing energy effectively (as fat) during periods of excess. This may be another survival mechanism that enables us to store energy when we are lucky enough to have excess food available.

Since major energy surpluses and deficits appear to activate homeostatic mechanisms, a possible means of making a desired change in weight and body composition is to avoid major energy-balance shifts. Exercise should be at the core of any desired body-composition change (i.e., an increase in lean mass and a decrease in fat mass, coupled with a small decrease in weight). But such a change might be easier to achieve if the energy deficit and energy surplus created are never too large during the day. Figures 12.2 and 12.3 show how eating patterns can affect body composition.

Energy surpluses and deficits are represented, respectively, by variations above and below the perfect energy-balance line (zero). In figure 12.3, when the line moves above zero, the athlete has consumed more energy than was expended. When the line moves below zero, the athlete has expended more energy than was consumed. Eating pattern 1 represents an athlete eating small meals frequently; there are no energy surpluses or deficits that exceed 400 calories. Eating pattern 2 represents infrequent eating, with excess calories (high-surplus energy peaks) consumed at each meal. Eating pattern 3 represents an athlete who spends the majority of the day in an energy-deficit state from not eating enough when the energy is needed, a condition that stimulates the breakdown of muscle tissue for energy. At the end of the day, a very large meal brings the athlete into energy balance, but much of this meal will be stored as fat. Within any given day, energy balance is important for both performance and body composition.

Weight is the best indicator of the adequacy of caloric intake, and body composition helps determine if the calories are being consumed in the proper amounts and at the correct intervals. See figures 12.2 and 12.3 for illustrations of how to optimally fuel your activity, and see chapters 16 to 18 for sample diet plans.

Since the standard three-meal-a-day schedule forces athletes to consume a large amount of energy at each meal to obtain the necessary energy, staying in energy balance is easier on a six-meal pattern. Frequent consumption of small meals to maintain a steady energy flow can be an important strategy in making the desired changes. Chapter 6 discusses the importance of meal timing.

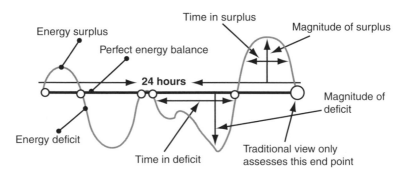

Figure 12.2 Sharp deviations in energy balance during the course of a day can affect body composition.

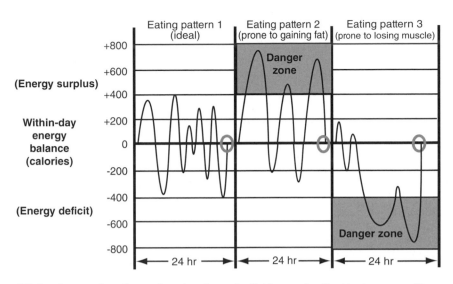

Figure 12.3 A person's eating pattern has the potential to greatly affect body composition.

BODY COMPOSITION

The purpose of body-composition assessment is to determine an athlete's distribution of fat-free mass and fat mass. A high ratio of fat-free mass to fat mass is typically synonymous with a high strength-to-weight ratio, which is typically associated with athletic success. However, there is no single ideal body composition for all athletes in all sports. Each sport has a range of lean mass and fat mass associated with it, and each athlete in a sport has an individual range that is ideal for her. Athletes trying to achieve an arbitrary body composition that is not right for them are likely to place themselves at health risk and will not achieve the performance benefits they seek. In fact, athletes nearly always perform less well when they try to achieve a weight or body composition that is inconsistent with their history and genetic makeup. Therefore, the key to body-composition assessment is to establish an acceptable range of fat-free mass and fat mass for the individual athlete. It is important to regularly monitor the fat-free mass and fat mass to ensure the stability or growth of the fat-free mass and a proportional maintenance or reduction of the fat mass. Just as much attention should be given to changes in fat-free mass (both in weight of fat-free mass and in the proportion of fat-free mass) as the attention traditionally given to body-fat percentage.

The fat mass and fat-free mass model of body composition assumes the combined weight of fat mass and fat-free mass equals total body weight. The assessment of body composition typically results in the prediction of body-fat percentage, or the proportion of total weight that is composed of fat. As an example, assuming an athlete weighs 150 pounds (68 kg) and has a body-fat percentage of 20 percent, the athlete has 30 pounds (150 × .20 = 30) (13.6 kg) of fat weight and 120 pounds (54.4 kg) of fat-free weight. If this same athlete were to experience a reduction in body-fat percentage to 15 percent while maintaining weight, this translates into 22.5 pounds (150 × .15 = 22.5) (10.2 kg) of fat weight and 127.5 pounds (57.8 kg) of fat-free weight. This increase of 7.5 pounds (3.4 kg) in fat-free weight and reduction in fat weight means the athlete is now smaller (pound for pound, lean mass takes up less space than fat mass because it has a higher density), which means he should be able to move more quickly and more efficiently (less drag) than before, despite being the same weight. However, if this 150-pound athlete were to maintain weight but increase fat mass while reducing lean mass, potential speed and efficiency of movement would be reduced. Weight, in the absence of knowledge of its components, is a poor measure for predicting athletic success and should not be used by itself for this purpose.

Body Composition and Performance

Athletic performance is, to a large degree, dependent on the athlete's ability to sustain power (both anaerobically and aerobically) and to overcome the resistance or drag associated with any physical activity. Both of these factors are interrelated with the athlete's body composition. In sports where a lean appearance is commonly expected (swimming, diving, gymnastics, figure skating), attainment of an "ideal" body composition often becomes a central theme of training. Besides the aesthetic and performance reasons for wanting to achieve an optimal body composition, there may also be safety reasons.

An athlete who is carrying excess weight may be more prone to injury when performing difficult skills than an athlete with a more desirable body composition. However, when athletes attempt to achieve an optimal body composition, their methods are often counterproductive. Diets and excessive training often result in such a severe energy deficit that, although total weight may be reduced, the constituents of weight also change, commonly with a lower muscle mass and a relatively higher fat mass. The resulting higher body-fat percentage and lower muscle mass inevitably result in even greater energy deficits. This downward energy intake spiral may be the precursor of eating disorders that place the athlete at serious health risk. Therefore, although achieving an optimal body composition is useful for high-level athletic performance, the processes athletes often use to attain an optimal body composition may reduce athletic performance, place athletes at a higher injury risk, increase health risks, and predispose them to eating disorders.

Athletes purposely trying to lose fat should be aware of the best physical activities to achieve this goal. Contrary to popular belief, low-intensity aerobic training, which is so often used as a fat-loss exercise regimen, is not particularly effective at achieving this goal. In a study specifically aimed at determining the relative fat-loss potential of different types of activity, it was found that high-intensity exercise training was significantly more effective at reducing total abdominal fat, and subcutaneous abdominal fat, than low-intensity exercise training.[16] High-intensity winter sports, for instance, are associated with a lower body-fat percentage and higher lean mass than are less intense activities.[17] Care must be taken, however, to avoid low blood sugar during high-intensity exercise, as low blood sugar is a predictor of high cortisol production, which is associated with a loss of fat-free mass, a loss of bone mass, and a higher body-fat percentage.[18] Maintenance of blood sugar during these high-intensity activities requires a conscious effort to consume a source of carbohydrate (typically a carbohydrate-containing sports beverage) at regular intervals during the activity.

In the minds of athletes, there is an inherent conflict between overcoming the resistance, or drag, associated with sport and having enough energy to sustain power output over the entire course of a competition or training session (see figure 12.4). Athletes view weight reduction (i.e., being smaller) as an effective means of overcoming resistance (imagine the position and profile a cyclist or speedskater assumes to reduce drag), and the common way to achieve weight reduction is to reduce caloric intake. However, having the capacity to sustain power output requires eating to at least a state of energy balance. It appears that

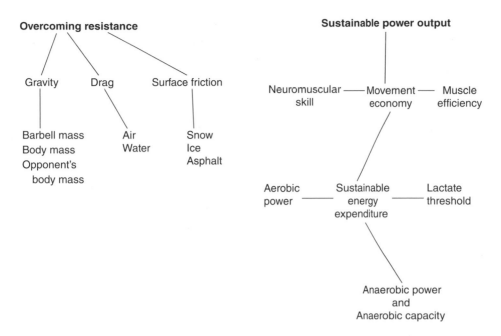

Figure 12.4 To train and compete successfully, an athlete must have enough energy to sustain the necessary power to overcome drag.

Reprinted, by permission, from D.R. Lamb, 1995, "Basic principles for improving sport performance," *GSSI Sports Science Exchange* #55 8(2). [Online]. Available: www.gssiweb.com/Article_Detail.aspx?articleid=28 [June 27, 2011].

many athletes believe that sustaining power output is not as important as reducing drag, resulting in the inadequate consumption of energy.

Many people have the unhealthy mind-set that food, regardless of the amount and type, is "fat producing." A much healthier (and from the point of view of an athlete, more appropriate) mind-set is that food is the provider of the fuel and nutrients associated with muscle energy.

Body-fat percentage should be thought of as having a general range for different sports, and it's OK for athletes to fall anywhere on that sport-specific range. Within some reasonable bounds, having a relatively low body-fat percentage may aid athletic performance by improving the strength-to-weight ratio: For a given weight, more of it is represented by lean mass that is power producing and less of it by fat mass that represents stored fuel. It also helps by lowering the resistance (or drag) an athlete has as he moves through the air, swims in water, or skates on ice; the smaller the body profile, the less resistance the body is likely to produce.

Less resistance is so important for some sports (typically the faster you go, the greater the importance of drag reduction) that performance techniques are based on reducing drag. After their initial strides off the starting line, for instance, speedskaters spend the entire race bent over to reduce wind resistance. Cyclists wear special streamlined helmets and clothing, position their bodies on the bicycle to reduce drag, and even strategize about the best time to sprint ahead of the cyclist in front of them. Going too soon can lead to premature exhaustion because it takes a great deal more energy (12 to 17 percent more) for the cyclist in the lead facing the air resistance to go the same speed. A gymnast who weighs

110 pounds (50 kg) and is 5 feet (152 cm) tall with a body-fat percentage of 15 percent will have a lower air resistance (i.e., less drag) tumbling through the air than a gymnast with the same weight and height but with a body-fat percentage of 20 percent. Figure skaters are increasingly required to perform jumps with more in-air revolutions to stay competitive. The greater the number of revolutions, the more difficult it is for a larger figure skater to complete the jump.

For some sports, however, drag may make little or no difference. It's hard to imagine how a lineman on a football team is concerned about air resistance. Nevertheless, even for this athlete, having a high strength-to-weight ratio makes a difference because the lineman who can move his mass more quickly and powerfully will knock over the lineman who moves more slowly. Even a powerlifter gains an advantage if, in meeting a weight category, more of the lifter's weight is composed of muscle and less is composed of fat. In sports where being aerodynamic helps, body composition makes a difference because, pound for pound, fat takes up more space than lean tissue does because it is less dense.

Body-Composition Estimation

It is extremely difficult to accurately determine body composition by weighing or looking at a person. There are many "thin" people who have lost so much lean mass that they actually have a relatively high body-fat percentage, and there are also many "large" people who are actually relatively lean. Even with modern equipment and sophisticated equations, it is extremely difficult to accurately measure body-fat percentage and to consistently repeat that measurement. We have no direct means of assessing body composition (the subject wouldn't survive if we tried), so all the techniques available to us are attempting to accurately estimate the fat mass or the fat-free mass. Each technique uses a different means of making this estimate, so cross-comparisons between techniques should not be made. As an example, athletes who have had body-fat percentage estimated via skinfolds should not compare the values from that method with values obtained by bioelectrical impedance analysis. The values obtained from these techniques are likely to be sufficiently different that, at the very least, the athlete will be confused. The common methods for assessing body composition include

- hydrostatic weighing (underwater weighing),
- skinfold measurements applied to prediction equations,
- bioelectrical impedance analysis (BIA),
- dual-energy X-ray absorptiometry (DEXA), and
- air displacement plethysmography.

Hydrostatic Weighing (Hydrodensitometry)

Hydrostatic weighing is the classic means of determining body composition. It uses what is known as Archimedes' principle,[19] which states that for an equal weight, lower-density objects have a larger surface area and displace more water than higher-density objects. From a body-composition standpoint, this principle is applied in the following way:

1. The subject is weighed on a standard scale to get a "land weight."
2. Using specialized equipment, the subject's lung volume is estimated (the subject blows into a tube).

3. The subject sits on a chair that is attached to a weight scale.

4. The chair and weight scale are positioned over water, and the chair is slowly lowered into the water.

5. When the subject is lowered into the water just below the chin, he is asked to fully exhale and completely lower his head into the water to be completely immersed.

6. While immersed, "underwater weight" is read off the scale that is attached to the chair the subject is sitting on.

Subjects weigh less in water than out of water because body fat (regardless of the amount present) makes the subject more buoyant. The difference between in-water weight and out-of-water weight reflects how much body fat the subject has. A very obese subject with a high level of body fat appears lighter in water relative to land weight. Lung volume is measured before taking the water weight, and there is an adjustment for the buoyancy that can be attributed to the air in the lungs. To minimize the lung–air effect, the subject is asked to exhale before full submersion, but there is always some remaining air in the lungs, referred to as residual volume.

Although there is some potential for error with hydrodensitometry related to a person's hydration status and residual volume, this technique is useful for determining the change in body composition over time if the technicians performing the measurements are good at precisely replicating the measurement procedure. It is also a useful means of determining the body composition of a population because the errors associated with the technique are likely to average themselves out over many measurements. However, people within that population would never be sure if their personal body-composition results were accurate. Good laboratories that do research in body composition have invested a great deal for the equipment needed to accurately do hydrostatic weighing. Further, they also invest in making sure they have highly qualified people to take the measurements.

Skinfolds

Skinfold calipers, which vary in cost from free to $500, are used to measure a double thickness of the fat layer under the skin. This fat layer (called subcutaneous fat) is hypothesized to represent approximately 50 percent of a person's total body fat. Therefore, if you can get a good estimate of the subcutaneous fat layer, you should be able to predict the total body-fat level. The prediction equations commonly used to determine body composition from skinfolds are based on the body-composition determinations derived from hydrodensitometry. It works something like this: You measure a group of people using hydrodensitometry to determine their body-fat percentages. Then you measure these same people with a series of skinfolds, which are used in statistics to predict the body-fat percentage obtained from hydrodensitometry. If the skinfolds, when applied to the newly created equation, can successfully predict the hydrodensitometry value, then you have a skinfold equation for predicting body-fat percentage.

A number of different equations are available for the general population, and several equations have been developed specifically for athletes. In general, using an equation that is more specific to the person you're measuring yields more accurate results. Also, equations that use more skinfold measurements are generally more accurate. For instance, one equation may require height, weight, age, triceps skinfold, and abdomen skinfold. Another equation may require height, weight, age, and skinfolds at the triceps, subscapular, midaxillary, suprailiac, abdomen, and midthigh sites.

It's important to say a word about the values that are derived from skinfold equations and used to predict body-fat percentage. Many of the equations used for athletes are actually meant for the general (i.e., nonathlete) population. Since many athletes are considerably leaner than the average nonathlete, the results derived from skinfold equations are unrealistically low. Many athletes come to the lab saying they have a body-fat percentage of 2 or 3 percent, and I know immediately that these are estimates from equations that have not been normalized on athletes. It's simply not possible to have such a low body-fat percentage. When these athletes are given the true value from a more realistic assessment (using either better, more population-specific equations or a more accurate technique), they don't usually respond positively when they receive the new number (usually somewhere between 8 and 18 percent). It's important for you to remember that when skinfold equations are used, the single number you get is not going to be perfectly accurate. However, that number can be used as a baseline to determine change over time if the same technique and same equation are used to get the second value. It is completely inappropriate to compare the first value with one that was obtained using a different set of skinfolds and a different equation.

Bioelectrical Impedance Analysis (BIA)

For those of you who know what to do if you're in a swimming pool and hear thunder nearby, you already know the principle behind bioelectrical impedance analysis (BIA). Water is a good conductor of electricity, and most body water is found in the lean mass. Fat, which has almost no water in it, is such a poor conductor of electricity that it actually impedes the electrical flow.

BIA equipment comes in two basic forms. In one form, the subject lies down and the right wrist and right ankle are fitted with electrodes, which produce an electrical current that runs from the wrist to the ankle. In another form, the subject stands on a platform with bare feet, and an electrical current runs from the right foot, up the right leg, down the left leg, and out the left foot. Regardless of the BIA equipment used, the principle behind the technique is the same. If you know the beginning level of energy (electricity) that enters the system and you can measure the level of energy that exits the system, you know how much of the energy has been impeded in the system. Since muscle is an efficient conductor of electricity (because of the water and electrolytes it contains) and fat is an efficient insulator of electricity, the greater the impedance, the greater the level of fat. If you start with 100 units of electricity going into your system, and 80 units of electricity come out of the system, you have more water and muscle than someone who has 100 units going in and 60 units coming out.

Of course, a number of adjustments to the prediction are necessary. The electrical current would run a longer distance in a taller person, so a taller person would automatically have a greater level of impedance. The ratio of weight to height is also important because it helps predict the distance the current is running and the composition of the tissues it is running through. Since body composition commonly changes with age (people become less lean and more fat as they get older), age is also an important predictor of body composition. At the initiation of the adolescent growth spurt, males and females begin to differentiate themselves on body composition, with females having relatively more fat than males do. So gender is also an important consideration in this prediction. Therefore, when performing a BIA, the variables age, height, weight, and gender are included in the equation that predicts body-fat percentage.

Although BIA has an excellent theoretical basis for making good body-composition predictions, several important protocols must be followed for the results to be accurate and repeatable. Since the technique is dependent on electrical conductivity through the lean mass, the hydration state of the subject can alter the results. If someone having a BIA test is not well hydrated, the electrical current will not be conducted through the lean mass as well, so the subject will appear to have more fat mass than she actually does. Therefore, it is critically important that the person being measured be in a well-hydrated state. It is generally believed that drinking alcohol, exercising, consuming large amounts of coffee, and spending time outside in hot and humid weather within 24 hours of a BIA test lead to sufficient dehydration that the results will not be accurate. Since serious athletes exercise most days, this technique may provide results that indicate more body fat than they really have. Therefore, athletes who are measured with this technique should wait until after a day of rest and should make certain they are well hydrated. An easy hydration check is to see if the urine is clear. The more clear the urine is, the better hydrated you are.

Some newer BIA equipment is capable of providing segmental body composition (arms, legs, abdomen) that is useful for determining muscular symmetry. The In Body 720 (from Biospace, Co. LTD), shown in figure 12.5, is an example of equipment using eight-mode BIA technology to perform segmental measurements; it also uses multiple frequencies and no empirical data.

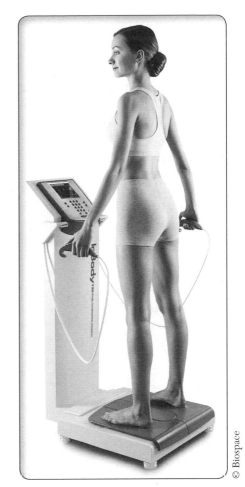

Figure 12.5 An eight-mode bioelectrical impedance device.

© Biospace

These newer BIA methods are also less sensitive to hydration state. A study using eight-mode BIA and DEXA determined no significant difference in body-fat estimation between these methods when applied to children.[20] However, persons with higher body fat may experience greater error in body-composition estimation using BIA than with DEXA.[21]

Dual-Energy X-Ray Absorptiometry (DEXA)

Dual-energy X-ray absorptiometry (DEXA) is the most accurate and most expensive means of determining body composition, and it is generally considered the current gold standard for this purpose. The information you can derive from a full-body scan on an athlete is invaluable, including bone density; body-fat percentage; lean body mass; fat mass; and the distribution of fat and lean tissue in the arms, trunk, and legs. DEXA output even provides the differences in lean mass and fat mass between the left and right sides. This information can be particularly important for athletes who wish to develop symmetrical bodies or who, because of the nature of the sport, need to produce the same muscular power in each leg or in each arm.

DEXA works by passing two X-ray beams through the subject and measuring the amount of X-ray absorbed by the tissue it has passed through. One beam is high intensity and one is low intensity, so the relative absorbance of each beam is an indication of the density of the tissue it has passed through. The higher the tissue density, the greater the reduction in X-ray intensity. Don't be frightened by all this talk of X-ray beams passing through your body. In fact, the amount of radiation energy that is used with DEXA is extremely small. You would need to have approximately 800 full-body DEXA scans before being exposed to the same amount of radiation received from one standard chest X-ray. In fact, the level of radiation is so low that DEXA is approved by the FDA as a screening device to predict body composition. Usually, X-ray devices are reserved as diagnostic instruments because of the amount of radiation they impart, but not so for DEXA.

The procedure for DEXA, which was originally developed to determine the density of bone, couldn't be easier. The subject lies on the DEXA table for approximately 20 minutes, and the pencil-beam X-rays pass through the subject and are interpreted by a mechanical arm above the subject. Because metal has such a high density, the subject is asked to remove all jewelry and must wear clothing that contains no metal. The resultant value is translated into a density value for bone, lean, and fat tissue. Because the density values are derived from a direct assessment of tissue density, this is as close as we can get to directly assessing tissue density (short of surgery). If you can find a lab with DEXA, the usual cost for a full-body scan is somewhere between $100 and $250.

Air Displacement Plethysmography

The Bod Pod (see figure 12.6) uses air displacement to determine body density. From body density, body-fat percentage can be predicted.

Using the same whole-body measurement principle as underwater weighing (hydrodensitometry), but with air displacement instead of water displacement, the Bod Pod measures a subject's mass and volume, from which whole-body density is determined. Using these data, body fat and lean muscle mass can then be calculated. This technique has been found valid and reliable for determining body composition, but it may slightly underestimate body-fat levels by 2 to 3 percent.[22]

The Bod Pod system has been used to assess athletes and requires minimal technical training for operation. An early study on collegiate football players determined that this method produced lower body-fat

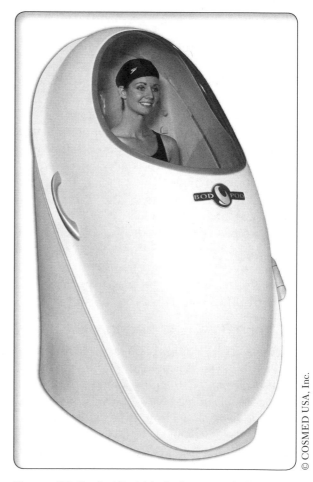

© COSMED USA, Inc.

Figure 12.6 Bod Pod (air displacement device for assessing body composition).

percentage results than either dual-energy X-ray absorptiometry or hydrostatic weighing.[23] The underprediction of body-fat percentage was also found when assessing adult females with the Bod Pod and with a four-compartment model.[24] A study of NCAA Division III wrestlers compared the Bod Pod with bioelectrical impedance analysis (leg to leg) and skinfolds. It was found that all the methods were correlated and that the Bod Pod and skinfolds could both be recommended for use with wrestlers.[25] A study assessing the Bod Pod and dual-energy X-ray absorptiometry with young women found that both techniques were valid for predicting body-fat percentage in this population.[26]

Changes in Body Composition

Body composition changes. We can influence that change by taking charge of what we eat and how we exercise. The general rule for lean mass (including bone mass) is "use it or lose it." We're wonderfully adaptive creatures, and we quickly adapt to our environments and our activities. We know, for instance, that the bones of astronauts quickly demineralize because the gravity-free environment of outer space eliminates the need for a strong skeleton. We would do quite well in that environment looking like a jellyfish, and the bones quickly adapt by releasing lots of calcium. The effect of this environment is so strong that astronauts must spend a significant amount of time doing exercise that places stress on the skeleton. Again, we're adaptive creatures, so placing this artificial stress on the bones helps keep them strong, even in a gravity-free environment. The same thing happens when people are bedridden because of an injury. Both bone and muscle masses are rapidly reduced because they simply aren't needed when you're lying in bed. The important thing to remember about our tissues is that they are alive and will do what's needed to adapt to their current situation. Even bone, which to the casual observer might appear to be a hard, rocklike, nonadaptive structure, is actually very much alive and changing all the time. Minerals move in and minerals move out, and this process leads to a constant remodeling of bone.

When you consider the influences on body composition, they boil down to the following:

• **Genetic predisposition.** This is everyone's bottom line, and no matter how hard you try, you can't change it. People have different inherited body types, and each type has a different predisposition toward accumulating more or less fat. Endomorphs (large trunk, short fingers, shorter legs) have a predisposition toward higher body-fat percentages, and ectomorphs (long legs, long fingers, shorter trunk) have a predisposition toward a slender build with less body fat. What you're born with can't change, so all you can hope to do is optimize what you've been given.

• **Age.** People generally develop a lower lean mass and higher fat mass after the age of 30. However, although this age-related change in body composition is normal, it isn't inevitable. It has been clearly shown that a good diet and regular activity can keep you lean. Since energy metabolism drops about 2 percent for each decade after age 30, it gets progressively more difficult to maintain a desirable weight and body composition. To maintain what you've got, you would have to make either a 2 percent increase in energy expenditure or a 2 percent decrease in energy intake each decade after 30 to match the drop in energy metabolism. Although this 2 percent difference seems small, it could make a major difference in your body composition. Consider that the average person consumes about 2,500 calories per day. If you need 2 percent less than this and don't make an adjustment, that represents a 50-calorie error of excess each day. Multiply that over 365 days and it represents

18,250 excess calories per year. Since an excess of 3,500 calories represents a 1-pound (.5 kg) weight gain, in the course of 1 year this small 50-calorie error would manifest itself as a weight gain of more than 5 pounds (2.3 kg). In 5 years, that's a weight gain of 25 pounds (11.4 kg), and in 10 years, that's a weight gain of a whopping 50 pounds (22.7 kg).

• **Gender.** All other things being equal, women have a higher body-fat percentage than do men. Nothing can be done to alter this, and there is certainly nothing wrong with it. The gender difference is just a manifestation of the different biological expectations of men and women. However, there are many women who have a lower body-fat percentage than some men because they exercise more and eat better. Therefore, despite this baseline difference, doing the right things can help you (regardless of your gender) optimize your body composition for your sport.

• **Menopause.** Studies now strongly suggest that menopause is associated with significant changes in body fatness, and estrogen, body fat, and menopause are all strongly influenced by a woman's energy balance. In one study of healthy women, it was found that estradiol (a major form of estrogen produced in the ovaries that is involved in uterine development) and body fat are strongly associated. Women with very low body fat and women with very high body fat both had decreased estradiol levels, and both estradiol and body fat were significantly influenced by energy balance.[27] It has also been found that both body fat and weight increase significantly in women becoming menopausal. It appears that all women tend to gain subcutaneous abdominal fat over time, but only those who are postmenopausal experience a significant increase in visceral fat.[28]

• **Type of activity.** Different types of activities place different stresses on the system, and as you would expect, the body responds differently to these stresses. Aerobic exercise is the standard for reducing body-fat percentage. However, there is good evidence that any type of activity (including anaerobic activity) will reduce body-fat percentage. High-intensity activity (such as performed by sprinters and weightlifters) may increase lean body mass and reduce body-fat percentage, so the impact on weight may be minimal. Nevertheless, this shift in body composition is still likely to make the person appear slightly smaller, since pound for pound, fat weight takes up more space than lean-mass weight. When energy expenditure (calories burned) is equivalent, both anaerobic and aerobic activity appear to lower body fat to the same extent, but it takes much longer to burn the same energy with aerobic activity. Aerobic activity also does not appear to have the same beneficial effect of increasing the fat-free mass.

• **Amount of activity.** Clearly, the more a person exercises, the greater the potential benefits in desirably altering body composition. However, activity must be supported by an adequate intake of energy. Increasing the time of activity without also increasing the amount of energy intake causes a breakdown of muscle mass to support energy needs. There is no question this would be an undesirable change in body composition for an athlete. In addition, although overtraining will not necessarily lead to a reduction in lean body mass, it causes an increase in muscle soreness and reduces muscular power and endurance. Therefore, the amount of activity should be carefully balanced with adequate energy intake and with adequate rest to ensure maintenance of muscle mass and athletic performance.

• **Nutrition.** Eating too much or too little can both negatively affect body composition. Eating too much, either over the course of a day or at one time, is likely to increase fat storage; eating too little will lower both lean (muscle) mass and fat mass. In addition, certain nutrients are important for metabolic processes. A failure to consume an adequate level of these nutrients (B vitamins, zinc, iron, and so on) may reduce your ability to properly burn fuel, thereby limiting your ability to burn fat through exercise.

Body-Composition Assessment Issues

Body composition has become an important part of athlete assessment. The amount of muscle and fat an athlete has can be predictive of performance, and bone mass assessment is important for understanding if developmental problems exist or if the athlete will face current or future risk for fracture. A periodic assessment of body composition also helps the athlete understand if the training regimen is causing the kinds of physical changes being sought. However, there are some important things to keep in mind when assessing body composition.

You can alter body composition by changing your diet and exercise, but these two should be considered together when making changes. Making dramatic changes in either direction is likely to cause unpredictable problems in your body composition. If you increase your training regimen, it is necessary to increase your energy intake to support the increase in energy expenditure. Putting yourself in a severe energy-deficit state by increasing exercise and maintaining or lowering energy intake is likely to lower metabolic rate, increase fat storage, and cause a breakdown of muscle to support energy needs. Eating too much is also likely to increase fat storage. It's best to maintain energy intake throughout the day, so athletes should be careful to consume enough energy to support exercise rather than make up for an energy deficit at the end of the day.

Athletes often compare body composition values with other athletes, but this comparison is not meaningful and may drive an athlete to change body composition in a way that negatively affects both performance and health. Health professionals involved in obtaining body-composition data should be sensitive to the confidentiality of this information. They should also explain to each athlete that differences in height, age, and gender are likely to result in differences in body composition, without necessarily any differences in performance. Strategies for achieving privacy and helping athletes put the information in the proper context include the following:

- Assess only one athlete at a time to limit the chance that the data will be shared.
- Give athletes information on body composition using phrases such as "within the desirable range" rather than a raw value, such as saying, "Your body-fat level is 18 percent."
- Provide athletes with information on how they have changed between assessments rather than offering the current value.
- Increase the focus on muscle mass, and decrease the focus on body fat.
- Use body-composition values as a means of explaining changes in objectively measured performance outcomes.

Most athletes would like their body-fat level to be as low as possible. However, athletes often try to seek a body-fat level that is arbitrarily low (so low that it has nothing to do with the norms in the sport or their own body-fat predisposition), and this can increase the frequency of illness, increase the risk of injury, lengthen the time for recovery after an injury, reduce performance, and increase the risk of an eating disorder. Body-composition values should be thought of as numbers on a continuum that are usual for a sport. If an athlete falls anywhere on that continuum, it is likely that factors other than body composition (e.g., training, skills acquisition) will be the major predictors of performance success.

Seeking arbitrarily low body-fat levels or weight is an issue in sports where making weight is a common expectation. Wrestlers in particular make dangerous efforts—sometimes leading to death—to lower body-fat levels and weight to be more competitive. Read more about this subject in the section on wrestling in chapter 13 (page 279).

Athletes who are assessed frequently (weight or skinfold measurements recorded regularly) are fearful of the outcome because the results are often (and inappropriately) used punitively. Real changes in body composition occur slowly, so there is little need to assess athletes every week, every two weeks, or even every month. Assessing body composition two to four times each year is an appropriate frequency to determine and monitor body-composition change. In some isolated circumstances when an athlete has been injured or is suffering from a disease, such as malabsorption, fever, diarrhea, or anorexia, it is reasonable for a doctor to recommend a more frequent assessment rate to control for changes in lean mass. Coaches who have traditionally obtained weight or body-composition values much more frequently (e.g., weekly, monthly) should shift their focus to a more frequent assessment of objective performance-related measures.

PATHOLOGIC WEIGHT CONTROL IN ATHLETES: EATING DISORDERS

It is unclear whether athletes in general are at greater risk of developing eating disorders than are the nonathlete population. In a study of both athletes and nonathletes, it was found that the risk for developing eating disorders was not related to whether or not the subjects were athletes.[3] A similar finding was observed in ethnically diverse urban female adolescent athletes and nonathletes; the athletes were not at higher risk for disordered eating.[29] This study also found that Hispanic and Caucasian urban adolescent females were at higher risk for eating disorders than were African-American urban adolescent females. However, athletes involved in sports that emphasize appearance or that have a weight requirement are clearly at a higher risk of developing an eating disorder, and the risk is higher in female athletes than in male athletes.[30]

A reduction in food intake that results in an energy deficiency, as seen in eating disorders, has a profound effect on multiple organ systems. Studies have found that a negative energy balance decreases leptin and increases ghrelin production, which disturbs normal appetite controls; increases cortisol, which catabolizes the fat-free mass; decreases plasma glucose, which influences central nervous system function; decreases insulin-like growth factor 1 (IGF-1), which is linked to lean-mass anabolism (the less IGF-1, the lower the lean mass); increases insulin-like growth factor binding protein 1 (IGFBP-1), which is inversely associated with IGF-1 (the higher the IGFBP-1, the greater the lean-mass breakdown); decreases fasting insulin, which is linked to lower plasma glucose; and decreases thyroid hormone (total T3), which is the body's attempt to lower energy metabolism in the face of an inadequate energy intake.[31-35] Food consumption that occurs when plasma glucose and insulin are low is likely to result in a hyperinsulinemic response, with a greater manufacture of fat from consumed foods. In brief, nothing good happens when a negative energy balance occurs. See table 12.4 for a summary of the effects of an inadequate energy intake on hormones.

Table 12.4 Effects of Energy Inadequacy on Hormones

Tissue/Organ	Hormone/Compound	Expected change
Adipocytes and Hypothalamus	Leptin	Decrease
Adrenal	Cortisol	Increase
Gastrointestinal tract	Ghrelin	Increase
Liver	Plasma glucose IGF-1[1] IGFBP-1[2]	Decrease Decrease Increase
Pancreas	Insulin	Decrease (fasting) Increase (eating)
Thyroid	Total T3[3]	Decrease

[a]Insulin-like growth factor 1

[b]Insulin-like growth factor binding protein 1

[c]Triiodothyronine

Data from endnotes 31-35.

There are clear differences in pubertal development in male and female artistic gymnasts, differences that are associated with adequacy of energy intake. Although female gymnasts display delayed menarche and delayed pubertal development, male gymnasts' developmental patterns appear normal.[36] But there are exceptions to the occurrence of developmental delays in female athletes. A study of British female synchronized swimmers (a subjectively scored sport where appearance is important) found that this group is relatively free of menstrual disturbances associated with eating disorders. None of the 23 national-team members who were assessed had amenorrhea, and only 3 of the 23 had oligomenorrhea.[37]

The traditional view of eating disorders suggests that a combination of genetic, social, and psychological factors creates the basis for their development (see figure 12.7). In athletes, however, there may be yet another important factor in the development of eating disorders involving a desire to perform well athletically. Because attainment of an ideal weight and body composition is critical for high-level sports performance, many athletes are predisposed to placing themselves on restrictive intakes. Restrictive intakes in athletes, particularly female athletes, are common. In a study of male and female collegiate athletes, 23 percent of the males and 62 percent of the females had inadequate energy intakes because they wanted to lose weight.[38] However, because restrictive intakes lower the metabolic mass, this makes it more difficult for athletes to eat normally without gaining weight, so they are forced into lower and lower caloric intakes that, ultimately, cause them to develop eating disorders. The most common eating disorders among these athletes are anorexia nervosa, bulimia, and anorexia athletica; in female athletes, these conditions often manifest themselves with low bone density and amenorrhea, referred to as the female athlete triad. Athletes and coaches should be sensitive to the warning signs of eating disorders, which include the following:[39]

- Preoccupation with food
- Preoccupation with weight
- Frequently stated concerns about being fat

- Frequent criticism about the eating patterns of teammates
- Going to the bathroom during or after meals
- Complaints about feeling cold
- Use of laxatives
- Frequently eating alone
- Additional exercise outside the normal training regimen

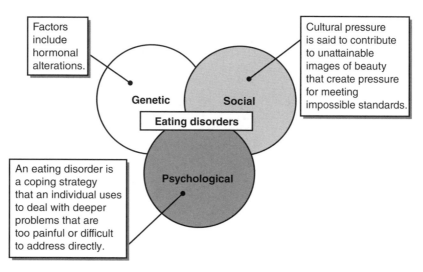

Figure 12.7 The various causes traditionally believed to contribute to an eating disorder.

Anorexia Nervosa and Anorexia Athletica

Anorexia nervosa and anorexia athletica are typified by restrained eating from a fear of becoming fat, with a resultant loss of weight that places these athletes at serious health risk. People with anorexia athletica may have abnormal exercise patterns, including the desire to exercise while injured and compulsive exercise beyond the normal training regimens. See table 12.5 for criteria associated with anorexia athletica.

The restrictive caloric intakes of anorexia are associated with lower bone density, a failure to reach a desirable peak bone density in adolescence, and an increased risk of stress fractures.[40] Although these conditions are serious in and of themselves, it should be remembered that mortality rates from anorexia nervosa have been reported as high as 18 percent, usually attributable to fluid and electrolyte abnormalities or suicide (see figure 12.8 for possible relationships between energy deficits and disordered eating).[41,42]

Hormone replacement therapy (i.e., estrogen replacement) is a strategy for dealing with the sequelae of amenorrhea, but it seems logical to either decrease the intensity and duration of exercise or increase the caloric intake, or both, to return athletes diagnosed with this condition to an energy-balanced state. To successfully achieve this, athletes must understand that proper eating can better optimize athletic performance and appearance by encouraging

Table 12.5 Criteria for Anorexia Athletica

Weight loss > 5% of expected body weight	Excessive fear of becoming obese
Delayed puberty (no menses by age 16—primary amenorrhea)	Restriction of caloric intake (diets < 1,200 cal)
Menstrual dysfunction (amenorrhea or oligomenorrhea)	Use of purging methods (vomiting, laxatives, and diuretics)
GI complaints	Binge eating
No medical illness explaining disorder	Compulsive exercising
Disturbance in body image	

Adapted, by permission, from J. Sundgot-Borgen, 1994, "Risk factors for the development of eating disorders in female elite athletes," *Medicine & Science in Sports & Exercise* 26(4): 414-419.

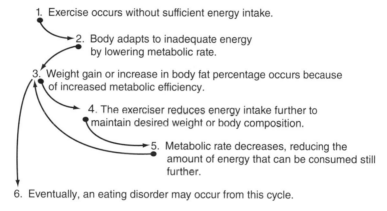

1. Exercise occurs without sufficient energy intake.
2. Body adapts to inadequate energy by lowering metabolic rate.
3. Weight gain or increase in body fat percentage occurs because of increased metabolic efficiency.
4. The exerciser reduces energy intake further to maintain desired weight or body composition.
5. Metabolic rate decreases, reducing the amount of energy that can be consumed still further.
6. Eventually, an eating disorder may occur from this cycle.

Figure 12.8 The possible relationship between energy deficits and eating disorders.

Reprinted, by permission, from D. Benardot and W.R. Thompson, 1999, "Energy from food for physical activity: Enough and on time," *ACSM's Health and Fitness Journal* 3(4): 14-18.

muscle-mass development while discouraging fat-mass development.[43] It is important that athletes understand the difference between wanting to be "thin" and needing to be "lean." See table 12. 6 for changes in body composition and hormones seen in anorexia nervosa.

Bulimia Nervosa

Bulimia nervosa is characterized by compulsive eating binges, during which people consume enormous quantities of foods, followed by purging episodes through vomiting or laxative intake to rid themselves of the consumed foods. The bingeing–purging cycles of bulimia nervosa are often referred to as gorge–purge syndrome. These athletes are often normal or near normal weight and, for this reason, may be more difficult to identify than those with anorexia nervosa. Symptoms include corrosion of teeth and gums (from frequent gastric acid exposure due to vomiting), edema, electrolyte abnormalities, dehydration, depression, and excessive bathroom visits.[25]

Table 12.6 Body Composition, Anorexia Nervosa, and Hormones

Variable	Increased	Decreased
Body composition		
BMI		XX
Fat mass		XX
Bone density		X
Bone formation		XX
Bone resorption	XX	
Bone marrow fat	X	
Hormones		
Estradiol		XX
Testosterone		X
IGF-1		XX
Growth hormone	X	
Insulin		X
Cortisol	X	
Appetite regulatory mediators		
Leptin		XX
Adiponectin	X	
Ghrelin	X	
PYY	X	

BMI = body mass index

IGF-1 = insulin-like growth factor 1

PYY = peptide YY

X = small change

XX = large change

Reprinted from *The American Journal of Medicine* 122(5), C.J. Rosen and A. Klibanski, "Bone, fat, and body composition: Evolving concepts in the pathogenesis of osteoporosis," 409-414, copyright 2009, with permission from Elsevier.

Eating Disorders and Sports Performance

Although many athletes initially experience an improvement in sports performance with weight loss, this improvement is generally short lived if it was due to a drastic reduction in food intake. A major decrease in food consumption depletes energy and can be indicative of an eating disorder. Lower plasma volume, impaired thermoregulation, and lower glycogen storage are all associated with eating disorders and can lower the levels of anaerobic and aerobic endurance.[44,45]

In addition, lowered food intake predisposes athletes to multiple micronutrient deficiencies that can lower athletic performance and increase the risk of injury. This is evidenced when examining the abnormal menstrual patterns that often accompany eating disorders. Females who have stopped menstruating have lower levels of calcium in their bones, increasing their risk for stress fractures. The menstrual abnormalities correlate to a negative balance of energy and are also associated with lower resting energy expenditure, which is typically the result of a decreased metabolic rate and lean mass.[46]

Body composition can be a useful tool in helping the athlete and coach understand the changes that are occurring as a result of training and nutrition factors. Health professionals involved in obtaining body-composition data should focus on using the same technique with the same prediction equations to derive valid comparative data over time. Care should be taken that body-composition values be used constructively as part of the athlete's total training plan. Ideally, the emphasis should be on a periodic (semiannually or quarterly) monitoring of the athlete's body composition to determine change of both the lean and fat mass. Many athletes are sensitive about body fat, so care should be taken to use body-composition values in a way that enables their constructive use in an athlete's general training plan. Athletes suspected of having an eating disorder should be quickly assessed and treated if necessary. It is likely that helping young athletes understand appropriate nutrition strategies for attaining a desirable body profile, weight, strength, and endurance will help reduce future eating disorder risk.

IMPORTANT POINTS

• The principles of energy thermodynamic theory are always at play. Consumption of more energy than is burned results in higher body weight (the excess energy is stored), and consumption of less energy than is burned results in lower body weight (some tissue is burned to supply the difference).

• Diet regimens that result in a lower body weight ultimately provide less energy than the athlete has burned. Severe diets are likely to cause a greater loss of lean mass, rather than fat mass, with a resultant increase in body-fat percentage.

• Infrequent eating is associated with higher per-meal intakes, higher insulin production, high fat storage, and high cortisol production that can result in a loss of muscle and bone mass.

• Frequent eating is associated with improved appetite control, lower insulin response, lower fat storage, and higher muscle mass.

• Higher muscle mass and lower fat levels make it easier for athletes to eat more food, take in more nutrients, and avoid increases in fat storage.

• Strategies for assessing body composition should not be used interchangeably, as the results they provide are likely to be different (based on the strategy used for assessment rather than true body-composition differences).

• The direction of change in both muscle mass and fat mass is more important than a single body-composition measurement. Athletes should compare themselves against themselves rather than other athletes and try to change body composition in a desirable direction.

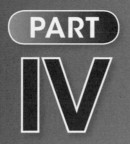

PART

IV

Nutrition Strategies for Specific Energy Systems

Anaerobic Metabolism for High-Intensity Bursts and Power

Athletes in power events, including weightlifting, gymnastics, baseball, football, hammer throw, sprinting, and shot put, must maximize their potential for success by improving muscular strength, speed, and power. Power development is a function of the maximum amount of energy a muscle can produce quickly and is largely dependent on the distribution and trained state of Type IIa and Type IIb muscle fibers. These muscle types can quickly produce power by simultaneously recruiting more fibers than Type I fibers are able to recruit; Type I fibers are more associated with endurance sports. Since athletes in power sports follow training regimens that increase their muscle mass, they have unique nutrition requirements for supporting or enlarging this mass. These athletes must consume enough energy so the nutrients, including protein, needed to support this larger mass are available for anabolic use and are not catabolized to meet energy requirements. In addition, eating strategies must be carefully planned so the consumed energy is available for muscular use at the time the muscles are in greatest need. Some power sports require "making weight," while others place a premium on gaining weight. However, the resultant weight loss or weight gain should always value the maintenance or increase of muscle mass.

Some athletes resort to vegetarianism as a strategy to make weight, and there may be certain positive health implications from a reduction in high-fat meats and an increased fruit and vegetable intake. However, athletes who turn to vegetarianism may also be at a higher risk for other unhealthy weight-reduction strategies.[1] Some of this difficulty rests with the source of nutrition information athletes rely on. There is good evidence that the most capable professionals for providing nutrition advice to athletes (registered dietitians) often take a back seat to athletic trainers and strength and conditioning coaches who are ill equipped to tackle the complexities of providing appropriate nutrition advice to athletes requiring both a high level of nutrients and energy and a low level of body fat.[2]

With that caveat aside, there is good evidence to suggest that adolescents involved in weight-related and power sports eat better and have better nutrient intakes than adolescents who are not involved in sport.[3] Put simply, while involvement in sport may carry certain nutrition risks, noninvolvement carries even higher risks for adolescents. Professional athletes may face different risks, depending on the sport. A recent report assessed 69 professional football players and professional baseball players to determine cardiovascular and metabolic risk factors. Baseball players had lower rates of obesity, hyperglycemia, and metabolic syndrome than football linemen.[4] All these factors have nutrition implications that should motivate players and those associated with sport to carefully consider if the way they eat might shorten their lives. Clearly, getting it right nutritionally both improves performance *and* reduces morbidity and mortality risks. This chapter presents the full spectrum of nutrition tactics power athletes can employ to meet the specific needs of their sports, whether it is to increase mass to be a more competitive lineman on a football team or to make weight for a wrestling competition.

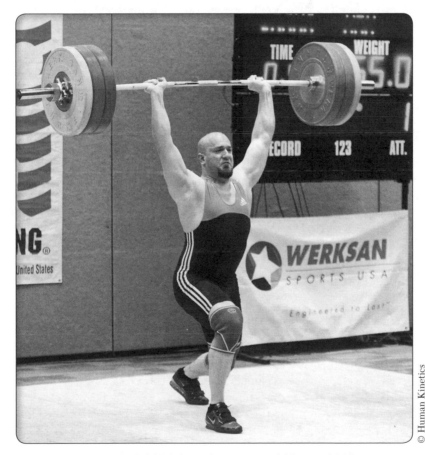

© Human Kinetics

Contrary to popular belief, high-intensity power activities are highly dependent on glycogen (carbohydrate).

NUTRITION TACTICS FOR POWER ATHLETES

Different activities place special metabolic requirements on muscle systems, and these differences alter the nutrition requirements for athletes involved in various types of sports. Sports that require a high level of power and speed over short distances have a high anaerobic component. Athletes in these sports are not interested in their ability to move efficiently over long distances for long periods of time; they want to be there first in short distances. When a baseball player steals a base, there is virtually nothing about that 4- to 5-second experience that requires aerobic efficiency. The sprint to the next base is entirely dependent on anaerobic metabolism, which is almost entirely dependent on phosphocreatine and glycogen as fuels. Bodybuilders need explosive power to train but almost never place continuous stress on the muscles for longer than 1.5 minutes, which is the approximate time limit for anaerobic activities.

There has been an evolution in the way athletes eat to support top athletic performance. Around AD 200, Diogenes Laertius wrote that the training diet of Greek athletes of the time consisted of dried figs, moist cheeses, and wheat products.[5] American Olympians at the Berlin Games of 1936 had a daily intake that included beefsteak, lots of butter, three eggs, custard, 1.5 liters of milk, and as much as they could consume of white bread, dinner rolls, fresh vegetables, and salads. With each successive Olympic Games, athletes have consumed certain foods and avoided other foods depending on the state of nutrition knowledge. Since the 1960s, however, there has been a purposeful scientific effort to learn what athletes need and why they need it. This scientific endeavor has led to a much-improved understanding of how muscles work for power and how they work for speed. The science of sports nutrition has also helped us understand the different nutrition demands associated with different types of activities. A failure to consider the nutrition implications of the activity will most certainly lead to problems in training and to performance outcomes that are below the capabilities of the athlete.

Our current knowledge of nutrition requirements for anaerobic activity is substantial, with the clear understanding of what it is that muscles use in this type of activity: phosphocreatine and glycogen. Of course, there is also a question of how to obtain and sustain the larger muscle mass typically needed by athletes involved in anaerobic activity, and the answer to this question is also known: more calories. However, despite the well-established nature of these facts, anaerobic athletes place an unyielding focus on protein intake to satisfy the phosphocreatine, glycogen, and muscle requirements of their activities.

ANAEROBIC METABOLIC PATHWAYS

Athletes have the capacity to obtain a limited amount of energy quickly without oxygen. Events that are predominantly anaerobic (i.e., they require maximal power and energy over a limited period of time) rarely last longer than 90 seconds because the anaerobic energy supply would be exhausted. In some anaerobic events, such as boxing, each round is followed by a period of rest to allow the cells to prepare for the next bout of intense work. What follows is a description of the anaerobic metabolic pathways.

Phosphocreatine (Phosphagen) System

Anaerobic metabolic processes supply ATP from phosphocreatine (PCr) and glycolysis without oxygen. The in-muscle concentration of preformed ATP is 25 to 33 percent of the concentration of PCr. The enzyme creatine kinase can break apart PCr into inorganic phosphate and creatine, with a resultant release of energy. The free inorganic phosphate is united with ADP to reform ATP. The breakdown of PCr is not reversible until energy is obtained from other sources (mainly through oxidative metabolic processes). The volume of energy that can be supplied by the breakdown of PCr is vast, and it can be produced instantaneously. However, the length of time this high volume of energy can be supplied is never greater than 10 seconds because of the limited amount of PCr stored in tissue. The formation of energy from PCr breakdown is directly linked to the intensity of exercise: The higher the exercise intensity, the greater the reliance on PCr breakdown as a source of energy. Athletes performing maximal exercise for 8 to 10 seconds (sprint, vault, jumps) must take a break of 2 to 4 minutes to allow for the regeneration of PCr before undertaking another maximal bout of exercise. Creatine monohydrate supplementation is popular because athletes want to increase the storage of PCr, with the hope of increasing both capacity and power.

Glycolysis (Glycolytic System)

Glycolysis refers to the anaerobic breakdown of glucose or glycogen for energy. As indicated in table 13.1, there is a delay of 5 to 10 seconds after the initiation of activity before the glycolytic system can supply energy to working tissues. The six-carbon glucose molecule is phosphorylated and broken into two three-carbon molecules (glyceraldehyde-3-phosphate, or G3P). Each molecule of G3P is converted into pyruvate with the formation of ATP. The glycolytic reaction creates two molecules of ATP for each molecule of glucose; it creates three molecules of ATP for each molecule of glucose if glycogen is the initial substrate. The pyruvate may be converted to acetyl-CoA for later storage as fat or conversion to lactate. In either case, the fat or lactate created from pyruvate can be oxidative sources of energy. As indicated in table 13.1, glycolysis has half the power to create energy as the PCr system but has three times the capacity. The combination of PCr and glycolysis can support predominantly anaerobic maximal work for approximately 90 seconds, often referred to as the anaerobic maximum.

Table 13.1 Capacity and Power of Anaerobic Systems for Producing ATP

System	Capacity (mmol ATP/kg)	Power (mmol ATP/kg)	Delay time
Phosphocreatine system	55-95	9.0	Instant
Glycolytic system	190-300	4.5	5-10 sec
Combined	250-370	11.0	—

Reprinted, by permission, from M. Gleeson, 2000, Biochemistry of exercise. In *Nutrition in sport*, edited by R.J. Maughan (Oxford: Blackwell Science), 22, 23.

SAMPLING OF SPORTS RELYING ON ANAEROBIC METABOLISM

Anaerobic sports require maximal effort over relatively short periods of time. Imagine a baseball player swinging the bat or running to first base; imagine a gymnast sprinting down the runway to perform a vault. In both of these cases the athlete is using mainly existing energy stores that are both limited and easily depleted. You could never imagine a baseball player running to first base, back to home, and back to first base over and over again for 30 minutes with the same power and speed shown while running to first base a single time because it is physiologically impossible to do so. Nor could you ever ask a gymnast to repeatedly perform the floor routine over and over again without a break because it would be impossible to do. What follows is a sampling of sports that have these special characteristics: extreme intensity, with breaks between each bout of intense effort.

Baseball and Softball

Baseball and softball are wonderful sports that require an almost equal combination of teamwork and individual effort. They are also highly *mental* games, requiring that the athletes stay constantly alert to make split-second judgments for the right play. It's safe to say that physically tired baseball and softball players are also likely to be mentally tired (glucose is the fuel for both the brain and muscles) and prone to bad judgment and poor physical performance.

David Halberstam, in his book *Summer of '49*, describes the 1949 pennant race between the Red Sox and Yankees.[6] A central theme of this book is how players get worn out during the long baseball season, with the outcome of the pennant race determined, to a degree, by the number of players who remain relatively fresh by the end of the year. Clearly, many factors contribute to wearing players down during a long season, including frequent travel, hard-fought games, and constant time-zone changes.[7]

Nutrition factors also come into play: Players who come to the playing field well fueled and hydrated will not only play better, they'll play better longer too.[8] The foods and fluids consumed over the long summer and fall season do make a difference in the outcome. When steak and beer are constantly on the menu, as was common for many baseball players in the past, it is predictable that physical and mental fatigue will eventually take its toll. Alcohol interferes with B-vitamin metabolism (and therefore energy metabolism) and also increases dehydration risk. Red meat is a useful means of supplying good-quality protein, iron, and zinc, but it should not be the focus of a baseball player's diet. What baseball players really need is plenty of bread, cereal, fruits, and vegetables to constantly provide carbohydrate to replace the glycogen used up in the quick and powerful actions of the game, as well as enough calories to support their muscle mass.

Softball players should also seriously consider whether food and beverage intakes dynamically match requirements. There is evidence that collegiate female softball players have numerous eating behaviors that could detract from optimal performance. One study found that meal skipping, delayed eating, and overeating when finally having a meal were common practices.[9] These players also had an excessively high intake of high-fat foods and insufficient intake of carbohydrate to replenish the fuels used in high-intensity activity.

Keeping all these factors in mind, baseball players must consider the following nutritionally relevant issues for their sport.

As primarily summer sports, baseball and softball are often played in a hot and humid environment. Optimally hydrated muscles are composed of more than 70 percent water, and it should be the athlete's goal to maintain this optimal hydration state. A failure to do so will lead to a progressive reduction in total body water, with a concomitant reduction in athletic performance. Evidence suggests that poor hydration makes an athlete more prone to injury by reducing mental function (poor hydration is associated with higher core temperatures that can reduce coordination) and by making muscles less resilient (thus increasing the risk of muscle tears and strains).

Baseball players (particularly pitchers) are known to experience a reduction in peak-torque arm strength between pre- and postseason measurements, with some of this power reduction caused by overuse injury to the pitching arm.[10] Reduced throwing power could also be due to reduced leg strength, which could negatively alter the throwing motion and exacerbate the risk of injury.[11] It seems likely that the degree to which the progressive reduction in power occurs could be reduced with a regular program of optimized hydration and energy intake.[12]

A study of baseball players strongly suggests that conditioning plays an important role in the ability of the athletes to maintain an optimal hydration state. At fixed exercise intensities, the better-conditioned baseball players were able to maintain body temperature with a lower sweat rate than that of players who were less fit.[13] Another study found that blood flow to the pitching arm (in pitchers) increased up to 40 pitches but steadily declined after that. By the 100th pitch, blood flow to the pitching arm was 30 percent below baseline.[14] The decrease in blood flow to the pitching arm matches a decrease in the general hydration state of the pitchers. Since it is established that blood volume is a key factor in the maintenance of athletic performance, the performance of pitchers may be strongly influenced by their ability to stay hydrated.

Given the possibility of frequent exposure to hot and humid environments, baseball and softball players should consider the following strategy for maintaining their hydration state:

1. During the preseason, weigh yourself before and after each game, and practice determining how much weight was lost. Then determine how much fluid should be consumed during a typical game—1 pint (16 ounces, or 480 ml) of fluid equals 1 pound (.5 kg) of body weight). The goal is to drink enough fluids to maintain body weight (±1 pound) during the game. Different people have different sweat rates, so your drinking schedule is likely to be different from those of your teammates.

2. Drink plenty of fluids before each game (a minimum of 16 ounces 1 hour before the game, followed by a constant sipping of fluids).

3. Use each opportunity between innings to consume fluids. Since baseball and softball both involve multiple bouts of high-intensity movements, the drain on stored glycogen is high. Therefore, fluids consumed should contain carbohydrate. Fluids containing a 6 to 7 percent carbohydrate solution are best both for replacing carbohydrate and for encouraging a fast fluid absorption.

4. Immediately after the game, eat and drink enough carbohydrate to reconstitute your glycogen stores and body water.

5. Avoid or limit the consumption of alcohol and caffeinated beverages. With sufficient intake, both alcohol and caffeine have a diuretic effect that could place an athlete in a negative water balance.

Baseball and softball require a combination of power and speed, both of which place a high reliance on phosphocreatine and carbohydrate (primarily glycogen) for muscular fuel. Phosphocreatine is synthesized from three amino acids (from protein), so an adequate intake of protein is necessary to ensure that sufficient phosphocreatine can be manufactured. However, the protein consumption must be part of an adequate total intake of energy (calories). It is easier for fully grown baseball and softball players to obtain sufficient energy (baseball players reach their peak at around age 28).[15] However, younger players must supply enough energy to support the activity plus enough energy to support growth. Inadequate energy intake causes the consumed protein to be burned as a fuel, making it unavailable for use as a substrate for the manufacture of other substances, such as creatine. With sufficient energy, even a modest protein intake of between 1.2 and 1.7 grams per kilogram is sufficient to support the synthesis of creatine and support a stable or growing muscle mass. In the context of an adequate energy intake, players should consume a diet that derives 60 to 65 percent of its energy from carbohydrate, 20 to 25 percent of its energy from fat, and 15 percent of its energy from protein.

Many games are played during the season, with several games played each week. This frequency of games and practices can easily lead to overtraining, with the associated problems of fatigue, weakness, and increased risk of illness. A key to limiting the impact of overtraining is adequate rest and the consumption of a high-carbohydrate diet to maintain muscle glycogen levels. It has been shown that daily practices or competitions will lead to a progressive reduction in muscle glycogen storage, with a related reduction in endurance and performance. Since baseball players are highly dependent on muscle glycogen as a fuel, a reduction in glycogen from inadequate carbohydrate intake would lead to a discernible lowering of performance with time.

Games typically last 2 to 3 hours. Normal blood glucose flux is approximately 3 hours. That is, from the time you finish eating a meal, blood glucose stays in the normal range for about 3 hours. After this, blood glucose falls below the normal range (80 to 120 milligrams per deciliter), a physiological event normally associated with hunger. In the exercising person, blood glucose is likely to fall below the normal range more quickly. Because blood glucose is an important factor in maintaining normal mental function, and it is also important for delivering fuel to muscles that have exhausted stored carbohydrate, baseball players should take steps to maintain blood glucose during the entire game by consuming a carbohydrate-rich beverage at every opportunity.

Pitchers work harder when they're pitching than other players on the team, which is why they are able to pitch effectively only every three to five games. Pitchers are better able to maintain muscular power (both in the legs and arms) by maximizing glycogen storage and hydration state before and during each game. The principle of carbohydrate loading (a general tapering of activity coupled with a high carbohydrate and fluid intake—refer to chapter 6 for more detailed information) can be followed with starting pitchers because they typically have several days between starts.

The weight and insulating effect of the equipment worn by catchers adds to their energy and fluid requirements. Catchers are constantly in motion, working with the pitcher, and since they tend to play on a more frequent rotation than starting pitchers, it's safe to say that, pound for pound, catchers have the highest energy and fluid requirements of any of the other positions.

Bodybuilding

Bodybuilders strive for a physique that is the extreme of high muscle mass and low body fat. The low body fat is a necessary adjunct to performance, which requires a high level of muscular definition to achieve a high score. A high body-fat level would mask the underlying muscle formation because approximately 50 percent of all body fat expresses itself subcutaneously. To achieve their muscle mass, bodybuilders must place a high level of repetitive stress (typically via free weights and muscle-resistance equipment) on each muscle group. This is never done aerobically (i.e., low-level muscular force over long time periods). Instead, bodybuilders rely on high-intensity repetitions that rarely last longer than 30 seconds per muscle group and never last longer than 1.5 minutes. In preparation for competition, bodybuilders couple this hard muscle training with the consumption of extra energy to support an enlargement of the muscle mass or reduction of the fat mass.[16] Diets of bodybuilders are often high in protein and protein-related supplements and creatine.[17]

Once the muscle mass is enlarged, bodybuilders go into a second training phase that involves a reduction in energy coupled with a small aerobic component.[18] This second phase is aimed at reducing body-fat levels (particularly subcutaneous fat) to allow for a greater visual muscle definition. During the week before competition, bodybuilders typically decrease total energy intake and increase carbohydrate intake to load the muscles with glycogen. Both fluids and sodium are typically restricted to aid in muscle definition. There is evidence that fluid restriction is dangerous, particularly in younger bodybuilders, where both low blood potassium and phosphorus have been observed.[19] There is also evidence that energy restriction immediately before competition causes a loss of lean body mass (muscle), suggesting that energy restriction is counterproductive.[17] Athletes in weight-related sports have a far greater prevalence of vomiting, abusing laxatives, taking diuretics, and taking steroids than nonathletes.[20] Perhaps no sport is as prone to nutrition misinformation as bodybuilding.

In a study evaluating advertisements in bodybuilding magazines, no scientific evidence was offered for 42 percent of the products for which beneficial nutrition claims were made. Only 21 percent of the advertised products had appropriate documentation to support their claims, and 32 percent of the products that had some scientific documentation were marketed in a misleading manner.[21] A study of male and female bodybuilders found widespread multidrug abuse (up to 40 percent of the subjects), and a majority of bodybuilders reported following regimens that led to severe dehydration.[22] In this same study, the female bodybuilders had extremely low calcium intakes and nutrition practices that placed them, as a group, at high risk for poor health. The New York City Department of Consumer Affairs indicated that more than half of all full-page advertisements for nutrition supplements in popular bodybuilding magazines were worthless and, perhaps, harmful, products.[23] College athletes may spend as much as $400 per month on supplements (consumer data for athletes at the professional level are not sufficient), which could otherwise have been spent much more wisely on fresh foods.[24]

Keeping all these factors in mind, bodybuilders must consider the following nutritionally relevant issues for their sport.

Bodybuilders strive for a high level of muscle mass, a goal that mandates a higher need for energy.   Although the total amount of protein needed to maintain this larger mass is slightly greater than what athletes with a stable muscle mass require, the proportion of protein provided by typically consumed foods is likely to satisfy need. Ideally, bodybuilders should consume between 1.5 and 1.7 grams of protein per kilogram of body weight, but this should be consumed in the context of adequate total energy consumption, where most of the energy is derived from carbohydrates.

Studies of bodybuilders strongly suggest that protein consumption is usually much higher than the body's capacity to use it anabolically (i.e., to use it to build tissue). Therefore, the excess protein is simply burned as a fuel or, in the case of excess total energy consumption, stored as fat. This has been confirmed by the findings in one study, which determined that bodybuilders had significantly higher protein intakes than did lean control subjects, and they also relied more heavily on protein as a fuel to meet the energy requirements of the muscles.[25] The belief that excess protein is a requirement for building muscle is pervasive among bodybuilders, but in truth, this extra protein is merely a source of needed calories that would be more efficiently provided through the non-nitrogenous energy substrates. The key to building muscle mass is to consume enough energy to support the larger mass. A bodybuilder now weighing 180 pounds (82 kg) who wishes to weigh 190 pounds (86 kg) should eat enough energy to support the larger mass. In doing so, the increase in calories should not come solely from protein but rather a proportionate increase in protein, carbohydrate, and fat where carbohydrates remain the major source of energy. Data from successful bodybuilders suggest that the ideal composition of diets should emphasize carbohydrate (55 to 60 percent of intake) and be relatively low in fat (15 to 25 percent of intake), with the remainder from protein (25 to 30 percent of intake).[26]

Bodybuilders strive for an extremely low fat mass. Body-fat percentage is, to a great degree, determined by a person's genetic makeup but can also be influenced by dietary and exercise habits. From a dietary standpoint, it is most important to consume only enough energy to meet physiological need because excess energy intake will manifest itself as stored fat. Dietary fat is the most concentrated source of energy, so consumption of excess fat may most easily create an excess total energy intake, and it is easily converted to stored fat. Carbohydrates are more efficiently burned as a fuel for high-intensity muscular work and are not as efficiently converted to fat for storage. For these reasons, fat intake should be kept relatively low (15 to 25 percent of total calories). This level of intake is below the general population recommendation that no more than 30 percent of total calories be provided from fat. The consumption of small and frequent meals is also a useful strategy because it helps suppress the manufacture of fat by lowering the insulin response to food. If you eat 1,500 calories in a single meal, the normal processing of so much energy at one time will inevitably lead to an important percentage of this intake being stored as fat. Were this 1,500-calorie meal to be consumed in two meals that are 3 hours apart (750 calories per meal), the energy could be more effectively processed without storing a significant proportion of it as fat. Therefore, eating the right amount of calories to maintain an energy-balanced state (something that is easier on a moderately low-fat diet) and eating small but frequent meals are both important strategies for obtaining a low body-fat percentage.

Bodybuilders commonly go through repetitive patterns of weight gain and weight loss in an attempt to build muscle and then reduce body-fat levels. The average reported weight loss experienced during the competitive season is 15 pounds (6.8 kg), and the average reported weight gain is 14 pounds (6.3 kg). This cyclic dieting leaves bodybuilders with a food preoccupation that leads to binge eating after competitions as well as psychological stress.[27] A much more logical approach to building muscle safely is to consume a moderate excess in calories (300 to 500 calories beyond current needs) from complex carbohydrate to support a larger muscle mass, coupled with activities that sufficiently stress the muscles to encourage their enlargement.

Bodybuilders appear to be excessively dependent on nutritional and quasi-nutritional products and ergogenic aids to achieve the desired body composition. Self-experimentation with ergogenic aids and nutritional products is common in many sports. However, bodybuilders are especially targeted by marketing efforts for these products. To make matters more complex, the placebo effect in nutrition is very real. That is, if an athlete believes a product will help him meet specific goals, then it probably will have some benefit even if there is no physiological or biological basis for this improvement. Ideally, athletes should consume products and foods that have a physiological and biological basis for achieving their goals. If the athletes also believe these products and foods work, they may realize an even greater benefit (i.e., the placebo effect).

It is also common for bodybuilders to rely on strategies that increase body-water loss to achieve the desired cut appearance. Dehydration is dangerous (numerous deaths occur yearly from dehydration, among both athletes and nonathletes) and diminishes athletic performance. With bodybuilders, even though it is important to have a cut appearance, achieving this through dehydration is an unacceptable strategy because it can lead to organ failure and death. Bodybuilders should achieve their desired appearance through hard work and the development of a relatively low level of body fat using the strategies discussed already.

Nutrient intake appears to be inadequate for many in this population. The focus on nutritional products (protein powders and shakes, amino acid supplements, creatine monohydrate supplements, and so on) rather than nutrient-rich foods may place bodybuilders at nutrition risk. Consumption of low-fat, high-carbohydrate, moderate-protein foods that provide adequate energy (calories) will ensure a good nutrient intake. An excessive reliance on supplements appears to provide an unnecessarily high protein intake and may not satisfy the nutrients most lacking in the diets of these athletes. Blindly consuming individual vitamin and mineral supplements is also not a useful strategy because athletes rarely know what specific nutrients are most needed. Consumption of a wide spectrum of foods that expose these athletes to all the nutrients is the best strategy, with supplements playing a role only where the adequate intake of energy substrates or nutrients is impossible.

Football (American)

Football is the epitome of an anaerobic sport, with the length of plays almost never exceeding 15 seconds, followed by a rest period between each play. However, when the ball is in play, the players are giving maximal muscular effort to move, or stop the movement of, the ball. Football players also carry the extra burden of heavy equipment, which adds to the energy requirement. The fuels most used in this type of activity are phosphocreatine and muscle glycogen, making the traditional steak and potato pregame meal less than ideal for ensuring an optimal storage of muscle glycogen because there is a relative overemphasis on protein (steak) and a relative underemphasis on carbohydrate (potato). Football players are in need of nutrition education, particularly on the use of dietary supplements.[28] This is particularly important when you consider the widespread use of ergogenic supplements among football players and that improper use of ergogenic aids may increase health risks.[29] Importantly, there is evidence that football players who are more knowledgeable in nutrition have a caloric intake that more closely matches requirement than those less knowledgeable.[30]

A study of college football players found that supplementing with creatine monohydrate had a performance-enhancing effect by improving lifting volume and repeated sprint performance.[31] Another study of football players found that creatine supplementation was useful for enhancing peak force and maximal strength.[32] However, findings from these and other studies should be reviewed carefully before embarking on a path of ergogenic aid supplementation because the total energy intake adequacy of the subjects in these studies was not evaluated. It is unclear, therefore, if the apparent benefit of creatine monohydrate supplementation would be sustained if the total energy intake of the football players was adequate.

In one of the few studies assessing the safety of long-term creatine supplementation, creatine monohydrate showed no long-term detrimental effects on kidney or liver function in the absence of other supplements.[33] In another study evaluating nutrient supplementation on athletic performance, football players who consumed chromium picolinate supplements for 9 weeks experienced no improvement in either body composition or strength when compared with a group of football players who did not supplement.[34] The stop-and-go nature of football, which vacillates between bouts of maximal effort and rest during a game, is also associated with a high level of body-water loss.

This loss of body fluid negatively affects cooling ability, athletic performance, and concentration.[35] A study of the consumption of carbohydrate-containing beverages among football players showed that these beverages were better able to maintain plasma volume than water alone.[36] Since maintenance of plasma volume is strongly associated with athletic performance, football players should consider consuming a well-designed sports beverage to maintain endurance and performance. Adequate fluid consumption before, during, and after games and practices should be an important part of the training regimen.

Football players at every level have recently been getting bigger and stronger each year and have a relatively positive body image when compared with other male athletes.[37] In a survey of high school All-American football teams from 1963 to 1971 and from 1972 to 1989, significant increases were found in the ratio of weight to height (body mass index) in the 1970s and 1980s that did not exist earlier.[38] In other words, football players are getting heavier (relative to their heights) at a rate much higher than existed before 1963.

Increased weight by itself may not be a good thing for football players. One study found that football linemen with higher body-fat percentages and higher body mass indexes had higher rates of lower-extremity injuries.[39] In another study, football players with higher body-fat levels had a 2.5 times higher relative risk of injury than those with lower body-fat levels.[40] In addition, an unexpectedly high rate of obesity was found among adolescent football players. Since body image is inversely related to body-fat percentage in male athletes (i.e., higher body fat is associated with poor body image), it is important to help athletes understand how to increase weight properly if higher weight is desirable.[41] Taken together, these findings strongly suggest that increasing lean (muscle) mass rather than simply increasing weight should be a priority for football players.

Many have questioned whether the recent increases in player size are due to improved preselection in a sport that attracts larger individuals, improved nutrition, or an increased reliance on anabolic steroid hormones. It is possible, of course, for all or any combination of these factors to contribute to the recent increases seen in body mass index. Football players appear to be eating better than their non-football-playing counterparts. In a study of junior high school and high school football players, it was found that, in general, their nutrient and energy intakes were better than those seen in the U.S. population of same-age boys.[42] Energy intakes, which are often below recommended levels in other sports, appeared to meet close to 94 percent of the requirement in the assessed football players. One nutrient found to be low in this study was zinc. In another study of football players, low zinc levels negatively affected maximal workloads. Since zinc is most easily obtained through the consumption of red meat, football players should consider a regular consumption of meat. However, meat consumption should not interfere with or replace the consumption of carbohydrate foods, which are essential for maintaining performance in stop-and-go activities. Vegetarians may be at higher risk for inadequate zinc intake, so they should be assessed by a qualified medical professional to determine if zinc supplements are warranted.

Weight loss is often an issue for lightweight football players. These players, who must maintain weight below a given threshold to be eligible to play, often display eating patterns that are unhealthy. In one study, 20 percent believed their weight-control practices frequently interfered with their thinking and other activities, and 42 percent had a pattern of dysfunctional eating. Almost 10 percent of those surveyed were practicing binge–purge (bulimic) eating behaviors.[43]

As with athletes in other professional sports, time-zone changes make a difference in performance outcomes. It has been found, for instance, that when games are played at night, travelling west coast teams have a clear advantage over eastern and central time-zone teams.[44] The west coast teams feel as if they're playing earlier in the day relative to the other teams, so they do not suffer from end-of-day fatigue to the degree that other teams do. West coast teams have a 75 percent and 68 percent winning percentage when playing central and east coast teams at home, respectively, and still maintain a high winning percentage even when playing in away games (approximately 68 percent). These data strongly suggest that football players who travel across time zones to play should do whatever it takes to return to normal circadian rhythms. Among the positive actions that players can take are eating small amounts of foods frequently and consuming plenty of fluids during travel.

Keeping all these factors in mind, football players must consider the following nutritionally relevant issues for their sport.

Football requires a high level of strength and speed of short duration but high frequency.   Football players are involved in activities that require repeated bouts of high effort interspersed with periods of rest. This type of activity requires a high level of carbohydrate to properly fuel the muscles. Therefore, football players should enter the game with their muscle glycogen levels full. However, even with muscle glycogen storage at its peak, a player cannot play an entire game without depleting muscle glycogen in specific muscle groups. Therefore, football players should take every opportunity to consume a carbohydrate-containing beverage during breaks in the game.

Linemen require a high mass. Although high mass affords linemen a clear advantage, the ability to move the mass quickly is equally important. Therefore, linemen should strive for a high level of muscle mass rather than just higher weight. To achieve this, consumption of a diet that meets the energy requirements plus 300 to 500 calories for the higher mass is needed, along with a relatively low intake of fat (less than 25 percent of total calories) and a moderate intake of protein (12 to 15 percent of total calories, or about 1.5 grams of protein per kilogram of body weight). This type of diet, coupled with exercise that places stress on the muscles, helps enlarge the muscle mass. Increasing total energy intake through the consumption of a high level of fatty foods greatly enables an increase in fat storage (and therefore mass), but fat does not contribute to strength. Thus, fatty foods negatively alter the strength-to-weight ratio and make it more difficult for a lineman to move quickly and powerfully off the line. A study assessing food intake in football players has found a distribution of energy substrates that is not ideal for supporting high-intensity work. This study determined that the 24 assessed football players consumed 45 percent of calories from carbohydrate, 17 percent from protein, and 38 percent from fat.[45]

Backfield defensive positions and pass receivers require high agility, speed, and quick reaction time.   High speed and agility require a relatively low level of body fat. Therefore, these football players should have an eating pattern that limits fat storage (i.e., a high-carbohydrate, low-fat intake consumed in small, frequent meals). Since multiple 40-yard sprints down the field to catch (or defend against) long passes will quickly deplete muscle glycogen storage, consumption of carbohydrate-containing beverages at natural breaks during the game is desirable. During hot and humid days, consuming these beverages will also enhance the ability to maintain a desirable hydration state.

Repeated high-intensity activity while wearing equipment (e.g., pads, helmet) translates into high sweat losses.   The fluid in sweat must be replaced to maintain optimal performance. To do this, consumption of sports beverages that contain a 6 to 7 percent carbohydrate solution is useful for maintaining the body's water level and replenishing carbohydrate fuel. Athletes typically place themselves in a state of voluntary underhydration, so there is every reason to set up a strategy that makes football players consciously consume fluids during every possible break in the game.

Gymnastics

The number of young gymnastics competitors continues to increase, so it is especially important that growth, weight, bone health, eating behavior, and other developmentally important factors be carefully monitored. In gymnastics, small athletes have become the norm, and gymnasts themselves commonly view this small body image as ideal. Weight is a prevailing theme in gymnastics, regardless of the gymnastics discipline. Even in men's gymnastics, it is suggested that controlling energy intake to achieve lower weight is an appropriate and desired approach if a gymnast is to achieve success.[46] However, growth in children is expected, so there should be a concomitant expectation of increasing weight. Not recognizing this fact, many young gymnasts try to achieve a low weight through unhealthy means. There is evidence that the delayed puberty and growth found in female gymnasts is most probably associated with an inadequate caloric intake.[47,48] Of course, inadequate caloric intake is associated with inadequate nutrient intake, and female gymnasts are at a particularly high risk of nonanemic iron deficiency, which could diminish health and performance.[49] Although it is true that lowering excess body fat will reduce body mass and, perhaps, lower the risk of traumatic injuries to joints, trying to achieve this through inappropriate means may also place the gymnast at risk.[50]

Elite-level gymnastics has four separate disciplines, including men's artistic gymnastics, women's artistic gymnastics, women's rhythmic gymnastics, and women's rhythmic group gymnastics. Although the total time spent in gymnastics practice is high for elite gymnasts (up to 30 hours of practice each week), the actual time spent in conditioning and skills training is considerably less. Gymnasts begin practice with a series of stretches and then initiate a series of basic skills on the floor mat as part of the warm-up routine. After warm-up, each gymnast takes a turn practicing one of the events. The time performing a skill in practice never exceeds that of the competition maximum and is usually a small fraction of it. Because practice involves repeated bouts of highly intense, short-duration activities, gymnasts rest between each practice bout to regenerate strength (i.e., regenerate phosphocreatine).

With the exception of the group competition in rhythmic gymnastics, none of the events within each of these disciplines lasts longer than 90 seconds. This maximal effort and short duration categorizes gymnastics as a high-intensity anaerobic sport. As anaerobes, gymnasts rely heavily on Type IIb (pure fast twitch) and Type IIa (intermediate fast twitch) muscle fibers.[51] These fibers, while capable of producing a great deal of power, are generally regarded as incapable of functioning at maximal intensity for longer than 90 seconds. Type II fibers have a low oxidative capacity, which limits fat usage as an energy substrate during gymnastics activity, and a poor capillary supply, which deprives these fibers of nutrient, oxygen, and carbon dioxide exchange during intensive work. Because of these factors, gymnastics is heavily dependent on phosphocreatine and carbohydrate (both glucose and glycogen) as fuels for activity.

A number of studies evaluating the nutrient intake of elite gymnasts have found inadequate intakes of energy, iron, and calcium.[52,53,54] Heavy gymnastics training and inadequate nutrient intake are implicated as causative factors in the primary amenorrhea experienced by many young gymnasts and may also contribute to the secondary amenorrhea experienced by older gymnasts. Although inadequate calcium intake is associated with poor bone development and increased risk of stress fractures, inadequate iron intake is associated with anemia, a risk factor in the development of amenorrhea (see table 12.1 in on page 234).[55]

Keeping all these factors in mind, gymnasts must consider the following nutritionally relevant issues for their sport.

Gymnasts are required to perform difficult tumbling and acrobatic skills that are easier for smaller people to do.

Artistic gymnasts are commonly small (30th percentile for height-to-age ratio) but extremely muscular (90th percentile for arm muscle circumference).[52] This tendency for small stature may be due to a self-selection in the sport (i.e., only those who are naturally small remain in the sport competitively because they tend to be more successful) or because of an inadequate nutrient intake. Both of these factors are possible, either together or separately. Gymnasts and gymnastics coaches know that the top gymnasts tend to be small, so many try to achieve this small size by reducing food intake. There are numerous problems with this strategy, not the least of which is the possibility of delayed growth, with resultant poor skeletal development. In the relatively few cases where this occurs because of an overzealous coach or a gymnast who has made severe cuts in food intake, the outcome may be grim, leading to life-threatening eating disorders. Luckily, however, the vast majority of gymnasts do very well in this sport, have a high self-esteem as a result of participating in this sport, thrive as adults, and have healthy families.

Unhealthy athletes do not remain competitive, so it's in everyone's interest to eat enough to sustain health and growth. Toward that end, gymnasts should think more about optimizing body composition rather than achieving an arbitrarily low weight. A difficulty arising from low-calorie dieting is that weight goes down more from a loss of muscle than from a loss of fat. At some point the muscle loss will inhibit the capacity of gymnasts to perform the required skills, and the downward spiral in the muscle-to-fat ratio may cause gymnasts to further reduce food intake. The progressive reduction in food intake can eventually lead to an eating disorder, with all the dangerous implications this involves.

Gymnasts are sensitive to the strength-to-weight ratio, both from appearance and performance standpoints.

It is impossible to avoid the reality that appearance is a factor in how highly a skill is scored. High strength enables gymnasts to more easily accomplish the required skill, and the appearance of effortlessness is a factor in the score (i.e., it enables an artistic gymnast to look more artistic). Gymnasts are constantly being reminded to smile while in competition, emphasizing that the performed skills are easily accomplished. The key is to be sufficiently conditioned and strong, factors requiring a stable muscle mass, so the skills can be completed with ease.

In a number of countries there is concern that gymnasts start learning skills too early, when they should be focusing on conditioning. A well-conditioned athlete can learn a skill more quickly and with a lower risk of injury. However, there are tremendous pressures on coaches to demonstrate that the gymnasts are making progress, and the best way to do this is to put them in junior competitions. A more balanced approach that focuses mainly on conditioning early in a gymnast's career while delaying the introduction of specific gymnastics skills may improve the skills acquisition learning curve later on. To improve conditioning, gymnasts must consume sufficient energy and nutrients to meet the combined demands of growth, maintenance, and improvement in musculature. The focus of gymnastics training should be on getting strong, with a relatively low body-fat percentage, rather than on staying (or getting) small, and this can be accomplished only through a training program that satisfies nutrition needs.

Gymnasts and many other female athletes have delayed menarche, which may play a role in bone health. Gymnasts failing to achieve menses by age 16 should see a doctor to determine the cause and, if needed, to seek a remedy. There are many possible causes for a delay or cessation of menses:

- Low body fat
- Poor iron status
- High physical stress
- High psychological stress
- High cortisol level (Cortisol is a hormone produced by the body to counteract the soreness created from activity; it is also produced when blood sugar drops below normal levels. It is commonly high in athletes and interferes with estrogen production.)
- Low energy intake

It is conceivable that gymnasts may have all these factors. Regardless of the causes, a delay in menstrual onset may negatively affect bone health and increase the later risk of early osteoporosis development. To reduce the risk of delayed menstrual onset, gymnasts should periodically assess both iron status and body composition to ensure a maintenance or enlargement of the muscle mass with age.

The competitive peak for female gymnasts is commonly reached at about age 16 to 18. With the exception of figure skating and diving, it is difficult to conceive of athletes who achieve this level of accomplishment at such a young age. For this to occur, a tremendous amount of time must be spent in conditioning and skills acquisition while the athlete is in the adolescent growth spurt. The combination of training and growth during these years places a tremendously high nutrition burden on the athlete that cannot be properly met without careful planning. However, with appropriate nutrition planning, it is possible to meet the combined needs of growth, physical activity, and tissue maintenance. Gymnasts who follow a sound nutrition program look better, perform better, enjoy the sport more, and stay in the sport longer.

Hockey

Regardless of whether it's played by men or women, hockey is a no-holds-barred, high-intensity, full-effort sport. If you watch hockey closely, you'll notice that the athletes play in shifts, rarely staying on the ice for more than 1.5 minutes before the next shift takes the ice and almost never skating continuously for longer than a minute. This system allows hockey players to play at full tilt for the entire time they're on the ice, while the bench time allows for the regeneration of phosphocreatine so the players are capable of more quick-burst activity when they return to the ice. This intense effort is highly anaerobic and, therefore, highly reliant on phosphocreatine and glycogen stores. It is possible to make positive changes in the diets of hockey players that can help them maintain weight during the off-season and improve anaerobic endurance during the season.[56]

Findings from a study of elite Swedish hockey players found that the distance skated, the number of shifts skated, the amount of time skated within shifts, and the skating speed all improved with carbohydrate loading.[57] Another study reached a similar conclusion, suggesting that hockey performance would be enhanced by carbohydrate ingestion.[58] It was concluded that individual performance differences among hockey players are directly related to muscle glycogen metabolism, a finding confirmed in a study of seven professional hockey players. In this study, 60 percent of the muscle glycogen in the quadriceps muscles was burned during a single game.[59] Since hockey players frequently skate in practice or play on successive days, it is possible for muscle glycogen to become depleted on an inadequate carbohydrate intake. Data from this study reveal that most players consume a diet high in protein and low in carbohydrate, a diet that is guaranteed to cause fuel-supply problems in muscles working anaerobically. Shifting away from a high-fat, high-protein intake toward one that is higher in carbohydrate is not easy, however, and may result in inadequate energy consumption because of the lower caloric density of carbohydrate compared with fat.

Another study confirmed that many hockey players consume a diet that is insufficient in calories, has poorly distributed energy substrates, and is deficient in a number of vitamins and minerals, including vitamins A, D, and E; calcium; magnesium; and zinc.[60] A study in which hockey players were placed on a special reduced-fat, reduced-protein, higher-carbohydrate intake resulted in an inadequate total energy intake.[61] Therefore, if a switch is made from a higher-fat diet to one that is lower in fat and higher in carbohydrate, care must be taken that the total energy intake is sufficient to meet the athlete's needs.

Keeping all these factors in mind, hockey players must consider the following nutritionally relevant issues for their sport.

Frequent games place a high demand on muscle glycogen, which requires the consumption of foods high in carbohydrate (60 to 65 percent of total energy) for glycogen replenishment. The strategies for optimizing glycogen storage must be considered. The pregame meal should consist almost entirely of carbohydrate foods that are mainly starch based, such as pasta, potatoes, rice, breads, and cereals. Fruits, vegetables, and high-bran foods (i.e., high in crude fiber) may increase gas production in the gut so should be avoided or consumed sparingly in the pregame meal. Every opportunity should be taken to provide carbohydrate-containing beverages during breaks in play and between periods. Postgame carbohydrate consumption in the first hour is critical to capitalize on the circulating glycogen synthetase.[62] The typical food intake not associated with games or training should focus on starch-based complex carbohydrate, but the during-game and immediately postgame intake should be more sugar-based simple carbohydrate.

Changing food intake to provide more carbohydrate may result in inadequate energy consumption. Surveys of hockey players strongly suggest that usual energy intakes tend to be high in fat, high in protein, and low in carbohydrate, an energy substrate distribution that does not adequately support the type of energy metabolic processes associated with hockey. However, because of the higher energy concentration of fat, it is easier for hockey players to obtain the total amount of energy they need. For the same weight of food, fat provides more than twice the caloric content of carbohydrate (9 calories per gram versus 4 calories per gram). Therefore, making a switch to foods that are lower in fat and higher in carbohydrate while maintaining the same eating frequency may create a negative energy balance that could also be detrimental to performance.[63] Inadequate energy intake in physically active people guarantees a catabolism of muscle, an outcome that reduces athletic performance in a power sport. A possible solution to this undesirable outcome is to make certain that hockey players increase their eating frequency to six times per day (breakfast, midmorning snack, lunch, midafternoon snack, dinner, evening snack) to create more eating opportunities while fat is being reduced and carbohydrate intake is being increased.

High-intensity activity causes body temperature to rise quickly, with a concomitant rise in sweat rate. This fact, plus the amount of equipment worn by hockey players, places them at high risk of dehydration. Following a good hydration plan is critical, therefore, for success. Hockey players should consume plenty of fluids before the game and take every opportunity to consume fluids during and after the game. Given the need for carbohydrates and the need for fluids, a good strategy is to consume a carbohydrate-containing beverage whenever possible. (See chapter 3 for additional information on hydration protocols.)

Track and Field (Sprints, Jumps, and Throws)

Track and field competition includes a number of events of short duration that rely on power through anaerobic energy. Sprints and hurdle events include races up to and including 400 meters, while field events include jumps and throws of short duration and maximal effort. There is evidence that male and female sprinters, jumpers, and throwers have less than optimal nutrition habits, with a majority having below-standard intakes of at least one vitamin or mineral.[64] There is also evidence that stress fracture risk, considered an outcome of inadequate energy and calcium intake, is high in track and field athletes.[65]

It is hard to imagine an overweight sprinter, strongly suggesting that aerobic activity is not necessary for lowering body fat. A study assessing the fat-lowering impact of high-intensity versus low-intensity activity found they were equally effective at lowering body fat.[66] Sprinting has been recommended as a normal component of interval training in many sports. Regardless of whether it's done for training or it makes up the sport itself (as in the 100-meter dash), sprinting has specific energy requirements that must be accounted for and satisfied to perform optimally. Sprints, which by their very nature rarely last longer than 10 seconds, primarily use the fuels phosphocreatine and glycogen. Muscles with an adequate storage of phosphocreatine can support high-intensity exercise for 8 to 10 seconds, making it likely that most athletes use primarily phosphocreatine for the entire duration of the sprint. A study assessing creatine monohydrate supplementation found it increased the muscular storage of phosphocreatine, promoted gains in fat-free mass (i.e., muscle), and improved sprint performance.[67] This is consistent with a number of studies in other sports that produced similar findings.[68] Carbohydrate intake also makes a difference in sprint performance. In a study evaluating the impact of high, moderate, and low carbohydrate intakes, the high carbohydrate intakes produced better initial sprint performance than did lower carbohydrate intakes.[69]

In some sports, a sprint may be the difference between winning or losing even when the majority of time is spent doing lower intensity activities. For instance, 10K runners and marathoners run almost the entire distance at the highest pace at which they are capable of sustaining aerobic metabolic processes. At the end of these races, however, the athletes go into a sprint pace (referred to as "the kick") that exceeds their oxidative capacity. A study emulating this high-pace aerobic running followed by an anaerobic kick found that a higher carbohydrate intake aided performance. Over 4 consecutive days, a high carbohydrate intake, when compared with a moderate carbohydrate intake, was more capable of maintaining muscle glycogen in athletes working at a high intensity of aerobic capacity (~75 percent of $\dot{V}O_2$max) followed by five 1-minute sprints.[70]

Keeping all these factors in mind, track and field athletes must consider the following nutritionally relevant issues for their sport.

Sprinting demands a large amount of phosphocreatine and carbohydrate fuels. By its very definition, a sprint requires the fastest possible movement over a short prescribed distance. Metabolic limitations control the maximum distance humans can sprint, and sprints never last longer than 1.5 minutes. During short sprints, there is a primary dependence on phosphocreatine as a fuel. It has been hypothesized that the ingestion of extra creatine, typically as a supplement in the form of creatine monohydrate, may improve phosphocreatine storage (refer to chapter 4 for more detailed information). This increased storage of phosphocreatine could increase the number of short all-out sprints an athlete is capable of performing and might also improve the maximal time muscles can rely mainly on phosphocreatine as a fuel. There is evidence that supplementing with creatine monohydrate does, in fact, improve both sprint frequency and sprint distance. However, inherent design weaknesses are present in some of these studies, so athletes should refrain from jumping on the creatine supplement bandwagon. For instance, these studies did not evaluate the energy intake adequacy of the athletes, so the inherent limits of synthesizing creatine without adequate energy may have been inhibiting performance, a problem that could be more easily and cheaply resolved through a greater energy intake, preferably from carbohydrate. Also, the issue of the safety of frequent and long-term creatine monohydrate ingestion has not yet been adequately addressed.

Creatine is a normal constituent of the diet and is plentiful in meat (beef, pork, poultry) and fish. Therefore, in the context of a high-carbohydrate diet, it seems useful for sprinters to consider consuming small amounts of lean meats regularly. Non-meat-eaters should take care to consume sufficient protein and calories so the synthesis of creatine can occur in the body. However, even more important than protein intake is satisfying total energy requirements so the athlete is capable of synthesizing all the creatine needed to sustain optimal performance. Pure sprinters may be inhibited by carbohydrate supercompensation, while endurance athletes may require carbohydrate supercompensation to support the end-of-race kick.

Pure sprinters must move their mass quickly over a relatively short distance, and the amount of mass that must be moved is a factor in how quickly it can be moved. Sprinters with high strength-to-weight ratios have advantages over those with lower strength-to-weight ratios. One of the effects of carbohydrate loading

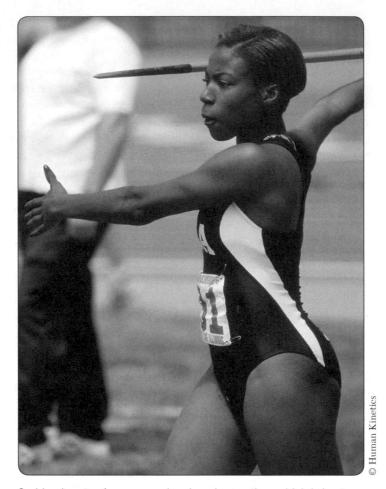

© Human Kinetics

Sudden bursts of power require phosphocreatine, which is best derived from a diet that satisfies both energy and protein needs.

(or supercompensation) is to force more carbohydrate (glycogen) into the muscles so it is available for muscular work. Glycogen is stored with water in a 1 to 3 ratio. That is, for each gram of glycogen stored, the body stores 3 grams of water. At times, athletes who undergo a carbohydrate-loading regimen mention that they feel stiff and heavy. Clearly, this is not the way a sprinter should feel at the beginning of a race, but it is a perfectly acceptable feeling for long-distance runners. Therefore, pure sprinters should regularly consume a high-carbohydrate intake that provides sufficient total calories but should avoid any carbohydrate-loading regimen that might force additional glycogen and water into the muscles.

Swimming (100 to 400 Meters)

Perhaps there is no other sport where so much time must be spent practicing to gain such incrementally small levels of improvement. Swimmers spend a considerable amount of time in the water to perfect techniques that will better overcome drag and to improve their capacity to sustain both aerobic and anaerobic energy production. In the shorter (sprint) distances where races are typically less than 2 minutes in length, the majority of energy is predominantly derived anaerobically from phosphocreatine and glycogen (see table 13.2). Although these sprint races are short, the amount of energy needed to sustain a high level of power output is tremendously high, and the majority of this energy (more than 55 percent) must come from glycogen and phosphocreatine. The time spent training has a high energy and nutrient cost that must be considered when developing a training plan.

A study of swimmers at a national developmental training camp found that the average energy intakes (5,221 calories for males; 3,573 calories for females) and nutrient intakes were adequate, but there was a large between-swimmer variation in intake.[71] This variation, coupled with a tendency for these swimmers to consume excessive amounts of fat and insufficient amounts of carbohydrate, suggests that a large proportion of swimmers may have dietary habits that do not optimally support training and competition needs. In addition, there is evidence of poor iron status among female collegiate swimmers, which could compromise training and exercise performance.[72] The desire for higher-fat foods from meats and dairy products has been tested in male swimmers, and it was found that they tend to like the sensory appeal of fat-containing animal products, even when undergoing a high level of exercise.[73]

High-level swimmers, often high school students and college-age adults, must spend a great deal of time in the pool to gain a speed improvement, which commonly translates into multiple training sessions each day. Swimmers typically practice in the early morning and late afternoon (before and after school), and they generally accept that they must get an hour or two of laps in before classes begin (often at 5 a.m.) to have a chance of improving. The problem, therefore, is ensuring that swimmers consume enough energy at the right time and in the right form to make it supportive of the training plan. Ideally, swimmers

Table 13.2 Relative Contribution of Aerobic and Anaerobic Energy Sources During Exercise of Different Lengths

Time	Anaerobic %	Aerobic %
0-30 sec	80	20
30-60 sec	60	40
60-90 sec	42	58
90-120 sec	36	64
120-180 sec	30	70
Expressed cumulatively		
0-60 sec	70	30
0-90 sec	61	39
0-120 sec	55	45
0-180 sec	45	55

Note: As the exercise time increases, power production decreases and a greater proportion of energy is derived aerobically. Aerobic metabolism is less reliant on glycogen and phosphocreatine because of an ability to metabolize fat for energy.

Adapted, by permission, from D.R. Lamb, 1995, "Basic principles for improving sport performance," *GSSI Sports Science Exchange* #55 8(2). [Online]. Available: www.gssiweb.com/Article_Detail.aspx?articleid=28 [June 27, 2011].

should make time between and during practices to consume a significant amount of high-carbohydrate foods. However, swimmers must do this in a way that ensures the stomach is empty before getting into the water. This means the focus, during practice and swim competitions, should be on carbohydrate-containing sports beverages. Having large amounts of solid foods shortly before getting into the water causes a fluid shift away from the muscles and into the GI tract and may cause cramping.

Keeping all these factors in mind, swimmers must consider the following nutritionally relevant issues for their sport.

Swimmers train for many hours and have an intensive training protocol.

Competitive swimmers work hard and long at getting better, and all that work translates into a tremendously high caloric need. Since swimmers often have an early-morning practice, it is important that they consume some carbohydrate immediately upon awakening to give the food or beverage enough time to leave the stomach before practice. A failure to consume a minimum of 100 to 200 calories (depending on body weight) of carbohydrate before practice may limit the benefits the athlete could derive from practice. Fluids (apple or grape juice or a sports beverage) are good to sip on during the trip to the pool. After the morning practice, swimmers should consume some high-carbohydrate breakfast foods (cereal, toast, bagel) that should be immediately available. This will help replenish the energy consumed during practice and begin the process of storing more energy for the afternoon practice. Also, because so much energy is needed, high school swimmers should seek approval from school administrators to consume a midmorning snack of 200 to 400 calories.

Swimmers who practice sprinting in the pool should be aware that phosphocreatine (a major fuel for sprints) is likely to become depleted in muscle cells, and it takes time to regenerate the phosphocreatine to get the cells ready for the next sprint. When total sprinting time meets or exceeds 2 minutes, there should be a recovery period of 4 minutes to allow cells time to replenish the depleted phosphocreatine. A failure to allow for this recovery period will force the swimmer to work at a lower intensity and for shorter periods on subsequent sprints. If that happens, the swimmer will be learning to sprint in a way that could adversely affect competitive times.[74]

Some swimmers believe body-weight reduction may be necessary to improve bathing suit appearance and reduce drag.

The paper-thin material used for racing suits makes it impossible for swimmers to hide their physiques. Since everyone wants to look good, swimmers may be motivated to reduce body weight. However, many swimmers could easily experience a reduction in performance if weight loss results in a loss of muscle with a secondary loss of power. If weight were lost in a way that reduces drag, there could be a performance benefit, but most weight-loss strategies backfire and hinder performance. Therefore, swimmers wishing to lose weight to either look better or go faster (or both) should do so only under the direct supervision of a qualified health professional. Also, the focus should be on fat reduction and muscle maintenance rather than weight reduction per se.

Swimmers rely heavily on glycogen and phosphocreatine, and sprinting performance is highly dependent on carbohydrate (to make stored glycogen) and phosphocreatine.

With sufficient total energy intake that focuses on carbohydrate (at least 30 calories of carbohydrate per kilogram of body weight) and the inclusion of an adequate amount of protein (about 1.2 to 1.7 grams per kilogram of body weight), there is every reason to believe that athletes can store enough glycogen and make enough phosphocreatine to properly fuel their muscles. However, there is tremendous motivation for athletes to consume creatine monohydrate supplements (a precursor to phosphocreatine) to gain a competitive edge. Although creatine monohydrate supplements may improve the number of high-intensity sprints a swimmer is able to do, swimmers should be aware that regular creatine consumption is associated with an increase in weight. Since this weight increase is likely to be from water, it could reduce buoyancy and increase drag. It is likely that a greater benefit could be achieved by creating opportunities to eat so as to ensure an optimal total energy intake.

Swimmers need to consume fluid.   It is difficult to imagine that, with so much water around, swimmers could be at risk for dehydration. The fact that swimmers work in a hypothermic environment (water is usually colder than air temperature) makes it easier for the excess heat generated from muscular work to be dissipated. However, there are other good reasons for swimmers to consider whether their hydration state is adequate. A poorly hydrated athlete may develop a lower blood volume that causes the heart to work harder to bring oxygen and nutrients to cells, and there is less volume in which to place metabolic by-products. Also, many competitions take place outside, where swimmers spend a great deal of time waiting for their events and where they can easily become overheated. Excess water storage could clearly cause a problem for swimmers by increasing weight and drag, but insufficient body water can influence performance and concentration. Therefore, a good rule of thumb is to constantly sip small amounts of water or sports beverage while avoiding strategies that could force an excess water storage (e.g., glycogen loading, creatine).

Wrestling

Wrestling has been around as a sport for thousands of years. Early sculpted artifacts and paintings from France, Egypt, and ancient Babylon show wrestlers involved in holds that are essentially the same as those used today. In the early Olympic Games in Greece, the wrestling competition was considered the premier event.[75] The basic strategy in all this time has not changed: Wrestlers attempt to force the shoulders of the opponent onto the mat to win the match. If neither wrestler is able to score such a fall, the winner is determined by officials, who use a point system that includes points for near falls, points for holding an opponent close to his back, and points for time controlling the opponent.

The techniques used by wrestlers to make weight (i.e., to achieve a weight that allows the wrestler to compete in the lowest possible weight class) have long been considered problematic. In 1996 the American College of Sports Medicine (ACSM) developed a position on weight loss in wrestlers:[76]

> *Despite a growing body of evidence admonishing the behavior, weight cutting (rapid weight reduction) remains prevalent among wrestlers. Weight cutting has significant adverse consequences that may affect competitive performance, physical health, and normal growth and development. To enhance the education experience and reduce the health risks for the participants, the ACSM recommends measures to educate coaches and wrestlers toward sound nutrition and weight control behaviors, to curtail weight cutting, and to enact rules that limit weight loss.*

Despite the ACSM's position warning of problems associated with techniques used to make weight, in 1997 the wresting community suffered the tragic deaths of three collegiate wrestlers who were practicing common weight-loss strategies. Jeff Reese, a University of Michigan junior, died of kidney and heart failure while working out in a rubber suit in a room heated to 92 degrees Fahrenheit (33 degrees Celsius) so he could qualify for a lower weight class. Billy Saylor (19 years old and three-time Florida State champion) of Campbell University and Joseph LaRosa (22 years old) of the University of Wisconsin also died while trying to lose a large amount of weight to qualify for a lower weight class.

The outrage resulting from these deaths led to serious examination of the rules encouraging the manipulation of normal weight and the techniques used (supplements, dehydration, fasting) to achieve a weight well below an athlete's natural weight to permit qualification in a lower weight class. An important outcome of this discussion has been an improvement in the information wrestling coaches have about weight loss, sport nutrition, training diets, dehydration, and body composition.

The National Collegiate Athletic Association (NCAA) regulates collegiate wrestling and has developed rules, also adopted by the National Association of Intercollegiate Athletics (NAIA), the National Junior College Athletic Association (NJCAA), and the National Collegiate Wrestling Association (NCWA), for organizing weight classifications. These rules have greatly reduced the motivation for making weight and have, therefore, had an impact on reducing health risks. The rules for weight classifications require the following:[77]

- *A wrestler must have weight assessed by a member of the institution's athletics medical staff (physician, athletic trainer, or registered dietitian) **before** the first official team practice.*

- *The weight assessed is then considered the wrestler's minimum weight class; the athlete may not compete below that weight class and may compete only at one weight class higher than the measured minimum weight.*

- *If a wrestler gains weight over the course of the wrestling season and wrestles at two levels above the minimum weight, she can no longer wrestle at the previously established minimum weight class.*

- *To ensure the athlete does not dehydrate to make the minimum weight classification, the athlete must also have a normal hydration state. To further diminish the chance of dehydration, the NCAA has banned the use of saunas and rubber suits. In addition, the weight allowance for each class has been increased from 1 pound to 2 pounds (from .5 kg to 1 kg).*

- *The weigh-in time has been moved from 24 hours before the match to 2 hours before the match. This lower time for recovery makes it far more difficult for an athlete to drop significant weight via dehydration with the hope of recovering before the match.*

A survey assessing weight-loss practices of college wrestlers determined that 40 percent of athletes were following the new NCAA rules and curbing their risky weight-loss practices.[78] Although this is a positive outcome, many wrestlers have maintained risky weight-loss behaviors. It was found that the majority of high school wrestlers in Michigan engaged in a minimum of one harmful weight loss method *each week* during the wrestling season. These methods include fasting and various means of losing weight through dehydration.[79] There is concern on many levels about the weight-loss techniques that are still commonly practiced by wrestlers. Some evidence suggests that undernutrition may lead to altered

ACSM's Position Stand on Weight Loss in Wrestlers

In its position stand, the American College of Sports Medicine makes the following recommendations:

1. Educate coaches and wrestlers about the adverse consequences of prolonged fasting and dehydration on physical performance and physical health.

2. Discourage the use of rubber suits, steam rooms, hot boxes, saunas, laxatives, and diuretics for making weight.

3. Adopt new state or national governing body legislation that schedules weigh-ins immediately before competition.

4. Schedule daily weigh-ins before and after practice to monitor weight loss and dehydration. Weight lost during practice should be regained through adequate food and fluid intake.

5. Assess the body composition of each wrestler before the season using valid methods for this population. Males 16 years and younger with a body fat below 7 percent or those over 16 years with a body fat below 5 percent need medical clearance before being allowed to compete. Female wrestlers need a body fat of 12 to 14 percent.

6. Emphasize the need for daily caloric intake obtained from a balanced diet high in carbohydrate (more than 55 percent of calories) and low in fat (less than 30 percent of calories), with adequate protein (15 to 20 percent of calories, 1.2-1.7 grams per kilogram of body weight) determined on the basis of RDA guidelines and physical activity levels. The minimal caloric intake for wrestlers of high school and college age should range from 1,700 to 2,500 calories per day, depending on weight; rigorous training may increase the requirement up to an additional 1,000 calories per day. Wrestlers should be discouraged by coaches, parents, school officials, and physicians from consuming less than their minimal daily needs. Combined with exercise, this minimal caloric intake will allow for gradual weight loss. After the minimal weight has been attained, caloric intake should be increased sufficiently to support the normal developmental needs of the young wrestler.

Reprinted, by permission, from R.A. Oppliger, H.S. Case, G.L. Landry, et al., 1996, "ACSM position stand: Weight loss in wrestlers," *Medicine & Science in Sports & Exercise* 28(10): 135-138.

growth hormone production in wrestlers, which could lead to permanent growth impairment if present over several seasons.[80] Another study determined that dietary restriction reduced protein nutrition and muscular performance.[81] These data are confirmed by findings indicating that weight loss by energy restriction significantly reduced the anaerobic performance of wrestlers. Those on a high-carbohydrate refeeding diet tended to recover their performance, while those with lower intakes of carbohydrate did not.[82]

Besides the obvious physiological changes that occur from rapid weight loss, there is good evidence that rapid weight loss in collegiate wrestlers causes an impairment of short-term memory, a fact that could affect scholastic achievement in these student athletes.[83] There is evidence that competing at a weight below the predicted minimum wrestling weight may be associated with greater success.[84] But there is also evidence that successful weight gain during this short period is important for success. In one study evaluating the relative weight gains of wrestlers, the heavier wrestler was successful 57 percent of the time.[85] There is also evidence that dehydration of as little as 3 percent impairs anaerobic endurance and anaerobic power, and a relatively minor 4 percent body-weight loss also impairs wrestling performance. It has been recommended, therefore, that wrestlers would do best if they competed after an exercise taper (to optimize glycogen stores), in a well-hydrated state, after ingesting a high-carbohydrate diet.[86]

Keeping all these factors in mind, wrestlers must consider the following nutritionally relevant issues for their sport.

Making weight is a hazard to both performance and health.   Ample evidence suggests that the weight cycling associated with making weight (i.e., weight loss to make weight followed by weight recovery for performance) is dangerous and can lead to glycogen depletion, a lower muscle mass, a lower resting energy expenditure, and an increase in body fat.[87] Should this occur with frequency, it is likely that the reduction in resting energy expenditure could make it more difficult for the athlete to achieve the desired weight through dietary restriction, leading the wrestler to take more draconian (and more dangerous) measures to achieve the desired weight outcome. Wrestlers and coaches should follow a reasonable model for achieving desired weight, such as that offered by the Wisconsin Interscholastic Athletic Association, to avoid health and performance difficulties.[88] This program develops reasonable goals for weight and provides nutrition education information to help wrestlers achieve desired weight reasonably and to understand the implications of improper weight-loss methods. In these weight-achievement guidelines, a cap is placed on the maximum amount of weight change that can occur during the course of a season, and a monitoring system has been added to ensure that sudden and dramatic weight change does not occur at any point in the season.

The anaerobic nature of wrestling implies a high need for good hydration to store carbohydrates.   Although there is an aerobic component to Olympic wrestling (matches may continue for 5 minutes without a break), high school wrestling is primarily an anaerobic sport (three 2-minute periods). The demand for carbohydrate in this type of activity is extremely high, and there is evidence that wrestlers perform better on high carbohydrate intakes. It is also of great concern that wrestlers commonly resort to dehydration as a means of achieving desired weight. Besides inhibiting carbohydrate storage (1 gram of glycogen requires 3 grams of water for storage), nothing could be more dangerous or more performance reducing than competing in a dehydrated state. Wrestlers should resist inducing dehydration because of the clear dangers (including organ failure, heatstroke, and death) associated with this strategy and should understand that well-hydrated athletes perform better than dehydrated ones.

Wrestlers and coaches should become better educated on the potential hazards of improper nutrition.   Trying to achieve an arbitrarily low weight in growing athletes is disease inducing rather than health enhancing (the ultimate goal of sport). It is not acceptable to place a young athlete in harm's way to achieve a falsely low weight goal, especially since the achieved weight has nothing to do with the weight at which the wrestler actually competes. Everyone involved in the sport should endorse the development of widely accepted weight-to-height norms that can be applied reasonably to wrestlers. Further, weight should be taken immediately before the competition rather than at a time that permits drastic and dangerous shifts in eating behaviors. Until the rules change, wrestlers and coaches should all be made aware of the hazards associated with the current procedures for making weight.

Speedskating

Speedskating has been an Olympic sport for men since 1924 and for women since 1960. The short-track races first became an official Olympic sport at the 1992 Olympic Games. Speedskaters typically train for 30 to 35 hours per week when preparing for competition.[89] These training volumes are associated with high energy requirements, regardless of the competitive distance. The cold-weather environment of some of the longer marathon speedskating races may contribute to the higher energy requirement by an additional 10 to 40 percent.[90] There is evidence that speedskaters who satisfy the higher energy intakes are also consuming higher micronutrient intakes as well, as would be expected.[91]

The difficulty of scheduling sufficient eating opportunities to satisfy the high energy requirement influences many speedskaters to take dietary supplements as an easy alternative to normal eating. A study assessing dietary supplement intake among elite athletes in 27 sports found that short-track speedskaters and long-track speedskaters had among the highest rates of dietary supplementation.[92] The highest-level athletes in this study reported that strength trainers, teammates, and family or friends were their top three sources of information regarding supplementation. However, it appears that much of the advice received from these sources was unrelated to the speedskaters' needs. In addition, the illegal substances found in many supplements could increase the risk of a positive doping test in speedskaters competing in sanctioned events.[93]

The training of speedskaters preparing for competition has been described as following a similar pattern as that of distance runners who are striving to improve their aerobic competence.[94] Forty percent of speedskater training includes distance running and cycling, 20 percent involves high-intensity interval training, 15 percent involves endurance or resistance training, and 25 percent involves training that emulates speedskating-specific motion.

Shorter speedskating distances (i.e., 500 to 1,500 meters) require a higher proportion of anaerobic metabolism, while longer distances (i.e., 5,000 and 10,000 meters) require more aerobic metabolism.[95] Particularly for the distances requiring a higher proportion of oxygen delivery, iron status is critically important. Some athletes try to optimize iron status by living in a high-altitude environment to stimulate the development of new red blood cells, but this strategy is useful only when sufficient iron stores are present.[96]

The historical data on speedskaters suggest that the nutrient intake of elite athletes has improved significantly. In 1983 speedskaters consumed an energy-dense diet, with 50 percent of the calories from fat and only 30 percent from carbohydrate. More recent dietary analyses suggest that carbohydrate intake increased to 60 percent of total calories, which is a level more closely in line with published recommendations.[97,98]

Keeping all these factors in mind, speedskaters must consider the following nutritionally relevant issues for their sport.

Satisfy the need for energy. Speedskaters have a high need for energy. Without sufficient energy, they would have difficulty sustaining adequate muscle mass and would compromise glycogen stores. Ideally, this high energy need should be met through increased eating opportunities that are strategically planned around the training regimen. Both the power and endurance components of speedskating place a high demand on carbohydrate fuel, which should be delivered at a level of 8 to 10 grams per kilogram of body weight, or approximately 65 percent of total calories consumed.

Ensure hydration needs are met. Sweat loss occurs in all environmental temperatures; a cold environment may also create a cold-induced diuresis that can further produce a hydration-compromised state. Any level of dehydration is likely to negatively affect performance, so speedskaters should ensure an adequate intake of fluid before, during, and after training. Dark urine, infrequent urination, or low urine volume are all suggestive of a poor hydration state. Ideally, speedskaters should begin a sipping protocol with a sports beverage (~6 percent carbohydrate and 150 to 200 milligrams of sodium per cup) immediately after the last meal of solid food before training. Skaters should take one or two mouthfuls every 10 to 15 minutes before training, followed by frequent sips of the same fluid at convenient intervals during training.

Eat and drink in a way that optimizes glycogen stores. Glycogen is best derived through the well-timed consumption of carbohydrate and fluid (1 gram of glycogen requires 3 grams of water). Dehydration makes glycogen storage a far more difficult task to achieve. Speedskaters should be concerned about both liver glycogen and muscle glycogen. The liver glycogen is primarily responsible for sustaining blood sugar and is dissipated in approximately 3 hours during the day when not exercising. However, exercise increases the demand for blood sugar dramatically, leading to exhausted liver glycogen stores and low blood sugar in as little as 30 minutes. Low blood sugar results in mental fatigue, which results in muscle fatigue. To sustain liver glycogen stores, it is important to take in carbohydrate (sipping on a sports beverage is a good strategy) as often as possible before and during exercise.

Optimal muscle glycogen storage requires the following: (1) a reduced utilization of the muscle glycogen through lower-intensity and lower-duration training and (2) a well-timed and adequate carbohydrate and fluid intake to support muscle glycogen storage. Consuming carbohydrate immediately postexercise is useful because this is when glycogen synthetase (the enzyme needed to convert glucose to glycogen) is most elevated. Consuming carbohydrate *during* exercise also helps diminish the degree to which muscle glycogen stores are used during exercise, making it easier to sustain higher glycogen stores on sequential days of exercise.

Ensure normal iron status. The metabolic oxygen needs of speedskaters are high, particularly for race distances that exceed 1,000 meters. Because of the long training protocols of most speedskaters, regardless of the distances they race, oxygen-carrying capacity is critically important. Given iron's importance in speedskating and the fact that iron deficiency is the single most prevalent nutrient deficiency, it makes sense for speedskaters to have an annual iron-status assessment. It is unlikely that a speedskater could train or compete at his best with a compromised iron status.

Provide ample time for eating and resting.   Speedskaters spend a great deal of time training, yet there is evidence that eating and resting are not an integral planned component of the training regimen. Inadequate food intake, insufficient eating opportunities (forcing excessive food consumption at single meals), and inadequate rest all diminish the potential for athletic improvement. Speedskaters should plan training days in a way that dynamically integrates food and beverage consumption with exercise.

Olympic Weightlifting

The International Weightlifting Federation (IWF) has established eight weight divisions for men and seven weight divisions for women, ranging from 56 kilograms (123 pounds) to greater than 105 kilograms (131 pounds) for men and from 48 kilograms (106 pounds) to greater than 75 kilograms (165 pounds) for women. Competitions involve the snatch (lifting the barbell above the head with arms straight in a single motion) and the clean and jerk (lifting the barbell above the head in two separate motions). The combined winner is the athlete who has lifted the greatest total weights in the snatch and the clean and jerk. When compared with other power athletes, Olympic lifers are significantly stronger than sprinters and produce significantly higher peak forces and power outputs than do powerlifters.[99]

Weightlifters tend to consume high levels of protein (2.5 grams per kilogram and above) and likely use this large protein intake to partially support the requirement for calories. Researchers have suggested that 1.0 gram per kilogram per day is likely sufficient for weightlifters who are in energy balance, and those consuming significantly above this level have negatively affected mood states.[100] A high level of protein intake is also likely to result in a high degree of metabolic nitrogenous waste that could result in dehydration and, over time, may be damaging to the renal tubules.[101]

A study assessing a mixture of creatine, protein, and carbohydrate found this mixture was superior to a protein and carbohydrate supplement for enlarging the muscle and improving strength (40 percent of the strength was attributable to muscle enlargement).[102] Another study found that whey protein was equivalent to creatine monohydrate in helping muscle enlargement and strength, suggesting that something other than creatine itself may be associated with strength gains.[103] A study assessing a protein supplement (unknown source) by itself determined that consumption of this supplement could not be clearly associated with improvements in muscular performance.[104] In addition, this study found that resting cortisol (a catabolic hormone) was significantly higher for the protein-supplemented group than the placebo group.

Caffeine consumption was found to enhance performance in short-term resistance activity when athletes exercise to the point of fatigue, and it may also result in a more positive mood state than when compared with a placebo.[105] The supplement betaine (derived from the amino acid glycine) has also been tested with weightlifters; 2 weeks of betaine supplementation improved muscle endurance and lowered muscle fatigue.[106] However, it is unlikely that this benefit would be observed in athletes consuming whole grains, shellfish, and fresh vegetables who naturally have high glycine and betaine concentrations.

Power athletes are known to take supplements with identified risks, including ephedra-containing dietary supplements.[107] Ephedra can cause serious cardiological and neurological problems. This is yet another example of athletes looking in the wrong place for performance enhancement. The potential benefits of most supplements disappear in athletes who consume sufficient energy from foods, particularly when the food is consumed in frequent small meals. A review of eating practices of Olympic weightlifters found some disturbing trends.[108] These athletes consider animal-derived protein as the most critical food consumed and ate more than twice as much meat and eggs as did triathletes. Lifters are frequent consumers of supplements for which there is no evidence to support an ergogenic benefit, and they frequently lower food intake before competition to lose weight and, perhaps, compete in a lower weight classification.

Body composition is an important factor in weightlifting performance, and lean body mass is strongly associated with performance in both the snatch and the clean and jerk. By contrast, body-fat percentage is negatively associated with performance in both the snatch and the clean and jerk.[109] These results clearly have implications for how and what weightlifters consume and also highlight why so many weightlifters seek supplemental means of attaining this desired body profile.

Keeping all these factors in mind, Olympic weightlifters must consider the following nutritionally relevant issues for their sport.

Maintaining weight at a competitive body composition is better than losing weight before competition and then regaining weight.

Athletes should find strategies that keep them at a competitive weight and body composition rather than go through cycles of weight loss to achieve the desired weight category. The cyclical reduction of weight is likely to have precisely the wrong effect on these athletes, who are so reliant on a high level of muscle and a low level of fat to perform at their best. Consumption of small, frequent meals that satisfy total energy needs and dynamically match energy intake with expenditure is most closely associated with a high lean mass and a low fat mass.

Food intake is always superior to reliance on supplements.

Foods are more likely to provide the wide array of needed nutrients and energy, are less expensive, and are not associated with potentially illegal substances (often not listed on the label of many supplements). Supplements do play a role for athletes who are, for whatever reason, unable to obtain sufficient food and nutrients. They are not a substitute, however, for good eating.

Protein is important, but it isn't everything.

Surveys of weightlifters strongly suggest an excessive reliance on and consumption of protein. It would be far better and safer for an athlete to satisfy energy requirements from a diet that provides protein at a level of no more than 2 grams per kilogram and carbohydrate at a level of no less than 6 grams per kilogram. This level of energy substrate distribution will help satisfy glycogen needs and provide more than enough protein to sustain or increase muscle mass.

Competition may be highly reliant on phosphocreatine for energy, but practices are long and rely heavily on muscle glycogen.

Athletes often mistake the metabolic needs of competition with the needs of training. In weightlifting, athletes require a high degree of phosphocreatine (PCr) to perform well. PCr can be optimized in muscle through an adequate energy and protein intake that avoids large energy deficits during the day. However, the demands of training, with many repetitions and long times in the gym, far exceed the capacity of PCr to supply the needed energy. Therefore, glycogen storage becomes increasingly important for repetitive high-intensity bouts of activity. Optimizing glycogen storage requires a relatively high carbohydrate intake that is strategically timed before, during, and after training.

Athletes in sports involving maximal power and speed should focus on consuming an adequate total energy intake, primarily from carbohydrate, so that sufficient glycogen can be synthesized and stored for muscular work. Since phosphocreatine and glycogen are the primary fuels for high-intensity activities, protein intake should also be sufficient (about 1.5 to 2.0 grams per kilogram of body weight) to ensure that creatine can be synthesized. There is increasing evidence that creatine supplementation can significantly improve performance in short-duration, high-intensity activity.[110] However, research design issues of many of these studies fail to clarify how athletes might perform with an adequate caloric consumption and if this might encourage a greater internal synthesis of creatine.

Many athletes across a wide-ranging spectrum of sports have unsatisfactory nutrition habits that should be corrected before embarking on a strategy of supplementation.[111] Fluid intake is also important because it helps maintain blood volume (a critically important factor in athletic performance), and inadequate fluid intake limits glycogen storage and also makes it difficult to maintain body temperature. Coaches tend to overvalue proteins, are excessive in recommending low-fat diets, and often use food myths rather than facts in making dietary recommendations to athletes.[112] Athletes should always adapt their carbohydrate and fluid needs to their sports, but in the case of high-intensity, short-duration activities, the needs are almost always high.[113]

IMPORTANT POINTS

• The higher the exercise intensity, the greater the reliance on carbohydrate as a fuel. However, the long duration of lower-intensity endurance sports makes carbohydrate equally important for high- and low-intensity activities.

• The storage capacity for carbohydrate (glycogen) and PCr is small compared with fat stores. Therefore, athletes involved in high-intensity sports that require quick bursts of power should have a strategy for optimizing carbohydrate storage as well as an exercise and eating pattern that optimizes PCr availability.

• Although power athletes often believe that high protein intake is essential for success, they may mistake the intake of protein with the requirement for calories needed to support a large muscle mass.

• Although many sports have competitions that require less than 90 seconds per exercise bout, practices for these sports often last for hours. Consuming a carbohydrate-containing sports beverage is useful during practices to ensure that glycogen stores are not depleted.

• Where multiple bouts of high-intensity exercise is typical of competitions (e.g., the rounds in a hammer throw event), athletes should take advantage of the natural breaks by consuming a beverage containing carbohydrate and electrolytes.

Aerobic Metabolism for Endurance

For endurance athletes, optimizing carbohydrate storage before competition, sustaining carbohydrate delivery during competition, and maintaining an optimal hydration state before and during competition are critical factors for achieving optimal performance. Surveys of endurance athletes indicate, on average, an inadequate consumption of calories, an overreliance on protein and fat, and an underreliance on carbohydrate needed for optimal performance. In addition, endurance athletes are only beginning to consider nutrition factors that will enhance muscle recovery after daily training sessions. Endurance athletes often train in ways that do not mimic competition (e.g., they rarely consume beverages every 3 miles [5 km] during training, although this is a standard protocol in long endurance runs), making it difficult for them to fully adapt to the competition environment. This chapter presents strategies for optimizing carbohydrate storage in preparation for training and competition, as well as hydration strategies that can sustain blood volume and sweat rates. In addition, the chapter provides a review of commonly available hydration and energy products to help endurance athletes recognize the best products in a variety of different training and competition environments.

NUTRITION TACTICS

Endurance events such as road cycling, long-distance swimming, marathon, triathlon, and the 10K run all require a high level of endurance and place a relatively low premium on anaerobic power. These events force competitors to perform at the margins of their maximal aerobic capabilities over long distances. As training, nutrition, and selection of athletes in endurance sports improve, records continue to fall. This suggests that doing the right things can and will result in moving the known envelope of speed in endurance events. The winner of the 2011 Boston Marathon, Geoffrey Mutai of Kenya, won in a world-record-breaking time of 2 hours, 3 minutes, and 2 seconds (that is a running speed of less than 4 minutes and 42 seconds per mile for 26.2 miles!). Despite this incredible speed, the athlete had to maintain this pace at a level that allowed a sufficient oxygen uptake to sustain, primarily, aerobic muscular metabolism. That is, the majority of all muscular work took place with fuel being burned in the presence of oxygen. This is an efficient means of obtaining energy, allowing the athlete to sustain muscular work for long periods of time.

Aerobic training does some wonderful things to an athlete's ability to use oxygen. The intermediary (Type IIa) fibers, which tend to behave more like fast-twitch (power) fibers than slow-twitch (endurance) fibers, dramatically increase in mitochondrial content and the enzymes involved in oxidative metabolism. The training impact on oxygen usage is well known. In studies looking at blood lactate concentration, trained athletes are far more capable of tolerating high levels of blood lactate than are untrained subjects doing the same intensity of work. The conversion of the behavior of the intermediary fibers results in an improvement in the athlete's aerobic endurance. The increased ability to use oxygen results in an improvement in the ability to burn fat as a primary fuel, reducing the reliance on carbohydrate.

Athletes in aerobic sports such as cross-country skiing and distance running have far higher maximal oxygen uptakes (>80 ml/kg/min) than do athletes in power sports such as weightlifting and speedskating (<60 ml/kg/min).[1] Since even the leanest athletes have a great deal of energy stored as fat, this increased ability to burn fat dramatically improves endurance. However, since carbohydrate is needed for the complete combustion of fat, carbohydrate is still the limiting energy source for endurance work because athletes have relatively low carbohydrate stores. This is clearly demonstrated by findings that athletes consuming a high-fat diet have a maximal endurance time of 57 minutes; on a normal mixed diet, their endurance rises to 114 minutes; and on a high-carbohydrate diet, their maximal endurance rises to 167 minutes.[2]

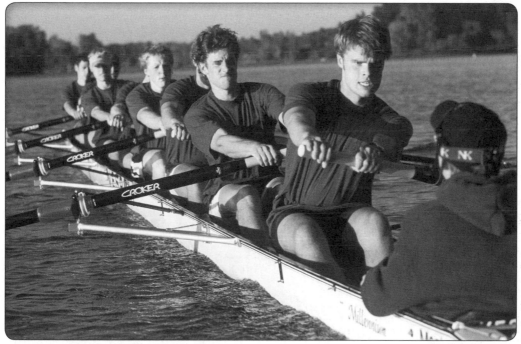

© Charlie Borland

For endurance athletes, there is no substitute for good aerobic conditioning and a high level of glycogen storage.

As we learn more about the interrelationship between sports and nutrition, nutrients that have rarely been considered are getting attention. One of these, choline (and its precursor, betaine), is now seen as potentially problematic for people who are chronically active. Choline, which is important for the synthesis of the neurotransmitter acetylcholine, is involved in cell-membrane signaling, in lipid transport, and in the reduction of homocysteine. Current studies show that endurance activity may result in a transient decrease in free-circulating blood choline.[3] As indicated in table 14.1, marathon running consistently results in a significant drop in circulating choline.

Many foods frequently and abundantly consumed in the past (e.g., liver, eggs) are now avoided by ever-increasing numbers of athletes. However, since these very foods provide the best delivery of choline in the diet, endurance athletes who avoid them are increasing the risk of choline deficiency from both ends (higher need and lower intake). Table 14.2 provides a summary of foods that are good sources of choline and identifies some supplements that can provide choline. As indicated in this table, vegetarian endurance athletes would have difficulty obtaining sufficient choline to satisfy the DRI of 425 milligrams per

Table 14.1 Effect of Endurance Activity on Blood Choline

Study	Sample gender	Activity	Duration (min)	Intensity (%$\dot{V}O_2$)	Baseline[t]/Pre[tt] vs. post (nmol/ml)	ρ (Statistical Significance)
Buchman et al., 1999	23 M + F	Marathon	Not given	Max effort	19.2[t] vs. 7.0	.005
Buchman et al., 2000	6 M + F	Marathon	156-348	Max effort	9.6[t] vs. 7.0	.09
Burns et al., 1988	10 M	Cycling	120	70% (105 min) + max effort (15 min)	Not given	>.05
Conlay et al., 1986	17*	Marathon	Not given	Max effort	10.1[tt] vs. 6.2	<.001
Deuster et al., 2002	13 M	Load carriage	~110	70%	8.5[tt] vs. 6.5	>.05
Pierard et al., 2004	21 M	Combat course	7,200	~35%	2.95% decrease[t]	<.01
Spector et al., 1995	10 M	Cycling	72	70%	8.5[t] vs. 10.0	>.05
Von Allwörden et al., 1993	4 M, 6 F	Cycling	120	35 km/hr	12.08[tt] vs. 10.04	<.01
Von Allwörden et al., 1993	10 M, 4 F	Cross country run	30-60	Max effort	14.51[tt] vs. 14.95	>.05
Warber et al., 2000	14 M	Load carriage	240	38%	8.14[tt] vs. 7.98	>.05

*Some subjects did not finish (DNF).

Reprinted, by permission, from J.T. Penry and M.M. Manore, 2008, "Choline: An important micronutrient for maximal endurance-exercise performance?," *International Journal of Sport Nutrition and Exercise Metabolism* 8(2): 191-203.

Table 14.2 Choline and Betaine Content of Selected Foods and Supplements

Food or supplement	Total choline (mg)	Total betaine (mg)
Chicken liver (2 oz; 60 g), pan fried	176	13
Large egg, hard boiled	158	.4
Pork chop (4 oz; 125 g), pan broiled	112	3
Chicken breast (4 oz; 125g), roasted	75	9
Beer, pint (16 oz; 480 ml)	47	38
Skim milk (8 oz; 240 ml)	37	4
Medium white potato, baked	22	.3
Firm tofu (2 oz; 60 g), nigari	16	.2
Spinach (2 oz; 60 g), unprepared	13	385
Whole-wheat bread (1 oz; 30 g), slice	7	98
Twinlab Choline Cocktail (choline bitartrate), 8 oz (240 ml) prepared	1,500	0
Twinlab choline bitartrate, 1 tablet	300	0
Jarrow Lecithin Mega-PC 35, 1 gel	114	0
Ultima Replenisher, 20 oz (600 ml) prepared	1	0
Twinlab betaine HCl, 1 tablet	0	648
Centrum, 1 multivitamin	0	0

Note: Adapted from the USDA database for the choline content of common foods (www.nal.usda.gov/fnic/foodcomp/Data/Choline/Cholne.pdf; June 23, 2007) and product labels of included supplements.

Reprinted, by permission, from J.T. Penry and M.M. Manore, 2008, "Choline: An important micronutrient for maximal endurance-exercise performance?," *International Journal of Sport Nutrition and Exercise Metabolism* 8(2): 191-203. Adapted from J.C. Howe, J.R. Williams, and J.M. Holden, 2004, *USDA database for the choline content of common foods* (www.nal.usda.gov/fnic/foodcomp/Data/Choline/Choline.pdf) and product labels of included supplements.

day for female adults and 550 milligrams per day for male adults. A supplement may increase endurance performance in athletes regularly involved in strenuous endurance activities.[1] A logical recommendation for nonvegetarian endurance athletes is to consume an egg or two (an excellent source of choline) daily and for vegetarians to give serious consideration to consuming a choline-containing supplement.

Dietary protein has also received more attention recently. An increasing body of evidence strongly suggests that skeletal muscle breakdown increases with endurance training or a single bout of endurance exercise. Athletes who consume foods immediately after endurance activity have a favorable synthesis of skeletal muscle protein.[4] The postendurance activity period is critically important for athletes, making it a time for serious planning. Carbohydrate should be consumed during this postexercise period at a rate of 1.2 grams per kilogram of body weight per hour over several hours, and mixing this with some high-quality protein appears to be useful from an exercise recovery standpoint.[5] Further, a good deal of beginning evidence suggests that the *amount* and *timing* of protein are important from a tissue utilization standpoint. The general recommendation of 1.2 to 1.7 grams of protein per kilogram of body weight per day is established and generally agreed to by several groups and is about double the nonathlete requirement of .8 gram per kilogram per day.[6,7] However, having excessive peaks and valleys in protein intake is not useful, even if the total amount consumed meets the recommendation. Using a guideline of a maximum of 30 grams of protein per timed intake, it is easy for someone to exceed the amount of protein that can be adequately processed at one time but still stay within the daily guidelines (see figure 14.1).

The types of protein or amino acid consumed may also have a role in endurance performance. A recent study indicated that adding a small amount of the amino acid beta-alanine to the diet (6 grams total in four separate 1.5-gram units in a dextrose solution) resulted in significant improvements in endurance performance and aerobic metabolism in college-age men.[8] Although one such study is not conclusive, other studies assessing whey protein (which has an excellent distribution of amino acids) found similar beneficial effects on muscle recovery and performance. Even milk, which has good-quality protein and other positive nutritional factors, appears to induce an exercise enhancement effect comparable

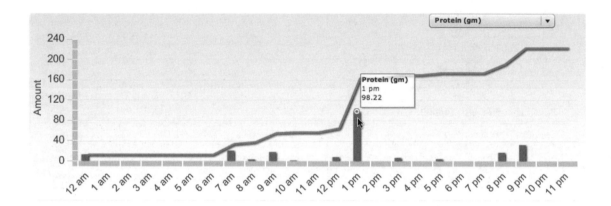

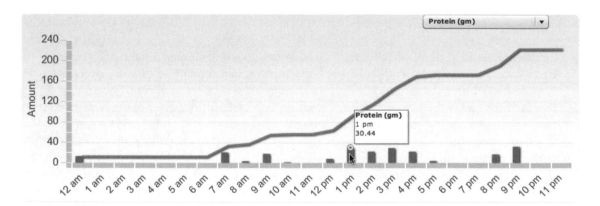

Figure 14.1 Timing and amount of protein consumed at one time are as important as meeting the total daily protein requirement. *(a)* Illustrates a protein intake of 98.22 g at 1 p.m. after an endurance run by an athlete who consumes 2.4 g/kg of protein per day. The total protein intake is more than sufficient, but the delivery of protein, with such a single high dose, would not be efficiently used and would not optimally help muscle mass recover. *(b)* Illustrates the same total protein consumption, but with the 98.22 g dose spread out over several hours, with a maximum dose not exceeding 30 g at a single feeding. This strategy is more likely to make more efficient use of the consumed protein and help sustain skeletal muscle.

to common carbohydrate and electrolyte sports beverages.[9] (Although the GI impact of milk is not likely to be as well tolerated over the course of an endurance event as are standard sports beverages.) Still, protein and endurance performance continue to be controversial, as a number of highly regarded scientists question how a level of protein beyond the current recommended amount could possibly increase endurance performance.[10]

The amount of carbohydrate consumed in the preexercise meal is likely to be a larger factor in improving the immune responses to an endurance performance run than the *type* of carbohydrate consumed (more is generally better).[11] Nevertheless, mixed sources of carbohydrate (e.g., glucose plus fructose rather than glucose alone) are far better during exercise; while the oxidation of glucose plateaus, the mixed-carbohydrate oxidation continues with increasing intake.[9]

How well an athlete adapts to training is also an important nutrition consideration. An increasing body of evidence supports the idea that initiating a 3- to 10-week endurance training program with periods of relatively low muscle glycogen stores or limited during-exercise carbohydrate consumption may more quickly improve the cellular capacity to use oxygen (and therefore help burn fat as a substrate). Since the availability of fat is far greater than the availability of carbohydrate (via stored glycogen), this faster adaptation toward improved fat metabolism has the potential of helping athletes achieve a faster improvement in cellular adaptation than would endurance performance.[12]

Fluid intake should not be overlooked as a primary ergogenic substance in endurance activity. A study of elite Kenyan endurance runners found that they remain well hydrated (as measured by body mass, urine osmolality, total body water, and daily fluid intake) from morning to night and from day to day with a free-flowing ad libitum fluid intake.[13] As a result, no runner showed any indication of being heat stressed during any period of the study.

Care must be taken, however, to not overdo a potentially good thing. Men supplemented with an oral dose of 1 gram (1,000 mg) of vitamin C per day had a significantly reduced endurance capacity, perhaps because the supplement prevented key cellular adaptations to exercise that would allow for training improvements.[14] On the other hand, getting *enough* of each nutrient and *enough* energy is critical for both performance and health. Restrained eating patterns in elite female endurance runners are the single biggest factor in low bone mass, and the longer the caloric restriction, the greater the problems associated with recovery of muscle mass and glucose tolerance.[15,16] Many endurance athletes fail to get enough nutrients or energy to get the most out of their training and to reduce injury risk. Studies assessing an Ironman triathlon, a simulated adventure race, and other ultraendurance cycling events all have found significant nutrition weaknesses in participating athletes.[17-19]

AEROBIC METABOLIC PATHWAYS

Aerobic metabolic pathways are the means we have for obtaining energy from fuels (carbohydrate, protein, and fat) in the presence of oxygen. See table 14.3 for average energy stores. The controlled release of energy during aerobic metabolism allows for a large amount of the energy in glucose to be stored as energy in ATP. The chemical reaction for the full oxidation of glucose produces energy, carbon dioxide, and water:

$$\text{Glucose} + 6\ O_2 + 38\ \text{ADP} + 39\ \text{phosphate} = >6\ CO_2 + 6\ H_2O + 38\ \text{ATP}$$

$$[\text{glucose} = C_6H_{12}O_6]$$

Table 14.3 Theoretical Average Energy Stores

	Mass (kg)	Energy (kcal)	Exercise time (min)
Liver glycogen	.08	306	16
Muscle glycogen	.40	1,529	80
Blood glucose	.01	38	2
Fat	10.5	92,787	4,856
Protein	12.0	48,722	2,550

Note: There is increasing evidence that muscle triglyceride is an important energy source for endurance activity. However, it appears to increase under conditions that compete with glycogen storage. Should an effective means be found for increasing both muscle triglyceride and glycogen, this would have positive implications for endurance performance.

Adapted, by permission, from M. Gleeson, 2000, Biochemistry of exercise. In *Nutrition in sport,* edited by R.J. Maughan (Oxford: Blackwell Science), 29.

In anaerobic metabolism, pyruvate is converted to lactate. However, in the presence of sufficient oxygen, pyruvate can be oxidized for energy in the mitochondria (often referred to as the energy factories of the cells). Glucose, a six-carbon molecule, is converted to two molecules of pyruvate, a three-carbon molecule. When pyruvate enters the mitochondria, it undergoes further conversion to a two-carbon molecule to form acetyl coenzyme A (commonly abbreviated to acetyl-CoA).[20] Acetyl-CoA can also be created from the beta-oxidation of fatty acids that reside in the mitochondria. During beta-oxidation, carbon is cleaved from the long carbon chains of fatty acids in two-carbon units. These two-carbon molecules form acetyl-CoA. The newly created acetyl-CoA from pyruvate or beta-oxidation of fats can be oxidized to carbon dioxide (CO_2) in the tricarboxylic acid cycle (TCA).[21] The critical aspect of the TCA cycle is producing hydrogen atoms for transport to the electron transport chain. It is in the electron transport chain that oxidative phosphorylation occurs to create ATP from ADP. With sufficient hydrogen to feed into the electron transport chain and enough oxygen for oxidative phosphorylation, the electron transport chain can continuously produce energy in the form of ATP.

If there is excess production of acetyl-CoA (i.e., inadequate oxidative enzymes to process the acetyl-CoA for energy or inadequate oxygen delivery), the excess can be converted to either fat for storage or to the amino acid alanine. Alanine can be converted by the liver to glucose or can be made part of larger protein structures (see figure 14.2).

Anaerobic metabolic processes have the capacity to provide ATP energy immediately but only for a short duration, while aerobic metabolic processes begin providing ATP energy more slowly but for long durations, provided there is sufficient substrate and oxygen available to the cells. We have large stores of energy we can call on to create ATP energy for muscular work (see table 14.3).

Of the energy stores available to us, fat is the most efficiently stored and provides the greatest mass from which we can derive ATP energy. Glycogen requires approximately 3 grams of water for storage, while fat storage is essentially anhydrous, making fat a more efficient form of energy storage. Muscle and liver glycogen stores represent a small fraction of the energy in fat stores but have the advantage of being able to be metabolized either anaerobically or aerobically, while fat can be metabolized only aerobically. Protein stores are from functional tissues that, under ideal conditions, would never be catabolized as a source of energy. Nevertheless, a small amount of protein (approximately 5 percent of total

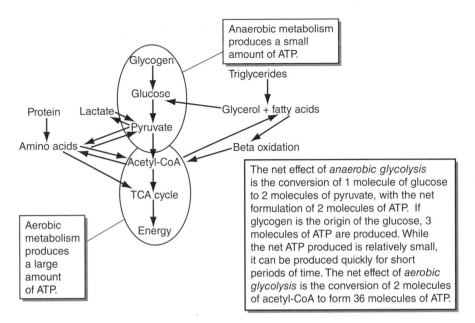

Figure 14.2 Substrate usage in energy pathways.

energy needs) does appear to be metabolized to meet energy requirements in most activities. In the absence of carbohydrate, protein stores are catabolized at a faster rate to provide a source of glucose (the amino acid alanine can be converted to glucose by the liver) and a source of acetyl-CoA and oxidative metabolism. However, this protein catabolism is not desirable and can be prevented with a regular supply of carbohydrates and adequate total energy consumption.

At the initiation of exercise, the majority of ATP is derived anaerobically. For highly intense, maximal-effort activities, the requirement for a high volume of energy mandates a continuous dependence on anaerobic processes. However, for lower-intensity activities the majority of ATP is initially provided anaerobically, but then the activity switches to aerobic metabolism to meet most ATP needs. Anaerobic and aerobic metabolic processes should be thought of as proceeding simultaneously, with the intensity of the activity determining the predominant metabolic pathway for the supply of ATP. High-intensity, maximal-effort activities rely more on anaerobic metabolism, while lower-intensity activities rely more on aerobic metabolism. Because far more energy is available to us aerobically (fat can be metabolized only aerobically), the high energy needs of endurance athletes force them to train muscles to be more aerobically competent. Cells of well-trained aerobic athletes have more mitochondria and more aerobic enzymes in the mitochondria, resulting in a higher capacity to derive energy aerobically.

CONSIDERATIONS FOR ENDURANCE SPORTS

Endurance sports are those in which the predominant form of energy metabolism is oxidative (it occurs in the presence of oxygen). Aerobic athletes must be capable of acquiring and delivering enough oxygen to the working muscles to support the physical work that is being done. Endurance work occurs at intensities below a person's maximal work capacity.

Working at a higher or maximal capacity exceeds the athlete's capacity to meet oxygen needs. Sprinters, who are working at maximal capacity, can run very fast but only for relatively short distances. Endurance athletes can't run as fast as sprinters but can go much longer distances because they are metabolizing energy using a much more clean-burning and energy-efficient oxidative system. To maintain the efficiency of their systems, endurance athletes should consider factors that can influence their aerobic capacity, including overtraining, overuse injuries, and dietary adequacy.

Overtraining

A world-class runner wrote the following in an e-mail communication:

> *I've just come off three weeks of particularly intense training. I went "hard" four days a week. I have plateaued and am now resting to allow my body to absorb all the good work I did but am still feeling a little bit lethargic. I sleep well but don't feel rested. My coach is concerned that I may have become anemic. As you know, my nutrition analysis has always come up good. Should I get some blood tests? Take iron? Take something else? I'm worried.*

These signs are typical of an overtrained athlete who is suffering the consequences. Overtraining has some well-established warning signs, including increased muscle soreness, delay of muscular recovery, inability to perform at the previous training load, poor-quality sleep, decreased vigor, swelling of lymph nodes, high illness frequency, and loss of appetite. Many of these signs are a result of working at a level harder than the body's capacity to adequately recover. Overtraining rarely leads to an improvement in performance and, in fact, commonly reduces performance as well as increases the likelihood that the athlete will become sick or injured.

A 26-year-old athlete who transferred to a more competitive team increased his training volume by 200 percent and after 2 months experienced continuous fatigue, tinnitus, palpitations, and insomnia. Nevertheless, he continued to play for 3 months but then became totally unfit, with sleepless nights and severe mental depression.[22] This is precisely what should never happen.

Overtraining is a problem for many athletes (10 to 20 percent of those who train intensively) and appears to be relatively common in endurance athletes. Among other factors that may increase the risk of developing this condition, a poor intake of carbohydrate and fluids is known to be a problem.[23] Overtraining syndrome is an untreated excessive training overload with inadequate rest, resulting in chronic decreases in performance and the ability to train. Other problems may result and may require medical attention. Factors associated with the development of overtraining syndrome include

- frequent competition, particularly if it involves quality efforts;
- monotonous training with insufficient rest;
- preexisting medical conditions (e.g., colds or allergies);
- poor diet, particularly inadequate intake of carbohydrate;
- dehydration;
- environmental stress (e.g., altitude, high temperatures, and humidity); and
- psychosocial stressors (e.g., work or school conflicts).

According to the American College of Sports Medicine, overtraining syndrome can be effectively eliminated through a logical training program that allows for adequate rest and recovery with proper nutrition and hydration.[23] Studies of marathon runners suggest that even athletes who consume a high-carbohydrate diet require 7 days after a marathon to return muscle glycogen to prerace levels.[24] A continuation of regular training before full muscle glycogen resynthesis will inevitably lead to performance degradation. Athletes must therefore understand that rest is a useful and necessary part of training, particularly after a hard and intensive training session. Athletes fearing that a reduction in training may diminish competitiveness may resist getting enough rest. Therefore, everyone in the athlete's training circle (family, coach, athletic trainer, and so on) should support the concept that overtraining is associated with reduced performance. Put simply, adequate rest and recovery time should be an integral part of the training plan.

Overuse Injuries

Overuse injuries occur when an athlete chronically repeats the same physical task; they may be particularly problematic in adolescent athletes experiencing rapid growth.[25] In its simplest and most benign form, a heel blister caused by the rubbing of an ill-fitting running shoe is an overuse injury. A more serious example is the constant pounding of legs on hard pavement that causes sufficient vibrational bone stress to induce a stress fracture. This is analogous to taking a wire clothes hanger and bending it repeatedly in the same place. After a while, the hanger develops a crack and eventually breaks. Because endurance athletes spend so many hours training, overuse injuries are a real concern.

A study of triathletes found that some developed skeletal injury early in the competition, which became worse as the competition progressed. These injuries to muscles may alter the use of energy substrates as the triathlon progresses and as the body heals after the competition.[26] Although protein breakdown and muscular damage occur during a race, well-trained athletes should experience no alteration in fitness provided nutrition status is maintained.[27] Adequately nourished athletes have a better capacity to heal the minor tissue damage that occurs during training and competition. Additionally, athletes who can maintain carbohydrate and fluid levels during exercise are likely to have better brain function, which translates into a smoother running style that is less prone to injury development. Loss of mental capacity, which can easily occur with either a carbohydrate or fluid storage deficit, causes a breakdown in coordination that can increase structural stresses that lead to injury.

Dietary Adequacy

Low glycogen stores reduce the time an athlete is capable of exercising, a fact that mandates the regular consumption of carbohydrate to maintain or replace glycogen.[28] This requires, ideally, a carbohydrate intake of between 7 and 10 grams per kilogram of body weight per day. As indicated in table 14.4, even for 100-pound (45 kg) athletes, this represents a substantial amount of calories from carbohydrate.

The timing of carbohydrate ingestion is also important and may influence glycogen storage and resynthesis. A study of highly trained male cross country runners found that food intake was generally adequate and well timed except for the period after competition. Although it is recommended that endurance athletes consume carbohydrate immediately after competition to encourage restoration of glycogen stores, these athletes delayed eating carbohydrate foods until, on average, 2.5 hours after competition.[29] A delay of this magnitude leads to poor glycogen replacement, and subsequent days of exercise showed the negative effect of reduced endurance.

A study of marathon runners found that a significant proportion of total energy intake occurs after 4:00 p.m. rather than earlier in the day when it's needed the most.[30] Delayed eating represents a missed opportunity for trained endurance athletes to maximize muscle glycogen storage after exercise.[31,32] There is no substitute for consuming sufficient energy and carbohydrate for endurance events. Supplements and ergogenic aids appear to be ineffective. The only strategy that works effectively is to eat enough and to eat at a time that is most useful for delivering energy to needy muscles or for maximizing glycogen storage. There is also evidence that endurance athletes must focus on glycogen storage activities about 1 week before a major competition.[33] A failure to do so can have a negative effect on the athlete's endurance capacity.

Endurance athletes, because of the time spent training and competing, may need to develop their own strategies for obtaining energy and fluids during the activity. This is not easy because consuming the wrong foods or fluids or consuming them at the wrong time will have a performance-decreasing effect. The "nervous stomach" many athletes experience just before a race makes the consumption of the right energy or fluid package even more difficult. Athletes should experiment to discover what sports beverages, carbohydrate gels, and other sources of energy and nutrients are well tolerated so they can use this information to optimize training sessions and achieve peak performances during competitions. Recommendations for the general athlete population may be a good starting point, but they are not enough to generate winning performances in tough competitive fields.

Each type of race alters slightly the proportion of carbohydrate and fat that is burned as fuel (more intensity equals proportionately more carbohydrate; lower intensity equals proportionately more fat), but it's the carbohydrate level that ultimately determines if the athlete will "hit the wall." That is, when the glycogen stores are depleted, the athlete will no longer be capable of maintaining a sufficiently strong pace. Since endurance events are long, every available opportunity must be capitalized on to ensure the athlete has enough food energy to continue the race and to store enough energy (glycogen) to do well during the next day of racing.

Table 14.4 Energy Intake for Endurance Athletes

	Grams per kg of body weight per day	Grams per pound of body weight per day	Calories per day for 100-pound (45 kg) athlete	Calories per day for 200-pound (90 kg) athlete
Carbohydrate	7.0-10.0	3.18-4.55	1,260-1,800	2,520-3,600
Protein	1.2-1.7	0.55-0.77	216-306	432-612
Fat	0.8-1.3	0.36-0.59	324-527	648-1,053
Total calories per day			1,800-2,633	3,600-5,265

Regardless of total body weight, eating a diet in the lower range for each energy substrate provides approximately 70% of calories from carbohydrate, 12% of calories from protein, and 18% of calories from fat; eating a diet in the upper range provides approximately 68% of calories from carbohydrate, 12% of calories from protein, and 20% of calories from fat.

Athletes should do whatever is necessary to take in sufficient energy and nutrients (bringing baggies filled with food to meetings, eating while walking to class, snacking while going to the car) or else the benefits derived from training will be wasted. Athletes who do not eat effectively become more easily fatigued and injured and are more likely to try unproven products touted as having ergogenic properties. There is no doubt whatsoever that a major reason athletes, whether they're cyclists, runners, or swimmers, turn to ergogenic aids and nutrient supplements is to overcome a failure in planning to eat enough and to eat on time. Maintaining hydration status is also important for operating at optimal physiological levels of efficiency. Endurance athletes should practice consuming fluids frequently, even in the absence of thirst, to reduce the chance of dehydration. Consumption of a carbohydrate-containing beverage with small amounts of sodium is useful for fluid absorption and for maintaining the drive to drink.

Nutrient Supplementation

Athletes who fail to consume sufficient carbohydrate or enough total energy are likely to be at increased risk of inadequate vitamin C, thiamin, riboflavin, niacin, calcium, magnesium, and iron intakes.[34] A study of marathon runners found that supplement usage (especially vitamins C and E, calcium, and zinc) was common. Forty-eight percent of the runners questioned reported using at least one supplement within the 3-day period surrounding the Los Angeles Marathon.[35] Other studies confirm that nonsupplemented marathon runners, soccer players, wrestlers, and basketball players have adequate serum concentrations of vitamin C and vitamin B_6, so supplementation of these vitamins does not appear to be warranted.[36,37] In a study evaluating the effectiveness of magnesium supplementation on marathon runners, the supplementation did not improve resistance to muscle damage during the race, did not enhance muscle recovery after the race, and did not improve running performance.[38]

Male marathon runners were evaluated to determine if the consumption of a commercial ergogenic supplement containing vitamins, minerals, amino acids, and unsaturated fatty acids was useful in improving performance. Results indicate that the ergogenic aid had no effect on oxygen consumption or any other important metabolic or physiological consideration that might be useful to endurance athletes.[39]

Nutrition Concerns for Female Endurance Athletes

Female endurance athletes must consume sufficient energy and nutrients to avoid amenorrhea (cessation of regular menstrual periods). Amenorrhea occurs for many reasons, including high physical stress, high psychological stress, inadequate energy intake, poor iron status, high cortisol levels, and low body-fat levels. It is conceivable that female endurance athletes have all of these factors working against them. Although some of these factors are clearly out of a woman's control, food intake is not one of those. Female athletes should do whatever is within their means to consume sufficient total energy with a balanced nutrient intake to support good health.

Amenorrhea is strongly associated with a loss in bone density and an increase in stress fracture risk. Additionally, low bone density during the running years places the athlete at higher osteoporosis risk later in life.

Nutrition Concerns for Ultra Events

Ultraendurance events have several working definitions, including all events that exceed the duration or distance of equivalent Olympic events and events that exceed either 4 or 6 hours in duration.[40,41] Included in ultraendurance competitions are cycling events such as the Tour de France; swimming, cycling, and running events such as the Hawaiian Ironman; ultradistance running events such as the South African Comrades Marathon; and distance swimming events such as swimming the English Channel. Regardless of the definition used, athletes involved in ultra events must be well conditioned and have long-term nutrition and hydration plans that can see them successfully through the entire event.

Some ultraendurance events create a caloric expenditure that ranges from 8,500 to 11,500 calories, a level that requires a great deal of meal planning to satisfy.[42]

Many of the same nutrition principles described for regular endurance events are critical for successful participation in an ultraendurance event, including

- adequate energy intake,
- sufficient carbohydrate intake before and during the event to sustain blood glucose and muscle carbohydrate status,
- fluid and electrolyte strategies that satisfactorily replace sweat loss, and
- a postexercise plan that quickly enables recovery in multiday ultra events.

Because sweat rates can range from as little as .3 liter up to 2.4 liters per hour, depending on the size of the athlete and the ambient temperature and humidity, it is difficult to provide a fluid intake recommendation for ultraendurance athletes, except to say that sufficient fluids should be consumed to make every attempt to sustain, but not increase, body weight. The goal is to prevent a body-fluid deficit that reduces weight by 2 percent or more, a level that measurably affects performance and heat stress risk.[43] Beverages containing 6 to 8 percent carbohydrate, plus sodium in the range of 150 to 200 milligrams per 240 milliliters, are useful for sustaining hydration and preventing hyponatremia (serum sodium concentration of less than 130 millimoles per liter). During the postexercise period, ultraendurance athletes should focus on replenishing both energy and fluids, with fluids consumed at a level of 16 to 24 ounces (510 to 720 ml) for every pound (.5 kg) lost during the activity.

Ultraendurance athletes typically fail to obtain sufficient carbohydrate to satisfy need. A study of female ultraendurance triathletes found that mean carbohydrate intake (3.15 grams per kilogram) was half of the minimum amount recommended (6 grams per kilogram).[44] There is also evidence that these athletes fail to adequately hydrate. A study of ultraendurance cyclists found a body-weight change pre- to postevent of approximately 4 percent (more than double the recommended maximum change).[45] The obvious conclusion from these findings is that many ultraendurance athletes have not trained in a way that provides the adaptations needed to adequately supply energy and fluids during competitive events, and the during-event strategy has failed to deliver sufficient energy and fluids.

SAMPLING OF SPORTS RELYING ON AEROBIC METABOLISM

Aerobic sports involve submaximal effort over long periods of time. The aerobic nature of these activities results in a steady creation of ATP energy in working muscles, allowing athletes to continue working for as long as there is sufficient fuel and for as long as the body does not become overheated (hydration state is important). Athletes who can rely more efficiently on fats and less on carbohydrate (glycogen) typically have better endurance because they have more fat fuel than glycogen fuel, which has limited stores. Because fats require a high amount of oxygen for efficient metabolism, the endurance athlete with the best oxygen system (e.g., most oxidative enzymes, best ability to carry oxygen to working cells) has the best endurance. What follows is a sampling of endurance sports and their special nutrition considerations.

Distance Running

Distance running is commonly thought of as any distance 10,000 meters (6.2 miles) or longer. To go these distances, runners place a premium on relying primarily on aerobic metabolic pathways during the majority of the run. Runners who are capable of doing this rely mainly on fat for the majority of fuel, enabling them to limit the usage of carbohydrate. Carbohydrate storage is finite, but fat storage is, from a practical standpoint, limitless. The higher reliance on fat enables long-distance runners to run very long distances. It also enables them to preserve carbohydrate for moments during the race when they require fast acceleration (e.g., at the end of the race or while passing another runner). According to one study, only 2 to 7 percent of the total energy burned in aerobic activity is derived anaerobically.[46] A small amount of carbohydrate is used even when maintaining aerobic activity, so distance runners must develop strategies for delivering carbohydrate during the run. A failure to do so will result in either low blood sugar or low muscle glycogen, both of which impair endurance by leading to premature muscle fatigue.

Keeping all these factors in mind, distance runners must consider the following nutritionally relevant issues for their sport.

Long-distance runners are at risk of amenorrhea, low bone density, and stress fractures. The distances these athletes run weekly to train may predispose them to stress fractures, despite the potential stimulating impact of running on skeletal mass.[47] Although stress fractures occur more frequently in women than in men, all runners should ensure their calcium intake is adequate to reduce the risk of fracture. Female runners are at higher risk of stress fractures because hard endurance training is often associated with cessation of the menstrual cycle. The reduced estrogen associated with amenorrhea is linked to lower bone density. Therefore, runners who experience either primary or secondary amenorrhea should seek appropriate medical advice to determine if reasonable steps can be taken to return to normal menstrual status.[48] Female runners should take the following steps to reduce the risk of osteoporosis:

- Consume calcium (1,500 milligrams per day) from food or a combination of food and supplements.
- Avoid overconsumption of protein because excess protein is associated with higher urinary calcium losses.
- Control the production of stress hormones (particularly cortisol) by maintaining hydration and blood sugar during exercise.
- Avoid overtraining, which is associated with amenorrhea.

Inadequate energy intake is a red flag that the intake of vitamins and minerals may also be low. A study comparing the nutrient intakes of trained female runners who were amenorrheic, oligomenorrheic, or menstruating normally found clear nutrition differences between these groups, despite being matched on height, weight, training distance, and body-fat percentage.[49] The runners who were not menstruating had zinc intakes well below the recommended level of intake and lower than those found in the runners who had normal menses. In addition, the runners who had normal menses had higher intakes of fat and a more adequate total energy consumption. This suggests that high-carbohydrate diets, which are preferred for optimal performance, make it more difficult to consume the needed level of energy because carbohydrate foods have a lower caloric density than high-fat foods. Therefore, athletes should concentrate on consuming more food when carbohydrates constitute the main energy source. A failure to menstruate normally is a strong risk factor in the development of weaker bones and resulting stress fractures. Female runners have good cause to be fully aware of the adequacy of their energy and nutrient intakes because almost no injury is more frustrating or potentially career ending than the development of frequent stress fractures. Endurance runs require enormous amounts of energy (a marathon requires about 2,900 calories); they cannot be adequately trained for or run without an adequate total energy consumption. Food intake strategies, including eating snacks between meals and consuming snacks or sports beverages before, during, and after exercise, are important for ensuring that fuel consumption matches need.

Surveys of distance runners confirm that total energy and carbohydrate intakes are below the recommended levels, suggesting that runners must make a concerted effort to consume the recommended amounts before, during, and after exercise.[50,51] In a case study assessing the nutrient intake of an ultraendurance runner during a race, it was found that if the pre-event and during-event guidelines for food and beverages are followed, then athletes will have sufficient energy and fluids to successfully complete the event.[52]

Tapering activity before a competition improves competition performance.[53] It does so by increasing glycogen stores, but it also makes the runner calmer, which gives the athlete an improved economy of running motion that enhances endurance. The importance of tapering exercise and of carbohydrate loading before an important event cannot be overemphasized.

Fluids are crucial.

Fluid consumption should be on a fixed time schedule (every 10 to 15 minutes) to avoid underhydration and thirst. Perhaps no single factor is more important for ensuring a long-distance runner's success than maintaining an optimal hydration state. Athletes should drink now, drink again in 10 to 15 minutes, and when they believe they've had enough, they should drink more. Of course, the type of beverage consumed is also important. See chapter 3 for more information on fluids and electrolytes.

A great deal of body heat is generated over the course of an endurance run, and this heat is liberated through sweat evaporation. Studies strongly suggest that a 6 to 7 percent carbohydrate solution with electrolytes is most effective for maintaining exercise endurance.[53] It has been firmly concluded that acute heat exposure is detrimental to muscular endurance.[54] Therefore, long-distance runners should develop the habit of frequent fluid consumption to maintain body-water status, whether they are thirsty or not. A fluid intake of .5 to 1 liter per hour is sufficient to prevent significant dehydration in most athletes in mild environmental conditions, but a greater intake of fluids is needed for athletes running at higher intensities or in more severe environmental conditions in order to avoid heat stress.[55]

Distance runners typically have relatively low body-fat levels.

Successful long-distance runners are commonly thin, and this body profile may be advantageous to them in dissipating heat during long runs.[56] However, some athletes may seek to achieve low body-fat levels through severe dieting. This inadequate energy intake is associated with amenorrhea, which is associated with a number of other difficulties including low bone density. Low body-fat levels are achieved best through a dynamic matching of energy intake and expenditure that removes large peaks and valleys in real-time energy balance.

A critical factor in the performance of all endurance athletes is iron status.   Evidence exists that endurance runners have reduced hemoglobin, hematocrit, and red blood cell counts when compared with strength and mixed-trained athletes.[57] Iron status is sufficiently important that one of the more common illegal ergogenic aids used by endurance runners is erythropoietin (EPO), which stimulates the production of red blood cells, thereby enhancing oxygen-carrying capacity. However, erythropoietin is associated with multiple deaths because it may cause a dangerously high increase in blood viscosity.

Iron is an essential oxygen-carrying component of hemoglobin (red blood cell iron), myoglobin (muscle cell iron), and ferrochromes (oxygen-carrying enzymes essential for making ATP) in the mitochondria. It appears that hemoglobin status is of highest priority, so iron from other cells is cannibalized to support a normal hemoglobin production when iron stores (ferritin) and intake are inadequate. Therefore, a standard blood test measuring hemoglobin may appear normal while other iron-containing cells are depleted. For this reason, it is important that blood tests in endurance athletes always include a measure of ferritin, which should be at a minimum of 20 nanograms per deciliter. Besides an inadequate dietary intake, which is most common in runners who do not eat red meat or who are vegetarians, there are several other common causes of low iron status in runners:[58-60]

- Excess iron loss in sweat
- Excess loss of blood through the GI tract
- Excess loss of blood in the urine (hematuria)
- Excess menstrual blood loss in female runners
- Poor absorption of iron
- Intravascular hemolysis

The issue of blood donations should also be considered because iron is so crucial to running success. Runners wishing to donate blood should first assess iron status. Normal hemoglobins and ferritins above 60 nanograms per milliliter after 5 days of hard training are the margin point for safely donating blood.[61] In addition, runners who do donate blood should not exercise with normal intensity for 3 to 6 weeks after the donation to allow for sufficient time to return blood volumes and iron status back to normal levels.

Triathlon

Muscular balance in the upper and lower body is important to successful triathletes because the three events each have a different muscular focus. Since all the major muscles are put to the test in triathlons, these athletes must consume enough total energy to ensure that the fuel capacity for each working muscle starts out full. Swimmers, for instance, have a much higher upper-body strength requirement than cyclists, while triathletes require balanced strength in all the muscles.[62] Perhaps this use of all the muscles is what makes the triathlon a sport with no preference for body type or shape, making it accessible to anyone who is willing to train hard in all three disciplines.[63]

Triathlons have different lengths, depending on the location and sponsor. An Olympic-distance triathlon consists of a 1.5-kilometer swim, a 40-kilometer cycle, and a 10-kilometer run. The most well-known Ironman competition in Hawaii includes a 2.4-mile swim; a 112-mile bike race; and a 26-mile, 385-yard run. A survey of nonelite triathletes indicates that even they have training loads that most people would find impossible to follow. This survey reveals that the average swimming distance per week for these triathletes is 8.8 kilometers, the cycling distance is 270 kilometers, and the running distance is 58.2 kilometers.[64] Still, it is important for triathletes to taper training before a competition. One study showed a statistically significant improvement in performance when triathletes reduced the total time spent training before an event.[65] Once again, rest before competition proves to be an effective adjunct to training.

Different sports induce athletes to consume different foods and, therefore, take in different levels of nutrients. Calcium intake was found to be lower in triathletes than in athletes participating in team sports such as volleyball and basketball. Of the athletes surveyed in a large French study with 10,373 subjects, calcium intakes were below the recommended level for the triathletes, and females had lower calcium intakes than did males.[66] This is bad news for athletes who place so much repetitive stress on the skeleton, which places them at increased risk for stress fractures.

Keeping all these factors in mind, triathletes must consider the following nutritionally relevant issues for their sport.

Maintenance of normal hydration is difficult.

Perhaps the most important performance-related factor for triathletes is creating a strategy for maintaining hydration state during this grueling event. Triathletes should find a well-tolerated sports beverage and develop a drinking schedule that results in the smallest possible weight loss by the end of the competition. Developing a workable drinking strategy of a carbohydrate and electrolyte beverage may be the single most important ergogenic act a triathlete can do.

There is concern that triathletes who wear wet suits during the swimming phase of the triathlon may predispose themselves to heat stress during the cycling and running portions of the race if the water temperature is warm. A study evaluating this issue found that a wet suit did not adversely affect body temperature during the cycling and running stages, provided the athlete maintained a good hydration state.[67] The importance of good hydration as it relates to triathlon performance is the theme of numerous studies, all of which state that hydration is one of two keys to a successful race (the other being maintenance of carbohydrate stores). Nevertheless, despite the importance of hydration, it appears that triathletes are rarely successful at maintaining good hydration during a competition, with a water-related weight loss that commonly exceeds 4 percent.[68]

Triathletes may also be predisposed to hyponatremia (low blood sodium level), which is a result of using replacement fluids (typically plain water) that contain no electrolytes.[69,70] An assessment of athletes completing an Ironman triathlon found that athletes lose an average of 5.5 pounds (2.5 kg) in body weight, and athletes with hyponatremia had fluid overload despite modest fluid intakes.[71] These findings imply that even modest consumption of fluids that contain no sodium may increase the risk of hyponatremia. Both body-water loss and hyponatremia are factors that influence performance, but these factors also place the athlete at health risk. Replacing fluids in the correct volume and of the right type is therefore critical for the athlete's safety and performance.[72]

Consumption of sufficient energy is needed.

The energy requirement for carbohydrate in a triathlete exceeds the body's ability to store it. Therefore, triathletes should develop a strategy for adequate consumption of carbohydrate energy during a race (typically 1 to 1.5 grams of carbohydrate per kilogram of body weight per hour).[73] To do this, athletes should find sports beverages that contain carbohydrate in a form and concentration that are well tolerated. Some triathletes can consume carbohydrate gels, bananas, or crackers during the cycle portion of the race (taken with a water chaser). If this is tolerated, it is an excellent way to boost the carbohydrate fuel level in the body before the beginning of the running portion of the race. Nutrition interventions capable of providing more fluids and carbohydrates to triathletes do work and lead to improvements in endurance performance.[74]

Triathletes run the risk of overtraining. Getting sufficient rest and tapering exercise before a race have been shown to be two of the best training strategies a triathlete can follow. By contrast, triathletes who increase the training frequency before an important race are not likely to do their best. Sufficient rest is just as important for a strong performance as sufficient training.

Planning a meal schedule for longer distances tends to take a back seat. The triathlon covers different distances, depending on whether it's a sprint, the Olympic distance, a long course, or an Ironman. The sprint can take as little as 45 minutes to complete, and an Ironman often takes longer than 10 hours. Regardless of the competition distance, triathletes train hard—and they find themselves juggling their training with work or school. Eating and drinking often take a back seat to all the other demands of life, yet they are critically important to the success an athlete can realize. The only solution is to sit down and develop a schedule that includes working, training, eating, resting, and drinking. All should be treated as having equal importance.

Many (if not most) triathletes have more than one workout each day, and some race weekly or every second week. This places a tremendous energy requirement on the athlete that is commonly not met. The more time an athlete takes to train, the less time there is to eat, so there is a natural conflict between the increased requirement for energy and the reduced time to supply what is needed. This problem makes a clear case for planning time for eating as much as planning time for training. If an athlete's training has a fixed schedule (it usually does) but the eating doesn't, the athlete will suffer.

Distance Swimming

Distance swimmers are unique people who must spend an enormous amount of time in the water to realize minuscule improvements in time. A key to performance appears to be the swimmer's capacity to go faster without increasing blood lactate levels or to go faster while utilizing a lower percentage of maximal aerobic capacity.[75] It appears that the endurance swimmer can work harder while maintaining a predominantly aerobic (oxidative) metabolic pathway. This translates into a terrific aerobic fitness, with the ability to maintain enough glycogen and oxygen in the system to ensure an efficient energy burn. Maintaining lower blood lactate concentrations may also be a function of maintaining a sufficient blood volume (lactate in a larger volume equals lower lactate concentration). Of course, this is largely dependent on adequate hydration and a good electrolyte status (sodium helps maintain blood volume).

Keeping all these factors in mind, distance swimmers must consider the following nutritionally relevant issues for their sport.

Swimmers often have lower bone densities. Swimmers tend to have lower bone densities when compared with other athletes.[76] The reason is easy to understand: Swimming produces less impact stress than does running. However, it may also be related to spending many hours doing laps in an indoor pool while other athletes are running outside, where they can increase their exposure to sunlight and manufacture more vitamin D, a difference that may be enough to influence bone development. For long-distance swimmers lucky enough to live in areas warm enough for outdoor pools, this is not an issue. A study of female swimmers found inadequate calcium intakes, a factor that could clearly contribute to lower bone mineral density.[77] Clearly, having sufficient calcium (1,500 milligrams per day) is critical for maintaining strong bones, but swimmers should also make an effort to satisfy vitamin D needs, particularly if they have few opportunities for sunlight exposure.

Replacement of fluids needs to be more prevalent during all-day events. The main focus for swimmers involved in a typical all-day meet is the replacement of adequate fluids to maintain blood volume and to provide a constant source of carbohydrate. It may not be the time in the water swimming that contributes to dehydration but the time out of the water (often in the sun) waiting for a turn to compete. Regardless of the source, a failure to drink sufficient fluids can lead to a serious performance detriment.

Consumption of carbohydrate during long competitions is critical for maintaining performance. Having a snacking plan is important to prevent hunger. Swimming competitions take many hours, making hunger an issue that must be addressed. It is a bad strategy to begin an endurance event in a hungry state. Athletes should sip on sports beverages and snack on crackers and other simple carbohydrate (mainly starchy) foods to get a constant trickle of carbohydrates into the system while they wait to compete.

Distance swimmers must eat enough to support the activity. Swimming long distances uses a tremendous amount of energy, a deficit that must be matched with an appropriate energy delivery from food. Swimmers often complain that they can't keep their weights up during the long competitive season, and that means they're burning muscle to meet their needs.

Cycling

A number of cycling endurance events take place over several days of competition. The Tour de France is notable for its extreme endurance demands on participating athletes, and each stage of the race places different physiological demands on the cyclists. They pedal approximately 4,000 kilometers (2,500 miles) over 3 weeks with only a single day of rest allowed! The energy expenditures are the highest values ever reported for athletes over a period longer than 7 days.[78] The cyclists consume approximately 62 percent of their energy from carbohydrate, 15 percent from protein, and 23 percent from fat. More than 49 percent of total energy consumption takes place between meals. Some days have long and hard hills, while other days have roads that are more level. Studies of Tour de France cyclists indicate they consume approximately 30 percent of their total daily energy intake in the form of carbohydrate-enriched beverages.[79] So much time during the day is spent on the bike, there is perhaps no other way to adequately consume sufficient energy.

There may be a connection between cycling and asthma. In studies of athletes at the 1996 Olympic Games in Atlanta, Georgia, athletes participating in cycling and mountain biking had the highest prevalence (45 percent) of asthma.[80] By contrast, 20 percent of the total U.S. team reported they had asthma. This suggests that asthma may be a contributing factor in determining the sport an athlete selects to participate in. For some athletes, it is possible that asthma might be triggered by an allergic response, and this could be an allergic response to food. Cyclists with asthma should be extremely careful about avoiding foods or other substances that could trigger an asthmatic response.

Keeping all these factors in mind, cyclists must consider the following nutritionally relevant issues for their sport.

Recovering at the end of each day of multiday events is necessary to sustain performance. The energy cost of multiday cycling events is enormous, and meal planning may make the difference between winning and losing. There is a clear requirement for carbohydrate, which conflicts with the huge requirement for energy because of carbohydrate's relatively low energy density. Although fats have a high energy density, they are not needed to the degree that carbohydrates are. Therefore, large amounts of carbohydrate should be consumed frequently, with the focus on starchy carbohydrate foods (e.g., pasta, bread, rice, potatoes).

Consumption of food and fluid during long rides. Cyclists have an advantage over other endurance athletes in that they can more easily carry fluids and foods on the bike frame or in jersey pockets. Since there is less bouncing while riding than while running, cyclists can consume solid foods without experiencing GI distress. Cyclists should take advantage of this on long rides by bringing along sports beverages to drink and some crackers, bananas, carbohydrate gel, or bread to eat. These high-carbohydrate foods should be well tolerated and can significantly boost the carbohydrate delivery to working muscles.

Training is very time and energy consuming. The longer athletes train, the more energy they need, but the less time is available to them to consume it. Therefore, cyclists should consider the training period as a time to take in a proportion of their daily caloric requirements. To do this, cyclists should find foods that are well tolerated, such as bananas and crackers, and bring them along during the ride. Sports beverages are also an important source of energy, so these should be consumed instead of plain water as a rehydration beverage. A failure to eat during training will inevitably lead to inadequate energy consumption and a decrease in performance.

Cross-Country Skiing

Cross-country skiing (XC skiing) is one of the Nordic ski events that is performed as a single event, but can also be part of events that include ski jumping and rifle target shooting in different combinations. XC skiing plus ski jumping is referred to as the Nordic combined, and XC skiing plus target shooting is referred to as the biathlon. The tremendously high oxidative capacity of XC skiers indicates this sport is among the most strenuous of all endurance sports, requiring athletes to have high maximal oxygen uptakes and also high anaerobic thresholds.[81] Typical races range from 1 to 30 kilometers (.6 to 19 miles), and there are also XC skiing marathons, which range from 54 to 160 kilometers (34 to 99 miles).

The energy expenditure per unit of time of XC skiing is among the highest of all athletic endeavors, requiring 9 to 13 calories per minute.[82] For males, the energy requirement for a typical 30 kilometer pursuit averages 8,500 calories, a level that is second only to an Ironman triathlon and ultraendurance running (e.g., a 600-mile race).[83] It is hard to imagine XC skiers sustaining any level of competitiveness without purposefully maintaining a chronic daily energy intake that fully satisfies the requirement for energy. The energy expenditure during a XC ski race is so high that skiers try to find ways to lower the work intensity. One study found that drafting (skiing behind another skier) significantly reduces heart rate and energy expenditure during a race.[84] Given the enormous energy requirement in this sport, such a strategy must be considered crucial for preserving sufficient glycogen to perform well at the end of the race—when skiers often sprint to the finish line.

A study assessing body composition and performance in XC skiers found that a higher lean mass resulted in faster races, and a higher body-fat level was associated with slower races.[85] Athletes who do not consume sufficient energy have difficulty maintaining the lean mass and typically have higher body-fat levels.

The stress hormone cortisol is significantly increased in ski racers after competition, and this is negatively associated with total energy intake[86] (the greater the energy intake, the lower the stress-hormone production). As would be expected, a negative relationship has been found between cortisol and the B vitamins and vitamin C. Skiers with the lowest intake of nutrients during the competition had the greatest cell damage and highest cortisol, both of which can negatively affect performance and increase injury risk. Another study confirmed that, given the enormous oxidative metabolism of XC skiers, iron status is critically important. However, athletes should not expect that iron supplements can successfully reverse iron deficiency or iron-deficiency anemia.[87] Iron status is something that must be preserved through proper eating over the long term and, once altered, takes a very long time to correct.

XC ski performance is significantly enhanced by preexercise carbohydrate intake.[88] Another study compared the effect of a carbohydrate and electrolyte sports beverage with water when consumed during XC ski training in elite collegiate skiers.[89] The plain water was not able to control fluid balance and led to plasma dilution and increased urinary output. The carbohydrate and electrolyte beverage, however, was better able to maintain plasma volume and resulted in lower urinary production. These findings emphasize the importance of maximizing carbohydrate availability in XC skiing and also demonstrate the importance of electrolyte (particularly sodium) consumption during physical activity to sustain sweat rates, energy delivery to muscles, and metabolic by-product removal from muscles.

Keeping all these factors in mind, XC skiers must consider the following nutritionally relevant issues for their sport.

The energy requirement in XC skiing is among the highest of any sport. It is inconceivable that an XC skier could continue training and competing without a nutrition plan that includes enough eating opportunities and time to consume the volume of food needed to satisfy the energy requirement of this sport.

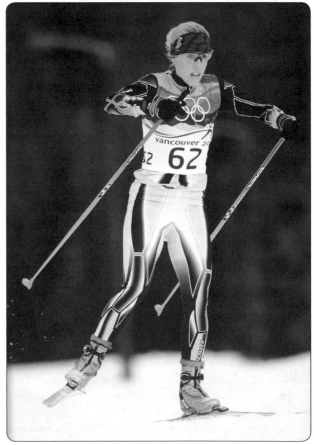

© Sport the Library

Cross-country skiing is one of the most strenuous endurance sports, requiring high levels of both aerobic conditioning and quality nutrient intake.

Distributing the energy in a way that dynamically matches requirement (i.e., within-day energy balance) is also important, since this strategy helps sustain or increase lean mass and lowers fat mass.

Maintain fluid balance. Water consumption does not satisfactorily sustain fluid balance and blood volume, while consumption of a carbohydrate and electrolyte sports beverage does. Given the intensity and duration of the competitions and training, the ideal beverage is likely to contain a 6 to 7 percent carbohydrate solution of mixed carbohydrates (i.e., glucose plus sucrose), plus a sodium concentration of between 150 and 200 milligrams per 240 ml (1 cup). Athletes should begin competition and training in a well hydrated state and, when possible, consume additional fluids during training and competition. XC skiers should also be prepared to consume large volumes of sports beverages and other fluids after exercise. A return to preexercise weight and clear urine is a sign that the hydration state has normalized.

Ensure normal iron status. Poor iron status will inhibit optimal oxygen delivery to working cells and compromise the metabolism of fat as an energy substrate. Poor fat metabolism increases the reliance on carbohydrate as a fuel, but since carbohydrate is poorly stored, this metabolic change will result in early fatigue. Recovering from poor iron status takes a very long time, during which athletes can expect subpar performances. Because of this, XC skiers should regularly (i.e., annually) assess their iron status (hemoglobin, hematocrit, and ferritin) to determine if they are at risk for deficiency *before* a deficiency actually occurs. This is particularly important for female XC skiers, who are likely to be at higher risk for iron deficiency.

Consuming carbohydrate before and during exercise enhances XC skiing performance. XC skiers should follow an eating pattern of a minimum of six eating opportunities per day to optimize glycogen stores, with sufficient time at each meal to contribute significantly to the energy need. Consumption of carbohydrate before XC skiing improves performance, and consuming a carbohydrate and electrolyte beverage during XC skiing also improves performance.

Rowing

Rowing has been a popular competitive sport for many years and is considered a growth sport. The race distance at world championships is 2,000 meters, which typically takes between 6 and 8 minutes to complete. Rowing races in U.S. high schools are typically 1,500 meters, and masters races (age 27 years and above) are typically 1,000 meters. The lightweight men's class and lightweight women's classes have weight limitations. Depending on the race, the lightweight cutoff for men is 72.7 or 75 kilograms (160 or 165 pounds), and the lightweight cutoff for women is 59.1 kilograms (130 pounds).[90]

The endurance capacity for rowers is among the highest of any athletes measured. Successful rowers and rowing teams also produce a tremendous amount of power. Rowing involves smooth repetitive motion, so injuries to bones, tendons, and muscles are rare. However, the repetitive motion does increase inflammation and delayed-onset muscle soreness (DOMS), and rowing over a distance of 2,000 meters creates significant blood oxidative stress.[91] This high stress level is even found in experienced and well-conditioned athletes.

Consumption of supplement buffers has been studied to determine if they can minimize the degree of oxidative stress and lactate concentration, but no benefit was shown.[92] Carbohydrate ingestion has also been tested to determine if stress factors were reduced. Using 15 elite female rowers as subjects, athletes received either carbohydrate or a placebo before, during, and after two separate 2-hour rowing bouts performed on consecutive days. Blood was collected before, immediately after, and 1.5 hours after rowing. The study found that carbohydrate reduced the level of certain stress factors (neutrophils, monocytes, phago-cytes, lymphocytes, and plasma interleukin-1).[93,94] An elite rower preparing for the 1995 World Rowing Championships was assessed to determine if consumption of a carbohydrate supplement provided twice during training was useful. The supplement was found to aid in maintaining blood glucose and also improved recovery heart rate. This particular athlete went on to win the gold medal at the championships.[95] Consumption of a regular high-carbohydrate intake at the level of 10 grams per kilogram per day, with a protein intake of 2 grams per kilogram per day, has also been tested on rowers. It was concluded that this type of diet promotes better muscle glycogen content and greater power output during training than a diet containing carbohydrate at the level of 5 grams per kilogram per day.[96]

Many athletes still select water rather than a carbohydrate and electrolyte beverage as their hydration solution. A study of lightweight rowers assessed the effect of water as the rehydration beverage during a maximal rowing trial. It was found that the water lowered plasma volume, lowered muscle glycogen utilization, and had a negative impact on rowing performance.[97]

Two separate studies have assessed the effect of caffeine on well-trained male and female rowers. Caffeine was provided to male rowers at the level of 6 milligrams per kilogram or 9 milligrams per kilogram 60 minutes before the start of a hard rowing workout (2,000 meters on a rowing ergometer). Both doses of caffeine enhanced performance when compared with the effect of a placebo.[98,99] Another assessment of caffeine's effect on performance was less clear. Using lower levels of caffeine (2, 4, or 6 milligrams per kilogram), it was found that individual differences in caffeine sensitivity made it impossible to demonstrate a perfor-mance enhancement.[100] This finding suggests that caffeine tolerance should be determined in athletes to better understand the appropriate ergogenic dose.

Body composition is an important factor for rowers in general and for lightweight rowers in particular. Ideally, rowers should strive for a relatively low fat mass and a relatively high fat-free mass, as this body profile is most clearly associated with performance success. Power production is closely linked to muscle mass and is closely associated with performance in rowers.[101-103] It has been found, however, that lightweight rowers engage in dietary restric-tions to achieve the desired weight cutoff, and this restriction limits the desired muscle mass development.[104]

Keeping all these factors in mind, rowers must consider the following nutritionally rel-evant issues for their sport.

Satisfy the high need for energy to sustain performance. The energy requirement for rowers is extremely high because of the training-associated utilization of energy. The likely temptation is to consume larger meals to satisfy this energy need, but a better strategy is to increase eating opportunities. This requires a level of meal planning that rowers may not be accustomed to, but eating more often has multiple advantages. These include an enhanced glycogen storage, a lower body-fat level, and a higher muscle mass (particularly if the protein dose is distributed throughout the meals and snacks).

Discussions with rowers suggest that the traditional early-morning training, often taking place before 6:00 a.m., is often done without a preexercise meal, and the foods available during competitions are rarely, if ever, available during training sessions. This implies that rowers are exercising in a state of low blood sugar (inevitable at wake-up) that is made worse by the training. The resultant higher cortisol response would detract significantly from the potential benefits that could be derived if the training took place with normal blood sugar. A simple strategy is to encourage rowers to consume at least enough easily digestible carbohydrate (250 to 400 calories) when they wake up to arrive at the training venue with normal blood sugar. A glass of apple juice with 2 slices of white-bread toast would be enough to do this, and the simple sugar and starch of these foods would likely be out of the stomach by the time of exercise if the athletes eat immediately upon waking up. Rowers should also have readily available snacks and drinks (e.g., chocolate milk, trail mix, energy bars) at the training site to be consumed immediately after exercise.

Maintain normal fluid balance. Studies on rowers and other athletes have demonstrated that consumption of a carbohydrate and electrolyte beverage is preferable to water. Water has the negative effect of lowering the plasma volume, which limits delivery of fluids to sweat glands and inhibits cooling. The lower plasma volume reduces delivery of needed nutrients to working muscles and removal of metabolic waste products from these muscles. Water also does nothing to maintain blood glucose, which is the primary fuel for the brain and an important fuel source for working muscles. A failure to maintain blood glucose leads to mental fatigue, which results in muscular fatigue regardless of the available fuel in working muscles. It is important for rowers to sip on sports beverages frequently before and during practice and not wait for thirst to occur before initiating drinking.

Consume a high level of carbohydrate. Carbohydrate intake is critically important for rowers. The recommended level of 10 grams per kilogram of carbohydrate is among the highest of all athletes, while the protein requirement (2 grams per kilogram) is similar to that of other athletes. Rowers must eat a great deal of food to satisfy the 10 grams per kilogram requirement. This is best achieved with frequent feedings of nutritious foods rather than a few larger meals. The small and frequent eating pattern helps optimize glycogen storage and has no adverse effect on body composition.

Ensure normal iron status. The high utilization of oxygen during training and rowing competitions mandates that rowers have an excellent iron status. Because poor iron status takes a great deal of time to reverse, serious rowers should have an iron test (hemoglobin, hematocrit, ferritin) annually to assess whether the dietary intake is satisfying the requirement. A ferritin level of less than 20 nanograms per deciliter should be considered one that places an athlete on the precipice of inadequacy. Athletes with low iron status should discuss the best strategy for improving iron values with their physicians.

Endurance athletes spend many hours training and have enormous energy needs. However, these training times make it difficult to consume the needed foods. Athletes should plan multiple eating breaks throughout the day (consuming something high in carbohydrate every 3 hours) to ensure an adequate total energy consumption. Fluid intake is also critically important, and endurance athletes should develop the habit of drinking frequently (every 10 to 15 minutes) regardless of thirst. A large body of evidence suggests that lower levels of either carbohydrate or fluids inhibit endurance. Nevertheless, when high-carbohydrate diets impair an athlete's capacity to consume sufficient energy because of their relatively low energy density, consuming a higher fat intake to help meet energy needs should be considered.[105] Except to satisfy energy needs, however, fat is not the most desirable energy substrate for endurance athletes.

Carbohydrate after exercise stimulates muscle protein synthesis more favorably than an equivalent amount of fat, so athletes should be careful not to consume fat at the expense of carbohydrate.[106] Under certain circumstances (see chapter 4), caffeine ingestion coupled with adequate hydration and regular carbohydrate intake may aid endurance performance.[107] However, because some studies raise doubts as to caffeine's effectiveness,[108] athletes should determine for themselves whether a small amount of caffeine ingested in long-duration events is useful for enhancing performance.

IMPORTANT POINTS

• Glycogen storage is best achieved through a diet that is adequate in calories and relatively high in carbohydrate, moderate in protein, and low in fat, with frequent fluid consumption.

• Failing to taper exercise before an endurance competition compromises both glycogen stores and hydration status, making optimal competition performance difficult.

• Athletes should practice hydrating and fueling themselves in a way that mimics competition. Failing to do this will inhibit the optimal adaptation to eating and drinking during a competition.

• Overtraining compromises performance because it typically leads to inadequate sleep, increased illness frequency, poor energy consumption, and inability to achieve optimal hydration.

• Endurance athletes should consider every fluid station as a critical opportunity to replenish lost fluids, sodium, and carbohydrate. A failure to consume enough fluid during an event dooms the athlete to poor performance.

• The nutrition strategies followed before, during, and after endurance activities are critically important for achieving continued high-level performance. For instance, a carbohydrate and protein mix immediately after endurance activity aids glycogen replenishment and reduces muscle soreness.

Metabolic Needs for Both Power and Endurance

Many sports, including basketball, soccer, tennis, golf, and figure skating, require a combination of power and endurance. The random intermittent fluctuations of exercise intensity in these sports result in a unique pattern of energy substrate utilization. Nutrition studies of athletes competing in these team sports indicate that a high carbohydrate intake (65 percent of total calories) results in improved performance. Nevertheless, surveys of soccer and basketball players have found that the typical intakes of these athletes provide a much lower carbohydrate level, suggesting there is great room for improvement. The periodic high bursts of activity in these sports also place a high reliance on phosphocreatine (PCr), signifying that protein (with adequate total calories) must also be consumed in amounts sufficient to synthesize the needed creatine, but surveys indicate that many of these athletes don't consume sufficient calories, which could impede creatine synthesis. Studies also show that performance in team sports could be enhanced with better hydration strategies. For instance, soccer players are often hyperthermic by the end of matches, where sweat losses can reach 3 to 4 liters.[1] It is impossible to imagine that this level of fluid loss could somehow be satisfied without a well-developed hydration strategy. However, team sport athletes consume about half of the fluid they require, based on measured sweat losses.[2]

The common practice of excessively relying on dietary supplements is not the answer to these profound dietary weaknesses. There appears to be a drop in the prevalence of supplement use in Olympic-level athletes between 2002 (81 percent) and 2009 (73 percent), perhaps from the well-founded fear of consuming contaminated products that would cause athletes to fail a dope test. Nevertheless, a majority of athletes continue to rely excessively on supplements for nourishment.[3, 4] In some sports, such as soccer, the prevalence of supplement use appears to be increasing.[5] One can only wonder how much better these athletes would have performed by following more sound nutrition practices. This chapter provides information on the nutrition requirements for team sport athletes, with techniques for optimizing glycogen storage and sustaining hydration state. In addition, strategies for achieving optimal nutrient intake during the precompetition, competition, and postcompetition periods are presented.

NUTRITION TACTICS FOR SPORTS REQUIRING POWER AND ENDURANCE

Team sports such as basketball, volleyball, rugby, team handball, and soccer all have combinations of high-intensity and lower-intensity activity interspersed throughout the competition. The mixed intensity of certain individual sports, such as figure skating and tennis, puts them into this category as well. These activity patterns differ from other sports, where the focus is either predominantly endurance or predominantly power or speed. There is nothing in artistic gymnastics training or competition that requires, for instance, a great deal of aerobic endurance; and marathon runners only rarely require the explosive power exhibited by gymnasts. Team sport athletes must focus on speed, power, *and* endurance. Soccer players must run the field at a controlled pace until a sudden opening requires a quick burst of speed. Basketball players may jog back and forth in a steady aerobic pace, but each player must have the capacity for a powerful jump to grab a rebound or for a quick sprint to make a defensive play.

The intermittent high and low intensity of team sports creates a requirement for energy that is derived from a combination of aerobic and anaerobic means. Although the anaerobic metabolic processes are solely reliant on existing stores of ATP, phosphocreatine (PCr), and muscle glycogen, the aerobic processes derive energy from muscle glycogen, blood glucose,

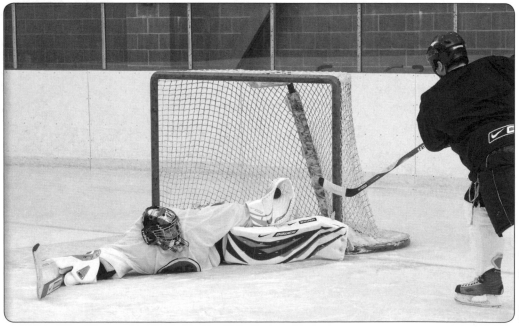

In hockey, frequent line changes help players replenish phosphocreatine, so they can perform at maximal intensity when back on the ice.

© Human Kinetics

fat, and to a lesser extent, protein. As indicated in figure 15.1, there is a heavy reliance on muscle glycogen for the majority of muscle energy during team sport activity, with nearly an equal reliance on fat and blood glucose for most of the remaining source of energy. Fat is almost never in short supply. However, the amount of glucose energy in blood is small and requires constant vigilance by the athlete to ensure a continuing source of glucose during the competition.

The heavy reliance on muscle glycogen and blood glucose to fulfill the energy needs of working muscles demands a high level of consumed carbohydrate before exercise and carbohydrate-containing sports beverages during exercise. In a study of the performance outcomes of a moderate (39 percent of total calories) versus high (65 percent of total calories) carbohydrate intake, the higher-carbohydrate diet significantly improved intermittent exercise performance.[6]

Repeated sprint work is enhanced by consumption of a carbohydrate and electrolyte beverage.[7] Although it has been long established that consumption of a carbohydrate and electrolyte beverage enhances submaximal endurance performance, only recent studies have clearly shown the benefits of these beverages during high-intensity, short-duration efforts such as those found in football and basketball. Subjects performed seven additional 1-minute cycling sprints at 120 to 130 percent of peak $\dot{V}O_2$ when they consumed a 6 percent carbohydrate and electrolyte beverage, as compared with a water placebo. This finding suggests that a dramatic improvement in sprint capability during the last 5 to 10 minutes of a basketball game is possible if players methodically consume a sports beverage. A similar study determined that sports drinks (i.e., carbohydrate and electrolyte beverages) can help maintain high-intensity efforts during high-intensity activities consisting of intermittent sprinting, running, and jogging.[8] Again, these findings have strong positive implications for sustaining high-intensity activity over the course of a typical basketball or soccer game.

The effects of consumption of the individual components of a sports beverage (electrolytes, water, or carbohydrate) and of the combination of all components have also been

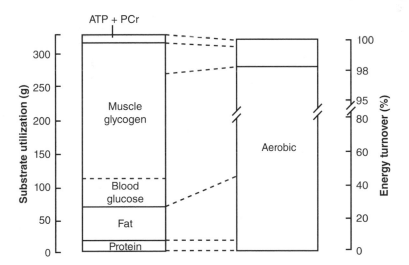

Figure 15.1 The relative anaerobic and aerobic substrate utilization in team sports, such as soccer.

From J. Bangsbo, "The physiology of soccer: With special reference to intense intermittent exercise," *Acta Physiologica Scandinavica* 151(Suppl 619): 1-155. © 1994 by Scandinavian Physiological Society. Reproduced with permission of Blackwell Publishing Ltd.

assessed. Compared with the electrolyte-only trial, performance during the water-only and carbohydrate-only trials was approximately 6 percent faster. However, the combination of carbohydrate and water caused a performance enhancement that was approximately 12 percent faster than the electrolyte trial and 5 to 6 percent faster than when water only or carbohydrate only was consumed.[9] These findings support the thesis that carbohydrate enhances water absorption and that the limited carbohydrate storage mandates consumption of carbohydrate during exercise. The high demands on circulating and stored carbohydrate during high-intensity work require a constant vigilance to ensure proper and speedy replacement. This study was based on earlier work that showed exercise performance improved significantly with higher levels of carbohydrate feedings.[10] It has also been found that the optimal level of carbohydrate concentration during exercise is a 6 to 7 percent solution, but no higher. This concentration is best for fluid absorption and also helps to efficiently deliver carbohydrate. An 8 percent carbohydrate solution causes a slower fluid absorption.[11]

A basketball player leaping for the ball and a soccer player sprinting toward the ball and jumping high to kick it are activities comparable to certain forms of strength training. A study of resistance-trained athletes found that athletes tended to perform more repetitions of the same weight when carbohydrate was consumed versus a water placebo. Blood glucose and lactate concentrations were higher with the carbohydrate trial, suggesting that more carbohydrate was available and used to sustain the high-intensity exercise.[12] A study of head-to-head comparisons of Gatorade, Powerade, and All Sport found that Gatorade stimulates fluid absorption faster than either Powerade or All Sport.[13] This difference can be attributed to both the type of carbohydrate and the concentration of carbohydrate in the beverages. Gatorade has a carbohydrate level that is consistent with the positive findings in virtually all the studies (6 percent) and contains an equal mixture of sucrose and glucose. Powerade and All Sport have higher carbohydrate concentrations, mainly from fructose. Free fructose has been shown to cause gastrointestinal (GI) distress, and it is also less efficient for sustaining blood glucose because it requires a secondary conversion in the liver after absorption.

Athletes who perform repeated or sustained high-power efforts experience a reduction in performance when they are

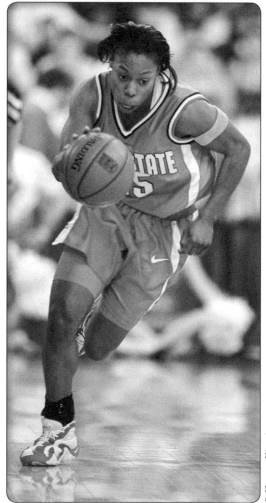

© Human Kinetics

Proper fueling before and during natural breaks in a basketball game can make a big difference in the second-half performance.

dehydrated.[14] A 6 percent carbohydrate solution aids in fluid delivery, a fact that should be considered when team sport athletes select a rehydration beverage. The fluid-consumption guidelines established by the American College of Sports Medicine are summarized in table 15.1.[15]

Several general nutrition guidelines—covering what to do before, during, and after exercise and competition—are important for virtually all athletes involved in sports that have intermittent periods of maximal intensity (see table 15.2). The two keys to these guidelines are fluids and carbohydrate in the context of a generally varied diet. Athletes should explore workable strategies to consume both fluids and carbohydrate at every opportunity. Recent findings tend to contradict the traditional and commonly followed belief that carbohydrate-containing beverages are useful only for endurance (aerobic) activities lasting longer than 60 minutes. The best predictors of athletic performance are maintenance of blood volume and maintenance of glycogen and glucose. What follows are some strategies that might be useful for achieving both enhanced hydration and improved maintenance of system carbohydrate in different sports.

Table 15.1 ACSM Fluid-Consumption Guidelines

Timing	Amount	Adaptation
2 hr before exercise	Drink 500 ml (.5 L, or approximately 17 oz).	None
During exercise	Drink 600 to 1,200 ml (.6 to 1.2 L or, approximately 20 to 40 oz) per hour.	Drink 150 to 300 ml (about 5 to 10 oz) every 15 to 20 min.
After exercise	Based on pre- and postexercise body-weight changes, drink enough fluid to restore body weight (16 oz of fluid = 1 lb of body weight; 1 L of fluid = 1 kg of body weight).	Drink 150% of the amount needed to restore body weight and satisfy postexercise fluid needs. This amount compensates for urine losses, which may induce hypohydration when only 100% of the weight-replacement fluid is consumed.

SAMPLING OF SPORTS RELYING ON A COMBINATION OF ANAEROBIC AND AEROBIC METABOLISM

Certain sports require a combination of aerobic and anaerobic metabolic processes. At times, these athletes work at maximal intensity (anaerobic), while at other times they work at submaximal intensity (aerobic). Imagine a soccer striker who is jogging to cover her area of the field, working to get an open position. At the moment the ball is passed to her, she sprints to the ball with maximal effort. This combination of anaerobic and aerobic effort has special nutrition considerations that are presented in the following sports.

Basketball

Basketball combines many of the best aspects of team cooperation and individual effort, with two guards, two forwards, and one center, all of whom play both defense and offense

Table 15.2 General Guidelines for Athletes in Sports With Intermittent High-Intensity Activity

General nutrition	• The ability to perform multiple bouts of high-intensity exercise is largely dependent on glycogen stores. Therefore, athletes should generally consume foods that will provide approximately 7-8 g/kg (3.2-3.7 g/lb) body weight of carbohydrate. • Protein status is also important for assuring optimal muscular recovery and synthesis of creatine. Therefore, athletes should consume approximately 1.5 g/kg (.7 g/lb) body weight of protein. • Fluids should be consumed liberally, as both muscle function and glycogen stores are dependent on maintaining a euhydrated state. • Adequate calories are essential for optimizing glycogen stores and for enabling optimal muscle function and recovery.
Preexercise or precompetition meal	• A relatively high carbohydrate meal that contains quality protein and is relatively low in fat should be completed approximately 2.5-3.0 hr prior to exercise. Ideally, the carbohydrates should be starchy (bread, pasta, potato, etc.) and low in fiber to avoid possible GI upset. • Fluids should be consumed liberally with the meal. Between the end of the meal and the beginning of exercise, the athlete should sip on a sports beverage (1-2 mouthfuls every 10-15 min) to sustain hydrated state and blood sugar.
During-exercise nourishment and hydration	Sports drinks with a 6-7% carbohydrate solution and a sodium concentration of approximately 100-150 mg/240 ml should be consumed liberally, with the goal of providing approximately 50 g of carbohydrate per hr to maintain blood sugar. The athlete should drink some sports beverage at every opportunity, which should be practiced to assure the athlete is fully aware of beverage consumption tolerance limits.
Postexercise or postcompetition replenishment	Immediately following exercise the athlete should consume approximately 200-400 calories (about 1.5 g/kg or .7 g/lb body weight of carbohydrate during the first 30 minutes following activity). This intake should be repeated every 2 hr for several hours. There is good evidence that high-quality protein (e.g., whey protein) added to the carbohydrate will reduce muscle soreness and improve muscle recovery. Therefore, including about 100-200 calories of protein (25-50 g) over the first several hours following exercise is desirable. Adequate fluids should be consumed to assure return to preactivity weight prior to exercising again. Consumption of chocolate milk during the postexercise period has been recommended because it provides the essential components (fluid, carbohydrate, and protein) in an easy to consume and good tasting form.

during the 32 (high school) or 48 (professional) minutes of the game. Basketball is played around the world by both men and women and has been a highly visible part of the Olympic Games since the 1936 Olympics in Berlin. Among the most impressive winning streaks in basketball was the 10 national championships (7 won consecutively) by the John Wooden–coached UCLA men's teams. In a conversation many years later, one of John Wooden's players shared that Wooden was brilliant at making sure his team was the best conditioned on the floor, and part of that conditioning regimen was making certain the players worked harder during practice than would be needed during any game against any opponent. But he also made certain all the players ate and rested well enough to be ready to give a 100 percent effort.

Studies of intermittent high-intensity sports imply there are clear ergogenic benefits for basketball players who consume the right foods and fluids before, during, and after the game. A study surveying the nutrition knowledge of college basketball coaches and coaches in other sports found that only 33 percent of the coaches were confident they responded correctly to questions related to nutrition.[16] In addition, this survey found that coaches believed college athletes had problems with the consumption of junk food, had generally poor eating habits, and generally consumed unbalanced diets. This poor-quality diet affects vitamin and mineral intake. There is a high prevalence of iron depletion, anemia, and iron-deficiency anemia among both male and female basketball players.[17] Poor iron status will clearly have a negative impact on aerobic work capacity and, therefore, basketball performance. A survey of male and female basketball players revealed that the diets of the female players were lacking in a number of nutrients, and there was an excessive reliance on nutrient supplements.[18] Neither of these findings give confidence that basketball players are taking appropriate steps to compete at their conditioned capacity.

Intense physical activity is associated with the increase of free radicals, such as peroxide, which are created from the oxidation of intercellular lipids. Studies continue to evaluate whether the consumption of antioxidant supplements, including alpha-tocopherol (vitamin E), beta-carotene (provitamin A), and ascorbic acid (vitamin C) might be useful in reducing the typical lipid peroxide production seen in basketball players during the season.[19,20] Although there appears to be some benefit, taking high doses of antioxidant supplements also raises some concerns. Of very real concern is the potential for supplement contamination that may place athletes at risk of unknowingly consuming banned substances.[21] The best alternative for reducing the production of free radicals is likely the regular consumption of fresh fruits and vegetables, which have high concentrations of both carbohydrates and antioxidants.

Keeping all these factors in mind, basketball players must consider the following nutritionally relevant issues for their sport.

Players should use the halftime to replenish fluids and carbohydrates. Basketball players have the advantage of a 10- to 20-minute halftime break. This is an excellent opportunity to sip on a sports beverage to replace lost fluids and carbohydrates. Some athletes find they do well by eating plain crackers and drinking water. However, players should be cautioned against consuming candy bars and other foods that, although they contain some carbohydrate sugar, are high in fat. Players really need carbohydrate and water, and consuming anything else detracts from their ability to take in what they need most (see table 15.3).

Players should use bench time to maintain hydration state. Players should take advantage of natural breaks in the game from official time-outs or substitutions by sipping on sports beverages, whether the players think they need it or not. Sipping on a carbohydrate-containing beverage should become part of the game plan, just as important as making the right defensive or offensive plays.

Frequent practices and games can wear a player out. Basketball players typically practice 6 days each week and often have two practices in a single day. Add to that a match schedule that has them playing at least one game during the week, and it's easy to see why a typical basketball season can wear a player out. In general, players should eat enough carbohydrate to ensure an adequate total energy intake and to support optimal glycogen storage. Optimizing glycogen storage is critical for basketball performance, and meeting

Table 15.3 Meeting Carbohydrate and Fluid Needs of Basketball Players

High-intensity training	For basketball players who train hard daily and need to maximize daily muscle glycogen recovery	7-10 g/kg body weight daily or 3.2-4.5 g/lb body weight daily (~500-700 g/day for a 155-lb [70 kg] player)	At least 10-12 cups/day (~2.5-3 L) plus fluids before, during, and after exercise
Moderate-intensity training	For basketball players who train less than 1 hr daily at a moderate intensity	5-7 g/kg body weight daily or 2.3-3.2 g/lb body weight daily	10-12 cups/day (~2.5-3 L) plus fluids before, during, and after exercise
Before exercise	To enhance fuel availability and prehydrate for a practice or game	1 g/kg body weight 1 hr before or 2 g/kg body weight 2 hr before or 3 g/kg body weight 3 hr before or 4 g/kg body weight 4 hr before	16 oz or 2 cups (~.5 L) (noncaffeinated, nonalcoholic) 2 hr before exercise
During exercise	To provide an additional source of carbohydrate fuel during moderate- and high-intensity basketball practices and games	30-60 g/hr	5-10 oz (150-300 ml) every 15 min to replace sweat losses
Recovery	To speed early recovery and rehydration after hard training or a game, especially during the season when there are back-to-back games and daily practices	1-1.5 g/kg body weight of high-glycemic carbohydrate beverages and foods immediately after exercise and every 2 hr after; total carbohydrate intake over the next 24 hr at 7-9 g/kg or approximately 500-600 g in 24 hr	~20 oz (~3 cups) per lb of body weight lost during exercise

Adapted, by permission, from J. Burns, J.M. Davis, D.H. Craig, and Y. Satterwhite, 1999, "Conditioning and nutrition tips for basketball," *GSSI Roundtable* #38 10(4). [Online]. Available: www.gssiweb.com/Article_Detail.aspx?articleid=2 [June 27, 2011].

total energy needs helps maintain muscle mass. A common complaint of coaches is they find it difficult to keep the weight of many players as high as they would like to, and this is a sure sign that the players are not eating enough to support the intense activity of practices and games. Teams that can make it through the season with muscle mass maintained are stronger and have better endurance than those who don't.

Playing as well in the second half as in the first half wins games.
Teams that can manage to sustain strength and endurance during the second half of the game tend to do better on the scoreboard than teams that don't. To do this, players should establish a pattern of frequent sipping on carbohydrate-containing beverages, whether they think they need to or not. Studies show that this frequent sipping pattern helps players keep their strength and endurance longer than if they drink water alone or fail to drink at all.

Figure Skating

Figure skating took its name from the figures that competitors were required to complete. These figures were, literally, outlined on the ice as two- or three-lobed figure eights that "figure" skaters had to skate over and match as closely as possible to receive a top score. In 1991, however, figures were removed from international competitive skating and eventually phased out of competition entirely, but the name "figure skating" has remained. Figure skaters aim to produce performances that are smooth, graceful, artistic, and seemingly effortless. The short, curved blades and toe picks of their skates permit these athletes to create intricate spins and perform explosive jumps. The sport has three separate events, and training is specialized for each of these: individual figure skating, pairs skating, and ice dancing. Singles skating is a single-gender competition (i.e., males compete against males, and females compete against females), and pairs skating and ice dancing are mixed-gender events.

In individual figure skating, there is an expectation of grace and effortlessness in the performance, but there is also a competitive premium placed on achieving difficult spins and jumps that favor stronger and smaller athletes. Since the density of air and the resistance of ice do not change for each athlete, large athletes have a greater ice resistance and are confronted with greater relative air resistance than are smaller competitors. Therefore, larger skaters require significantly greater strength to do the same skills as smaller skaters. Each successive group of top flight figure skaters appears to be gradually getting smaller with each international competition.

In pairs skating, the male partner is usually considerably larger and stronger than the female. For anyone who has seen a pairs competition, the reason is obvious: The male must lift and throw his female partner frequently during the competition, and this is easier if he's lifting someone smaller. Finding the right physical match is difficult, and poorly matched pairs skaters have difficulty performing at the top level even if they are superb individual skaters.

In ice dancing, there is a much smaller premium on a large male and smaller female because there are no throws or overhead lifts in the competition, and being closer in size helps with the synchronization of the difficult dance skills. Given the intricacy of foot movement and grace found in ice dancing, the sport is well named. The constant movement coupled with a lower power requirement makes this the most aerobic of the three skating disciplines.

Studies have found that figure skaters possess an average aerobic capacity but have the ability to produce high power peaks.[22] That is, when they need to, they can call on their muscles to instantly produce a tremendous amount of power. Studies also indicate that young female skaters consume diets that are relatively high in fat and protein and relatively low in carbohydrate, calcium, and iron.[23] Dietary supplement intake in figure skaters is high, with 65 percent of the male skaters and 76 percent of the female skaters reporting regular supplement intake (mainly multivitamins and multiminerals).[24] The top three reported reasons for taking the supplements were to prevent illness, provide more energy, and make up for an inadequate diet.

Although there has been a long-standing concern that competitive figure skaters do not consume sufficient energy, a recent study suggests this concern may be unfounded for most skaters.[25] However, there remains a proportion of skaters who may be at risk for certain disordered eating patterns, and when this occurs, nutrient intake is likely to be low. The distribution of calories throughout the day in figure skaters does appear to be problematic, an issue that skaters should correct to optimize physical performance and mental concentration.[26]

As with any elite sport, injuries occur. The rate of injuries among pairs skaters is particularly alarming. In one study, female senior pairs skaters reported an average of 1.4 serious injuries over a 9-month period, while other skaters had injury rates averaging .5 serious injuries over this same time period.[27] Most of these are lower-extremity injuries that might be related to boot design, but other researchers suggest that injuries might be related to poor conditioning.[28]

Keeping all these factors in mind, figure skaters must consider the following nutritionally relevant issues for their sport.

Many skaters restrict calories because appearance on the ice is important.

Optimal weight is best achieved through the consumption of a low-fat, moderate-protein, high-complex-carbohydrate diet plus a good exercise and conditioning program. Although dieting is counterproductive, evidence suggests this is the weight-management strategy of choice among skaters. The consumption of adequate energy from carbohydrate is important for both performance and achievement of a desirable body composition. Inadequate energy intake may predispose the skater to nutrient deficiencies; low energy expenditure; and high body-fat levels that can increase the risk of injury, create ill health, and reduce athletic performance.

Figure skating jumps require sufficient phosphocreatine and muscle glycogen stores.

Adequate energy intake from carbohydrate, interspersed with a regular intake of meats (to provide creatine or sufficient protein to make creatine), is important for skaters. For vegetarian skaters, ensuring an adequate total protein and total energy consumption is critical for maintaining muscle mass and synthesizing creatine. The quick burst of muscular activity associated with the jumps required in competitive figure skating is not possible without sufficient storage of phosphocreatine and muscle glycogen. For ice dancing competitions, the fuel requirement involves more muscle glycogen than phosphocreatine, so these athletes are likely to do better with slightly less protein (or meat), but they still require an adequate total energy intake to perform well.

Practices are considerably longer than performances.

Although skating performances last only several minutes, practices may last for an hour or longer, may occur more than once each day, and may be very early in the morning or very late at night (ice time is hard to find). Practice schedules mandate that skaters must alter eating patterns to satisfy their practice needs. For very early morning practices, skaters should eat and drink something (even a slice of toast and a small glass of juice is better than nothing) before taking to the ice to be certain that muscles are well fueled. For late-night practices, a small dinner 2 hours before practice followed by another small dinner immediately after practice will help ensure that muscles are well fueled. Skating while "on empty" will not help the muscles become more conditioned and may actually be counterproductive in inducing a training benefit. At the very least, skaters should sip on sports beverages between the time of the last meal and practice, and even take some sips during practice if the opportunity arises.

There are clear benefits to ensuring a normal hydration state. A study of elite figure skaters found that plasma electrolyte concentrations were suggestive of a poor hydration state.[29]

Soccer, Lacrosse, and Field Hockey

The popularity of soccer worldwide is enormous, and its popularity in the United States is on the rise. Soccer is a wonderful sport from a fitness standpoint because the average distance covered by a typical player during a match is approximately 6 miles (10 km).[30] In addition, soccer players appear to have significantly greater bone mineral densities—likely from all the running stresses placed on the bones—than do age- and weight-matched controls.[31,32] Although much of the activity is aerobic, a large proportion is anaerobic as players sprint for the ball. There is less activity in the second half of a typical soccer game compared with the first, likely the result of unsustained muscle glycogen stores. It was suggested long ago that the ingestion of carbohydrate immediately before, during, and after a game may play an important role in reducing player fatigue during a game.[30] Following this strategy would sustain available glucose and glycogen to working muscles.

In studies of professional soccer players' nutrient consumption, their energy and nutrient intake was similar to that of the general population, despite having a far higher energy and nutrient requirement.[33,34] Although the recommended training diet for soccer players should include 55 to 65 percent carbohydrate, 12 to 15 percent protein, and less than 30 percent fat,[35] the athletes in this and other surveys consumed foods that were considerably lower in carbohydrate and higher in fat.[36] A survey of NCAA Division I female soccer players found that their carbohydrate consumption did not meet the minimum recommendations to promote glycogen repletion (7 to 10 grams per kilogram), but protein and fat intakes were above the recommended level.[37] It is generally believed that playing soccer places a high demand on glycogen stores, so glycogen depletion could cause premature fatigue and reduced performance during a match.[38]

The ergogenic benefit of carbohydrate for sports such as soccer was confirmed in a study assessing the combined and separate benefits of carbohydrate and chromium ingestion during intermittent high-intensity exercise to fatigue. Data from this study confirmed the benefit of carbohydrate but did not support the benefit of chromium.[39] Of course, adequate energy intake, estimated to be approximately 4,000 calories for males and 3,200 calories for females, is also important. Without sufficient energy intake, glycogen will become depleted regardless of the makeup of the diet. In addition, inadequate caloric intake makes optimal synthesis of phosphocreatine (needed for sudden, quick-burst activity) difficult. This point is emphasized in a study that demonstrated a performance benefit of creatine supplementation in young soccer players, a finding that would be unlikely with adequate energy consumption.[40] Although not yet well researched from a nutrition perspective, the nature of play in lacrosse and field hockey is sufficiently similar to soccer that it could be assumed the nutrition demands are also similar. However, player knowledge and practices tend to vary widely by sport, so it is unclear if athletes in these sports have higher or lower nutrition risks.

Keeping all these factors in mind, soccer players must consider the following nutritionally relevant issues for their sport.

Because play in soccer is continuous, it's difficult for players to consume fluids. Since soccer players may not have an opportunity to regularly consume fluids during a game, pregame hydration status is particularly important. Whenever possible (between periods and during official breaks), players should consume a sports beverage to rehydrate and to replace carbohydrates. A study of soccer players found a wide variability in voluntary fluid intake patterns, with the conclusion that most players fail to adequately hydrate.[41] Surveys suggest the consumption of carbohydrate is less than optimal for soccer players, yet an adequate carbohydrate consumption that provides 55 to 65 percent of total calories is important to assure high level performance. Players should make a conscious effort to improve carbohydrate intake.

In one study on field hockey players, sweat losses were similar to that seen in soccer, but hydration practices tended to more adequately satisfy fluid needs. With regular substitutions and an apparent good understanding of optimal hydration practices, players were able to sustain hydration state.[42]

Pregame glycogen storage is critical. Soccer players spend a great deal of time running up and down the field, placing a tremendous drain on muscle glycogen. Players who begin the game with more stored glycogen will experience an endurance advantage. To achieve a higher glycogen storage, players should consistently consume plenty of carbohydrate and fluids and also focus mainly on carbohydrate during the pregame meal (see table 15.4).

Table 15.4 Fuel and Fluids for Soccer

Time	Recommendation
During routine training	• Consume 8-10 g of carbohydrate per kg of body weight per day, or roughly 55-65%. • Drink sufficient fluids to sustain weight. Dark urine is a sign of dehydration.
Pregame	• Eat a high-carbohydrate meal of familiar, easy-to-digest foods 3-4 hr before match play. • Avoid high-fat (especially fried) foods. • Avoid high-fiber foods because they cause GI distress and gas. • Avoid solid foods just before the game because they are digested too slowly. • Nervous players should consider sipping on liquid meals.
During the game	• Consume a carbohydrate and electrolyte sports beverage at every opportunity. • At halftime drink enough sports beverage to maintain pregame weight.
Postgame	• Consume some carbohydrate-containing beverages and foods (fruit juices, bread, pasta, etc.) immediately after the game to help replace glycogen. Also consuming some protein at this time, such a whey protein added to fruit juice, has been shown to reduce muscle soreness and enhance muscle recovery. • Consume 24 oz (720 ml) of fluid (preferably sports beverage) for every pound of weight lost over a 2- to 3-hr period after the game. • In 24 hr consume enough fluid and food to return weight to pregame level.

Adapted, by permission, from J. Lea, D. Richardson, H. O'Malley, Y. Satterwhite, and M. Macedonio, 2000, "Conditioning and nutrition tips for basketball," *GSSI Roundtable* #38 11(1). [Online]. Available: www.gssiweb.com/Article_Detail. aspx?articleid=77 [June 27, 2011].

Rugby

Rugby, also referred to as *rugby football*, *Australian football*, *rugby union*, or simply *football* in much of the world (although this can be confused with soccer, which is also referred to as *football* in much of the world), has earlier origins than either American or Canadian football, which are modifications of traditional rugby. Depending on the league, rugby is played with different numbers of players (typically between 7 and 15 per side). Players can gain ground only by running with the ball or kicking the ball, which looks much like an American oval football. There is more continuous play than play stoppage in rugby than in football, placing a high degree of importance on endurance. The muscular nature of the game, particularly in the "ruck" or "maul" after a tackle, also requires a high degree of strength. Therefore, the combination of moderate- to long-duration exercise, coupled with repeated bouts of high-intensity exercise, characterizes rugby as a stop-and-go sport that requires a combination of endurance and power. Rugby players must have a high aerobic capacity but must also have a well-developed glycolytic capacity and the ability to use and resynthesize phosphocreatine (PCr).

Like athletes in many sports, rugby players often emphasize protein intake for the purpose of optimizing muscle size and strength and to achieve a relatively low body-fat level. Despite this belief, it appears that the maximal utilization of muscle synthesis after training occurs at a relatively small intake level of 20 to 25 grams (80 to 100 calories) of high-quality protein.[43] There is also no evidence to suggest that higher protein intakes are associated with improved body composition in rugby players. The emphasis on protein is misplaced, since the combination of power and endurance in rugby places a high need on dietary carbohydrate intake. Studies have shown a significant depletion of muscle glycogen during a rugby match, with many athletes having subpar performances during the last half of a match due to inadequate glycogen stores.[44, 45] Higher carbohydrate intakes of approximately 8 grams per kilogram per day have been shown to improve performance in intermittent running to fatigue.[46]

The postgame replenishment protocol followed by rugby players is an important consideration because, if appropriate strategies are followed, players can experience improved performance in subsequent games or training. This is particularly important when there is a short time between matches. One study demonstrated that consumption of a high-carbohydrate diet after competition was successful at replenishing glycogen stores.[47] Despite the importance of postgame nutrition replenishment, the strategy most used to improve recovery of elite rugby players after training and matches is stretching and ice or cold-water immersion.[48] In the ideal world, these strategies would be coupled with fluid, carbohydrate, and protein consumption. Alcohol consumption may inhibit optimal glycogen restoration.

Some evidence suggests that training with a relatively low muscle glycogen content improves fuel metabolism adaptation.[49] This suggests that training with inadequate glycogen may enhance the adaptation to training. Playing a match after this training protocol, but with muscle glycogen stores full, may have a performance-enhancing effect and is referred to as the train low, compete high strategy. However, the potential for greater muscle soreness and dehydration with this protocol (glycogen requires water for storage) may compromise the potential benefits.

Hydration state is clearly important for rugby players and has been shown to be associated with early fatigue and a deterioration of football-related skills.[50] There are opportunities for rugby players to consume fluids during breaks in play, during halftime, and when players are substituted. In fact, it is allowable for trainers to run to the players on the field with fluid bottles during pauses in the game. Despite the importance of adequate hydration and ample opportunities for players to drink fluids, there is evidence that they may fail to drink enough.[51,52] Data suggest fluid losses during a rugby match are in the range of 600 to 1,400 milliliters per hour, while intake levels rarely approach this level.[53]

Many athletes in different sports are interested in ergogenic aids, and rugby players are no different. Of the ergogenic aids that have been assessed in team sport athletes, the two that may have some benefit are creatine monohydrate and caffeine.[54,55] However, as indicated in the chapter on ergogenic aids, adequate caloric intake with sufficient carbohydrate may diminish the benefit of creatine supplementation. Sodium bicarbonate ($NaHCO_3$) has also been tested on rugby players to determine if it would enhance anaerobic potential by improving lactic acid buffering. Although there was a measurable improvement in blood lactate concentration in the supplemented group of rugby players, there was no measurable impact on exercise performance.[56] In addition, a significant proportion of the players complained of severe GI symptoms after ingestion of the sodium bicarbonate. These symptoms would negatively affect any potential benefit this supplement might have.

Of particular concern regarding supplementation with ergogenic aids is that many of the nutrition recommendations given to players come from coaches with limited nutrition knowledge. A study of New Zealand premier rugby coaches found that most of the coaches provided nutrition advice to their players (83.8 percent), but they responded correctly to only 55.6 percent of nutrition knowledge questions.[57] Clearly, a better way must be found to supply players with appropriate information that will enhance performance, reduce injury risk, and sustain health.

Keeping all these factors in mind, rugby players must consider the following nutritionally relevant issues for their sport.

Learning the basis of nutrition recommendations will encourage athletes and coaches to follow sound nutrition practices. A poor level of nutrition knowledge among players and coaches results in poor food choices. Educational opportunities for these players and associated staffs should be established to help players understand the basic elements of good sport nutrition, coupled with counseling that individualizes the dietary plan for each player.[58] Players should come to understand that supplements and ergogenic aids are not appropriate substitutes for the regular consumption of good food.

Carbohydrate and sodium-containing sports beverages are important for performance. Players should consume a relatively high carbohydrate intake to enter training and competition with full liver and muscle glycogen stores. This will reduce fatigue and help athletes sustain blood sugar for the beginning of the game. Sustaining blood sugar is an important strategy for maintaining skills and mental acuity and for preventing CNS-mediated muscular fatigue. Opportunities for consuming carbohydrate- and sodium-containing fluids during training and matches should not be missed. Regular consumption of sports beverages will help maintain blood sugar and blood volume and, by doing so, will minimize premature fatigue.

Post-game recovery is important to assure optimal performance the following day. Post-training and match intake should be well planned so there is little time between the end of play and the availability of foods and beverages. The focus should be on starch-based carbohydrate, high-quality protein (such as whey protein), and ample fluids.

Alcohol consumption should be avoided, because it interferes with optimal performance. There is evidence in the literature that alcohol consumption by some rugby players may be sufficiently high and frequent that it compromises athletic performance. Players should make every attempt to minimize alcohol consumption, particularly during the competitive season.

Tennis

It is generally agreed that tennis has both aerobic and anaerobic components, but the majority of the energy supply appears to come from anaerobic systems.[59,60] This heavy reliance on the anaerobic metabolic system is likely why carbohydrate supplementation improves the stroke quality during the final stages of a tennis match.[61] Since long-lasting, high-intensity exercise is highly dependent on carbohydrate as a fuel, it makes perfect sense for tennis players to ensure that carbohydrate is available to the muscles.

Although carbohydrate consumption may be of concern, it appears that collegiate tennis players (Division I) have been well coached to consume sufficient fluids in hot environments. In a study evaluating fluid and electrolyte balance during multiday match play in a hot environment, the athletes successfully maintained overall balance, resulting in no occurrence of heat illness.[62]

It also appears, from data on young tennis players, that the adequacy of energy intake is better than that seen in other sports (gymnastics and swimming). It is well established that menstrual onset is, to a great degree, dependent on adequate energy intake. In general, females experience the first menses at around the age of 13. Females who have energy deficits may have up to a 2-year delay in the age of menarche. Tennis players, however, appear to have only a slight delay (13.2 years) in the age of menarche, suggesting that energy consumption is good.[63] Typically, there is less concern in tennis about making weight. The focus is on conditioning, regardless of where the weight ends up, and there is evidence that college women tennis players are no more at risk of eating disorders than any other young woman.[64]

Keeping all these factors in mind, tennis players must consider the following nutritionally relevant issues for their sport.

Tennis is commonly played outside, where the reflective temperature from the court is higher than the environmental temperature. This excessive heat coupled with the high-intensity intermittent sprints of tennis can quickly increase body temperature. Players should be aware of the signs of heat disorders (thirst, fatigue, vision problems, inability to speak normally) and take quick action if they, a partner, or an opponent appears to have any heat-related symptoms (see table 15.5).

Tennis players should use the natural breaks after each odd game when opponents change sides to replenish fluids and carbohydrates. These natural breaks in a tennis match are, perhaps, why tennis players are in relatively good hydration state during and after a match. However, because carbohydrate supplementation has been found to improve end-of-game strokes, players should make certain the beverage consumed contains carbohydrate. These sports beverages, if sipped during a match, will help ensure that high-intensity activity can be maintained for a longer period of time.

Table 15.5 Heat Disorder Symptoms

Heat cramps	Muscle spasms that occur involuntarily during or after exercise, typically in the muscles that did most of the work during the exercise.
Heat exhaustion	Weak and rapid heart rate with low blood pressure, headache, dizziness, and severe weakness. Body temperature is not elevated to dangerous levels, but sweat rate may be reduced, increasing the risk of high body temperature. Blood volume is typically low. At this stage, the athlete should stop exercising, go to a shady area or cool building, and consume fluids to rehydrate.
Heatstroke	A failure of the body's ability to maintain temperature. Characterized by a failure to sweat. Circulatory system collapse may lead to death. Immediate steps should be taken to cool the body by applying ice, placing the person in cold water, or applying alcohol rubs. This is an emergency condition, so medical assistance should be called immediately.

Volleyball

Typical volleyball matches average 1 hour 15 minutes to 2 hours in length. The skills and techniques used in volleyball require high and frequent vertical jumps, sudden changes of direction, skilled passing, deft and brave defending, and superhuman digs to keep balls from hitting the court. The duration of the sets plus the quickness of movements means all the energy metabolic systems come into play: the phosphocreatine (PCr) system for high-intensity, quick-burst activity; anaerobic activity for prolonged power production during the 10 to 15 seconds of each point; and aerobic metabolism to satisfy the energy requirements between points. The quick-burst power production of volleyball strongly implies the need for optimizing glycogen and creatine stores, both of which require regularly satisfying total energy needs from a predominantly high carbohydrate intake.

A study of volleyball players found that longer years of training were associated with more oxidative stress.[65] Other studies suggest that, in adolescents, typical volleyball practice is associated with a greater tissue-promoting (i.e., anabolic) than tissue-decreasing (i.e., catabolic) effect, but it does result in a higher production of inflammatory markers (notably interleukin-6) associated with oxidative stress.[66] In an attempt to determine if specific dietary modifications might reduce the potential for oxidative harm, volleyball athletes were placed on either a typical Mediterranean diet (high in vegetables, fish, and olive oil) or a high-protein, low-calorie diet supplemented with 3 grams per day of fish oil.[67] Fish oil has been found in some studies to exert an anti-inflammatory effect. After 2 months, the group with the low-calorie, high-protein fish oil diet had a greater potential for cellular harm, suggesting that the classical Mediterranean diet would be the better choice. In essence, low calorie intakes, regardless of their quality, create athletic difficulties.

Attempts to improve the dietary intakes of volleyball players have not fared well.[68,69] Providing general feedback may not be as useful as feedback that addresses how volleyball players could modify intake at specific times of the day to ensure a desirable within-day energy balance and an optimal nutrient intake. These studies illustrate the difficulty of making individual recommendations for change without addressing the global realities of a player's environment. Most players can modify their diets for a short period, but the environmental influences on diet (e.g., training table, eating schedules) must also be changed to ensure that dietary modifications can be more permanent. Ultimately, the environment must be structured in a way that helps ensure each athlete's diet is good. Athletes will inevitably have eating behaviors most typical of the group and environment they are in. Dietary assessments of elite adolescent female volleyball players strongly suggest there is room for dietary improvements. Many of these players are at risk for menstrual dysfunction and consume a level of energy and nutrients that would result in jeopardized performance.[70] These concerns appear to be consistent regardless of country. The greater the energy inadequacy, the greater the likelihood of menstrual irregularities in female athletes.[71,72] Another study found that one-third of those assessed had low serum ferritin levels, indicating high risk for the development of anemia.[73]

The dietary intake issue in volleyball players has important implications for coaches, who often have no formal training in sport nutrition. To make matters worse, many coaches weigh athletes or assess body composition and use this information punitively to encourage athletes to lose weight.[74] Athletes often interpret this by placing themselves on restrictive intakes that lower nutrient intake, lower energy intake, increase dysmenorrhea risk, increase stress fracture risk, and increase body fat as a proportion of remaining weight. One study found a high level of body fatness among volleyball players that might be attributable to the degree of restrained eating that they practice.[75] The focus on weight alone also has implications for the use of nonprescription weight-loss products. A study of collegiate athletes found that more volleyball players (23.6 percent) used diuretics than either softball players (3.6 percent) or basketball players (1.0 percent).[76] This study also found that more volleyball players used laxatives (18.8 percent, compared with 1.8 percent for softball players and 1.0 percent for basketball players).

Fluid intake is important for all athletes but particularly for athletes performing in hot and humid outdoor environments. Beach volleyball players, therefore, should consider the importance of consuming sufficient fluids to maintain sweat rates and prevent changes in cardiovascular dynamics. One study of voluntary fluid intake of beach volleyball players during an official tournament found a wide variation in fluid intake, with an average intake that was inadequate.[77]

Keeping all these factors in mind, volleyball players must consider the following nutritionally relevant issues for their sport.

Volleyball practices and games increase oxidative stress.   There is increasing interest in antioxidant supplements because they potentially reduce oxidative stress. However, trials with antioxidants in a number of settings and with a number of different subjects have provided mixed results. The food delivery of antioxidant nutrients (i.e., a nonsupplemental delivery) does provide benefits in reducing oxidative stress. Greater consumption of foods that deliver vitamin C, vitamin E, and beta-carotene (i.e., fresh fruits and vegetables) is likely to be the best strategy. Since these same foods are high in water content, fiber, and carbohydrate, they bring other beneficial aspects to the diet that cannot be matched by supplements.

High body-fat levels in volleyball players is a concern.   Evidence suggests that many volleyball players have more body fat than other athletes. Besides influencing oxidative stress (higher body-fat levels are associated with higher oxidative stress), high body-fat levels negatively affect the strength-to-weight ratio and the capacity to jump high and move quickly. The common strategy followed by many volleyball players is to place themselves (either through a coach's encouragement or on their own) on a diet that is severely deficient in both energy and nutrients. The ultimate outcome is a gradual loss of lean mass, a higher fat mass, higher risk of dysmenorrhea, and increased risk of stress fractures. The best strategy is to lose fat while maintaining or increasing lean mass. This can be achieved with a proper distribution of energy and nutrients throughout the day, avoiding large peaks or valleys in energy delivery that cause greater fat storage or an increase in muscle loss. Frequent eating of smaller meals is a much more effective strategy than low-calorie dieting.

Hydration should become a natural and planned activity. Ideally, volleyball players should find a sports beverage they find palatable during training and competition and learn through trial and error the amount of fluid they can consume at fixed intervals. It is particularly important for beach volleyball players to become accustomed to drinking in a pattern that prevents thirst throughout practice and competition. After training or competition, a special effort should be made to consume carbohydrate beverages, including some with protein, to maximize glycogen storage and reduce postexercise muscle soreness. Away from the playing venue, athletes should drink plenty of water with meals and always have a sports beverage available to consume between meals.

Volleyball players should take a look at how they eat before, during, and after practice and competition. There is no substitute for food, and an inadequate consumption of food cannot be replaced by the intake of nutrient supplements. Although eating real food takes planning and time, it's worth it. The nature of volleyball play suggests a high requirement for carbohydrate (60 to 65 percent of total calories) but also enough total calories so that muscle tissues can use consumed proteins to synthesize creatine. By its nature, inadequate energy intake is a catabolic event that breaks down tissue, inhibits tissue repair, makes glycogen storage difficult, and inhibits muscle recovery.

Golf

Golf was last played at the Olympics in 1924, but it will once again be an official Olympic sport at the 2016 Summer Games in Rio de Janeiro.[78] A typical 18-hole round of golf requires players to walk at least 5.6 miles (9 km) and lasts approximately 4 hours, a duration that could result in both low blood sugar and dehydration that would negatively influence coordination and concentration. The hydration concern is real, particularly if the golf round is played in a hot and humid environment.

Strategies to counteract the negative effects of dehydration have been tested. Twenty male golfers consumed beverages containing caffeine, a carbohydrate and electrolyte beverage with caffeine, or a flavor-matched placebo containing no energy or caffeine. The carbohydrate and electrolyte sports drink with caffeine significantly improved putting performance and increased feelings of alertness.[79] Another study found that the ingestion of adequate amounts of fluids during a simulated 18-hole golf match had clear benefits on mental and physiological function.[80]

Caffeine is increasingly being recognized in the literature as having beneficial effects on physical, cognitive, and psychomotor functioning. In an assessment designed to specifically address physical and cognitive performance during long-duration activity, caffeine improved endurance performance and complex cognitive ability during and after exercise.[81] This is a particularly important finding for a sport such as golf, where the ability to concentrate would play a large role in success.

Allowing dehydration to occur and blood sugar to drop has another disadvantage: It could increase injury risk. According to one study, lower self-awareness of the environment could increase injury risk in golfers, and low blood sugar and dehydration play a role.[82] Reducing golf injuries is an important issue: In 2007 the U.S. Consumer Product Safety Commission reported that 52,861 golfers presented to emergency departments with an injury, and another study estimated that 60 percent of professionals and 40 percent of amateurs sustain a golf injury each year.[83] Although many of these injuries are golf-swing specific, it is hard to imagine nutrition doesn't play an important role in these and other injuries. Dehydration, for instance, is associated with reduced flexibility that could predispose an athlete to muscle injury. Although less frequently seen in the golf literature, stress fractures of the ribs do occur, mainly on the golfer's lead swing side, and stress fractures are also known to have a nutrition component.[84] Athletes with better calcium and vitamin D dynamics have higher bone densities that are more resistant to stress fracture.

The Royal Canadian Golf Association estimates that players expend 2,000 to 2,500 calories during a typical 18-hole round of play.[85] Ideally, this level of energy should be provided in a rationally distributed meal plan that provides at least some of the energy during the round.

Keeping all these factors in mind, golfers must consider the following nutritionally relevant issues for their sport.

It is necessary to consume adequate energy to avoid large energy deficits. Golfers should find ways to prevent energy deficits that could compromise attention and weaken the swing. Ideally, a golfer should finish a small to moderate pregame meal that is high in carbohydrate about 2 to 3 hours before play. For the period between the last meal and play, the golfer should maintain a sipping protocol with a sports beverage or some fruit juice to maintain blood sugar. An alternative would be an energy bar consumed with water, about 90 minutes after the pregame meal. The postgame meal is also important for replacing the energy used during golf and replenishing glycogen stores. Having a 200- to 400-calorie snack available to eat before heading for the clubhouse is a good idea, followed by frequent small meals after the locker room routine. The goal is to develop a plan so there is never more than 3 hours between eating opportunities (either a snack or meal), with fluids consumed liberally whenever food is consumed.

A pattern for consuming snacks and sports beverages can help sustain blood sugar and prevent dehydration. Golf rounds last a long time and are often played in direct sunlight. Fluids are needed to maintain blood volume, sweat rates, and mental function. The best fluids contain sodium (~50 to 100 milligrams per cup) and sugars (~6 to 7 percent carbohydrate) and should be sipped on a fixed schedule to prevent dehydration. Water, although commonly consumed, is not likely to optimize the potential benefits of drinking because it contains no sodium (blood volume and sweat rates will drop) and no sugars (central nervous system function will drop). There is now evidence that a small amount of caffeine in the hydration beverage is useful, as caffeine is a central nervous system stimulant that can help maintain mental acuity.

Golfers should avoid consuming alcohol during a round of play. Although alcohol is commonly consumed on golf courses, it is probably the worst substance golfers can have if they are serious about their game. Alcohol quickly lowers blood sugar, negatively affects central nervous system function, increases urinary production, and increases dehydration risk. It's hard to imagine anything worse. Golfers should know that the central nervous system effect of alcohol can be measured for several days after its consumption.

Regular consumption of carbohydrate will optimize glycogen stores. The golf swing, to a large degree, is glycogen dependent. Glycogen stores are best optimized through the regular consumption of relatively high-carbohydrate foods, through the consumption of plenty of fluids, and by avoiding activities that are glycogen depleting (such as intense exercise the day before a round of golf). The food consumed immediately after exercise is important and should be high in carbohydrates and high in fluids.

Sports that require a combination of power and endurance have only recently received the same level of scientific attention that endurance sports have enjoyed for many years. Studies on these sports indicate that carbohydrate consumption is useful for enhancing performance even if the activity lasts less than 1 hour. This is an important finding because it was traditionally thought that water was an appropriate hydration beverage for activities lasting less than 1 hour, whereas carbohydrate-containing sports beverages were appropriate for activities lasting longer than 1 hour. We now know that even for these shorter activities, carbohydrate consumption is performance enhancing. Since many of these sports (basketball, soccer, tennis) place an enormous caloric drain on the system, athletes should develop eating strategies (i.e., to eat enough) that encourage maintenance of muscle mass during long and arduous seasons.

IMPORTANT POINTS

• Maintaining a diet high in complex carbohydrate, moderate in protein, and low in fat will help build and sustain glycogen stores. Fluids are needed to achieve a good hydration state and to store glycogen.

• During the precompetition period and after the pregame meal, athletes should consume starchy, easily digested snacks, such as crackers, with fluids. If not well tolerated, athletes should sip frequently on a sports beverage.

• During competition, athletes should consume a 6 to 7 percent carbohydrate sports beverage with between 100 and 200 milligrams of sodium per cup. When play takes place in a hot and humid environment, the higher level of sodium and additional fluids should be consumed to sustain the sweat rate and blood volume.

• All breaks (both timed breaks such as halftime and breaks that occur as a result of time-outs) should be used as an opportunity to replenish fluids and carbohydrate. Each player should have an identifiable container of his beverage ready and easily available. This is particularly important in soccer, where exertion is continuous, with little stop in action.

• After exercise, athletes should immediately (before the shower) consume fluids and a carbohydrate and protein mix to replenish glycogen stores and aid muscle recovery. Glycogen synthetase is elevated after physical activity, so immediately providing fluids and carbohydrate is a successful strategy to replenish depleted glycogen stores.

• When competition takes place in a hot and humid environment, athletes should have a system for cooling down quickly if heat disorder symptoms occur. This need not be complicated—a kiddy pool filled with ice water next to the field is sufficient.

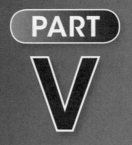

PART V

Nutrition Plans for Specific Sports

Sports Requiring Power and Speed

Power athletes are naturally focused on maximizing their strength-to-weight ratio so as to generate the greatest power at the lowest weight. To do this requires an eating strategy that enables a maintenance or increase of the muscle mass, coupled with the lowest possible body-fat percentage. Ideally, power athletes should sustain a protein intake of between 1.2 and 1.7 grams per kilogram of body weight, with the lower value for athletes seeking to sustain muscle mass and the higher value for athletes seeking to increase muscle mass. It is important to consider these two facts: (1) Most athletes (vegetarians are an exception) consume ample quantities of protein from food alone, often at levels well above 2.0 grams per kilogram of weight; and (2) a higher level of protein consumption by itself will not contribute to a larger muscle mass unless the higher protein intake is coupled with sufficient energy to satisfy energy need. Many athletes actually help to satisfy total energy requirements through consumption of protein, but the levels of protein consumed (> 1.7 g/kg) are often far higher than can be used anabolically. Athletes must also distribute both calories and protein in a way that sustains energy balance and the amino acid pool throughout the day, preventing large peaks and valleys in both. In essence, athletes should consume enough calories to sustain the current weight and muscle mass, plus enough additional calories to support a larger weight and muscle mass. This typically amounts to an additional 300 to 400 calories per day, coupled with enough of the right kind of resistance activity to stimulate the need for a larger mass.

A number of sports require the achievement of a specific competition weight (boxing, wrestling, and horse racing are notable examples), while other sports mandate the production of a high level of power at the lowest possible weight for both appearance and performance factors (e.g., gymnastics, figure skating, and diving). There is good evidence that these athletes often follow eating strategies that either restrict calories or induce dehydration to achieve the desired weight. Neither of these strategies is appropriate or healthful. Restrained eating is likely to cause a significant catabolism of the lean body mass, which negatively influences the strength-to-weight ratio, and dehydration causes negative performance outcomes. Because restrained eating and induced dehydration are counterproductive to the athletes' ultimate goals, may be dangerous, and may lead to more serious eating disorders, they are inappropriate strategies for power athletes to follow. Instead, athletes should consider eating strategies that optimize performance and hydration state. To do so requires a meal pattern that includes six or more eating opportunities. This is a distinct separation from the usual three-meals-per-day eating pattern and, because of this, may be difficult to accomplish (people tend to eat in the way most around them eat). Nevertheless, the rewards of having smaller and more frequent meals are real. Athletes who practice eating smaller and more frequent meals and who drink frequently are likely to feel better and do better, a fact that is likely to encourage them to continue eating in this way.

ABOUT THE EATING PLANS

This chapter includes seven eating plans for intakes of 2,100, 2,300, 2,700, 3,100, 3,400, 3,700, and 4,600 calories. To help athletes understand how to best integrate an eating plan into their exercise schedules, the plans include differently timed practice sessions. The foods are consumed around the practice sessions in a way that helps sustain energy balance throughout the day (± 400 calories) and also helps distribute protein and other nutrients throughout the day. Rather than viewing energy balance just at the end of the day, the eating plans include information on the number of hours spent in a catabolic state (i.e., energy balance is below 0) or in an anabolic state (i.e., energy balance is above 0). An anabolic:catabolic ratio of 1 should result in weight and body-composition stabilization; a ratio of >1 should allow the athlete to increase muscle mass; and a ratio of <1 should help the athlete lower body-fat percentage. The goal is to provide a *guide* for eating that gives athletes a starting point for developing the best possible eating strategy that is specific to their needs.

It is important to note that the caloric level of these diets is for illustration only and is not likely to be perfect for anyone. Weight stability and a healthy body-fat level are the best guides that an appropriate number of calories are being consumed at the right times. Athletes should find a caloric intake level and intake pattern that works for them as individuals. It is also important to note that fluid intakes are likely to be much higher than the fluids listed here. Athletes should consume ample quantities of water with meals and may also need to consume more sports beverages during bouts of physical activity. Athletes should drink enough to sustain optimal body water, an indication of which is nearly clear urine.

Table 16.1 2,100-Calorie Plan for a 5'0" (152 cm), 100 lb (45 kg) 17-Year-Old-Female Power/Speed Athlete

Energy-balance graph

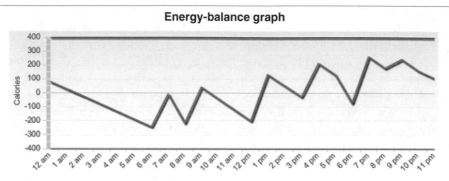

Hours anabolic (calories > 0) = 12; hours catabolic (calories < 0) = 12; anabolic:catabolic ratio = 1.0

Energy Substrate Distribution

Total Calories: 2,127		Carbohydrate %: 69		Protein %: 15	Fat %: 16

Hour	Activity	Food	Amount	Calories
7-8 a.m.	Important to consume carbohydrate to support liver glycogen and blood sugar before exercise.	Bagel, cinnamon raisin	1 small (3 in, 7.5 cm)	156
		Jam	1 tbsp	56
		Grapefruit juice	8 oz (240 ml)	102
8-9 a.m.	Vigorous, high-intensity exercise; important to consume sports beverage during exercise to sustain blood volume and blood sugar, 60 min.	Sports drink	8 oz (240 ml)	62
9-10 a.m.	Breakfast should be consumed immediately after the postexercise cool-down.	Cereal, Corn Flakes	1 cup	101
		Cereal, All Bran	1/4 cup	25
		Blueberries	1 cup	84
		Flaxseed, ground	1 tbsp	53
		Milk, 1% fat	8 oz (240 ml)	102
		Water	As desired	0
10 a.m.-1 p.m.	Any relaxed walking, sitting, household, or school activities.	Water	As desired	0
1-2 p.m.	Lunch should provide ample quantities of carbohydrate and fluids.	Beans, refried, fat free	1/4 cup	46
		Cheese, cheddar	1 tbsp	61
		Salsa	1/4 cup	17
		Flour tortillas, soft taco, 8 in (20 cm)	1 tortilla	146
		Carrots, baby, raw	1/2 cup	42
		Pear	1 medium	103
		Water	As desired	0
2-4 p.m.	Any relaxed walking, sitting, household, or school activities.	Water	As desired	0
4-5 p.m.	Snack is important to ensure energy balance does not drop excessively.	Pretzels, hard, salted	3/4 oz (23 g)	79
		Yogurt, fruit, low fat	1 cup	243

Hour	Activity	Food	Amount	Calories
5-6 p.m.	Any relaxed walking, sitting, household, or school activities.	Water	As desired	0
6-7 p.m.	Sports drinks that contain carbohydrate and sodium are useful in returning to normal hydration state before the next day's exercise.	Sports drink	8 oz (240 ml)	62
7-9 p.m.	Dinner should be nourishing with a wide variety of vegetables and lean protein.	Chicken breast, roasted, no skin	3 oz (90 g)	147
		Potato, baked, no skin	1 medium	145
		Sour cream	2 tbsp	46
		Green beans, boiled	1 cup	44
		Cabbage, raw	1 cup	18
		Vegetable oil (canola)	1 tsp	41
		Vinegar	1 tbsp	3
		Water	As desired	0
9-10 p.m.	A presleep snack is useful for ensuring that the next day begins within the desirable energy-balance bounds.	Pudding, vanilla	4 oz (125 g)	143
		Water	As desired	0

Totals for selected nutrients

Total kcal	2,127	Iron (mg)	19.4	Vit C (mg)	176.7	Vit B$_{12}$ (mcg)	7.39
Carbohydrate (g)	381	Calcium (mg)	1,243	Vit B$_1$ (mg)	1.87	Folic acid (DFE)	621.5
Protein (g)	82	Zinc (mg)	9.05	Vit B$_2$ (mg)	2.46	Vit A (RAE)	1,457
Fat (g)	39	Magnesium (mg)	365.7	Niacin (mg)	28.4	Vit D (IU)	156
Sodium (mg)	3,242	Potassium (mg)	3831	Vit B$_6$ (mg)	3.65	Vit E (mg)	4.91

Note: This type of exercise regimen might be typical of an intermediate figure skater who is involved in intensive training to improve power for better jumps. A review of the energy-balance graph indicates that athletes of this weight and height who undergo this level of physical training and eat in the pattern described will sustain a good energy balance state throughout the day. This type of energy balance is associated with the ability to sustain a relatively low body-fat percentage while sustaining muscle mass.

Source: Energy balance and nutrient intake values were derived using NutriTiming®. The energy balance graph is copyrighted by NutriTiming LLC and is used with permission.

Table 16.2 2,300-Calorie Plan for a 5'5" (165 cm), 125 lb (57 kg) 17-Year-Old Female Power/Speed Athlete

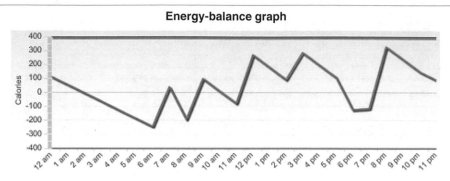

Energy-balance graph

Hours anabolic (calories > 0) = 15; hours catabolic (calories < 0) = 9; anabolic:catabolic ratio = 1.67

Energy Substrate Distribution

Total Calories: 2,316 **Carbohydrate %:** 65 **Protein %:** 17 **Fat %:** 18

Hour	Activity	Food	Amount	Calories
7-8 a.m.	Preexercise snack; important to ensure normal blood sugar during the morning exercise session.	Bread, raisin, toasted	2 slices	172
		Jam	1 tbsp	48
		Grape juice with vitamin C	8 oz (240 ml)	152
8-9 a.m.	Intense 60 min exercise; important to consume at least 8 oz of carbohydrate and sodium sports drink to support blood sugar and blood volume.	Sports drink	8 oz (240 ml)	62
9-10 a.m.	This high-carbohydrate breakfast should be consumed immediately after the postexercise cool-down.	Cereal, oatmeal	1 cup cooked	159
		Milk, 1% fat	8 oz (240 ml)	102
		Walnuts	1/3 oz (10 g)	61
		Raisins, seedless	2 tbsp	90
10 a.m.-12 p.m.	Normal daily activities typical of desk work, walking, school, and light household chores.	Water	As desired	0
12-1 p.m.	Lunch; provides a balance of high-quality protein and fresh (high-carbohydrate) vegetables; fluids should be consumed liberally with all food consumption.	Turkey, white meat, rotisserie	3 oz (90 g)	95
		Bread, multigrain	2 slices	189
		Mustard, prepared, yellow	1 tsp	3
		Lettuce, romaine	1 inner leaf	1
		Carrots, baby, raw	1 cup	84
		Apple, with skin	1 medium	65
		Water	As desired	0
1-3 p.m.	Normal daily activities typical of desk work, walking, school, and light household chores.	Water	As desired	0
3-4 p.m.	Important for sustaining blood sugar and ensuring that liver glycogen is normal in advance of the afternoon workout.	Cheese, mozzarella, part-skim milk	1 oz (30 g)	72
		Crackers, rye	1 oz (30 g)	108
		Grapes, seedless	1 cup	104

Hour	Activity	Food	Amount	Calories
4-5 p.m.	Normal daily activities typical of desk work, walking, school, and light household chores.	Water	As desired	0
5-6 p.m.	A 30 min warm-up before exercise session is desirable.	Water	As desired	0
6-7 p.m.	Intense 60 min exercise; important to consume at least 8 oz of carbohydrate and sodium sports drink to support blood sugar and blood volume.	Sports drink	8 oz (240 ml)	62
7-8 p.m.	Postexercise hydration; there is evidence that chocolate milk is an excellent postexercise beverage for both glycogen recovery and reduced muscle soreness.	Chocolate milk, low fat	8 oz (240 ml)	158
8-9 p.m.	Balanced dinner should be consumed immediately after the postexercise cool-down.	Spinach, boiled	1 cup cooked	41
		Rice, brown, long-grain, cooked	3/4 cup	162
		Salmon, broiled	4 oz (125 g)	234
		Tomatoes, cherry	1 cup	27
		Orange	1 medium	65
		Water	As desired	0
9-10 p.m.	Normal daily activities typical of desk work, walking, school, and light household chores.			

Totals for selected nutrients

Total kcal	2,316	Iron (mg)	33.8	Vit C (mg)	232.2	Vit B$_{12}$ (mcg)	5.52
Carbohydrate (g)	393	Calcium (mg)	1,645	Vit B$_1$ (mg)	2.5	Folic acid (DFE)	819.4
Protein (g)	101	Zinc (mg)	12.8	Vit B$_2$ (mg)	3.1	Vit A (RAE)	3,483
Fat (g)	47	Magnesium (mg)	626	Niacin (mg)	31.34	Vit D (IU)	126.9
Sodium (mg)	3,040	Potassium (mg)	5,245	Vit B$_6$ (mg)	3.78	Vit E (mg)	6.19

Note: This food plan represents the intake of a 200 m or 400 m sprinter who has practice in the early morning and another practice in the late afternoon, both of equal intensity. Eating as this plan describes will have the athlete spending more time in an anabolic state (energy balance above 0 calories) than in a catabolic state (energy balance below 0 calories) while maintaining a good (±400 calories) energy-balance state throughout the day. The greater time in an anabolic state would be necessary to help this athlete enlarge the muscle mass if coupled with vigorous training (as is described).

Source: Energy balance and nutrient intake values were derived using NutriTiming®. The energy balance graph is copyrighted by NutriTiming LLC and is used with permission.

Table 16.3 2,700-Calorie Food Plan for a 5'10″ (178 cm), 150 lb (68 kg) 19-Year-Old Male Pairs Figure Skater

Energy-balance graph

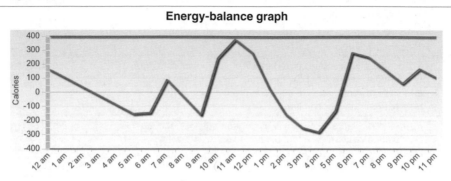

Hours anabolic (calories > 0) = 14; hours catabolic (calories < 0) = 10; anabolic:catabolic ratio = 1.4

Energy Substrate Distribution

Total calories: 2,704   **Carbohydrate %:** 62   **Protein %:** 13   **Fat %:** 25

Hour	Activity	Food	Amount	Calories
6-7 a.m.	Important to consume immediately upon waking to prevent low blood sugar.	Orange juice	12 oz (360 ml)	164
7-8 a.m.	Small breakfast to begin day's activities.	Cereal, Shredded Wheat, with sugar	1.5 cups	275
		Milk, 1%	8 oz (240 ml)	102
		Coffee	1 cup	2
		Milk, 1% for coffee	1 oz (30 ml)	13
8-10 a.m.	Typical school activities.	Water	As desired	0
10-11 a.m.	Important to have snack to maintain energy balance and blood sugar.	Trail mix with chocolate chips, salted nuts, and seeds	3/4 cup	530
11 a.m.-12 p.m.	Lunch prepared at home and brought to school.	Turkey sandwich:		
		Turkey breast, no skin	3 oz (90 g)	134
		Mustard, prepared	1 tsp	3
		Tomato slices	2 slices	16
		Whole grain bread	2 regular slices	138
		Water	As desired	0
12-1 p.m.	School	Water	As desired	0
1-2 p.m.	Sport-specific on-ice training to go over routines; involves frequent lifting of partner and multiple jumps and spins.	Sports drink	12 oz (360 ml)	94
2-3 p.m.	Off-ice training involves going over choreography with partner and coach, involving jumps, leaps, and lifts.	Sports drink	12 oz (360 ml)	94
3-4 p.m.	Light 30 min solitary jog to help athlete focus on goals	Sports drink	8 oz (240 ml)	62

Hour	Activity	Food	Amount	Calories
4-5 p.m.	Cool-down; immediate consumption of sports drink after jog.	Sports drink	8 oz (240 ml)	62
5-6 p.m.	Postexercise snack; milk shake provides protein and carbohydrate to prepare muscles for next day, to reduce muscle soreness, and to sustain energy balance.	Vanilla milk shake	8 oz (240 ml)	246
6-7 p.m.	Dinner consists of foods desired by athlete, plus water.	Stewed beef	1 cup	215
		Carrots, boiled	1 cup	55
		Potato, boiled, no skin	1 medium	118
		Cranberry juice	8 oz (240 ml)	118
		Water	As desired	0
7-10 p.m.	Relaxed activities including homework, discussions with friends and family, and household chores.	Sports drink	8 oz (240 ml)	62
		Water	As desired	0
10-11 p.m.	Snack and bedtime; important to consume this snack to ensure maintenance of blood sugar and energy balance.	Honeydew melon	1 cup	64
		Ice cream, vanilla (regular)	1/2 cup	137

Totals for selected nutrients

Total kcal	2,704	Iron (mg)	14.96	Vit C (mg)	230	Vit B_{12} (mcg)	5.23
Carbohydrate (g)	436	Calcium (mg)	980	Vit B_1 (mg)	2.48	Folic acid (DFE)	539.83
Protein (g)	92	Zinc (mg)	14.4	Vit B_2 (mg)	3.41	Vit A (RAE)	1,982
Fat (g)	76	Magnesium (mg)	544.9	Niacin (mg)	32.88	Vit D (IU)	142.5
Sodium (mg)	3,113	Potassium (mg)	5,403	Vit B_6 (mg)	3.64	Vit E (mg)	6.74

Note: This young pairs skater must balance being small enough to manage the difficult individual skills of skating (spins, jumps) but also strong enough to do multiple lifts with his 115 lb (52 kg) female partner. This diet maintains a good energy balance throughout the day, and it also maintains an anabolic:catabolic hourly ratio of 1.0, which should enable this athlete to sustain muscle mass and weight. Working food and activity into a school day is particularly difficult for many young athletes and requires planning.

Source: Energy balance and nutrient intake values were derived using NutriTiming®. The energy balance graph is copyrighted by NutriTiming LLC and is used with permission.

Table 16.4 3,100-Calorie Food Plan for a 5'11" (180 cm), 170 lb (77 kg) 27-Year-Old Male Power/Speed Athlete

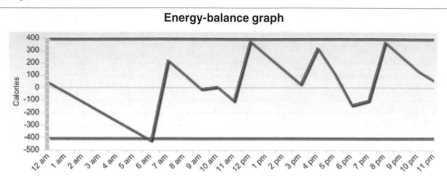

Energy-balance graph

Hours anabolic (calories > 0) = 14; hours catabolic (calories < 0) = 10; anabolic:catabolic ratio = 1.4

Energy Substrate Distribution

Total calories: 3,065   **Carbohydrate %:** 59   **Protein %:** 19   **Fat %:** 23

Hour	Activity	Food	Amount	Calories
7-8 a.m.	Hearty breakfast needed to ensure sufficient glycogen storage (both muscles and liver) to help replenish the previous day's glycogen loss and prepare for the evening's practice.	Cereal, Cheerios	1.5 cups	154
		Strawberries	1 cup	49
		Milk, 1% fat	8 oz (240 ml)	102
		English muffin, multigrain, toasted	1 muffin	156
		Peanut butter, chunk style	2 tbsp	188
		Orange juice	8 oz (240 ml)	110
8-10 a.m.	Any regular daytime activity that does not elevate the heart rate.	Water	As desired	0
10-11 a.m.	Morning snack; snack important for sustaining within-day energy balance.	Banana	1 medium	134
11 a.m.-12 p.m.	Any regular daytime activity that does not elevate the heart rate.	Water	As desired	0
12-1 p.m.	Nourishing lunch; athlete should consume water liberally whenever food is consumed.	Beef, roasted, thinly sliced	4 oz (125 g)	133
		Bread, multigrain	3 slices	207
		Mustard, prepared, yellow	1 tsp	3
		Mayonnaise	1/2 tsp	52
		Lettuce, romaine	2 leafs	2
		Pretzels, hard	1 oz (30 g)	106
		Apple, with skin	1 large	98
1-4 p.m.	Any regular daytime activity that does not elevate the heart rate.	Water	As desired	0

Hour	Activity	Food	Amount	Calories
4-5 p.m.	Preactivity snack followed by warm-up; snack should be consumed early in the hour; late in the hour the warm-up should begin for the late-afternoon practice.	Almonds, roasted	1 oz (30 g)	163
		Yogurt, fruit, low fat	8 oz	243
5-6 p.m.	Intense practice; fluids providing carbohydrate, sodium, and potassium are important to sustain high-intensity activity.	Sports drink	16 oz (480 ml)	125
		Coconut water	16 oz (480 ml)	91
6-7 p.m.	Intense practice; fluids providing carbohydrate, sodium, and potassium are important to sustain high-intensity activity.	Sports drink	16 oz (480 ml)	125
		Coconut water	8 oz (240 ml)	46
7-8 p.m.	Consumption of a carbohydrate drink that has good-quality protein is important for exercise recovery.	Chocolate milk, low fat	8 oz (240 ml)	190
8-9 p.m.	Dinner; water should be consumed liberally with all food consumption.	Chicken breast, roasted, no skin	5 oz (150 g)	245
		Sweet potato, baked in skin	1 large	162
		Margarine-like spread	1 tbsp	85
		Zucchini, raw	1 cup	20
		Dinner roll, whole wheat	1 roll	76
		Water	As desired	0
9-10 p.m.	Any regular daytime activity that does not elevate the heart rate.			

Totals for selected nutrients

Total kcal	3,065	Iron (mg)	32.16	Vit C (mg)	310	Vit B_{12} (mcg)	8.23
Carbohydrate (g)	462	Calcium (mg)	1,799	Vit B_1 (mg)	2.99	Folic acid (DFE)	1,234
Protein (g)	146	Zinc (mg)	22.6	Vit B_2 (mg)	4.32	Vit A (RAE)	2,529
Fat (g)	79	Magnesium (mg)	790	Niacin (mg)	53.57	Vit D (IU)	226.9
Sodium (mg)	4,692	Potassium (mg)	7,577	Vit B_6 (mg)	4.81	Vit E (mg)	15.82

Note: This represents the exercise and food intake for a wall climber who has 2 hr of intense late-afternoon practice. The food (energy) intake matches energy expenditure, so the athlete stays in a good within-day energy balance that allows him to spend more time in an anabolic state than a catabolic state. This intake and energy expenditure should allow the athlete to improve lean mass while sustaining a relatively low body-fat level.

Source: Energy balance and nutrient intake values were derived using NutriTiming®. The energy balance graph is copyrighted by NutriTiming LLC and is used with permission.

Table 16.5 3,400-Calorie Food Plan for a 6'2" (188 cm), 200 lb (91 kg) 21-Year-Old Male Power/Speed Athlete

Energy-balance graph

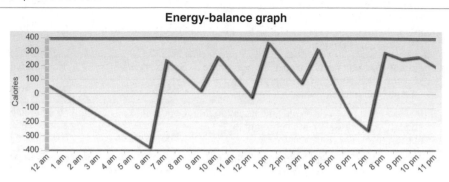

Hours anabolic (calories > 0) = 15; hours catabolic (calories < 0) = 9; anabolic:catabolic ratio = 1.67

Energy Substrate Distribution

Total calories: 3,397		Carbohydrate %: 62	Protein %: 19		Fat %: 19

Hour	Activity	Food	Amount	Calories
7-8 a.m.	Breakfast that provides calories, protein, and carbohydrate to support muscle glycogen and muscle recovery.	Eggs, scrambled	2 large eggs	199
		Bagel, egg	4 oz (90 g)	240
		Bacon, Canadian style	2 oz	69
		Orange juice	16 oz (480 ml)	219
8-10 a.m.	Any relaxed walking, sitting, household, or school activities.	Water	As desired	0
10-11 a.m.	Morning snack; snack is important to maintain blood sugar and provide an ongoing source of carbohydrate.	Cantaloupe, raw	1 cup	60
		Strawberries, raw	1 cup	49
		Yogurt, fruit, low fat	8 oz	243
11 a.m.-1 p.m.	Any relaxed walking, sitting, household, or school activities.	Water	As desired	0
1-2 p.m.	A nourishing lunch that is relatively low in fat to support speedy gastric emptying.	Beef, roasted, eye of round	2 oz (60 g)	120
		Rice, white, long-grain	1/4 cup	49
		Beans, refried, traditional style	1/2 cup	108
		Cheese, cheddar	1 oz (30 g)	114
		Flour Tortillas, soft taco, 8 in (20 cm)	1 tortillas	146
2-4 p.m.	Any relaxed walking, sitting, household, or school activities.	Water	As desired	0
4-5 p.m.	Afternoon snack and warm-up; this snack should be consumed early in the hour, with the warm-up beginning during the last 15 min of the hour.	Cheese, mozzarella, part-skim milk	2 oz (60 g)	142
		Pretzels, hard, salted	1 oz (30 g)	106
		Grapes	1 cup	104

Hour	Activity	Food	Amount	Calories
5-6 p.m.	Intense practice with a large volume of fluid loss through sweat; beverages help support muscle glycogen and fluid balance; coconut water has about the same sodium and carbohydrate and slightly more potassium than many sports beverages and is a good alternative to commercial sports beverages.	Sports drink	16 oz (480 ml)	125
		Coconut water	8 oz (240 ml)	46
6-7 p.m.		Sports drink	16 oz (480 ml)	125
		Coconut water	16 oz (480 ml)	91
7-8 p.m.	Postexercise snack; chocolate milk is an effective postexercise beverage.	Chocolate milk, low fat	8 oz (240 ml)	158
8-9 p.m.	Nourishing, well-balanced dinner.	Shrimp, cooked in moist heat	6 oz	168
		Rice, brown, long-grain, cooked	1 cup	216
		Collards, boiled, with salt	1 cup	49
		Dinner roll, whole wheat	1 roll	114
		Margarine spread (about 48% fat)	2 tsp	42
		Mango	1 cup	107
9-10 p.m.	Any relaxed walking, sitting, household, or school activities.	Sports drink	8 oz (240 ml)	63
10-11 p.m.	Evening snack; this snack helps ensure that liver glycogen can support blood sugar throughout the night of sleep.	Ice cream, lite vanilla (low fat)	1/2 cup	125

Totals for selected nutrients

Total kcal	3,397	Iron (mg)	28.70	Vit C (mg)	457	Vit B_{12} (mcg)	7.55
Carbohydrate (g)	530	Calcium (mg)	2,315	Vit B_1 (mg)	2.70	Folic acid (DFE)	759.4
Protein (g)	167	Zinc (mg)	19.78	Vit B_2 (mg)	3.39	Vit A (RAE)	1,884
Fat (g)	73	Magnesium (mg)	725.71	Niacin (mg)	27.49	Vit D (IU)	67.3
Sodium (mg)	5,709	Potassium (mg)	7,031	Vit B_6 (mg)	3.07	Vit E (mg)	9.17

Note: This food plan represents the intake for an American football player with 2 hr of late-afternoon practice. The food intake is matched to energy expenditure so that the athlete stays in good within-day energy balance (±400 calories) and maintains more hours in an anabolic state than in a catabolic state. This type of intake should enable the athlete to support muscle mass and maintain a low body-fat percentage.

Source: Energy balance and nutrient intake values were derived using NutriTiming®. The energy balance graph is copyrighted by NutriTiming LLC and is used with permission.

Table 16.6   3,700-Calorie Food Plan for a 6'0" (183 cm), 190 lb (86 kg) 22-Year-Old
Male Power/Speed Athlete

Energy-balance graph

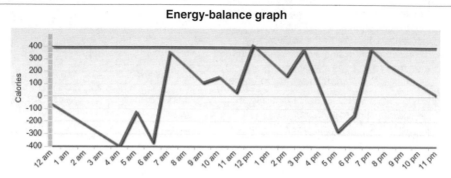

Hours anabolic (calories > 0) = 15; hours catabolic (calories < 0) = 9; anabolic:catabolic ratio = 1.67

Energy Substrate Distribution

Total calories: 3,676   **Carbohydrate %:** 61   **Protein %:** 15   **Fat %:** 24

Hour	Activity	Food	Amount	Calories
5-6 a.m.	Should be consumed as soon as the athlete wakes up (before dressing, driving to pool).	Apple juice with vitamin C	12 oz (360 ml)	171
		Bread, whole wheat, toasted	2 slices	171
		Jam	1 tbsp	56
6-7 a.m.	A moderately intense swim practice.	Sports drink	16 oz (480 ml)	125
7-8 a.m.	Breakfast should be available as soon as the athlete has completed the cool-down.	Cereal, granola	1 cup	443
		Milk, 1% fat	8 oz (240 ml)	102
		English muffin, whole grain	1 muffin	156
		Blueberries	1 cup	84
		Orange juice	8 oz (240 ml)	110
		Peanut butter, chunk style, with salt	1 tbsp	94
		Bread, whole wheat, toasted	1 slice	77
8 a.m.-12 p.m.	Any relaxed walking, sitting, or household activities.	Water	As desired	0
12-1 p.m.	This hearty lunch will help the athlete sustain a good within-day energy balance.	Ham, roasted, lean	3 oz (90 g)	140
		Cheese, Swiss	1 oz (30 g)	108
		Mustard, prepared, yellow	1 tsp	3
		Lettuce, romaine, shredded	.5 cup	4
		Roll, hard (Kaiser type)	1 roll	167
		Apple, with skin	1 large	85
1-3 p.m.	Any relaxed walking, sitting, or household activities.	Water	As desired	0

Hour	Activity	Food	Amount	Calories
3-4 p.m.	Preexercise snack; this is an important snack before the 2 hr swim practice; it should be consumed early in the hour.	Grapes	1 cup	62
		Crackers, wheat, regular	1 oz (30 g)	134
		Cheese, mozzarella, part-skim milk	2 oz (60 g)	142
4-5 p.m.	Swim practice creates a high energy expenditure and, even though the athlete is in the water, a good deal of water loss; the sports drinks are important for sustaining blood volume and blood sugar during this long practice.	Sports drink	16 oz (480 ml)	125
5-6 p.m.		Sports drink	16 oz (480 ml)	125
6-7 p.m.	Postexercise replenishment; important to help replenish some muscle glycogen used during practice.	Chocolate milk, low fat	8 oz (240 ml)	190
		Vanilla wafers, regular	5 wafers	147
7-8 p.m.	This hearty dinner will help the athlete replenish some of the energy used during practice and help prepare him for the next day.	Steak, porterhouse, lean, broiled	4 oz (125 g)	321
		Potato, baked	1 medium potato	145
		Sour cream	1 tbsp	23
		Broccoli, boiled	1 large stalk	84
		Pineapple, fresh	1 cup chunks	82
8-9 p.m.	Any relaxed walking, sitting, or household activities.	Water	As desired	0

Totals for selected nutrients

Total kcal	3,676	Iron (mg)	21.4	Vit C (mg)	543	Vit B_{12} (mcg)	6.40
Carbohydrate (g)	572	Calcium (mg)	1,848	Vit B_1 (mg)	3.07	Folic acid (DFF)	716.2
Protein (g)	142	Zinc (mg)	18.6	Vit B_2 (mg)	3.10	Vit A (RAE)	777
Fat (g)	101	Magnesium (mg)	479.2	Niacin (mg)	32.45	Vit D (IU)	227
Sodium (mg)	4,431	Potassium (mg)	5,507	Vit B_6 (mg)	3.2	Vit E (mg)	7.7

Note: This power swimmer has 2 practices daily: a 1 hr practice early in the morning at 6 a.m. and a 2 hr practice in the late afternoon. Failure to nutritionally support this level of intensity with the right amount and timing of nutrient intake will result in inevitable symptoms of overtraining and failure of the athlete. This plan incorporates food and beverage intake to support both practices and does so while maintaining a good within-day energy balance. Importantly, this eating plan allows the athlete to spend more time in an anabolic state than a catabolic state, which should enable good support of muscle while sustaining a relatively low body-fat percentage. Water should be consumed liberally throughout the day, particularly with food consumption.

Source: Energy balance and nutrient intake values were derived using NutriTiming®. The energy balance graph is copyrighted by NutriTiming LLC and is used with permission.

Table 16.7 4,600-Calorie Food Plan for a 6'4" (193 cm), 230 lb (104 kg) 20-Year-Old Male Lineman

Energy-balance graph

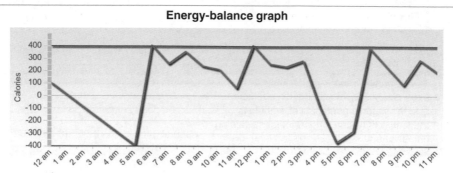

Hours anabolic (calories > 0) = 17; hours catabolic (calories < 0) = 7; anabolic:catabolic ratio = 2.43

Energy Substrate Distribution

Total calories: 4,603   **Carbohydrate %:** 64   **Protein %:** 15   **Fat %:** 21

Hour	Activity	Food	Amount	Calories
6-7 a.m.	Important to consume breakfast as soon as the athlete wakes up (before dressing, driving to practice).	Yogurt, fruit, low fat	8 oz	243
		Toast, multigrain	4 slices	276
		Strawberry jam	2 tbsp	111
		Eggs, hard boiled	2 large	156
		Orange juice	12 oz (360 ml)	164
7-8 a.m.	Preparation for morning football practice.	Water	As desired	
8-9 a.m.	Warm-up; should be consumed early in the hour.	Protein/energy bar	1 bar	322
		Water	As desired	0
9-11 a.m.	Intense practice for 1 hr 45 min; last 15 min is cool-down; the sports beverage should be sipped on throughout the practice.	Sports beverage	48 oz (1.5 L)	381
11 a.m.-12 p.m.	This hearty lunch will help the athlete sustain a good within-day energy balance; athlete should be encouraged to consume plenty of water with lunch.	Ham, roasted, lean	3 oz (90 g)	140
		Cheese, Swiss	1 oz (30 g)	108
		Mustard, prepared, yellow	1 tsp	3
		Lettuce, romaine, shredded	.5 cup	4
		Roll, hard (Kaiser type)	1 roll	167
		Apple, with skin	1 large	85
		Water	As desired	0
12-1 p.m.	Relaxed activities.	Water	As desired	0
1-3 p.m.	Any relaxed walking, studying, sitting, or household activities.	Grapes	1 cup	62
		Wheat crackers	1 oz	134

Hour	Activity	Food	Amount	Calories
3-5 p.m.	Slightly less intense than the morning practice; the sports beverage should be sipped on regularly throughout the practice.	Sports beverage	32 oz (960 ml)	250
5-6 p.m.	Postexercise nourishment; important for this to be consumed immediately after practice.	Chocolate milk, low fat	16 oz (480 ml)	190
6-7 p.m.	Snacking is an important strategy for maintaining energy balance and replenishing glycogen stores.	Vanilla wafers, regular	5 wafers	93
		Water	As desired	0
7-8 p.m.	This hearty dinner will help the athlete replenish some of the energy used during practice in preparation for the next day.	Steak, porterhouse, lean, broiled	6 oz (175 g)	481
		Potato, baked	1 medium potato	145
		Sour cream	1 tbsp	23
		Broccoli, boiled	1 large stalk	84
		Pineapple, fresh	1 cup chunks	82
8-9 p.m.	Any relaxed walking, sitting, or household activities.	Water	As desired	0
9-10 p.m.	Snack and sleep at 10 p.m.; early sleep because of the early-morning practice.	Popcorn, air popped	4 cups	124
		Apple juice	16 oz (480 ml)	228

Totals for selected nutrients

Total kcal	4,603	Iron (mg)	30.6	Vit C (mg)	661	Vit B_{12} (mcg)	15.9
Carbohydrate (g)	740	Calcium (mg)	2,410	Vit B_1 (mg)	4.9	Folic acid (DFE)	1,345
Protein (g)	174	Zinc (mg)	28.4	Vit B_2 (mg)	5.8	Vit A (RAE)	1,085
Fat (g)	110	Magnesium (mg)	707	Niacin (mg)	54.8	Vit D (IU)	306
Sodium (mg)	4,720	Potassium (mg)	6,901	Vit B_6 (mg)	5.9	Vit E (mg)	107

Note: This is a collegiate football player (lineman) with 2 practices daily. These practices are energy draining and predispose athletes to dehydration because there is little time to return to a hydrated state before the 2nd practice. This diet plan manages to provide sufficient energy through a combination of frequent eating and nearly constant drinking. The athlete who follows this plan will sustain a desirable energy balance and, because more time is spent in an anabolic state than in a catabolic state, is in a position to enlarge the muscle mass.

Source: Energy balance and nutrient intake values were derived using NutriTiming®. The energy balance graph is copyrighted by NutriTiming LLC and is used with permission.

Sports Requiring Endurance

Endurance athletes, including distance runners, triathletes, distance swimmers, cyclists, cross-country skiers, and rowers, spend long hours in training and competition. The high volume of training they do underlies the importance they place on consumption of adequate calories to fuel the activity and sufficient fluids to sustain body temperature. Although endurance-trained athletes have a superb capacity to burn fat as a source of energy and use fat as the *primary* source of energy during endurance events, it is their ability to stay well hydrated and store carbohydrate, as glycogen, that is the critical factor in endurance competitions. All athletes have a phenomenally high capacity to store fat (and have all the necessary aerobic enzymes to metabolize it), but there is an inherent limit to how much glycogen (stored carbohydrate) a human can store. Since this stored carbohydrate enables a more complete oxidation of fat for energy and is the primary fuel for higher-intensity work (e.g., the high-speed kick successful endurance runners employ at the end of a race), endurance athletes can't afford to let glycogen run out. This is precisely the reason so many endurance athletes consume large volumes of pasta and other carbohydrate foods before a race.

However, *how* the carbohydrate is provided can influence how well the glycogen is stored. Although endurance athletes can effectively process carbohydrates into stored glycogen, this process takes time and water. Water is necessary because for every gram of stored glycogen, 3 grams of water are needed. Because there is a limit to how quickly a cell can convert excess glucose to stored glycogen, endurance athletes should focus on consuming carbohydrate frequently over the course of several days rather than relying solely on a belly-busting high-carbohydrate meal on the day before an event.

ABOUT THE EATING PLANS

This chapter includes five eating plans for intakes of 1,900 (lacto-ovo vegetarian), 2,000 (gluten free), 2,300, 2,800, and 4,500 calories. To help athletes understand how to best integrate an eating plan into their exercise schedules, the plans include differently timed practice sessions. The foods are consumed around the practice sessions in a way that helps sustain energy balance throughout the day (± 400 calories) and also helps distribute protein and other nutrients throughout the day. Rather than viewing energy balance just at the end of the day, the eating plans include information on the number of hours spent in a catabolic state (i.e., energy balance is below 0) or in an anabolic state (i.e., energy balance is above 0). An anabolic:catabolic ratio of 1 should result in weight and body composition stabilization; a ratio of >1 should allow the athlete to increase muscle mass; and a ratio of <1 should help the athlete lower body-fat percentage. The goal is to provide a *guide* for eating that gives athletes a starting point for developing the best possible eating strategy for them.

It is important to note that the caloric level of these diets is for illustration only and is not likely to be perfect for anyone. Weight stability and a healthy body-fat level are the best guides that an appropriate number of calories is being consumed at the right times. Athletes should find a caloric intake level and intake pattern that works for them as individuals. It is also important to note that fluid intakes are likely to be much higher than the fluids listed here. Athletes should consume ample quantities of water with meals and may also need to consume more sports beverages during bouts of physical activity. Athletes should drink enough to sustain optimal body water, an indication of which is nearly clear urine.

Table 17.1   1,900-Calorie Food Plan for a 5'2" (157 cm), 120 lb (54 kg) 18-Year-Old
Female Endurance Athlete (Lacto-Ovo Vegetarian)

Energy-balance graph

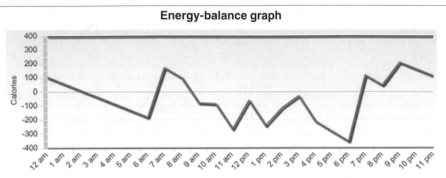

Hours anabolic (calories > 0) = 10; hours catabolic (calories < 14) = 13; anabolic:catabolic ratio = 0.74

Energy Substrate Distribution

Total calories: 1,902   **Carbohydrate %:** 62   **Protein %:** 15   **Fat %:** 23

Hour	Activity	Food	Amount	Calories
7-8 a.m.	Important to consume this breakfast before showering and dressing.	Cranberry juice	8 oz (240 ml)	111
		Scrambled egg	1 large egg	100
		Milk, 1% fat	8 oz (240 ml)	102
		Cereal, Multigrain Cheerios	1 cup	114
8-9 a.m.	Warm-up.	Water	As desired	0
9-11 a.m.	A sports drink during training sustains blood sugar and central nervous system function, provides a source of energy to working muscles, and helps sustain blood volume and sweat rate.	Sports drink	8 oz (240 ml)	65
		Water	As desired	0
11 a.m.-12 p.m.	Cool-down.	Water	As desired	0
12-1 p.m.	This snack should be consumed as soon after exercise as possible; water should be consumed liberally whenever foods are consumed.	Nutri-Grain cereal bar, fruit filled	1 bar	139
		Yogurt, plain, skim milk	1 cup	137
1-2 p.m.	Relaxed activities.	Water	As desired	0
2-3 p.m.	The midafternoon snack is needed to sustain energy balance and to continue to replenish glycogen stores.	Ranch dressing	2 oz	172
		Carrots, baby, raw	5 large	26
		Cake, pound, fat free	2 oz (60 g)	158
3-4 p.m.	Warm-up.	Water	As desired	0
4-5 p.m.	A light skills training that helps the athlete work on technique without being exhaustive; fluids can be consumed as needed.	Water	As desired	0
5-7 p.m.	Any relaxed activities, including walking, light housework, and desk work.	Water	As desired	0

Hour	Activity	Food	Amount	Calories
7-9 p.m.	A hearty dinner is important for satisfying energy needs and should contain plenty of carbohydrate.	Milk, 1% fat	8 oz (240 ml)	102
		Salad dressing	1 tbsp	72
		Vegetable salad	1.5 cups	33
		Pasta, cooked	6 oz (175 g)	224
		Marinara sauce	1/2 cup	111
9-10 p.m.	This is an important time to have a snack to ensure sufficient liver glycogen stores to sustain blood sugar through the night.	Chocolate milk, low fat	12 oz (360 ml)	236

Totals for selected nutrients

Total kcal	1,902	Iron (mg)	29.35	Vit C (mg)	106	Vit B$_{12}$ (mcg)	11.84
Carbohydrate (g)	295	Calcium (mg)	2,005	Vit B$_1$ (mg)	2.92	Folic acid (DFE)	1,185
Protein (g)	72	Zinc (mg)	26.29	Vit B$_2$ (mg)	5.31	Vit A (RAE)	1,683
Fat (g)	49	Magnesium (mg)	296.6	Niacin (mg)	35.8	Vit D (IU)	285.7
Sodium (mg)	2,428	Potassium (mg)	3,494	Vit B$_6$ (mg)	3.76	Vit E (mg)	18.8

Note: This endurance athlete has a moderately intensive running regimen in the morning for 90 min, followed by a shorter and less intense training regimen in the early afternoon. While calorically balanced, her food plan causes her to spend more time in a catabolic than anabolic state, which should result in achieving one of her goals of losing some body fat. Importantly, the daily diet manages to keep her in a good within-day energy balance, which should also help sustain her lean mass. Her protein intake, while moderate, still fulfills her needs by providing 1.33 g of protein per kilogram of body weight.

Source: Energy balance and nutrient intake values were derived using NutriTiming®. The energy balance graph is copyrighted by NutriTiming LLC and is used with permission.

Table 17.2 2,000-Calorie Food Plan for a 5'1" (155 cm), 110 lb (50 kg) 25-Year-Old Female Cyclist (Gluten-Free Intake)

Energy-balance graph

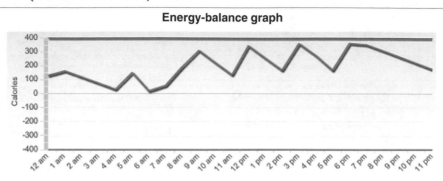

Hours anabolic (calories > 0) = 24; hours catabolic (calories < 0) = 0; anabolic:catabolic ratio = >1 (no hr catabolic)

Energy Substrate Distribution

Total calories: 2,019   **Carbohydrate %:** 61   **Protein %:** 18   **Fat %:** 21

Hour	Activity	Food	Amount	Calories
6-7 a.m.	Breakfast early in hour, 30 min of stretching followed by a 30 min bike ride; important to start the day with enough calories to satisfy activity.	"Food for Life" brown rice gluten-free bread	2 slices	219
		Cytomax	2.25 scoops	226
7-8 a.m.	An additional 30 min bike ride, followed by stretching exercises; a small amount of high-quality protein with resistance activity encourages enlargement of muscle mass.	Whey protein isolate (gluten free)	1 scoop	78
8-9 a.m.	A hearty breakfast; note the nontraditional foods consumed to sustain gluten-free intake.	Egg, boiled	1 large	70
		Baked potato, with skin	1 small	116
		Peppers, sweet, red, raw	1 cup sliced	30
		Spinach, raw	1/2 oz (25 g)	3
		Yogurt, plain, skim milk	6 oz (175 g)	95
9-10 a.m.	Snack at 9:50 a.m.; workplace activity.	Strawberries, fresh, raw	1/3 cup	18
		Blueberries, fresh, raw	1/4 cup	20
		Mango, fresh, raw	1/4 cup	26
		Coconut, shredded	1 tbsp	47
10-11 a.m.	Workplace activity.	Water	As desired	0
11 a.m.-12 p.m.	Workplace activity.	Water	As desired	0

Hour	Activity	Food	Amount	Calories
12-1 p.m.	Lunch; it is unlikely that a gluten-free lunch would be available at the workplace, so this must be planned in advance and brought to work in a cooler to avoid spoilage.	Water chestnuts, Chinese	4 nuts	44
		Broccoli, raw	3/4 cup	24
		Carrots, baby, raw	1/6 cup	16
		Chicken, light meat, roasted,	1 oz (30 g)	49
		Almonds	2 tsp (10 g)	58
		"Food for Life" brown rice gluten-free bread	1 slice	110
		Water	As desired	0
1-3 p.m.	Workplace activity.	Water	As desired	0
3-4 p.m.	Midafternoon snack; this is an important snack while at work to sustain energy balance and blood sugar.	Amy's black bean vegetable soup	1 can	279
4-5 p.m.	Drive home, stretch, and strength activities.	Water	As desired	0
5-6 p.m.	This predinner snack is important to obtain needed nutrients and to sustain the desired anabolic state to help build muscle.	Spinach, raw	1 oz (50 g)	12
		Carrots, raw	8 large (100 g)	41
6-8 p.m.	This traditional dinner is composed entirely of gluten-free foods—there can be *no* exceptions in sustaining a gluten-free intake.	Tomatoes, red cherry	1/2 cup	14
		Salmon, pink, canned	2 oz (60 g)	79
		Gluten-free Caesar dressing	1 tbsp	75
		Food for Life brown rice gluten-free bread	3/4 slice	82
		Peppers, sweet, red, raw	1/2 cup (75 g)	23
		Amy's lentil soup	1/4 can	89
8-9 p.m.	Relaxed activities.	Water	As desired	0
9-10 p.m.	The evening snack is important to sustain blood sugar throughout the night.	Peppers, sweet, red, raw	1/3 cup (60 g)	19
		Cashew nuts, dry roast, with salt	1/3 oz (10 g)	57

Totals for selected nutrients

Total kcal	2,019	Iron (mg)	15.78	Vit C (mg)	659	Vit B$_{12}$ (mcg)	4.11
Carbohydrate (g)	313	Calcium (mg)	935	Vit B$_1$ (mg)	.70	Folic acid (DFE)	461
Protein (g)	92	Zinc (mg)	6.15	Vit B$_2$ (mg)	1.54	Vit A (RAE)	2,777
Fat (g)	47	Magnesium (mg)	324	Niacin (mg)	16.08	Vit D (IU)	355
Sodium (mg)	1,019	Potassium (mg)	3,662	Vit B$_6$ (mg)	2.32	Vit E (mg)	14.9

Note: This athlete has celiac disease that was undiagnosed and resulted in a significant loss of muscle mass. After the diagnosis of celiac disease, the athlete has been maintaining a gluten-free diet and has adjusted her exercise and eating schedule to enable an enlargement of the muscle mass. The greater amount of time spent in an anabolic state (zero hours spent catabolic) is the energy balance profile for someone wishing to increase lean mass. This athlete has a very early workout for 1 hr followed by typical daily activities the rest of the day, with multiple eating opportunities to maintain an anabolic profile throughout the day.

Source: Energy balance and nutrient intake values were derived using NutriTiming®. The energy balance graph is copyrighted by NutriTiming LLC and is used with permission.

Table 17.3 2,300-Calorie Food Plan for a 5'0" (152 cm), 100 lb (45 kg) 20-Year-Old Female Figure Skater

Energy-balance graph

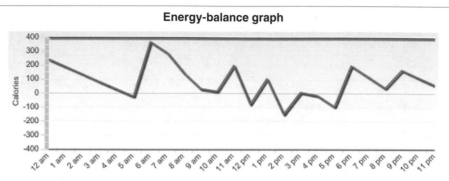

Hours anabolic (calories > 0) = 19; hours catabolic (calories < 0) = 5; anabolic:catabolic ratio = 3.80

Energy Substrate Distribution

Total calories: 2,280   **Carbohydrate %:** 68   **Protein %:** 10   **Fat %:** 22

Hour	Activity	Food	Amount	Calories
6-8 a.m.	Breakfast; consumption of some food before the morning workout is critically important for maintaining blood sugar and energy balance during the subsequent exercise.	2 slices toasted whole wheat	2 slices	90
		1 large egg, fried	1 large egg	97
		1 slice American cheese, low fat	1 oz	51
		Sweetened ice tea with lemon flavor	12 oz (360 ml)	126
8-9 a.m.	Warm-up, 30 min.			
9-10 a.m.	Snack, then 50-min exercise.	Grapes, red	1 cup	104
		Sports drink	8 oz (240 ml)	63
10-11 a.m.	Cool-down; consumption of a rehydration beverage after exercise is important for returning to a hydrated state and replenishing used glycogen stores.	Sports drink	8 oz (240 ml)	63
11 a.m.-12 p.m.	Lunch should be consumed early in the hour to allow sufficient time for gastric emptying before skills practice at 12:10.	Tofu, dried-frozen (koyadofu)	1 piece (2/3 oz)	82
		Beans, snap, green, boiled, with salt	1/2 cup	22
		Yogurt, fruit, low fat	4.4 oz (125 g)	135
		Grapes, red	1 cup	104
		Plum	1 medium	30
		Water	As desired	0
12-1 p.m.	Skills practice for 50 min.	Water	As desired	0

Hour	Activity	Food	Amount	Calories
1-2 p.m.	The frequent exercise schedule requires that the athlete take every available opportunity to consume snacks and fluids.	Granola bar with fruit	2.5 oz (70 g)	264
		Water	As desired	0
2-3 p.m.	Weight training for 60 min.	Sports drink	8 oz (240 ml)	63
3-4 p.m.	A snack after a workout, particularly carbohydrate (bread and apple) and good-quality protein (cheese), is important for glycogen recovery and for reducing muscle soreness.	Bread, whole wheat	2 slices	133
		Cheese, processed, American	1 slice	105
		Apple, with skin	1 medium	57
		Water	As desired	0
4-6 p.m.	Preparation for dinner.	Water	As desired	0
6-7 p.m.	This high-carbohydrate dinner is desirable for athletes who must recover glycogen for the next day of activity.	Spaghetti	1.25 cups	275
		Meatballs	2 oz	60
		Marinara sauce	1/3 cup	39
7-9 p.m.	Relaxed activities.	Water	As desired	0
9-10 p.m.	Evening snack; relax.	Grapes, red	2 cups	208

Totals for selected nutrients

Total kcal	2,280	Iron (mg)	15.9	Vit C (mg)	93	Vit B$_{12}$ (mcg)	1.91
Carbohydrate (g)	398	Calcium (mg)	837	Vit B$_1$ (mg)	1.82	Folic acid (DFE)	369
Protein (g)	59	Zinc (mg)	7.59	Vit B$_2$ (mg)	2.36	Vit A (RAE)	757
Fat (g)	58	Magnesium (mg)	2.71	Niacin (mg)	17.85	Vit D (IU)	0.00
Sodium (mg)	3,508	Potassium (mg)	3,165	Vit B$_6$ (mg)	2.03	Vit E (mg)	2.50

Note: This day is typical of a figure skater who has multiple skating sessions involving warm-ups, skating, jumps and lifts, and weight training. The food intake is spaced in a way that keeps the athlete in a good within-day energy balance throughout the day to ensure a good maintenance of the muscle mass and a low body-fat percentage. This eating and exercise plan results in a high anabolic-to-catabolic ratio, enabling this athlete to sustain or increase muscle mass while reducing the chance for increasing body-fat percentage.

Source: Energy balance and nutrient intake values were derived using NutriTiming®. The energy balance graph is copyrighted by NutriTiming LLC and is used with permission.

Table 17.4   2,800-Calorie Food Plan for a 5'9" (175 cm), 140 lb (64 kg) 27-Year-Old Male Endurance Athlete

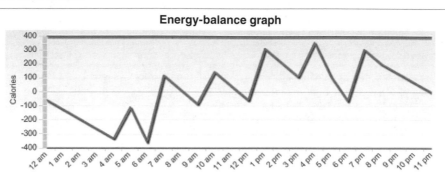

Hours anabolic (calories > 0) = 14; hours catabolic (calories < 0) = 10; anabolic:catabolic ratio = 1.4

Energy Substrate Distribution

Total calories: 2,801   **Carbohydrate %:** 66   **Protein %:** 19   **Fat %:** 15

Hour	Activity	Food	Amount	Calories
5-6 a.m.	Preexercise meal (consumed immediately upon awakening); failure to consume energy before morning exercise may predispose the athlete to low blood sugar and a low energy balance that could make maintenance of muscle mass difficult.	Bread, whole wheat, toasted	2 slices	171
		Jam	1 tbsp	39
		Apple juice, unsweetened, with vitamin C	8 oz (240 ml)	114
6-7 a.m.	Morning run, 60 min.	Sports drink	12 oz (360 ml)	94
7-8 a.m.	As early as possible, even during the cooldown and stretch, athlete should consume fluids (orange juice and milk) to enhance glycogen replacement and enable better muscle recovery.	Orange juice	8 oz (240 ml)	109
		Oatmeal cereal, cooked	1 cup	159
		Milk, 1% fat	8 oz (240 ml)	102
		Strawberries	1 cup	49
		Egg, whole, poached	1 large	71
		Bread, whole wheat, toasted	1 slice	88
		Margarine, Harvest Soft (80% fat)	1 tsp	34
		Water	As desired	0
8-9 a.m.	Prepare for work.	Water	As desired	0
9-10 a.m.	Normal work activities.	Water	As desired	0
10-11 a.m.	Morning snack; small frequent meals make sustaining good energy balance much easier and may also lower body-fat percentage.	Bagel, egg	1 small	192
		Cream cheese, low fat	1 tbsp	30
		Cranberry juice cocktail	8 oz (240 ml)	111
11 a.m.-12 p.m.	Normal work activities.	Water	As desired	0
12-1 p.m.	Normal work activities.	Water	As desired	0

Hour	Activity	Food	Amount	Calories
1-2 p.m.	Lunch at place of work; this lunch may not easily be obtained at work so will need to be brought to work in a cooler to maintain freshness.	Tuna, light, canned in water	3 oz (90 g)	97
		Oil and vinegar dressing	1 tbsp	72
		Celery	1/4 cup	4
		Lettuce, romaine	2 cups	16
		Tomato, fresh	1/2 cup	13
		Corn, canned	1/2 cup	83
		Beans, kidney, canned	1/4 cup	54
		Dinner roll, wheat	1 roll	76
		Cantaloupe, cubed	1 cup	60
		Water	As desired	0
2-3 p.m.	Normal work activities.	Water	As desired	0
3-4 p.m.	Normal work activities.	Water	As desired	0
4-5 p.m.	The midafternoon snack is important for maintaining energy balance within narrow bounds.	Yogurt, fruit, low fat	1 cup	243
		Pretzels, hard, salted	1 oz (30 g)	106
5-6 p.m.	Afternoon run, 60 min.	Sports drink	12 oz (360 ml)	94
6-7 p.m.	Continuation of run for 30 min.	Sports drink	6 oz (180 ml)	47
7-8 p.m.	This is a hearty dinner but is relatively low in fat, making it easier to deliver desired energy in a filling meal.	Chicken, light meat, roasted, no skin	4 oz (125 g)	196
		Broccoli, boiled	1 cup	84
		Carrots, boiled	1/4 cup	14
		Celery	1/2 cup	8
		Peppers, sweet, red, raw	1/2 cup	23
		Onions, sweet, raw	1/2 cup	39
		Rice, brown, medium grain, cooked	1/2 cup	109
		Water	As desired	0
8-9 p.m.	Relaxed activities.	Water	As desired	0

Totals for selected nutrients

Total kcal	2,801	Iron (mg)	33.3	Vit C (mg)	689	Vit B_{12} (mcg)	5.91
Carbohydrate (g)	473	Calcium (mg)	1,424	Vit B_1 (mg)	2.97	Folic acid (DFE)	1,173
Protein (g)	136	Zinc (mg)	13.74	Vit B_2 (mg)	3.23	Vit A (RAE)	2151
Fat (g)	46	Magnesium (mg)	561	Niacin (mg)	53.7	Vit D (IU)	143.88
Sodium (mg)	3,101	Potassium (mg)	5,613	Vit B_6 (mg)	4.11	Vit E (mg)	10.38

Note: This diet satisfies the needs of an endurance athlete with a morning and afternoon run. It is critically important for this runner to consume a small, easy-to-digest breakfast before the morning run to ensure normal energy dynamics. The anabolic-to-catabolic energy balance should enable the athlete to easily sustain or even increase muscle mass. Water should be consumed throughout the day as desired, but particularly with food.

Source: Energy balance and nutrient intake values were derived using NutriTiming®. The energy balance graph is copyrighted by NutriTiming LLC and is used with permission.

Table 17.5 4,500-Calorie Food Plan for a 5'11" (180 cm), 160 lb (73kg) 24-Year-Old Male Distance Runner

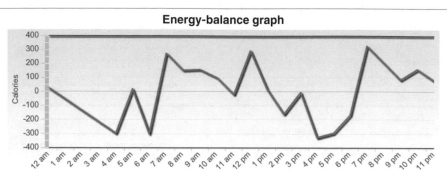

Energy-balance graph

Hours anabolic (calories > 0) = 13; hours catabolic (calories < 0) = 11; anabolic:catabolic ratio = 1.18

Energy Substrate Distribution

Total calories: 4,475 **Carbohydrate %:** 64 **Protein %:** 17 **Fat %:** 19

Hour	Activity	Food	Amount	Calories
5-6 a.m.	Wake-up and prerun nourishment; should be consumed as soon as possible after waking to ensure time for gastric emptying before the morning run.	Bread, whole wheat, toasted	2 slices	153
		Jam	1 tbsp	56
		Apple juice	12 oz (360 ml)	171
6-7 a.m.	A relatively intense run lasting the entire hour.	Sports beverage	16 oz (480 ml)	125
8-9 a.m.	Cool-down followed by breakfast which should include plenty of fluids and should be high in carbohydrate.	Granola cereal, whole grain	1 cup	443
		Milk, 1% fat	8 oz (240 ml)	102
		English muffin, toasted	1/2 muffin	78
		Blueberries	1 cup	84
		Orange juice	8 oz (240 ml)	110
9 a.m.-12 p.m.	Normal daily activities; beverage should be readily available to allow for sips at regular intervals to help athlete return to hydrated state, recover glycogen, and maintain blood sugar.	Sports beverage	24 oz (720 ml)	189
12-1 p.m.	Lunch during early part of the hour; liberal amounts of water should be consumed with foods.	Roast beef sandwich	1 sandwich	477
		Roast beef	5 oz (150 g)	316
		American cheese, regular	1 oz (30g)	106
		Lettuce	1 leaf	4
		Mayonnaise	1/2 tbsp	51
		Water	As desired	0
1-2 p.m.	Weightlifting for 30 min during last half of hour (moderate weights with many repetitions).	Sports beverage	16 oz (480 ml)	127

Hour	Activity	Food	Amount	Calories
2-4 p.m.	Cool-down and stretching, followed by normal activities; midafternoon snack is important for maintaining energy balance and blood sugar.	Apple, with skin	1 medium	65
		Wheat crackers	1 oz (30 g)	134
		Cheese, mozzarella, part-skim milk	2 oz (60 g)	142
		Water	As desired	0
4-5 p.m.	Intense 1 hr run, with sipping on sports beverage that mirrors actual drinking frequency at competition.	Sports beverage	16 oz (480 ml)	125
5-6 p.m.	Postrun cool-down and replenishment; a protein and carbohydrate beverage after a workout reduces muscle soreness and helps replenish glycogen stores.	Chocolate milk	16 oz (480 ml)	315
6-7 p.m.	Household activities and snack; frequent snacking is necessary to supply sufficient energy to maintain energy balance.	Saltine crackers	9 crackers	177
		Milk, 1% fat	12 oz (360 ml)	154
7-10 p.m.	Hearty dinner to satisfy nutrient and energy needs should be consumed between 7 and 8 p.m.	Chicken, roasted, light meat	6 oz (175 g)	363
		Potato, baked	1 medium	145
		Sour cream	1 tbsp	23
		Broccoli, boiled	1 cup	84
10-11 p.m.	Snack and bedtime; evening snack before bedtime is important to prevent low blood sugar during the night and maintain energy balance.	Grapes, fresh	1.5 cups	156

Totals for selected nutrients

Total kcal	4,475	Iron (mg)	24.64	Vit C (mg)	491	Vit B_{12} (mcg)	7.65
Carbohydrate (g)	655	Calcium (mg)	2,403	Vit B_1 (mg)	2.72	Folic acid (DFE)	747.8
Protein (g)	194	Zinc (mg)	19.0	Vit B_2 (mg)	4.25	Vit A (RAE)	1,130
Fat (g)	77	Magnesium (mg)	513.3	Niacin (mg)	52.01	Vit D (IU)	317
Sodium (mg)	4,948	Potassium (mg)	6,581	Vit B_6 (mg)	4.3	Vit E (mg)	6.6

Note: This competitive distance runner has two long and intense training runs plus does weights between the two runs. This level of activity accounts for the high energy need (~4,500 calories), which can be provided only through frequent meals and snacks and nearly constant sipping on sports beverages. The athlete wishes to enlarge his muscle mass to improve the end-of-race sprints, and his anabolic-to-catabolic ratio of >1 suggests he should be able to achieve this with this eating and exercise pattern.

Source: Energy balance and nutrient intake values were derived using NutriTiming®. The energy balance graph is copyrighted by NutriTiming LLC and is used with permission.

Sports Requiring Combined Power and Endurance

Sports requiring a combination of power and endurance, including soccer, golf, figure skating, tennis, volleyball, and basketball, require the ultimate balance in conditioning and often have an additional requirement for a high level of skill that is sport specific. The nutrition demands on athletes involved in team sports are high, with a need for sufficient calories to endure long and frequent practices and enough fluids to sustain hydration state. Unlike many other sports, team sports often have natural breaks during practices and competitions that should be considered by participating athletes as a golden opportunity to replenish carbohydrate stores and fluids. The ideal training regimen is one that gives athletes constant practice in understanding how much fluid they can tolerate during these breaks so that drinking during competitions will be performance enhancing rather than performance detracting. Humans are highly adaptable to food and nutrient intake, so practicing fluid consumption should lead to an enhanced capacity to consume more fluids over time without any GI distress.

Given what we now know to be true from well-designed research studies, athletes who drink plain water during the natural breaks in practice and competition are missing a valuable opportunity to sustain blood volume, sustain sweat rates, and sustain carbohydrate delivery to working muscles. Only carbohydrate- and electrolyte-containing beverages have the potential of fulfilling these during-exercise needs, while plain water alone may actually be counterproductive. Consumption of anything else, such as protein bars, simply detracts from what working muscles really need: carbohydrate and fluid. There is a time for meal-replacement bars that contain vitamins, minerals, and protein, but halftime during a basketball game is not one of those times. In some cases, athletes have adapted to eating a banana, crackers, or bread during halftime, but these should be well practiced *before* a competition to be certain they are well tolerated and leave the stomach before the game restarts.

ABOUT THE EATING PLANS

This chapter includes five eating plans for intakes of 2,300, 2,500, 2,400 (injury recovery), 2,800, and 3,800 calories. To help athletes understand how to best integrate an eating plan into their exercise schedules, the plans include differently timed practice sessions. The foods are consumed around the practice sessions in a way that helps sustain energy balance throughout the day (± 400 calories) and also helps distribute protein and other nutrients throughout the day. Rather than viewing energy balance just at the end of the day, the eating plans include information on the number of hours spent in a catabolic state (i.e., energy balance is below 0) or in an anabolic state (i.e., energy balance is above 0). An anabolic:catabolic ratio of 1 should result in weight and body composition stabilization; a ratio of >1 should allow the athlete to increase muscle mass; and a ratio of <1 should help the athlete lower body-fat percentage. The goal is to provide a *guide* for eating that gives athletes a starting point for developing the best possible eating strategy for them.

It is important to note that the caloric level of these diets is for illustration only and is not likely to be perfect for anyone. Weight stability and a healthy body fat level are the best guides that an appropriate number of calories is being consumed at the right times. Athletes should find a caloric intake level that works for them as individuals. It is also important to note that fluid intakes are likely to be much higher than the fluids listed here. Athletes should consume ample quantities of water with meals and may also need to consume more sports beverages during bouts of physical activity. Athletes should drink enough to sustain optimal body water, an indication of which is nearly clear urine.

Table 18.1 2,300-Calorie Food Plan for a 5'7" (170 cm), 132 lb (60 kg) 19-Year-Old Female Combined Power and Endurance Athlete

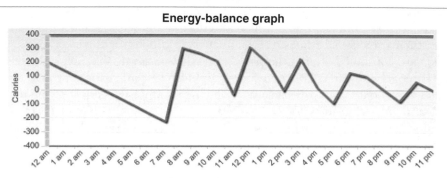

Energy-balance graph

Hours anabolic (calories > 0) = 16; hours catabolic (calories < 0) = 8; anabolic:catabolic ratio = 2.0

Energy Substrate Distribution

Total calories: 2,295   **Carbohydrate %:** 49   **Protein %:** 22   **Fat %:** 30

Hour	Activity	Food	Amount	Calories
8-9 a.m.	Wake-up activities (shower, dress); although many athletes do not consume breakfast before the morning workout, it is important to do so to maintain blood sugar and energy balance.	Eggs, scrambled	2 eggs	199
		Bread, wheat, toasted	2 slices	150
		Peanut butter, smooth, with salt	2 tbsp	188
		Milk, nonfat (skim)	8 oz (240 ml)	83
9-10 a.m.	Preparation for exercise.	Water	As desired	0
10 a.m.-12 p.m.	Warm-up followed by 45 min practice; This intense workout leaves little opportunity for drinking, but the athlete should take whatever opportunities there are to sip on a sports beverage.	Sports drink	8 oz (240 ml)	63
12-1 p.m.	Lunch consumed early in the hour to ensure an empty stomach at the time of the afternoon practice at 2 p.m.	Tuna salad (canned tuna in water, with mayonnaise)	1 cup	383
		Crackers, wheat, low salt	1 oz (30 g)	134
		Salad, vegetable	1.5 cups	33
		Water	As desired	0
2-3 p.m.	Warm-up followed by 45-min practice that begins at 2:15 p.m.	Sports drink	8 oz (240 ml)	63
3-4 p.m.	Relaxed activities; the energy bar and water are important for replenishing fluids and for glycogen and muscle recovery.	Marathon bar	1 bar	322
		Water	As desired	0
4-5 p.m.	Moderate exercise for 45 min.	Sports drink	8 oz (240 ml)	63
5-6 p.m.	Stretch for 15 min followed by weightlifting at 6 p.m.			

Hour	Activity	Food	Amount	Calories
6-7 p.m.	15 min of light weightlifting at the top of the hour, followed by dinner.	Milk, nonfat (skim)	8 oz (240 ml)	83
		Chicken breast, baked or grilled	1.5 oz	66
		Corn on the cob with butter	1 ear	155
		Salad, vegetable	2.5 cups	58
		Creamy Caesar dressing	1 tbsp	48
		Water	As desired	0
7-10 p.m.	Relaxed household activities	Water	As desired	0
10-11 p.m.	Relaxed household activities; evening snack is important for maintaining energy balance throughout the night and preventing low blood sugar.	Popcorn, air popped	3 cups	93
		Cranberry juice cocktail	8 oz (240 ml)	111
11 p.m.	Sleep.			

Totals for selected nutrients

Total kcal	2,295	Iron (mg)	22.23	Vit C (mg)	198	Vit B_{12} (mcg)	12.02
Carbohydrate (g)	282	Calcium (mg)	1,408	Vit B_1 (mg)	2.76	Folic acid (DFE)	982
Protein (g)	126	Zinc (mg)	15.4	Vit B_2 (mg)	3.89	Vit A (RAE)	796
Fat (g)	77	Magnesium (mg)	489	Niacin (mg)	49.71	Vit D (IU)	271.22
Sodium (mg)	3,273	Potassium (mg)	3,369	Vit B_6 (mg)	3.85	Vit E (mg)	108.1

Notes: This represents the typical exercise schedule and intake of a young female basketball player attending summer basketball camp. Fluid intake should be liberal and sufficient to maintain a well-hydrated state. The anabolic-to-catabolic energy-balance ratio of 2.0 should enable this athlete to increase muscle mass and strength while avoiding an increase in body-fat percentage.

Source: Energy balance and nutrient intake values were derived using NutriTiming®. The energy balance graph is copyrighted by NutriTiming LLC and is used with permission.

Table 18.2   2,500-Calorie Food Plan for a 5'2" (157 cm), 110 lb (50 kg) 20-Year-Old Female Combined Power and Endurance Athlete

Energy-balance graph

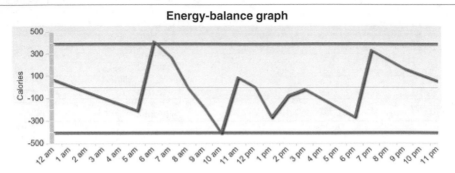

Hours anabolic (calories > 0) = 12; hours catabolic (calories < 0) = 12; anabolic:catabolic ratio = 1.0

Energy Substrate Distribution

Total calories: 2,513   **Carbohydrate %:** 42   **Protein %:** 33   **Fat %:** 25

Hour	Activity	Food	Amount	Calories
6-7 a.m.	Breakfast is important to consume before morning practice; wake-up time should be adjusted to allow for consumption of enough food to maintain energy balance and prevent low.	Blueberries	1 cup	84
		Sausage patty	3 oz (90 g)	348
		Egg whites, cooked	1 cup	117
		Chocolate milk, low fat	8 oz (240 ml)	158
		Water	As desired	0
7-8 a.m.	Wake-up activities (shower, dress) and then warm-up for 25 min.	Tea, brewed (no sugar)	9 oz (270 ml)	3
8-9 a.m.	Moderately high-intensity exercise for 60 min (team practice, drills); coconut water is an appropriate sports beverage substitute (contains sodium, potassium, and carbohydrate) for indoor (i.e., temperature controlled) environments.	Coconut water (as sports beverage)	8 oz (240 ml)	47
9-10 a.m.	Moderately high-intensity exercise for 45 min (team practice, drills).	Coconut water (as sports beverage)	8 oz (240 ml)	47
10-11 a.m.	Moderate-intensity exercise (skills practice) for 30 min.	Water	As desired	0
11 a.m.-12 p.m.	This lunch contains a good balance of carbohydrate and protein yet is relatively low in fat.	Cottage cheese, 1% fat	1 cup	163
		Jam (no sugar added)	1 tbsp	18
		Soy protein isolate (powder to put in a drink)	1 oz (30 g) powder	106
		Banana	1 small	134
		Strawberries	1 cup	49
		Soy milk	8 oz (240 ml)	70
		Chicken breast, grilled	2 oz (60 g)	44
		Water	As desired	0

Hour	Activity	Food	Amount	Calories
12-1 p.m.	Relaxed activities	Water	As desired	0
1-2 p.m.	Warm-up for 15 min, followed by resistance activity for 45 min.	Coconut water (as sports beverage)	8 oz (240 ml)	47
2-4 p.m.	Afternoon snack at 2:30 p.m.; this meal provides plenty of carbohydrate and protein, but with relatively low fat, to satisfy needs.	Peanut butter, smooth, with salt	1 tbsp	94
		Whole wheat bread	1 slice	69
		Ketchup	2 tbsp	10
		Ham patty, grilled	1 oz (30 g)	98
		Corn, sweet, boiled, with salt	1 ear	96
		Tomatoes, red, fresh	1 cup	27
		Water	As desired	0
4-7 p.m.	Typical school activities, including homework and attending meetings.	Water	As desired	0
7-8 p.m.	Dinner; this meal mixes needed carbohydrate and relatively low-fat protein foods.	Chicken, light meat, roasted/diced, no skin	1 cup	242
		Crackers, whole wheat	10 crackers	178
		Yogurt, fruit, low fat	4.4 oz container (125 g)	135
		Fruit juice	10 oz (300 ml)	129
8-9 p.m.	Relaxed activity, including homework and planning for the next day's activities.	Water	As desired	0

Totals for selected nutrients

Total kcal	2,513	Iron (mg)	16.1	Vit C (mg)	1519	Vit B_{12} (mcg)	10.21
Carbohydrate (g)	272	Calcium (mg)	1,572	Vit B_1 (mg)	1.82	Folic acid (DFE)	329
Protein (g)	216	Zinc (mg)	27.7	Vit B_2 (mg)	8.30	Vit A (RAE)	3,861
Fat (g)	72	Magnesium (mg)	557	Niacin (mg)	87.27	Vit D (IU)	119
Sodium (mg)	5,071	Potassium (mg)	6,586	Vit B_6 (mg)	7.77	Vit E (mg)	5.28

Note: This is a typical exercise and intake schedule for a collegiate field hockey player in preseason training. Although this represents a relatively high protein intake, it is well distributed throughout the day to optimize tissue protein utilization. Even so, by distributing the right foods at the right time, the athlete can maintain a good energy balance throughout the day. The even anabolic and catabolic hours are indicative of someone who is able to maintain the current weight and body composition.

Source: Energy balance and nutrient intake values were derived using NutriTiming®. The energy balance graph is copyrighted by NutriTiming LLC and is used with permission.

Table 18.3 2,400-Calorie Food Plan for a 6'2" (188 cm), 188 lb (85 kg) 29-Year-Old Male Tennis Player Recovering From an Injury

Energy-balance graph

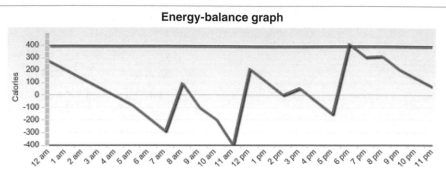

Hours anabolic (calories > 0) = 15; hours catabolic (calories < 0) = 9; anabolic:catabolic ratio = 1.67

Energy Substrate Distribution

Total calories: 2,456   **Carbohydrate %:** 30   **Protein %:** 34   **Fat %:** 37

Hour	Activity	Food	Amount	Calories
8-9 a.m.	Wake-up and breakfast; breakfast is important to consume before morning practice to ensure maintenance of energy balance and blood sugar.	Bagel, oat bran	1 small	145
		Butter, with salt	1 tsp	36
		Potatoes, hash brown	1 serving	63
		Eggs, fried	3 large	270
		Water	As desired	0
9-10 a.m.	Wake-up activities (shower, dress), then 30 min warm-up at 9:30 a.m.	Water	As desired	0
10-11 a.m.	45-min tennis drills (light) followed by snack.	Clif bar (Mojo peanut butter and jelly)	1 bar	220
		Water	As desired	0
11 a.m.-12 p.m.	30-min tennis stroke practice (light).	Sports beverage, if needed	8 oz (240 ml)	63
12-1 p.m.	This lunch is relatively high in protein but maintains a low fat level; plenty of fluids should be consumed to aid digestion and hydration.	Cheese, mozzarella, part-skim milk	1 oz (30 g)	72
		Cheese, American, nonfat	3.25 slices	101
		Beef tenderloin, lean, broiled	4 oz (125 g)	234
		Cactus tortillas	4 tortillas	200
		Avocado	1/2 avocado	114
		Water	As desired	0
1-3 p.m.	Relaxed activities around the house; water consumed as desired.	Water	As desired	0

Hour	Activity	Food	Amount	Calories
3-4 p.m.	A midafternoon snack is important for maintaining energy balance; good-quality protein, if distributed throughout the day, may also help in muscle recovery.	Chocolate flavored whey protein and milk drink	12 oz	160
4-6 p.m.	Relaxed activities and dinner preparation.	Water	As desired	0
6-7 p.m.	This is a hearty and filling dinner, although it maintains a relatively low calorie level by keeping the fat level relatively low.	Zucchini squash, chopped	1 cup	20
		Rice, brown, cooked	1/3 cup	32
		Chicken, light meat, roasted, no skin	2 oz (60 g)	98
		Egg, large, hard-boiled	1/2 egg	36
		Edamame, prepared	1/2 cup	95
		Beef tenderloin, lean, broiled	6 oz (125 g)	350
		Chicken broth	8 oz (240 ml)	36
		Water	As desired	0
7-9 p.m.	Relaxed activities.	Water	As desired	0
9-10 p.m.	Evening snack; snack should be consumed between 9 and 10 p.m. to ensure maintenance of blood sugar during the night.	Kiwi fruit	2 fruits	111

Totals for selected nutrients

Total kcal	2,456	Iron (mg)	18.1	Vit C (mg)	225.1	Vit B_{12} (mcg)	8.44
Carbohydrate (g)	178	Calcium (mg)	1,540	Vit B_1 (mg)	1.28	Folic acid (DFE)	679
Protein (g)	200	Zinc (mg)	26.1	Vit B_2 (mg)	2.60	Vit A (RAE)	612
Fat (g)	98	Magnesium (mg)	407.6	Niacin (mg)	41.41	Vit D (IU)	62.8
Sodium (mg)	3,711	Potassium (mg)	3,557	Vit B_6 (mg)	3.41	Vit E (mg)	13.5

Note: This represents the exercise and food intake pattern of a tennis player who is recovering from an injury. The level of physical activity is dramatically reduced from the activity when playing on the tour, so the energy intake is also reduced to match. Although the protein intake may be slightly higher than the typical requirement, the additional protein may aid in injury healing and muscle recovery. The anabolic-to-catabolic ratio (1.67) should enable muscle recovery.

Source: Energy balance and nutrient intake values were derived using NutriTiming®. The energy balance graph is copyrighted by NutriTiming LLC and is used with permission.

Table 18.4 2,800-Calorie Food Plan for a 5'8" (173 cm) 145 lb (66 kg) 21-Year-Old Male Elite Figure Skater

Energy balance

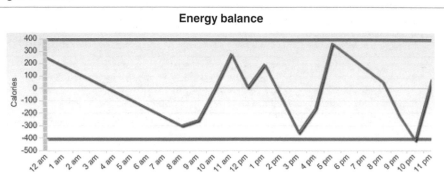

Hours anabolic (calories > 0) = 12; hours catabolic (calories < 0) = 12; anabolic:catabolic ratio = 1.0

Energy Substrate Distribution

Total calories: 2,782   **Carbohydrate %:** 63   **Protein %:** 16   **Fat %:** 20

Hour	Activity	Food	Amount	Calories
9-10 a.m.	Wake-up activities (shower, dress); orange juice should be consumed as soon as athlete awakens to prevent a below-desirable energy balance.	Orange juice	8 oz (240 ml)	110
10-11 a.m.	Breakfast immediately follows showering and dressing.	Cereal, oatmeal	1.75 cups	271
		Milk, nonfat (skim)	8 oz (240 ml)	83
11 a.m.-12 p.m.	This preexercise snack, consumed early in the hour, will help provide energy needed for the exercise that follows.	Marathon bar	1 bar	322
		Sports drink	8 oz (240 ml)	63
12-1 p.m.	Warm-up and light exercise.	Water	As desired	0
1-2 p.m.	Moderate-intensity drills for 30 min, followed by lunch.	Bread, whole wheat, toasted	2 slices	153
		Peanut butter, smooth, with salt	2 tbsp	188
		Water	As desired	0
2-3 p.m.	Full practice (high intensity) for 60 min; although practice takes place in a relatively cool environment (ice rink), the athlete still sweats and uses blood sugar as an energy substrate; the sports drink will help prevent low blood sugar, which could compromise mental acuity and also result in premature muscular fatigue.	Sports drink	8 oz (240 ml)	63
3-4 p.m.	Full practice (high intensity) for an additional 30 min (90 min total), followed by cool-down.	Sports drink	8 oz	63
4-5 p.m.	Relaxed household activities	Water	As desired	0

Hour	Activity	Food	Amount	Calories
5-6 p.m.	This dinner is nicely balanced, with relatively high carbohydrate and a small amount of high-quality protein.	Spaghetti	1 cup	220
		Tomato basil sauce	1/2 cup	111
		Cheese, Parmesan, grated	1/3 cup	81
		Ribeye steak, lean, broiled	3 oz (90 g)	299
		Coffee, brewed from grounds	1 cup	2
		Coffee cream	2 tbsp	50
		Sugar	1 tsp	15
		Apple	1 large	130
		Water	As desired	0
6-9 p.m.	Relaxed household activities and preparation for the next day.	Water	As desired	0
9-10 p.m.	Warm-up and light on-ice exercise.	Water	As desired	0
10-11 p.m.	Moderately intense skills practice for 20 min, followed by snack.	Gelatin desert	2 cups	299
		Pear	1 large	155
		Grapes, red	1 cup	104
		Water	As desired	0

Totals for selected nutrients

Total kcal	2,782	Iron (mg)	32.7	Vit C (mg)	220	Vit B_{12} (mcg)	9.84
Carbohydrate (g)	438	Calcium (mg)	1,147	Vit B_1 (mg)	3.79	Folic acid (DFE)	261.8
Protein (g)	111	Zinc (mg)	29.3	Vit B_2 (mg)	4.83	Vit A (RAE)	2,822
Fat (g)	62	Magnesium (mg)	447	Niacin (mg)	57.82	Vit D (IU)	106.9
Sodium (mg)	2,930	Potassium (mg)	4,167	Vit B_6 (mg)	5.3	Vit E (mg)	105.5

Notes: This represents the intake of an elite male figure skater in training for competition. Although he's not of a large stature, the high-intensity activity increases his energy requirement substantially. The carbohydrate and protein intakes are appropriate for an athlete undergoing this level of training and is distributed in a way that will sustain muscle mass and body-fat percentage. The relatively late practice is due to ice availability, which often forces skaters to train either early in the morning or late at night.

Source: Energy balance and nutrient intake values were derived using NutriTiming®. The energy balance graph is copyrighted by NutriTiming LLC and is used with permission.

Table 18.5   3,800-Calorie Food Plan for a 6'3" (191 cm), 190 lb (86 kg) 21-Year-Old Female Collegiate Volleyball Player

Energy-balance graph

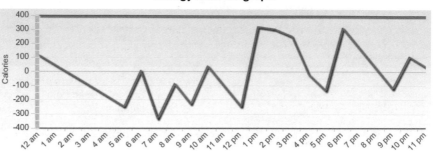

Hours anabolic (calories > 0) = 12; hours catabolic (calories < 0) = 12 ; anabolic:catabolic ratio = 1.0

Energy Substrate Distribution

Total calories: 3,807   **Carbohydrate %:** 66   **Protein %:** 14   **Fat %:** 21

Hour	Activity	Food	Amount	Calories
6-7 a.m.	Important for athlete to have something to eat as soon as possible after waking up to prepare for exercise session at 7 a.m.	Raisin toast	2 slices	172
		Honeydew melon	2 cups	127
		Sports drink	8 oz (240 ml)	63
7-8 a.m.	Weight-room workout; sipping on sports beverage during a workout is important for sustaining blood sugar and hydration state.	Sports drink	12 oz (360 ml)	94
8-9 a.m.	Cool-down and breakfast; chocolate milk should be consumed immediately upon completion of workout.	Chocolate milk, low fat	8 oz (240 ml)	158
		Coffee	2 cups	5
		Bread, multigrain, toasted	2 slices	138
		Margarine	1 tsp	36
		Jam	1 tbsp	39
		Egg, hard boiled	1 egg	105
9-10 a.m.	Normal daytime activities.	Water	As desired	0
10-11 a.m.	Midmorning snack is important to maintain blood sugar and energy balance.	Sports drink	16 oz (480 ml)	127
		Bagel, egg	1 medium	288
11 a.m.-1 p.m.	Normal daytime activities.	Water	As desired	0
1-2 p.m.	Lunch is high in carbohydrate, moderate in protein, and low in fat; athlete should drink liberal amounts of water with the meal.	Milk, skim	8 oz (240 ml)	83
		Cereal, whole grain	1 cup	175
		Bagel, egg	1 small	192
		Chicken, white meat, no skin	3.25 oz (90 g)	156
		Orange juice	8 oz (240 ml)	110
		Water	As desired	0

Hour	Activity	Food	Amount	Calories
2-4 p.m.	Sports beverage should be sipped consistently in this 2 hr period to ensure a well-hydrated state going into volleyball practice.	Sports drink	28 oz (840 ml)	221
4-6 p.m.	Intense 2 hr practice; every opportunity should be taken to consume sports beverage; the chocolate milk should be consumed immediately after practice.	Sports drink	32 oz (960 ml)	250
		Chocolate milk, low fat	8 oz (240 ml)	158
6-7 p.m.	Dinner; the calorie total may appear high, but the energy-balance graph indicates this is necessary to achieve good energy balance.	Beef steak, broiled	4 oz (125 g)	381
		Potato, baked	1 medium	160
		Sour cream	1 tbsp	23
		Green beans	1 cup	25
		Butter	1 tbsp	100
		Water	As desired	0
7-10 p.m.	Normal school activities for a collegiate athlete.	Sports drink	6 oz (180 ml)	47
10-11 p.m.	The evening snack is necessary to ensure energy balance and maintenance of blood sugar during the night.	Popcorn, air popped	5 cups	155
		Orange juice	16 oz (480 ml)	219

Totals for selected nutrients

Total kcal	3,807	Iron (mg)	25.8	Vit C (mg)	375	Vit B_{12} (mcg)	8.01
Carbohydrate (g)	635	Calcium (mg)	1,375	Vit B_1 (mg)	3.3	Folic acid (DFE)	804.3
Protein (g)	132	Zinc (mg)	17.9	Vit D_2 (mg)	4.0	Vit A (RAE)	1,078
Fat (g)	88	Magnesium (mg)	555.6	Niacin (mg)	31.1	Vit D (IU)	108.3
Sodium (mg)	4,257	Potassium (mg)	6,621	Vit B_6 (mg)	3.25	Vit E (mg)	3.35

Note: This athlete has two workouts per day, one in the morning in the weight room and a 2 hr team volleyball practice in the afternoon. She is a tall and powerful athlete who wishes to sustain her muscle mass, and with this diet she should be able to do this (her anabolic-to-catabolic ratio is 1.0, suggesting she should be stable in both weight and body composition). The focus is on carbohydrate (66% of total intake), with ample fluids to ensure replenishment of muscle glycogen used in volleyball-specific explosive muscle movement.

Source: Energy balance and nutrient intake values were derived using NutriTiming®. The energy balance graph is copyrighted by NutriTiming LLC and is used with permission.

Appendix:
Institute of Medicine's Dietary Reference Intakes for Macronutrients

Dietary Reference Intakes: Macronutrients

Nutrient	Function	Life stage group	RDA/ AI* g/d	AMDR	Selected food sources	Adverse effects of excessive consumption
Carbohydrate— total digestible	RDA based on its role as the primary energy source for the brain; AMDR based on its role as a source of kilocalories to maintain body weight.	Infants			Starch and sugar are the major types of carbohydrates. Grains and vegetables (corn, pasta, rice, potatoes, breads) are sources of starch. Natural sugars are found in fruits and juices. Sources of added sugars are soft drinks, candy, fruit drinks, and desserts.	While no defined intake level at which potential adverse effects of total digestible carbohydrate was identified, the upper end of the adequate macronutrient distribution range (AMDR) was based on decreasing risk of chronic disease and providing adequate intake of other nutrients. It is suggested that the maximal intake of added sugars be limited to providing no more than 25% of energy.
		0-6 mo	60*	ND[b]		
		7-12 mo	95*	ND		
		Children				
		1-3 y	**130**	45-65		
		4-8 y	**130**	45-65		
		Males				
		9-13 y	**130**	45-65		
		14-18 y	**130**	45-65		
		19-30 y	**130**	45-65		
		31-50 y	**130**	45-65		
		50-70 y	**130**	45-65		
		>70 y	**130**	45-65		
		Females				
		9-13 y	**130**	45-65		
		14-18 y	**130**	45-65		
		19-30 y	**130**	45-65		
		31-50 y	**130**	45-65		
		50-70 y	**130**	45-65		
		>70 y	**130**	45-65		
		Pregnancy				
		≤18 y	**175**	45-65		
		19-30 y	**175**	45-65		
		31-50 y		45-65		
		Lactation				
		≤18 y	**210**	45-65		
		19-50 y	**210**	45-65		
		31-50 y	**210**	45-65		

Nutrient	Function	Life stage group	RDA/ AI* g/d	AMDR	Selected food sources	Adverse effects of excessive consumption
Total fiber	Improves laxation, reduces risk of coronary heart disease, assists in maintaining normal blood glucose levels.	Infants			Includes dietary fiber naturally present in grains (such as found in oats, wheat, or unmilled rice) and functional fiber synthesized or isolated from plants or animals and shown to be of benefit to health.	Dietary fiber can have variable composition and therefore it is difficult to link a specific source of fiber with a particular adverse effect, especially when phytate is also present in the natural fiber source. It is concluded that as part of an overall healthy diet, a high intake of dietary fiber will not produce deleterious effects in healthy individuals. While occasional adverse gastrointestinal symptoms are observed when consuming some isolated or synthetic fibers, serious chronic adverse effects have not been observed. Due to the bulky nature of fibers, excess consumption is likely to be self-limiting. Therefore, a UL was not set for individual functional fibers.
		Infants				
		0-6 mo	ND			
		7-12 mo	ND			
		Children				
		1-3 y	19*			
		4-8 y	25*			
		Males				
		9-13 y	31*			
		14-18 y	38*			
		19-30 y	38*			
		31-50 y	38*			
		50-70 y	30*			
		>70 y	30*			
		Females				
		9-13 y	26*			
		14-18 y	26*			
		19-30 y	25*			
		31-50 y	25*			
		50-70 y	21*			
		>70 y	21*			
		Pregnancy				
		≤18 y	28*			
		19-30 y	28*			
		31-50 y	28*			
		Lactation				
		≤18 y	29*			
		19-30 y	29*			
		31-50 y	29*			

NOTE: The table is adapted from the DRI reports; see www.nap.edu. It represents recommended dietary allowances (RDAs) in **bold type** and adequate intakes (AIs) in ordinary type followed by an asterisk (*). RDAs and AIs may both be sued as goals for individual intake. RDAs are set to meet the needs of almost all (97 to 98%) individuals in a group. For healthy breastfed infants, the AI is the mean intake. The AI for other life stage and gender groups is believed to cover the needs of all individuals in the group, but lack of data prevents being able to specify with confidence the percentage of individuals covered by this intake.

[a]Acceptable macronutrient distribution range (AMDR)[a] is the range of intake for a particular energy source that is associated with reduced risk of chronic disease while providing intakes of essential nutrients. If an individual consumes in excess of the AMDR, there is a potential for increasing the risk of chronic diseases and insufficient intakes of essential nutrients.

[b]ND = not determinable due to lack of data of adverse effects in this age group and concern with regard to lack of ability to handle excess amounts. Source of intake should be from food only to prevent high levels of intake.

Data from Food and Nutrition Board, Institute of Medicine of the National Academies, 2005, *Dietary reference intakes for energy, carbohydrate, fiber, fat, fatty acids, cholesterol, protein, and amino acids.* Adapted with permission from the National Academies Press, Copyright 2005, National Academy of Sciences.

Dietary Reference Intakes: Macronutrients

Nutrient	Function	Life stage group	RDA/AI* g/d	AMDR	Selected food sources	Adverse effects of excessive consumption
Total fat	Energy source and when found in foods is a source of n-6 and n-3 polyunsaturated fatty acids. Its presence in the diet increases absorption of fat-soluble vitamins and precursors such as vitamin A and provitamin A carotenoids.	Infants			Butter, margarine, vegetable oils, whole milk, visible fat on meat and poultry products, invisible fat in fish, shellfish, some plant products such as seeds and nuts, and bakery products.	While no defined intake level at which potential adverse effects of total fat was identified, the upper end of AMDR is based on decreasing risk of chronic disease and providing adequate intake of other nutrients. The lower end of the AMDR is based on concerns related to the increase in plasma triacylglycerol concentrations and decreased HDL cholesterol concentrations seen with very low fat (and thus high carbohydrate) diets.
		0-6 mo	31*			
		7-12 mo	30*			
		Children				
		1-3 y		30-40		
		4-8 y		25-35		
		Males				
		9-13 y		25-35		
		14-18 y		25-35		
		19-30 y		20-35		
		31-50 y		20-35		
		50-70 y		20-35		
		>70 y		20-35		
		Females				
		9-13 y		25-35		
		14-18 y		25-35		
		19-30 y		20-35		
		31-50 y		20-35		
		50-70 y		20-35		
		>70 y		20-35		
		Pregnancy				
		≤18 y		20-35		
		19-30 y		20-35		
		31-50 y		20-35		
		Lactation				
		≤18 y		20-35		
		19-50 y		20-35		
		31-50 y		20-35		

Nutrient	Function	Life stage group	RDA/AI* g/d	AMDR	Selected food sources	Adverse effects of excessive consumption
n-6 poluyun-saturated fatty acids (linoleic acid)	Essential compo-nent of structural membrane lipids, involved with cell signaling, and precursor of eico-sanoids. Required for normal skin function.	Infants			Nuts, seeds, and vegetable oils such as soybean, saf-flower, and corn oil	While no defined intake level at which potential adverse effects of *n*-6 polyunsatu-rated fatty acids was identified, the upper end of the AMDR is based on the lack of evidence that demonstrates long-term safety and human in vitro studies that show increased free radical for-mation and lipid peroxidation with higher amounts of *n*-6 fatty acids. Lipid peroxidation is thought to be a component of the development of atherosclerotic plaques.
		0-6 mo	4.4*	ND[b]		
		7-12 mo	4.6*	ND		
		Children				
		1-3 y	7*	5-10		
		4-8 y	10*	5-10		
		Males				
		9-13 y	12*	5-10		
		14-18 y	16*	5-10		
		19-30 y	17*	5-10		
		31-50 y	17*	5-10		
		50-70 y	14*	5-10		
		>70 y	14*	5-10		
		Females				
		9-13 y	10*	5-10		
		14-18 y	11*	5-10		
		19-30 y	12*	5-10		
		31-50 y	12*	5-10		
		50-70 y	11*	5-10		
		>70 y	11*	5-10		
		Pregnancy				
		≤18 y	13*	5-10		
		19-30 y	13*	5-10		
		31-50 y	13*	5-10		
		Lactation				
		≤18 y	13*	5-10		
		19-30 y	13*	5-10		
		31-50 y	13*	5-10		

NOTE: The table is adapted from the DRI reports; see www.nap.edu. It represents recommended dietary allowances (RDAs) in **bold type** and adequate intakes (AIs) in ordinary type followed by an asterisk (°). RDAs and AIs may both be sued as goals for individual intake. RDAs are set to meet the needs of almost all (97 to 98%) individuals in a group. For healthy breastfed infants, the AI is the mean intake. The AI for other life stage and gender groups is believed to cover the needs of all individuals in the group, but lack of data prevents being able to specify with confidence the percentage of individuals covered by this intake.

[a]Acceptable macronutrient distribution range (AMDR)[a] is the range of intake for a particular energy source that is associated with reduced risk of chronic disease while providing intakes of essential nutrients. If an individual consumes in excess of the AMDR, there is a potential for increasing the risk of chronic diseases and/or insufficient intakes of essential nutrients.

[b]ND = Not determinable due to lack of data of adverse effects in this age group and concern with regard to lack of ability to handle excess amounts. Source of intake should be from food only to prevent high levels of intake.

Data from Food and Nutrition Board, Institute of Medicine of the National Academies, 2005, *Dietary reference intakes for energy, carbohydrate, fiber, fat, fatty acids, cholesterol, protein, and amino acids.* Adapted with permission from the National Academies Press, Copyright 2005, National Academy of Sciences.

Dietary Reference Intakes: Macronutrients

Nutrient	Function	Life stage group	RDA/AI* g/d	AMDR	Selected food sources	Adverse effects of excessive consumption
n-3 polyunsaturated fatty acids (α-linolenic acid)	Involved with neurological development and growth. Precursor of eicosanoids.	Infants			Vegetable oils such as soybean, canola, and flax seed oil, fish oils, fatty fish, with smaller amounts in meats and eggs	While no defined intake level at which potential adverse effects of n-3 polyunsaturated fatty acids was identified, the upper end of AMDR is based on maintaining the appropriate balance with n-6 fatty acids and on the lack of evidence that demonstrates long-term safety, along with human in vitro studies that show increased free radical formation and lipid peroxidation with higher amounts of polyunsaturated fatty acids. Lipid peroxidation is thought to be a component of in the development of atherosclerotic plaques.
		0-6 mo	0.5*	ND[b]		
		7-12 mo	0.5*	ND		
		Children				
		1-3 y	0.7*	0.6-1.2		
		4-8 y	0.9*	0.6-1.2		
		Males				
		9-13 y	1.2*	0.6-1.2		
		14-18 y	1.6*	0.6-1.2		
		19-30 y	1.6*	0.6-1.2		
		31-50 y	1.6*	0.6-1.2		
		50-70 y	1.6*	0.6-1.2		
		>70 y	1.6*	0.6-1.2		
		Females				
		9-13 y	1.0*	0.6-1.2		
		14-18 y	1.1*	0.6-1.2		
		19-30 y	1.1*	0.6-1.2		
		31-50 y	1.1*	0.6-1.2		
		50-70 y	1.1*	0.6-1.2		
		>70 y	1.1*	0.6-1.2		
		Pregnancy				
		≤18 y	1.4*	0.6-1.2		
		19-30 y	1.4*	0.6-1.2		
		31-50 y	1.4*	0.6-1.2		
		Lactation				
		≤18 y	1.3*	0.6-1.2		
		19-50 y	1.3*	0.6-1.2		
		31-50 y	1.3*	0.6-1.2		

NOTE: The table is adapted from the DRI reports; see www.nap.edu. It represents recommended dietary allowances (RDAs) in **bold type** and adequate intakes (AIs) in ordinary type followed by an asterisk (°). RDAs and AIs may both be sued as goals for individual intake. RDAs are set to meet the needs of almost all (97 to 98%) individuals in a group. For healthy breastfed infants, the AI is the mean intake. The AI for other life stage and gender groups is believed to cover the needs of all individuals in the group, but lack of data prevents being able to specify with confidence the percentage of individuals covered by this intake.

[a]Acceptable macronutrient distribution range (AMDR)[a] is the range of intake for a particular energy source that is associated with reduced risk of chronic disease while providing intakes of essential nutrients. If an individual consumes in excess of the AMDR, there is a potential for increasing the risk of chronic diseases and/or insufficient intakes of essential nutrients.

Nutrient	Function	Life stage group	RDA/AI* g/d	AMDR	Selected food sources	Adverse effects of excessive consumption
Saturated and trans fatty acids and cholesterol	No required role for these nutrients other than as energy sources was identified; the body can synthesize its needs for saturated fatty acids and cholesterol from other sources.	Infants			Saturated fatty acids are present in animal fats (meat fats and butter fat) and coconut and palm kernel oils. Sources of cholesterol include liver, eggs, and foods that contain eggs such as cheesecake and custard pies. Source of trans fatty acids include stick margarines and foods containing hydrogenated or partially hydrogenated vegetable shortenings.	There is an incremental increase in plasma total and low-density lipoprotein cholesterol concentrations with increased intake of saturated or trans fatty acids or with cholesterol at even very low levels in the diet. Therefore, the intakes of each should be minimized while consuming a nutritionally adequate diet.
		0-6 mo	ND			
		7-12 mo	ND			
		Children				
		1-3 y				
		4-8 y				
		Males				
		9-13 y				
		14-18 y				
		19-30 y				
		31-50 y				
		50-70 y				
		>70 y				
		Females				
		9-13 y				
		14-18 y				
		19-30 y				
		31-50 y				
		50-70 y				
		>70 y				
		Pregnancy				
		≤18 y				
		19-30 y				
		31-50 y				
		Lactation				
		≤18 y				
		19-30 y				
		31-50 y				

[b]ND = Not determinable due to lack of data of adverse effects in this age group and concern with regard to lack of ability to handle excess amounts. Source of intake should be from food only to prevent high levels of intake.

Data from Food and Nutrition Board, Institute of Medicine of the National Academies, 2005, *Dietary reference intakes for energy, carbohydrate, fiber, fat, fatty acids, cholesterol, protein, and amino acids.* Adapted with permission from the National Academies Press, Copyright 2005, National Academy of Sciences.

Dietary Reference Intakes: Macronutrients

Nutrient	Function	Life stage group	RDA/AI* g/d	AMDR	Selected food sources	Adverse effects of excessive consumption
Protein and amino acids	Serve as the major structural component of all cells in the body and function as enzymes, in membranes, as transport carriers, and as some hormones. During digestion and absorption dietary proteins are broken down to amino acids, which become the building blocks of these structural and functional compounds. Nine of the amino acids must be provided in the diet; these are termed indispensable amino acids. The body can make the other amino acids needed to synthesize specific structures from other amino acids.	Infants			Proteins from animal sources, such as meat, poultry, fish, eggs, milk, cheese, and yogurt, provide all nine indispensable amino acids in adequate amounts, and for this reason are considered complete proteins. Proteins from plants, legumes, grains, nuts, seeds, and vegetables, tend to be deficient in one or more of the indispensable amino acids and are called incomplete proteins. Vegan diets adequate in total protein content can be complete by combining sources of incomplete proteins that lack different indispensable amino acids.	While no defined intake level at which potential adverse effects of protein was identified, the upper end of AMDR is based on complementing the AMDR for carbohydrate and fat for the various age groups. The lower end of the AMDR is set at approximately the RDA.
		0-6 mo	9.1*	ND[b]		
		7-12 mo	**11.0**	ND		
		Children				
		1-3 y	**13**	5-20		
		4-8 y	**19**	10-30		
		Males				
		9-13 y	**34**	10-30		
		14-18 y	**52**	10-30		
		19-30 y	**56**	10-35		
		31-50 y	**56**	10-35		
		50-70 y	**56**	10-35		
		>70 y	**56**	10-35		
		Females				
		9-13 y	**34**	10-30		
		14-18 y	**46**	10-30		
		19-30 y	**46**	10-35		
		31-50 y	**46**	10-35		
		50-70 y	**46**	10-35		
		>70 y	**46**	10-35		
		Pregnancy				
		≤18 y	**71**	10-35		
		19-30 y	**71**	10-35		
		31-50 y	**71**	10-35		
		Lactation				
		≤18 y	**71**	10-35		
		19-50 y	**71**	10-35		
		31-50 y	**71**	10-35		

NOTE: The table is adapted from the DRI reports; see www.nap.edu. It represents recommended dietary allowances (RDAs) in **bold type** and adequate intakes (AIs) in ordinary type followed by an asterisk (*). RDAs and AIs may both be sued as goals for individual intake. RDAs are set to meet the needs of almost all (97 to 98%) individuals in a group. For healthy breastfed infants, the AI is the mean intake. The AI for other life stage and gender groups is believed to cover the needs of all individuals in the group, but lack of data prevents being able to specify with confidence the percentage of individuals covered by this intake.

[a]Based on 1.5 g/kg/day for infants, 1.1 g/kg/day for 1-3 y, .95 g/kg/day for 4-13 y, .85 g/kg/day for 14-18 y, .8 g/kg/day for adults, and 1.1 g/kg/day for pregnant (using pre-pregnancy weight) and lactating women.

[b]Acceptable Macronutrient Distribution Range (AMDR)[a] is the range of intake for a particular energy source that is associated with reduced risk of chronic disease while providing intakes of essential nutrients. If an individual consumes in excess of the AMDR, there is potential of increasing the risk of chronic diseases and insufficient intakes of essential nutrients.

[c]ND = Not determinable due to lack of data of adverse effects in this age group and concern with regard to lack of ability to handle excess amounts. Source of intake should be from food only to prevent high levels of intake.

Data from Food and Nutrition Board, Institute of Medicine of the National Academies, 2005, *Dietary reference intakes for energy, carbohydrate, fiber, fat, fatty acids, cholesterol, protein, and amino acids.* Adapted with permission from the National Academies Press, Copyright 2005, National Academy of Sciences.

Dietary Reference Intakes: Macronutrients

Nutrient	Function	IOM/FNB 2002 scoring pattern[a]	Mg/g protein	Adverse effects of excessive consumption
Indispensable amino acids:	The building blocks of all proteins in the body and some hormones. These nine amino acids must be provided in the diet and thus are termed indispensable amino acids. The body can make the other amino acids needed to synthesize specific structures from other amino acids and carbohydrate precursors.			Since there is no evidence that amino acids found in usual or even high intakes of protein from food present any risk, attention was focused on intakes of the L-form of these and other amino acids found in dietary protein and amino acid supplements. Even from well-studied amino acids, adequate dose-response data from human or animal studies on which to base a UL were not available. While no definite intake level at which potential adverse effects of protein was identified for any amino acid, this does not mean that there is no potential for adverse effects resulting from high intakes of amino acids from dietary supplements. Since data on the adverse effects of high levels of amino acid intakes from dietary supplements are limited, caution may be warranted.
Histidine		Histidine	18	
Isoleucine		Isoleucine	25	
Leucine		Leucine	55	
Lysine		Lysine	51	
Methionine & cysteine		Methionine & cysteine	25	
Phenylalanine & tyrosine		Phenylalanine & tyrosine	47	
Threonine		Threonine	27	
Tryptophan		Tryptophan	7	
Valine		Valine	32	

NOTE: The table is adapted from the DRI reports; see www.nap.edu.

[a]Based on the amino acid requirements derived from preschool children (1-3 y): (EAR for amino acid ÷ EAR for protein), where EAR for protein = .88 g/kg/d.

Data from Food and Nutrition Board, Institute of Medicine of the National Academies, 2005, *Dietary reference intakes for energy, carbohydrate, fiber, fat, fatty acids, cholesterol, protein, and amino acids.* Adapted with permission from the National Academies Press, Copyright 2005, National Academy of Sciences.

Endnotes

Chapter 1

1 Hultman E, Nilsson LH. Liver glycogen in man: Effects of different diets and muscular exercise. In: Pernow B, Saltin B, eds. *Muscle Metabolism During Intense Exercise.* London: Plenum Press; 1971:143-151.

2 Hultman E, Greenhaff PL. Carbohydrate metabolism in exercise. In: Maughan RJ, ed. *Nutrition in Sport.* London: Blackwell Science; 2000:90-91.

3 Glucogenic amino acids have carbon chains that can be converted to glucose. In humans, the glucogenic amino acids are glycine, serine, valine, histidine, arginine, cysteine, proline, alanine, glutamate, glutamine, aspartate, asparagines, and methionine. Amino acids that are both glucogenic and ketogenic included isoleucine, threonine, phenylalanine, tyrosine, and tryptophan. (The ketogenic amino acids produce ketones rather than glucose.)

4 Pate TD, Brunn JC. Fundamentals of carbohydrate metabolism. In: HIckson JF, Wolinsky I, eds. *Nutrition in Exercise and Sport.* Boca Raton, FL: CRC Press; 1989:37-49.

5 Karlsson J, Saltin B. Diet, muscle glycogen, and endurance. *Journal of Applied Physiology.* 1971; 31(2):203-206.

6 Felig P, Wahren J. Amino acide metabolism in exercising man. *Journal of Clinical Investigation.* 1971; 50:2703-2714.

7 Sahlin K, Katz A, Broberg S. Tricarboxylic cycle intermediates in human muscle during submaximal exercise. *Amercian Journal of Physiology.* 1990; 259:834C-841C.

8 Fitts RH. Cellular mechanisms of muscle fatigue. *Physiological Reviews.* 1994; 74:49-94.

9 The branched-chain amino acids are leucine, isoleucine, and valine.

10 Newsholme EA, Catell LM. Amino acids, fatigue and immunodepression in exercise. In: Maughan RJ, ed. *Nutrition in Sport.* London: Blackwell Science; 2000:156-158.

11 Davis JM, Alderson NL, Welsh RS. Serotonin and central nervous system fatigue: Nutritional considerations. *American Journal of Clinical Nutrition.* 2000;72(2)(suppl):573S-578S.

12 Davis JM, Zhao Z, Stock HS, Mehl KA, Buggy J, Hand GA. Central nervous system effects of caffeine and adenosine on fatigue. *American Journal of Physiology: Regulatory, Integrative and Comparative Physiology.* 2003;284(2):399R-404R.

13 Institute of Medicine. *Dietary Reference Intakes for energy, carbohydrate, fiber, fat, fatty acids, cholesterol, protein and amino acids.* Food and Nutrition Board. Washington, DC: National Academies Press; 2002.

14 Position of the American Dietetic Association, Dietitians of Canada, and the American College of Sports Medicine. Nutrition and athletic performance. *Journal of the American Dietetic Association.* 2000;100:1543-1556.

15 USDA/HHS. Nutrition and your health: Dietary Guidelines for Americans. *Home and Garden Bulletin.* no. 232. Washington DC: Government Printing Office; 2000.

16 Costill DL, Sherman WM, Fink WJ, Maresh C, Witten M, Miller JM. The role of dietary carbohydrate in muscle glycogen synthesis after strenuous running. *American Journal of Clinical Nutrition.* 1981;34:1831-1836.

17 Sherman WM. Metabolism of sugars and physical performance. *American Journal of Clinical Nutrition.* 1995;62(suppl):228S-241S.

18 Burke LM, Kiens B, Ivy JL. Carbohydrates and fat for training and recovery. *Journal of Sports Sciences.* 2004;22:15-30.

19 Liu S, Willett WC. Dietary glycemic load and atherothrombotic risk. *Current Atherosclerosis Reports.* 2002;4(6):454-461.

20 Coutts A, Reaburn P, Mummery K, Holmes M. The effect of glycerol hyperhydration on Olympic distance triathlon performance in high ambient temperatures. *International Journal of Sport Nutrition and Exercise Metabolism.* 2002;12(1):105-119.

21 Magal M, Webster MJ, Sistrunk LE, Whitehead MT, Evans RK, Boyd JC. Comparison of glycerol and water hydration regimens on tennis-related performance. *Medicine and Science in Sports and Exercise.* 2003;35(1):150-156.

22 Bucci L. *Nutrients as Ergogenic Aids for Sports and Exercise.* Boca Raton, FL: CRC Press; 1993:20.

23 Mickleborough TD, Murray RL, Ionescu AA, Lindley MR. Fish oil supplementation reduces severity of exercise-induced bronchoconstriction in elite athletes. *American Journal of Respiratory and Critical Care Medicine.* 2003;168:1181-1189.

24 Brilla LF, Landerholm TE. Effect of fish oil supplementation and exercise on serum lipids and aerobic fitness. *Journal of Sports Medicine.* 1990;30(2):173.

25 Huffman DM, Altena TS, Mawhinney TP, Thomas TR. Effect of n-3 fatty acids on free tryptophan and exercise fatigue. *European Journal of Applied Physiology.* 2004;92(4/5):584-591.

26 Lenn J, Uhl T, Mattacola C, Boissonneault G, Yates J, Ibrahim W, Bruckner G. The effects of fish oil and isoflavones on delayed onset muscle soreness. *Medicine and Science in Sports and Exercise.* 2002;34(10):1605-1613.

27 Simopoulos AP. Omega-3 fatty acids and athletics. *Current Sports Medicine Reports.* 2007;6:230-236.

28 Coyle EF. Fat metabolism during exercise. *Sports Science Exchange.* 1995; 8(6):59-65.

29 Kiens B, Helge JW. Adaptations to a high fat diet. In: Maughan RJ, ed. *Nutrition in Sport.* London: Blackwell Science; 2000:192-202.

30 Bach AS, Babayan VK. Medium-chain triglycerides: An update. *American Journal of Clinical Nutrition.* 1982;36(5):950-962.

31 Seaton TB, Welle SL, Warenko MK, Campbell RG. Thermic effect of medium-chain and long-chain triglycerides in man. *American Journal of Clinical Nutrition.* 1986;44(5):630-634.

32 Geliebter A, Torbay N, Bracco EF, Hashim SA, Van Itallie TB. Overfeeding with medium-chain triglyceride diet results in diminished deposition of fat. *American Journal of Clinical Nutrition.* 1983;37(1):1-4.

33 Scalfi L, Coltorti A, Contaldo F. Postprandial thermogenesis in lean and obese subjects after meals supplemented with medium-chain and long-chain triglycerides. *American Journal of Clinical Nutrition.* 1991;53(5):1130-1133.

34 Angus DJ, Hargreaves M, Dancey J, Febbraio MA. Effect of carbohydrate or carbohydrate plus medium-chain triglyceride ingestion on cycling time trial performance. *Journal of Applied Physiology.* 2000;88(1):113-119.

35 Lambert EV, Goedecke JH, Zyle C, Murphy K, Hawley JA, Dennis SC, Noakes TD. High-fat diet versus habitual diet prior to carbohydrate loading: Effects of exercise metabolism and cycling performance. *International Journal of Sport Nutrition and Exercise Metabolism.* 2001;11(2):209-225.

36 Misell LM, Lagomarcino ND, Schuster V, Kern M. Chronic medium-chain triacylglycerol consumption and endurance performance in trained runners. *Journal of Sports Medicine and Physical Fitness.* 2001;41(2):210-215.

37 Kern M, Lagomarcino ND, Misell LM, Schuster V. The effect of medium-chain triacylglycerols on the blood lipid profile of male endurance runners. *Journal of Nutritional Biochemistry.* 2000;11(5):288-292.

38 Kasai M, Nosaka N, Maki H, Suzuki Y, Takeuchi H, Aoyama T, Ohra A, Harada Y, Okazaki M, Kondo K. *Journal of Nutritional Science and Vitaminology*. 2002;48(6):536-240.

39 St-Onge MP, Ross R, Parsons WD, Jones PJ. Medium-chain triglycerides increase energy expenditure and decrease adiposity in overweight men. *Obesity Research*. 2003;11(3):395-402.

40 Jukendrup AE, Saris WHM, Schrauwen P, Brouns F, Wagermakers AJM. Metabolic availability of medium-chain triglycerides coingested with carbohydrate during prolonged exercise. *Journal of Applied Physiology*. 1995;79:756-762.

41 Cwik, V. Disorders of lipid metabolism in skeletal muscle. *Neurologic Clinics*. 2000;18:167-184.

42 Meredith CN, Zackin MJ, Frontera WR, Evans WJ. Dietary protein requirements and body protein metabolism in endurance-trained men. *Journal of Applied Physiology*. 1989;66(6):2850-2856.

43 Butterfield GE, Calloway DH. Physical activity improves protein utilization in young men. *British Journal of Nutrition*. 1984;51:171-184.

44 Butterfield G, Cady C, Moynihan S. Effect of increasing protein intake on nitrogen balance in recreational weight lifters. *Medicine and Science in Sports and Exercise*. 1992;24:71S.

45 Hoffman JR, Falvo MJ. Protein: Which is best? *Journal of Sports Science and Medicine*. 2004;3(3):118–130.

46 Schaafsma G. The protein digestibility-corrected amino acid score. *Journal of Nutrition*. 2000;130:1865S-1867S.

47 USDA/HHS. *Dietary Guidelines for Americans, 2010*. Washington, DC: Government Printing Office; 2010.

48 Tarnopolsky MA, MacDougall JD, Atkinson SA. Influence of protein intake and training status on nitrogen balance and lean body mass. *Journal of Applied Physiology*. 1988;64(1):187-193.

49 Position of the American Dietetic Association, Dietitians of Canada, and the American College of Sports Medicine. Nutrition and Athletic Performance. *Journal of the American Dietetic Association*. 2009;109:509-527.

50 Steen SN. Precontest strategies of a male bodybuilder. *International Journal of Sport Nutrition*. 1991;1:69-78.

51 Kleiner SM, Bazzarre TL, Ainsworth BE. Nutritional status of nationally ranked elite body-builders. *International Journal of Sport Nutrition*. 1994;4:43-69.

52 Gibala M. Regulation of skeletal muscle amino acid metabolism during exercise. *International Journal of Sport Nutrition and Exercise Metabolism*. 2001;11:87-108.

53 Gibala MJ. Dietary protein, amino acid supplements, and recovery from exercise. *GSSI Sports Science Exchange*. 2002;15(4):1-4.

54 Kumar V, Atherton P, Smith K, Rennie MJ. Human muscle protein synthesis and breakdown during and after exercise. *Journal of Applied Physiology*. 2009;106:2026-2039.

55 Paddon-Jones D, Rasmussen BB. Dietary protein recommendations and the prevention of sarcopenia: Protein amino acid metabolism and therapy. *Current Opinions in Clinical Nutrition and Metabolic Care*. 2009;12(1):86-90.

56 Tipton KD, Elliott TA, Cree MG, Aarsland AA, Sanford AP, Wolfe RR. Stimulation of net muscle protein synthesis by whey protein ingestion before and after exercise. *American Journal of Physiology and Endocrinological Metabolism*. 2007;292:71E-76E.

57 Cermak NM, Solheim AS, Gardner MS, Tarnopolsky MA, Gibala MJ. Muscle metabolism during exercise with carbohydrate ingestion. *Medicine and Science in Sport and Exercise*. 2009;41(12):2158-2164.

58 Howarth KR, Moreau NA, Phillips SM, Gibala MJ. Coingestion of protein with carbohydrate during recovery from endurance exercise stimulates skeletal muscle protein synthesis in humans. *Journal of Applied Physiology*. 2009;106:1394-1402.

59 Howarth KR, Phillips SM, MacDonald MJ, Richards D, Moreau NA, Gibala MJ. Effect of glycogen availability on human skeletal muscle protein turnover during exercise and recovery. *Journal of Applied Physiology*. 2010;109(2):431-438.

60 Burd NA, West DWD, Staples AW, Atherton PJ, Baker JM, Moore DR, Holwerda AM, Parise G, Rennie MJ, Baker SK, Phillips SM. Low-load high volume resistance exercise stimulates muscle protein synthesis more than high-load low volume resistance exercise in young men. *PloS ONE*. 2010;5(8):12033E.

61 Key TJ, Appleby PN, Rosell MS. Health effects of vegetarian and vegan diets. *Proceedings of the Nutrition Society*. 2006;65:35-41.

62 Craig WJ, Mangels AR. Position of the American Dietetic Association: Vegetarian diets. *Journal of the American Dietetic Association*. 2009;109(7):1266-1282.

63 Venderley AM, Campbell WW. Vegetarian diets: Nutritional considerations for athletes. *Sports Medicine*. 2006;36(4):293-305.

64 Borrione P, Grasso L, Quaranta F, Parisi A. Vegetarian diet and athletes. *Sport- und Präventivmedizin*. 2009;20-24.

65 Nichols DL, Sanborn CF, Essery EV. Bone density and young athletic women: An update. *Sports Medicine*. 2007;37(11):1001-1014.

66 Renda M, Fischer P. Vegetarian diets in children and adolescents. *Pediatrics in Review*. 2009;30:1E-8E.

67 Lemon PW. Effects of exercise on dietary protein requirements. *International Journal of Sport Nutrition*. 1998;8(4):426-447.

68 Maughan R. The athlete's diet: Nutritional goals and dietary strategies. *Proceedings of the Nutrition Society*. 2002;6(1):87-96.

69 Zawadzki KM, Yaspelkis BB, Ivy JL. Carbohydrate-protein complex increases the rate of muscle glycogen storage after exercise. *Journal of Applied Physiology*. 1992;72(5):1854-1859.

70 Roy BD. Milk, the new sports drink? A review. *Journal of the International Society of Sports Nutrition*. 2008;5:15.

71 Shirreffs SM, Watson P, Maughan RJ. Milk as an effective post-exercise rehydration drink. *British Journal of Nutrition*. 2007;98:173-180.

72 Thomas K, Morris P, Stevenson E. Improved endurance capacity following chocolate milk consumption compared with 2 commercially available sports drinks. *Applied Physiology and Nutrition Metabolism*. 2000;34.78-82.

73 Cockburn E, Hayes PR, French DN, Stevenson E, St. Clair Gibson A. Acute milk-based protein-CHO supplementation attenuates exercise-induced muscle damage. *Applied Physiology and Nutrition Metabolism*. 2008;33(4):775-783.

74 Hartman JW, Tang JE, Wilkinson SB, Tarnopolsky MA, Lawrence RL, Fullerton AV, Phillips SM. Consumption of fat-free fluid milk after resistance exercise promotes greater lean mass accretion than does consumption of soy or carbohydrate in young, novice, male weightlifters. *American Journal of Clinical Nutrition*. 2007;86:37.

Chapter 2

1 Osmolality is the number of particles per unit of water. The greater the number of particles, the greater the osmolality. High-osmolar solutions slow gastric emptying and may also cause an infusion of fluids into the intestines to lower the osmolar concentration before absorption. Both of these effects impede efficient delivery of fluid and fluid contents to working muscles. Some sports beverages control osmolality by including carbohydrate at a concentration that does not exceed 7 percent and by keeping sodium chloride concentration at 200 milligrams per cup or less.

2 Maughan RJ, Depiesse F, Geyer H. The use of dietary supplements by athletes. *Journal of Sports Sciences*. 2007:103S-113S.

3 Gleeson M, Nieman DC, Pedersen BK. Exercise, nutrition and immune function. *Journal of Sports Sciences*. 2004;22:115-125

4 Nieman DC. Marathon training and immune function. *Sports Medicine*. 2007;37(4/5):412-415.

5 Nieman DC, Henson DA, McAnulty SR, McAnulty LS, Morrow JS, Ahmed A, Heward CB. Vitamin E and immunity after the Kona Triathlon World Championship. *Medicine and Science in Sports and Exercise.* 2004;36(8):1328-1335

6 Maughan RJ. Contamination of dietary supplements and positive drug tests in sport. *Journal of Sports Sciences.* 2005;23(9):883-889.

7 Miller ER, Pastor-Barriuso R, Dalal D, Riemersma RA, Appel LJ, Guallar E. Meta-analysis: High-dosage vitamin E supplementation may increase all-cause mortality. *Annals of Internal Medicine.* 2005;142:37-46.

8 Bernstein AL. Vitamin B$_6$ in clinical neurology. *Annals of the New York Academy of Sciences.* 1990;585:250-260.

9 Institute of Medicine. *Dietary Reference Intakes: The Essential Guide to Nutrient Requirements.* Washington DC: National Academies Press; 2006.

10 Loosli Ar, Benson J, Gillien DM, Bourdet K. Nutritional habits and knowledge in competitive adolescent female gymnasts. *The Physician and Sports Medicine.* 1986;14:18.

11 Short SH, Short WR. Four-year study of university athletes' dietary intake. *Journal of the American Dietetic Association.* 1983;82:632.

12 Steen SN, McKinney S. Nutritional assessment of college wrestlers. *The Physician and Sports Medicine.* 1986;14:101.

13 Keys A, Henschel AF, Michelsen O, Brozek JM. The performance of normal young men on controlled thiamin intakes. *Journal of Nutrition.* 1943;26:399.

14 Chen JD, Wang JF, Li KJ, Zhao YW, Wang SW, Jiao Y, Hou XY. Nutritional problems and measures in elite and amateur athletes. *American Journal of Clinical Nutrition.* 1989;49:1084-1089.

15 Zaleman I, Guarita HV, Juzwiak CR, Crispim CA, Antunes HKM, Edwards B, Tufik S, de Mello MT. Nutritional status of adventure racers. *Nutrition.* 2007;(23):404-411.

16 Diaz E, Ruiz F, Hoyos I, Zubero J, Gravina L, Gil J, Irazusta J, Gil SM. Cell damage, antioxidant status, and cortisol levels related to nutrition in ski mountaineering during a two-day race. *Journal of Sports Science and Medicine.* 2010;(9):338-346.

17 Belko AZ, Obarzanek E, Kalkwarf JH, Rotter MA, Bogusz S, Miller D, Haas JD, Roe DA. Effects of exercise on riboflavin requirements of young women. *American Journal of Clinical Nutrition.* 1983;37:509-517.

18 Belko AZ, Obarzanek MP, Rotter BS, Urgan G, Weinberg S, Roe DA. Effects of aerobic exercise and weight loss on riboflavin requirements of moderately obese, marginally deficient young women. *American Journal of Clinical Nutrition.* 1984;40:553.

19 Belko AZ, Meredith MP, Kalkwarf HJ, Obarzanek E, Weinberg S, Roach R, McKeon G, Roe DA. Effects of exercise on riboflavin requirements: Biological validation in weight-reducing young women. *American Journal of Clinical Nutrition.* 1985;41:270.

20 Tremblay A, Boiland F, Breton M, Bessette H, Roberge AG. The effects of a riboflavin supplementation on the nutritional status and performance of elite swimmers. *Nutrition Research.* 1984;4:201.

21 Manore M, Thompson J. *Sports Nutrition for Health and Performance.* Champaign, IL: Human Kinetics.

22 Borrione P, Grasso L, Quaranta F, Parisi A. FIMS position statement: Vegetarian diet and athletes. *Sport- und Präventivmedizin.* 2009:20-24.

23 Lukaski HC. Vitamin and mineral status: Effects on physical performance. *Nutrition.* 2004;20:632-644.

24 Carlson LA, Havel RJ, Ekelund LG, Holmgren A. Effect of nicotinic acid on the turnover rate and oxidation of the free fatty acids of plasma in man during exercise. *Metabolism: Clinical and Experimental.* 1963;12:837.

25 Bergstrom J, Hultman E, Jorfeldt L, Pernow B, Wahnen J. Effect of nicotinic acid on physical working capacity and on metabolism of muscle. *Journal of Applied Physiology.* 1969;26:170.

26 Hilsendager D, Karpovich PV. Ergogenic effect of glycine and niacin separately and in combination. *Research Quarterly.* 1964;35:389.

27 Huskisson E, Maggini S, Ruf M. The role of vitamins and minerals in energy metabolism and well-being. *Journal of International Medical Research.* 2007;35:277-289.

28 Dalton K, Dalton MJT. Characteristics of pyridoxine overdose neuropathy syndrome. *Acta Neurologica Scandinavica.* 1987;76:8-11.

29 Schaumberg H, Kaplan J, Windebank A, Vick N, Ragmus S, Pleasure D, Brown MJ. Sensory neuropathy from pyridoxine abuse. *New England Journal of Medicine* 1983;309:445-448.

30 Manore MM. Vitamin B-6 and exercise. *International Journal of Sport Nutrition.* 1994;4:89-103.

31 Fogelholm M, Ruokonen I, Laakso JT, Vuorimaa T, Himberg JJ. Lack of association between indices of vitamin B-1, B-2, and B-6 status and exercise-induced blood lactate in young adults. *International Journal of Sport Nutrition.* 1993;3:165-176.

32 Guilland JC, Penarand T, Gallet C, Boggio V, Fuchs F, Klepping J. Vitamin status of young athletes including the effects of supplementation. *Medicine and Science in Sports and Exercise.* 1989;21:441-449.

33 Telford RD, Catchpole EA, Deakin V, McLeay AC, Plank AW. The effect of 7 to 8 months of vitamin/mineral supplementation on the vitamin and mineral status of athletes. *International Journal of Sport Nutrition.* 1992;2:123-134.

34 Suboticanec K, Stavljenic A, Schalch W, Buzina R. Effects of pyridoxine and riboflavin supplementation on physical fitness in young adolescents. *International Journal for Vitamin and Nutrition Research.*1990;60:81-88.

35 Delitala G, Masala A, Alagna S, Devilla L. Effect of pyridoxine on human hypophyseal trophic hormone release: A possible stimulation of hypothalamic dopaminergic pathway. *Journal of Clinical Endocrinology and Metabolsm.* 1976;42:603-606.

36 Dunton N, Virk R, Young J, Leklem J. Effect of vitamin B-6 supplementation and exhaustive exercise on vitamin B-6 metabolism and growth hormone. Abstract. *FASEB Journal.* 1992;6:1374A.

37 Moretti C, Fabbri A, Gnessi L, Bonifacio V, Fraioli F, Isidori A. Pyridoxine (B$_6$) suppresses the rise in prolactin and increases the rise in growth hormone induced by exercise. *New England Journal of Medicine.* 1982;307(7):444-445.

38 Dreon DM, Butterfield GE. Vitamin B-6 utilization in active and inactive young men. *American Journal of Clinical Nutrition.* 1986;43:816-824.

39 Albert MJ, Mathan VI, Baker SJ. Vitamin B-12 synthesis by human small intestinal bacteria. *Nature.* 1980;283:781-782.

40 Ryan A. Nutritional practices in athletics abroad. *The Physician and Sports Medicine.* 1977;5:33.

41 U.S. Senate. *Proper and Improper Use of Drugs by Athletes.* June 18 and July 12-13 hearings. Washington, DC: U.S. Government Printing Office; 1973.

42 Montoye HJ, Spata PJ, Pincney V, Barron L. Effects of vitamin B-12 supplementation on physical fitness and growth of young boys. *Journal of Applied Physiology.* 1955;7:589.

43 Tin-May Than, Ma-Win-May, Khin-Sann-Aung, Mya-Tu, M. The effect of vitamin B-12 on physical performance capacity. *British Journal of Nutrition.*1978;40:269.

44 Read M, McGuffin S. The effect of B-complex supplementation on endurance performance. *Journal of Sports Medicine and Physical Fitness.* 1983;23:178.

45 Sharabi A, Cohen E, Sulkes J, Garty M. Replacement therapy for vitamin B$_{12}$ deficiency: Comparison between the sublingual and oral route. *British Journal of Clinical Pharmacology.* 2003;56(6):635-638.

46 McNulty, H. 1995. Folate requirements for health in different population groups. *British Journal of Biomedical Science.* 52:110-112.

47 Baily LB. Folate requirements and dietary recommendations. In: Baily LB, ed. *Folate in Health and Disease*. New York: Dekker; 1995:123.

48 Wycoff KF, Ganji V. Proportion of individuals with low serum vitamin B-12 concentrations without macrocytosis is higher in the post folic acid fortification period than in the pre folic acid fortification period. *American Journal of Clinical Nutrition*. 2007;86(4):1187-1192.

49 Figucriredo JC, Grau MV, Haile RW, Sandler RS, Summers RW, Bresalier RS, Burke CA, McKeown-Eyssen GE, Baron JA. Folic acid and risk of prostate cancer: Results from a randomized clinical trial. *Journal of the National Cancer Institute*. 2009;101(6):432-435.

50 Mason JB, Dickstein A, Jacques PF, Haggarty P, Selhub J, Dallal G, Rosenberg IH. A temporal association between folic acid fortification and an increase in colorectal cancer rates may be illuminating important biological principles: A hypothesis. *Cancer Epidemiology, Biomarkers and Prevention*. 2007;16(7):1325-1329.

51 Matter M, Stittfall T, Graves J, Myburgh K, Adams B, Jacobs P, Noakes TD. The effect of iron and folate therapy on maximal exercise performance in female marathon runners with iron and folate deficiency. *Clinical Science*. 1987;72Z:415-420.

52 Weight LM, Noakes TD, Labadarios D, Graves J, Jacobs P, Berman PA. Vitamin and mineral status of trained athletes including the effects of supplementation. *American Journal of Clinical Nutrition*. 1988;47:186-192.

53 Davies MB, Austin J, Pantridge DA. *Vitamin C: Its Chemistry and Biochemistry*. Cambridge: Royal Society of Chemistry; 1991.

54 Institute of Medicine. *Dietary Reference Intakes for Vitamin C, Vitamin E, Selenium, and Carotenoids*. Food and Nutrition Board. Washington DC: National Academies Press; 2000.

55 Hickson JF, Wolinsky I, eds. *Nutrition in Exercise and Sport*. Boca Raton, FL: CRC Press; 1989:121.

56 Bramich K, McNaughton L. The effects of two levels of ascorbic acid on muscular endurance, muscular strength, and V\od\O₂max. *International Clinical Nutrition Revue* 1987;7:5.

57 Schwartz PL. Ascorbic acid in wound healing: A review. *Journal of the American Dietetic Association*. 1970;56:497.

58 Kanter MM. Free radicals, exercise, and antioxidant supplementation. *International Journal of Sport Nutrition*. 1994;4:205-220.

59 Herbert V. Does mega-C do more good than harm, or more harm than good? *Nutrition Today* 1993;Jan/Feb.28-32.

60 Peake JM. Vitamin C: Effects of exercise and requirements with training. *International Journal of Sport Nutrition and Exercise Metabolism*. 2003;13:125-151.

61 Institute of Medicine. *Dietary Reference Intakes for Vitamin A, Vitamin K, Arsenic, Boron, Chromium, Copper, Iodine, Iron, Manganese, Molybdenum, Nickel, Silicon, Vanadium, and Zinc*. Food and Nutrition Board. Washington DC: National Academies Press; 2002.

62 Institute of Medicine. *Dietary Reference Intakes for Calcium, Phosphorus, Magnesium, Vitamin D, and Fluoride*. Food and Nutrition Board. Washington DC: National Academies Press; 2000.

63 Benson J, Gillien DM, Bourdet K, Loosli AR. Inadequate nutrition and chronic calorie restriction in adolescent ballerinas. *The Physician and Sports Medicine*. 1985;13-79.

64 Cohen JL, Potosnak L, Frank O, Baker H. A nutritional and hematological assessment of elite ballet dancers. *The Physician and Sports Medicine*. 1985;13:43.

65 Welsh PK, Zager KA, Endres J, Poon SW. Nutrition education, body composition and dietary intake of female college athletes. *The Physician and Sports Medicine*. 1987;15:63

66 Nelson-Steen S, Mayer K, Brownell KD, Wadden TA. Dietary intake of female collegiate heavy weight rowers. *International Journal of Sports Nutrition*. 1995;5:225.

67 Neuman I, Nahum H, Ben-Amotz A. Prevention of exercise-induced asthma by a natural isomer mixture of beta-carotene. *Annals of Allergy and Asthma Immunology*. 1999;82:549-553.

68 Khanna S, Atalay M, Laaksonen DE, Gul M, Roy S, Sen CK. Alpha-lipoic acid supplementation: Tissue glutathione homeostasis at rest and after exercise. *Journal of Applied Physiology*. 1999;86:1191-1196.

69 Murray R, Horsun CA II. Nutrient requirements for competitive sports. In: Ira Wolinsky, ed. *Nutrition in Exercise and Sport*. 3rd ed. Boca Raton, FL: CRC Press; 1998:550.

70 Schubert L, DeLuca HF. Hypophosphatemia is responsible for skeletal muscle weakness of vitamin D deficiency. *Archives of Biochemistry and Biophysics*. 2010;500(2):157-161.

71 Cannell JJ, Hollis BW, Sorenson MB, Taft TN, Anderson JJ. Athletic performance and vitamin D. *Medicine and Science in Sports and Exercise*. 2009;41(5):1102-1110.

72 Hamilton B. Vitamin D and human skeletal muscle. *Scandinavian Journal of Medicine and Science in Sports*. 2010;20(2):182-190.

73 Williams MH. Dietary supplements and sports performance: Minerals. *Journal of the International Society of Sports Nutrition*. 2005;2:43-49.

74 Williams MH. Dietary supplements and sports performance: Introduction and vitamins. *Journal of the International Society of Sports Nutrition*. 2004;1:1-6

75 Barr SI, Prior JC, Vigna YM. Restrained eating and ovulatory disturbances: Possible implications for bone health. *American Journal of Clinical Nutrition*. 1994;59:92-97.

76 Chesnut CH. Theoretical overview: Bone development, peak bone mass, bone loss, and fracture risk. *American Journal of Medicine*. 1991;91(suppl 5B):2-4.

77 Heaney RP. Effect of calcium on skeletal development, bone loss, and risk of fractures. *American Journal of Medicine*. 91(suppl 5B):23-28.

78 Benardot D. 1997. Unpublished data from USOC research project on national-team gymnasts. Georgia State University. Laboratory for Elite Athlete Performance.

79 Neville HE, Ringel SP, Guggenheim MA, Wehling CA, Starcevich JM. Ultra-structural and histochemical abnormalities of skeletal muscle in patients with chronic vitamin E deficiency. *Neurology*. 1983;33:483

80 Miller ER III, Pastor-Barriuso RP, Dalal D, Riemersma RA, Appel LJ, Guallar E. Meta-analysis: High-dosage vitamin E supplementation may increase all-cause mortality *Annals of Internal Medicine*. 2005;142(1):37-46.

81 Talbot D, Jamieson J. An examination of the effect of vitamin E on the performance of highly trained swimmers *Canadian Journal of Applied Sport Sciences*. 1977;2:67.

82 Bunnell RH, DeRitter E, Rubin SH. Effect of feeding polyunsaturated fatty acids with a low vitamin E diet on blood levels of tocopherol in men performing hard physical labor. *American Journal of Clinical Nutrition*. 1975;28:706.

83 Sharman IM, Down MG, Sen RN. The effect of vitamin E and training on physiological function and athletic performance in adolescent swimmers. *British Journal of Nutrition*.1971;26:265.

84 Sharman IM, Down MB, Norgan NG. The effects of vitamin E on physiological function and athletic performance of trained swimmers. *Journal of Sports Medicine*.1976;16:215.

85 Brady PS, Brady LJ, Ullrey DE. Selenium, vitamin E, and the response to swimming stress in the rat. *Journal of Nutrition*. 1979;109:1103.

86 Dillard CJ, Liton RE, Savin WM, Dumelin EE, Tappel AL. Effects of exercise, vitamin E, and ozone on pulmonary function and lipid peroxidation. *Journal of Applied Physiology*. 1978;45:927.

87 Shephard RJ, Campbell R, Pimm P, Stuart D, Wright GR. Vitamin E, exercise, and the recovery from physical activity. *Journal of Applied Physiology*. 1974;33:119-126.

88 Bügel S. Vitamin K and bone health. *Proceedings of the Nutrition Society*. 2003;62:839-843.

89 Weber P. Vitamin K and bone health. *Nutrition.* 2001;17:880-887.

90 Feskanich D, Weber P, Willett WC, Rockett H, Booth SL, Colditz GA. Vitamin K intake and hip fractures in women: A prospective study. *American Journal of Clinical Nutrition.* 1999;69:74-79.

91 Booth SL, Tucker KL, Chen H, Hannan MT, Gagnon DR, Cupples LA, Wilson PWF, Ordovas J, Schaefer EJ, Dawson-Hughes B, and Kiel DP.Dietary vitamin K intakes are associated with hip fracture but not with bone mineral density in elderly men and women. *American Journal of Clinical Nutrition.* 2000;71:1201-1208.

92 Booth SL, Pennington JA, Sadowski JA. Food sources and dietary intakes of vitamin K-1 (phylloquinone) in the American diet: Data from the FDA Total Diet Study. *Journal of the American Dietetic Association.* 1996;96:149-154.

93 Lukaski HC. Micronutrients (magnesium, zinc, and copper): Are mineral supplements needed for athletes? *International Journal of Sport Nutrition.* 1995;5:74S-83S.

94 Benardot D. Nutrition for gymnasts. In: Marshall NT, ed. *The Athlete Wellness Book.* Indianapolis, IN: USA Gymnastics; 1999:12-13.

95 Lotz M, Zisman E, Bartter FC. Evidence for a phosphorus-depletion syndrome in man. *New England Journal of Medicine.* 1968;278:409-415.

96 National Research Council. *Recommended Dietary Allowances.* 10th ed. Washington, DC: National Academy of Sciences; 1989.

97 Bucci L. *Nutrients as Ergogenic Aids for Sports and Exercise.* Boca Raton, FL: CRC Press; 1993.

98 Keller WD, Kraut HA. Work and nutrition. *World Review of Nutrition and Dietetics.* 1959;3:65.

99 Cade R, Conte M, Zauner C, Mars D, Peterson J, Lunne D, Hommen N, Packer D. Effects of phosphate loading on 2,3-diphosphoglycerate and maximal oxygen uptake. *Medicine and Science in Sports and Exercise.* 1984;12:263.

100 Duffy DJ, Conlee RK. Effects of phosphate loading on leg power and high intensity treadmill exercise. *Medicine and Science in Sports and Exercise.* 1986;18:674.

101 Shils ME. Magnesium. In: Shils ME, Olson JA, Shike M, eds. *Modern Nutrition in Health and Disease.* 8th ed. Philadelphia: Lea & Febiger; 1993:164-184.

102 Steinacker JM, Grunert-Fuchs M, Steininger K, Wodick RE. Effects of long-time administration of magnesium on physical capacity. *International Journal of Sports Medicine.* 1987;8:151.

103 Golf SW, Bohmer D, Nowacki PE. Is magnesium a limiting factor in competitive exercise? A summary of relevant scientific data. In: Golf S, Dralle D, Vecchiet L, eds. *Magnesium.* London: Libbey; 1993:209-220.

104 Brilla LR, Haley TF. Effect of magnesium supplementation on strength training in humans. *Journal of the American College of Nutrition.* 1992;11:326-329.

105 Terblanche S, Noakes TD, Dennis SC, Marais D, Eckert M. Failure of magnesium supplementation to influence marathon running performance or recovery. *International Journal of Sport Nutrition.* 1992;2(2):154-164.

106 Hickson JF, Schrader J, Trischler LC. 1986. Dietary intake of female basketball and gymnastics athletes. *Journal of the American Dietetic Association.* 86:251-254.

107 Lukaski HC. Prevention and treatment of magnesium deficiency in athletes. In: Vecchiet L, ed. *Magnesium and Physical Activity.* Carnforth, UK: Parthenon; 1995:211-226.

108 Volpe SL. Magnesium and athletic performance. *ACSM's Health & Fitness Journal.* 2008;12(1):33-35.

109 Table salt is 40 percent sodium and 60 percent chloride. To obtain 1.5 grams of sodium, a person would require an intake of approximately 3.8 grams of table salt.

110 Institute of Medicine. *Dietary Reference Intakes: Electrolytes and Water.* Washington, DC: National Academies Press; 2010.

111 Pivarnik JM. Water and electrolytes during exercise. In: Hickson JF, Wolinsky I, (Editors) N*utrition in Exercise and Sport.* Boca Raton, FL: CRC Press; 1989:185-200.

112 Maughan RJ (Ed), "IOC Encyclopaedia of Sports Medicine: Nutrition in Sports". Blackwell Science Ltd: Oxford, England; 2000.

113 Clarkson P. Vitamins, iron, and trace minerals. In: Lamb D, Williams M, eds. *Ergogenics: Enhancement of Performance in Exercise and Sport.* Indianapolis: Benchmark Press; 1991.

114 Shaskey DJ, Green GA. Sports haematology. *Sports Medicine.* 2000;29(1):27-38.

115 Selby GB, Eichner ER. Endurance swimming, intravascular hemolysis, anemia, and iron depletion. *American Journal of Medicine.* 1986;81:791-794.

116 Waller M, Haymes E. The effects of heat and exercise on sweat iron loss. *Medicine and Science in Sports and Exercise.* 1996;28:197-203.

117 Brune M, Magnusson B, Persson H, Hallberg L. Iron losses in sweat. *American Journal of Clinical Nutrition.* 1986;43:438-443.

118 Baska RS, Moses FM, Graeber G, Kearney G. Gastrointestinal bleeding during an ultramarathon. *Digestive Diseases and Sciences.* 1990;35:276-279.

119 Balaban EP. Sports anemia. *Clinical Sports Medicine.* 1992;11(2):313-325.

120 Gleeson M, Nieman DC, Pedersen BK. Exercise, nutrition and immune function. *Journal of Sports Sciences.* 2004;22(1):115-125.

121 Cook JD, Finch CA, Smith NJ. Evaluation of the iron status of a population. *Blood.* 1976;48:449-455.

122 Wolinsky I, Driskell JA. *Sports Nutrition: Vitamins and Trace Elements.* Boca Raton, FL: CRC Press; 1997:148.

123 Lampe JW, Slavin JL, Apple FS. Iron status of active women and the effect of running a marathon on bowel function and gastrointestinal blood loss. *International Journal of Sports Medicine.* 1991;12:173-179.

124 Haymes EM, Spillman DM. Iron status of women distance runners, sprinters, and control women. *International Journal of Sports Medicine.* 1989;10:430-433.

125 Stephenson LS. Possible new developments in community control of iron-deficiency anemia. *Nutrition Reviews.* 1995;53(2):23-30.

126 Zoller H, Vogel W. Iron supplementation in athletes: First do no harm. *Nutrition.* 2004;20(7/8):615-619.

127 Zotter H, Robinson N, Zorzoli M, Schattenberg L, Saugy M, Mangin P. Abnormally high serum ferritin levels among professional road cyclists. *British Journal of Sports Medicine.* 2004;38(6):704-708.

128 Gleeson M, Lancaster GI, Bishop NC. Nutritional strategies to minimize exercise-induced immunosuppression in athletes. *Canadian Journal of Applied Physiology.* 2001;26(suppl):23S-35S.

129 Dressendorfer RH, Sockolov R. Hypozincemia in runners. *The Physician and Sports Medicine.* 1980;8:97-100.

130 Haralambie G. Serum zinc in athletes during training. *International. Journal of Sports Medicine.* 1981;2:135-138.

131 Singh A, Deuster PA, Moser PB. Zinc and copper status of women by physical activity and menstrual status. *Journal of Sports Medicine and Physical Fitness.* 1990:30:29-35.

132 Krotkiewski M, Gudmundsson M, Backstrom P, Mandroukas K. Zinc and muscle strength and endurance. *Acta Physiologica Scandinavica.* 1982;116:309-311.

133 Koury JC, de Olilveria AV Jr., Portella ES, de Olilveria CF, Lopes GC, Donangelo CM. Zinc and copper biochemical indices of antioxidant status in elite athletes of different modalities. *International Journal of Sport Nutrition and Exercise Metabolism.* 2004;14(3):358-372.

134 Brun JF, Dieu-Cambrezy C, Charpiat A, Fons C, Fedou C, Micallef JP, Fussellier M, Bardet L, Orsetti A. Serum zinc in highly trained adolescent gymnasts. *Biological Trace Element Research.* 1995;47(1-3):273-278.

135 Fischer PWF, Giroux A, L'Abbe MR. Effect of zinc supplementation on copper status in adult man. *American Journal of Clinical Nutrition*. 1984;40:743-746.

136 Hooper PL, Visconti L, Garry PJ, Johnson GE. Zinc lowers high-density lipoprotein cholesterol levels. *Journal of the American Medical Association*. 1980;244:1960-1961.

137 Spencer H. 1986. Minerals and mineral interactions in human beings. *Journal of the American Dietetic Association*. 86:864-867.

138 Wilborn CD, Kerksick CM, Campbell BI, Taylor LW, Marcello BM, Rasmussen CJ, Greenwood MC, Almada A, Kreider RB. Effects of zinc magnesium aspartate (ZaMA) supplementation on training adaptations and markers of anabolism and catabolism. *Journal of the International Society of Sports Nutrition*. 2004;1(2):12-20.

139 Zamora AJ, Tessier F, Marconnet P, Margaritis I, Marini JF. Mitochondria changes in human muscle after prolonged exercise, endurance training, and selenium supplementation. *European Journal of Applied Physiology*. 1995;71(6):505-511.

140 Tessier F, Margaritis I, Richard M-J, Moynot C, Marconnet P. Selenium and training effects on the glutathione system and aerobic performance. *Medicine and Science in Sports and Exercise*. 1995;27(3):390-396.

141 Lukaski HC, Hoverson BS, Gallagher SK, Bolonchuk WW. Physical training and copper, iron, and zinc status of swimmers. *American Journal of Clinical Nutrition*. 1990;53:1093-1099.

142 Evans GW. The effect of chromium picolinate on insulin controlled parameters in humans. *International Journal of Biosocial Research*. 1989;11:163.

143 Clancy SP, Clarkson PM, DeCheke ME, Nosaka K, Freedson PS, Cunningham JJ, Valentine JJ. Effects of chromium picolinate supplementation on body composition, strength, and urinary chromium loss in football players. *International Journal of Sport Nutrition*. 1994;4:142.

144 Hasten DL, Rome EP, Franks BD, Hegsted M. Effects of chromium picolinate on beginning weight training students. *International Journal of Sport Nutrition*. 1992;2:343.

145 Stearns D, Wise J, Paterno S, Wetterhahn. Chromium (III) picolinate produces chromosome damage in Chinese hamster ovary cells. *FASEB Journal*. 1995;9:1643-1648.

Chapter 3

1 Poortmans J. Exercise and renal function. *Sports Medicine*. 1984;1:125-153.

2 Zambraski EJ. Renal regulation of fluid homeostasis during exercise. In: Gisolfe CV, Lamb CV, eds. *Perspectives in Exercise Science and Sports Medicine, Volume 3: Fluid Homeostasis During Exercise*. Carmel, IN: Benchmark Press; 1990:247-280.

3 It is necessary to excrete metabolic by-products. This excretion can take place via the production of dilute or concentrated urine, depending on hydration state.

4 Sawka MN, Latzka WA, Montain SJ. Effects of dehydration and rehydration on performance. In: Maughan RJ, ed. *Nutrition in Sport*. London: Blackwell Science; 2000:216-217.

5 Maughan RJ. Water and electrolyte loss and replacement in exercise. In: Maughan RJ, ed. *Nutrition in Sport*. London: Blackwell Science; 2000:226.

6 Leithead CS, Lind AR. *Heat Stress and Heat Disorders*. London: Casell; 1964.

7 Maughan RJ. Thermoregulation and fluid balance in marathon competition at low ambient temperature. *International Journal of Sports Medicine*. 1985;6:15-19.

8 Costill DL. Sweating: Its composition and effects on body fluids. *Annals of the New York Academy of Sciences*. 1977;301:160-174.

9 Kenney WL. Body fluid and temperature regulation as a function of age: In: Lamb DR, Gisolfi CV, Nadel ER, eds. *Perspectives in Exercise Science and Sports Medicine, Volume 8: Exercise in Older Adults*. Indianapolis: Benchmark Press; 1995:305-352.

10 Hubbard RW, Szlyk PC, Armstrong LE. Influence of thirst and fluid palatability on fluid ingestion during exercise. In: Gisolfi CV, Lamb DR, eds. *Perspectives in Exercise Science and Sports Medicine, Volume 3: Fluid Homeostasis During Exercise*. Indianapolis: Benchmark Press; 1990:39-95.

11 Fitzsimons JT. Evolution of physiological and behavioural mechanism in vertebrate body and homeostasis. In: Ramsay DJ, Booth DA, eds. *Thirst: Physiological and Psychological Aspects*. ILSI Human Nutrition Reviews. London: Springer-Verlag; 1990:3-22.

12 Rehrer NJ. Factors influencing fluid bioavailability. *Australian Journal of Nutrition and Dietetics*. 1996;53(suppl 4):8S-12S.

13 Davis JM, Burgess WA, Slentz CA, Bartoli WP, Pate RR. Effects of ingesting 6% and 12% glucose-electrolyte beverages during prolonged intermittent cycling in the heat. *European Journal of Applied Physiology*. 1988;57:563-569.

14 Rehrer JN, Beckers EJ, Brouns F, ten Hoor F, Saris WHM. Exercise and training effects on gastric emptying of carbohydrate beverages. *Medicine and Science in Sports and Exercise*. 1989;21:540-549.

15 American College of Sports Medicine. Position paper: Nutrition and athletic performance. *Medicine and Science in Sports and Exercise*. 2009;41(3):709-731.

16 Rehrer JN, Brouns F, Beckers EJ, Saris WHM. The influence of beverage composition and gastrointestinal function on fluid and nutrient availability during exercise. *Scandinavian Journal of Medicine and Science in Sports*. 1994;4:159-172.

17 Noakes TD, Rehrer NJ, Maughan RJ. The importance of volume in regulating gastric emptying. *Medicine and Science in Sports and Exercise*. 1991;23:307-313.

18 Sun WM, Houghton LA, Read NW, Grundy DG, Johnson AG. Effect of meal temperature on gastric emptying of liquids in man. *Gut*. 1988;29:302-305.

19 Costill DL, Saltin B. Factors limiting gastric emptying. *Journal of Applied Physiology*. 1974;37:679-683.

20 Ryan AJ, Navarne AE, Gisolfi CV. Consumption of carbonated and noncarbonated sports drinks during prolonged treadmill exercise in the heat. *International Journal of Sport Nutrition*. 1991;1:225-239.

21 Lambert GP, Bleiler TL, Chang R, Johnson AK, Gisolfi CV. Effects of carbonated and noncarbonated beverages at specific intervals during treadmill running in the heat. *International Journal of Sport Nutrition*. 1993;3:177-193.

22 Wolf S. The psyche and the stomach. *Gastroenterology*. 1981;80:605-614.

23 Bar-Or O. Children's responses to exercise in hot climates: Implications for performance and health. *GSSI Sports Science Exchange* .1994;7(2):1-4.

24 Gisolfi CV, Summers R, Schedl H. Intestinal absorption of fluids during rest and exercise. In: Gisolfi CV and Lamb DR, eds. *Perspectives in Exercise Science and Sports Medicine, Volume 3: Fluid Homeostasis During Exercise*. Carmel, IN: Benchmark Press; 1990:39-95.

25 Maughan RJ, Noakes TD. Fluid replacement and exercise stress: A brief review of studies on fluid replacement and some guidelines for the athlete. *Sports Medicine*. 1991;12:16-31.

26 Kenney WL. Heat flux and storage in hot environments. *International Journal of Sports Medicine*. 1998;19:92S-95S.

27 Kenefick R, Mahmood NV, Mattern CQ, Kertzer R, and Quinn TJ. Hypohydration adversely affects lactate threshold in endurance athletes. *Journal of Strength and Conditioning Research*. 2002;16:38-43.

28 Naghii M. The significance of water in sport and weight control. *Nutrition and Health*. 2000;14:127-132.

29 Bergeron M. Averting muscle cramps. *The Physician and Sportsmedicine*. 2002;30(11):14.

30 Bergeron M. Sodium: The forgotten nutrient. *GSSI Sports Science Exchange*. 2000;13(3):1-4.

31 Wharam PC, Speedy DB, Noakes TD, Thompson J, Reid SA, Holtzhausen L-M. NSAID use increases the risk of developing hyponatremia during an Ironman triathlon. *Medicine and Science in Sports and Exercise.* 2006;38(4):618-622.

32 Craig S. Hyponatremia in emergency medicine. *eMedicine Journal.* www.emedicine.com/EMERG/topic275.htm. Accessed January 20, 2005.

33 Bergeron MF. Exertional heat cramps: Recovery and return to play. *Journal of Sport Rehabilitation.* 2007;16:190-196.

34 USA Track & Field is the national governing body (NGB) for the following events: track and field, long-distance running, and race walking.

35 Noakes T. The hyponatremia of exercise. *International Journal of Sport Nutrition.* 1992;2:205-228.

36 Gisolfi C. Fluid balance for optimal performance. *Nutrition Revue.* 1996;54:159S-168S.

37 Rehrer N. Fluid and electrolyte balance in ultra-endurance sport. *Sports Medicine.* 2001;31:701-715.

38 Speedy D, Noakes TD, Schneider C. Exercise-associated hyponatremia: A review. *Emergency Medicine.* 2001;13:17-27.

39 Mayo Clinic staff. Low blood sodium in endurance athletes. MayoClinic.com. www.mayoclinic.com. Accessed July 28, 2003.

40 Hargreaves M. Physiological benefits of fluid and energy replacement during exercise. *Australian Journal of Nutrition and Dietetics.* 1996;53(suppl 4):3S-7S.

41 Burke LM. Rehydration strategies before and after exercise. *Australian Journal of Nutrition and Dietetics.* 1996;53(suppl 4):22S-26S.

42 Nadel ER, Mack GW, Nose H. Influence of fluid replacement beverages on body fluid homeostasis during exercise and recovery. In: Gisolfi CV, Lamb DR, eds. *Perspectives in Exercise Science and Sports Medicine, Volume 3: Fluid Homeostasis During Exercise.* Carmel, IN: Benchmark Press; 1990:181-205.

43 Kristal-Boneh E, Glusman JG, Shitrit R, Chaemovitz C, Cassuto Y. Physical performance and heat tolerance after chronic water loading and heat acclimation. *Aviation, Space and Environmental Medicine.* 1995;66:733-738.

44 Sawka MN, Montain SJ, Lazka WA. Body fluid balance during exercise: Heat exposure. In: Buskirk ER, Puhl SM, eds. *Body Fluid Balance: Exercise and Sport.* Boca Raton, FL: CRC Press; 1996:143-161.

45 Lyons TP, Riedesel ML, Meuli LE, Chick TW. Effects of glycerol-induced hyperhydration prior to exercise in the heat on sweating and core temperatures. *Medicine and Science in Sports and Exercise.* 1990;22:477-483.

46 Montner P, Stark DM, Riedesel ML, Murata G, Robergs R, Timms M, Chick TW. Pre-exercise glycerol hydration improves cycling endurance time. *International Journal of Sports Medicine.* 1996;17:27-33.

47 Shirreffs SM, Armstrong LE, Cheuvront SN. Fluid and electrolyte needs for preparation and recovery from training and competition. *Journal of Sports Sciences.* 2004;22(1):57-63.

48 Lyle DM, Lewis PR, Richards DAB, Richards R, Bauman AE, Sutton JR, Cameron ID. Heat exhaustion in the *Sun-Herald* City to Surf Fun Run. *Medical Journal of Australia.* 1994;161:361-365.

49 McConnell G, Burge CM, Skinner SL, Hargreaves M. Ingested fluid volume and physiological responses during prolonged exercise in a mild environment. Abstract. *Medicine and Science in Sports and Exercise.* 1995;27:19S.

50 Walsh RM, Noakes TD, Hawley JA, Dennis SC. Impaired high-intensity cycling performance time at low levels of dehydration. *International Journal of Sports Medicine.* 1994;15:392-398.

51 Maughan RJ, Fenn CE, Leiper JB. Effects of fluid, electrolyte and substrate ingestion on endurance capacity. *European Journal of Applied Physiology.* 1989;58:481-486.

52 Mitchell JB, Costill DL, Houmard JA, Fink WJ, Pascoe DD, Pearson DR. Influence of carbohydrate dosage on exercise performance and glycogen metabolism. *Journal of Applied Physiology.* 1989;67:1843-1849.

53 Tsintzas OK, Liu R, Williams C, Campbell I, Gaitanos G. The effect of carbohydrate ingestion on performance during a 30-km race. *International Journal of Sport Nutrition.* 1993;3:127-139.

54 Coggan AR, Coyle EF. Reversal of fatigue during prolonged exercise by carbohydrate infusion or ingestion. *Journal of Applied Physiology.* 1987;63:2388-2395.

55 Coyle EF, Hagberg JM, Hurley BF, Martin WH, Ehami AA, Holloszy JO. Carbohydrate feeding during prolonged strenuous exercise can delay fatigue. *Journal of Applied Physiology.* 1983;55:230-235.

56 Coyle EF, Coggan AR, Hemmert MK, Ivy JL. Muscle glycogen utilization during prolonged, strenuous exercise when fed carbohydrate. *Journal of Applied Physiology.* 1986;61:165-172.

57 Tsintzas OK, Williams C, Boobis L, Greenhaff P. Carbohydrate ingestion and glycogen utilization in different muscle fibre types in man. *Journal of Physiology.* 1995;489:243-250.

58 Hargreaves M, Costill DL, Coggan AR, Fink WJ, Nishibata I. Effect of carbohydrate feedings on muscle glycogen utilization and exercise performance. *Medicine and Science in Sports and Exercise.* 1984;16:219-222.

59 Yaspelkis BB, Patterson JG, Anderla PA, Ding Z, Ivy JL. Carbohydrate supplementation spares muscle glycogen during variable-intensity exercise. *Journal of Applied Physiology.* 1993;75:1477-1485.

60 Below PR, Mora-Rodriquez R, Gonzalez-Alonso J, Coyle EF. Fluid and carbohydrate ingestion independently improve performance during 1 h of intense exercise. *Medicine and Science in Sports and Exercise.* 1995;27:200-210.

61 Nicholas CW, Williams C, Lakomy HKA, Phillips G, Nowitz A. Influence of ingesting a carbohydrate-electrolyte solution on endurance capacity during intermittent, high intensity shuttle running. *Journal of Sports Sciences.* 1995;13:283-290.

62 Simard C, Tremblay A, Jobin M. Effects of carbohydrate intake before and during an ice hockey match on blood and muscle energy substrates. *Research Quarterly for Exercise and Sport.* 1988;59:144-147.

63 Coyle EF, Coggan AR, Hemmert MK, Ivy JL. Muscle glycogen utilization during prolonged, strenuous exercise when fed carbohydrate. *Journal of Applied Physiology.* 1986;61:165-172.

64 Murray R, Paul GL, Seifert JG, Eddy DE, Halaby GA. The effects of glucose, fructose, and sucrose ingestion during exercise. *Medicine and Science in Sports and Exercise.* 1989;21:275-282.

65 Owen MD, Kregel KC, Wall PT, Gisolfi CV. Effects of ingesting carbohydrate beverages during exercise in the heat. *Medicine and Science in Sports and Exercise.* 1986;18:568-575.

66 Murray R, Paul GL, Seifert JG, Eddy DE, Halaby GA. The effects of glucose, fructose, and sucrose ingestion during exercise. *Medicine and Science in Sports and Exercise.* 1989;21:275-282.

67 Bjorkman O, Sahlin K, Hagenfeldt L, Wahren J. Influence of glucose and fructose ingestion on the capacity for long-term exercise in well-trained men. *Clinical Physiology.* 1984;4:483-494.

68 Mason WL, McConell GK, Hargreaves M. Carbohydrate ingestion during exercise: Liquid vs. solid feedings. *Medicine and Science in Sports and Exercise.* 1993;25:966-969.

69 A 1 percent carbohydrate solution is 1 gram of carbohydrate per 100 milliliters of water. One liter of water is 1,000 milliliters, so consumption of 1 liter of a 6 percent carbohydrate solution will provide 240 calories from carbohydrate (6 \x\ 4 kilocalories per gram \x\ 10).

70 Coggan AR, Coyle EF. Reversal of fatigue during prolonged exercise by carbohydrate infusion or ingestion. *Journal of Applied Physiology.* 1987;63:2388-2395.

71 Coyle EF, Montain SJ. Benefits of fluid replacement with carbohydrate during exercise. *Medicine and Science in Sports and Exercise.* 1992;24(suppl):324S-330S.

72 Wagenmakers AJM, Brouns F, Saris WHM, Halliday D. Oxidation rates of orally ingested carbohydrates during prolonged exercise in men. *Journal of Applied Physiology.* 1993;75:2774-2780.

73 Broad EM, Burke LM, Gox GR, Heeley P, Riley M. Body weight changes and voluntary fluid intakes during training and competition sessions in team sports. *International Journal of Sport Nutrition.* 1996;6:307-320.

74 Noakes TD, Adams BA, Myburgh KH, Greff C, Lotz T, Nathan M. The danger of inadequate water intake during prolonged exercise. *European Journal of Applied Physiology.* 1988;57:210-219.

75 Rothstein A, Adolph EF, Wills JH. Voluntary dehydration. In: Adolph EF, ed. *Physiology of Man in the Desert.* New York: Interscience; 1947:254-270.

76 Carter JE, Gisolfi CV. Fluid replacement during and after exercise in the heat. *Medicine and Science in Sports and Exercise.* 1989;21:532-539.

77 Gonzalez-Alonso J, Heaps CL, Coyle EF. Rehydration after exercise with common beverages and water. *International Journal of Sports Medicine.* 1992;13:399-406.

78 Maughan RJ, Leiper JB. Sodium intake and post-exercise rehydration in man. *European Journal of Applied Physiology.* 1995;71:311-319.

79 Maughan RJ, Leiper JB, Shirreffs SM. Restoration of fluid balance after exercise-induced dehydration: Effects of food and fluid intake. *European Journal of Applied Physiology.* 1996;73:317-325.

80 Osmolarity is largely determined by the number of molecules contained in a given volume of fluid. The size of the molecules does not have an impact on osmolarity, just the number of molecules. A polymer contains many carbohydrate units in a single molecule, thereby giving it a lower osmolar impact than the same number of carbohydrate units dispersed in the solution individually.

81 Triplett D, Doyle JA, Rupp JC, Benardot D. An isocaloric glucose-fructose beverage's effect on simulated 100-km cycling performance compared with a glucose-only beverage. *International Journal of Sport Nutrition and Exercise Metabolism.* 2010;20:122-131.

82 Pfeiffer B, Stellingwerff T, Zaltas E, Jeukendrup AE. Carbohydrate oxidation from a carbohydrate gel compared to a drink during exercise. *Medicine and Science in Sports and Exercise.* 2011;43(2): 327-334.

83 Peake J, Peiffer JJ, Abbiss CR, Nosaka K, Laursen PB, Suzuki K. Carbohydrate gel ingestion and immunoendocrine responses to cycling in temperate and hot conditions. *International Journal of Sport Nutrition and Exercise Metabolism.* 2008;18:229-246.

Chapter 4

1 Greenhaff PL, Casey A, Short AH, Harris R, Soderlund K, Hultman E. Influence of oral creatine supplementation of muscle torque during repeated bouts of maximal voluntary exercise in man. *Clinical Science.* 1993;84:565-571.

2 Harris RC, Soderlund K, Hultman E. Elevation of creatine in resting and exercised muscle of normal subjects by creatine supplementation. *Clinical Science.* 1992;83:367-374.

3 Maughan RJ. Creatine supplementation and exercise performance. *International Journal of Sport Nutrition.* 1995;5:94-101.

4 Campbell WW. Synergistic use of higher-protein diets or nutritional supplements with resistance training to counter sarcopenia. *Nutrition Reviews.* 2007;65(9):416-422.

5 Paddon-Jones D, Sheffield-Moore M, Urban RJ, Sanford AP, Aarsland A, Wolfe RR, Ferrando AA. Essential amino acid and carbohydrate supplementation ameliorates muscle protein loss in humans during 28 days bedrest. *Journal of Clinical Endocrinology and Metabolism.* 2004;89:4351-4358.

6 Butterfield G, Cady C, Moynihan S. Effect of increasing protein intake on nitrogen balance in recreational weight lifters. *Medicine and Science in Sports and Exercise.* 1992;24:71S.

7 Maughan RJ, Depiesse F, Geyer H. The use of dietary supplements by athletes. *Journal of Sports Sciences.* 2007;25(1):103S-113S.

8 Ahrendt DM. Ergogenic aids: Counseling the athlete. *American Family Physician.* 2001;63(5):913-922.

9 Gurley BJ, Gardner SF, White LM, Wang PL. Ephedrine pharmacokinetics after the ingestion of nutritional supplements containing ephedra sinica (ma huang). *Therapeutic Drug Monitoring.* 1998;20:439-445.

10 Watson S. How to evaluate vitamins and supplements. WebMD Medical Reference. WebMD.com. Accessed May 1, 2011.

11 Maughan RJ. Dietary supplements: Contamination may cause failed drug tests. GSSI Hot Topic. 2001; May.

12 Nagle FJ, Bassett DR. Energy metabolism. In: Hickson JF, Wolinsky I, eds. *Nutrition in Exercise and Sport.* Boca Raton, FL: CRC Press; 1989:87-106.

13 Costill DL, Hargreaves M. Carbohydrate nutrition and fatigue. *Sports Medicine.* 1992;13(2):86

14 Valeriani A. The need for carbohydrate intake during endurance exercise. *Sports Medicine.* 1991;12(6):349.

15 Tarnopolsky MA, Atkinson SA, Phillips SM, MacDougall JD. Carbohydrate loading and metabolism during exercise in men and women. *Journal of Applied Physiology.* 1995;78:1360-1368.

16 Coyle EF. Effects of glucose polymer feedings on fatigability and the metabolic response to prolonged strenuous exercise. In: Fox EL, ed. *Ross Symposium on Nutrient Utilization During Exercise.* Columbus, OH: Ross Laboratories; 1983:4-11.

17 Berning JR, Leenders MM, Ratliff K, Clem KL, Troup JP. The effects of a high carbohydrate pre-exercise meal on the consumption of confectioneries of different glycemic indices. *Medicine and Science in Sports and Exercise.* 1993;25(5):125S.

18 Anantaraman R, Carmines AA, Gaesser GA, Weltman A. The effects of carbohydrate supplementation on maximal effort endurance performance. *Medicine and Science in Sports and Exercise.* 1994;26(5):34S.

19 Coyle EF. Timing and method of increased carbohydrate intake to cope with heavy training, competition and recovery. *Journal of Sports Sciences.* 1991;9:18-37.

20 Roy BD, Tarnopolsky MA, MacDougall JD, Fowles J, Yarasheski KE. The effect of oral glucose supplements on muscle protein synthesis following resistance training. *Medicine and Science in Sports and Exercise.* 1996;28(5):769S.

21 Branch JD, Schwarz WD, Van Lunen B. Effect of creatine supplementation on cycle ergometer exercise in a hyperthermic environment. *Journal of Strength and Conditioning Research.* 2007;21(1):57-61

22 Watson G, Casa DJ, Fiala KA, Hile A, Roti MW, Healy JC, Armstrong LE, Maresh CM. Creatine use and exercise heat tolerance in dehydrated men. *Journal of Athletic Training.* 2006;41(1):18-29.

23 Greenhaff PL. Creatine and its application as an ergogenic aid. *International Journal of Sport Nutrition.* 1995;5:100S-110S.

24 Greenhaff PL, Casey A, Short AH, Harris R, Soderlund K, Hultman E. Influence of oral creatine supplementation on muscle torque during repeated bouts of maximal voluntary exercise in man. *Clinical Science.* 1993;84:565-571.

25 Tarnopolsky MA. Caffeine and creatine use in sport. *Annals of Nutrition and Metabolism.* 2010;57(suppl 2):1S-8S.

26 Becque MD, Lochmann JD, Melrose DR. Effects of oral creatine supplementation on muscular strength and body composition. *Medicine and Science in Sports and Exercise.* 2000;32:654-658.

27 Volek JS, Rawson ES. Scientific basis and practical aspects of creatine supplementation for athletes. *Nutrition.* 2004;20:609-614.

28 Engelhardt M, Neumann G, Berbalk A, Reuter I. Creatine supplementation in endurance sports. *Medicine and Science in Sports and Exercise.* 1998;30(7):1123-1129.

29 Kozak CJ, Benardot D, Cody M, Doyle JA, Thompson WR. The effect of creatine monohydrate supplementation on anaerobic power and anaerobic endurance in elite female gymnasts. Master's thesis, Georgia State University; 1996.

30 Koenig C, Benardot D, Cody M, Thompson W. The influence of creatine monohydrate and carbohydrate supplements on repeated jump height. *Medicine and Science in Sports and Exercise.* 2004;36(5):347S.

31 Koenig CA, Benardot D, Cody M, Thompson WR. Comparison of creatine monohydrate and carbohydrate supplementation on repeated jump height performance. *Journal of Strength and Conditioning Research.* 2008;22(4):1081-1086.

32 Harris RC, Soderlund K, Hultman E. Elevation of creatine in resting and exercised muscle of normal subjects by creatine supplementation. *Clinical Science.* 1992;83:367-374.

33 Walker JB. Creatine biosynthesis, regulation, and function. *Advanced Enzymology.* 1979;50:117-142.

34 Robergs RA. Glycerol hyperhydration to beat the heat? *Sportscience Training and Technology.* 1988; January.

35 Montner P, Stark DM, Riedesel ML, Murata G, Robergs RA, Timms M, Chick TW. Pre-exercise glycerol hydration improves cycling endurance time. *International Journal of Sports Medicine.* 1996;17:27-33.

36 Montgomery DL, Beaudin PA. Blood lactate and heart rate response of young females during gymnastic routines. *Journal of Sports Medicine.* 1982;22:358-365.

37 Hyland PJ, MacConnie SE, Meigs RA. The effect of sodium bicarbonate ingestion on work output during a 2,000 meter rowing ergometer time trial. *Medicine and Science in Sports and Exercise.* 1993;25(5):1085S.

38 Webster MJ, Webster MN, Crawford RE, Gladden LB. Effect of sodium bicarbonate ingestion on exhaustive resistance exercise performance. *Medicine and Science in Sports and Exercise.* 1993;25(5):1086S.

39 Avedisian L, Guerra A, Wilcox A, Fox S. The effect of selected buffering agents on performance in the competitive 1600 meter run. *Medicine and Science in Sports and Exercise.* 1995;27(5):133S.

40 Butterfield G, Cady C, Moynihan S. Effect of increasing protein intake on nitrogen balance in recreational weight lifters. *Medicine and Science in Sports and Exercise.* 1992;24:71S.

41 Tarnopolsky MA, MacDougall JD, Atkinson SA. Influence of protein intake and training status on nitrogen balance and lean body mass. *Journal of Applied Physiology.* 1988;64(1):187-193.

42 Spriet LL. Caffeine and performance. *International Journal of Sport Nutrition.* 1995;5:84S-99S.

43 Bucci L. *Nutrients as Ergogenic Aids for Sports and Exercise.* Boca Raton, FL: CRC Press; 1993.

44 Ganio MS, Klau JF, Casa DJ, Armstrong LE, Maresh CM. Effect of caffeine on sport-specific endurance performance: A systematic review. *Journal of Strength and Conditioning Research.* 2009;23(1):315-324.

45 Cox GR, Desbrow B, Montgomery PG, Anderson ME, Bruce CR, Macrides TA, Martin DT, Moquin A, Roberts A, Hawley JA, Burke LM. Effect of different protocols of caffeine intake on metabolism and endurance performance. *Journal of Applied Physiology.* 2002;93:990-999.

46 Graham TE, Spriet LL. Performance and metabolic responses to a high caffeine dose during prolonged exercise. *Journal of Applied Physiology.* 1991;71:2292-2298.

47 Silver MD. Use of ergogenic aids by athletes. *Journal of the American Academy of Orthopaedic Surgeons.* 2001;9(1):61-70.

48 Kalmar JM, Cafarelli E. Effects of caffeine on neuromuscular function. *Journal of Applied Physiology.* 1999;87:801-808.

49 Graham TE, Battram DS, Dela F, El-Sohemy A, Thong FSL. Does caffeine alter muscle carbohydrate and fat metabolism during exercise? *Applied Physiology and Nutrition Metabolism.* 2008;33:1311-1318.

50 Tarnopolsky MA. Caffeine and endurance performance. *Sports medicine.* 1994;18:109-125.

51 Jackman M, Wendling P, Friars D, Graham J. Metabolic catecholamine, and endurance responses to caffeine during intense exercise. *Journal of Applied Physiology.* 1996;81:1658-1663.

52 Armstrong LE, Douglas C, Maresh CM, Ganio MS. Caffeine, fluid-electrolyte balance, temperature regulation, and exercise-heat tolerance. *Exercise and Sport Sciences Reviews.* 2007;35(3):135-140.

53 Paluska SA. Caffeine and exercise. *Current Sports Medicine Reports.* 2003;2(4):213-219.

54 Kanter MM, Williams MH. Antioxidants, carnitine, and choline as putative ergogenic aids. *International Journal of Sport Nutrition.* 1995;5:120S-131S.

55 Clarkson PM. Nutrition for improved sports performance: Current issues on ergogenic aids. *Sports Medicine.* 1996;21:393-401.

56 Juhnson WA, Landry GL. Nutritional supplements: Fact vs. fiction. *Adolescent Medicine.* 1998;9:501-513.

57 Oostenbrug GS, Mensink RP, Hardeman MR, DeVries T, Brouns F, Hornstra G. Exercise performance, red blood cell deformability, and lipid peroxidation: Effects of fish oil and vitamin E. *Journal of Applied Physiology.* 1997;83(3):746-752.

58 Raastad T, Hostmark AT, Stromme SB. Omega-3 fatty acid supplementation does not improve maximal aerobic power, anaerobic threshold and running performance in well-trained soccer players. *Scandinavian Journal of Medicine and Science in Sports.* 1997;7:25-31.

59 Tartibian B, Maleki BH, Abbasi A. The effects of ingestion of omega-3 fatty acids on perceived pain and external symptoms of delayed onset muscle soreness in untrained men. *Clinical Journal of Sport Medicine.* 2009;19(2):115-119.

60 Babayan VK. Medium-chain triglycerides: Their composition, preparation, and application. *Journal of the American Oil Chemists' Society.* 1967;45:23.

61 Bach AS, Babayan VK. Medium-chain triglycerides: An update. *American Journal of Clinical Nutrition.* 1982;36:950.

62 Misell LM, Lagomarcino ND, Schuster V, Kern M. Chronic medium-chain triacylglycerol consumption and endurance performance in trained runners. *Journal of Sports Medicine and Physical Fitness.* 2001;41(2):210-215.

63 Horowitz JF, Mora-Rodriguez R, Byerley LO, Coyle EF. Preexercise medium-chain triglyceride ingestion does not alter muscle glycogen use during exercise. *Journal of Applied Physiology.* 2000;88(1):219-225.

64 Goedecke JH, Elmer-English R, Dennis SC, Schloss I, Noakes TD, Lambert EV. Effects of medium-chain triaclyglycerol ingested with carbohydrate on metabolism and exercise performance. *International Journal of Sport Nutrition.* 1999;9(1):35-47.

65 Avakian EV, Sugimoto BR. Effect of Panax ginseng extract on blood energy substrates during exercise. *Federal Proceedings.* 1980;39:287.

66 Morris AC, Jacobs I, Klugerman A, McLellan, TM. No ergogenic effect of ginseng extract ingestion. *Medicine and Science in Sports and Exercise.* 1994;26(5):35S.

67 Egert S, Wolffram S, Bosy-Westphal A, Boesch-Saadatmandi C, Wagner AE, Frank J, Rimbach G, Mueller MJ. Daily quercetin supplementation dose-dependently increases plasma quercetin concentrations in healthy humans. *Journal of Nutrition.* 2008;138:1615-1621.

68 Jin F, Nieman DC, Shanely RA, Knab AM, Austin MD, Sha W. The variable plasma quercetin response to 12-week quercetin supplementation in humans. *European Journal of Clinical Nutrition.* 2010;64:692-697.

69 Davis JM, Carlstedt CJ, Chen S, Carmichael MD, Murphy EA. The dietary flavonoid quercetin increases V\od\O$_2$max and endurance capacity. *International Journal of Sport Nutrition and Exercise Metabolism*. 2010;20:56-62.

70 Davis JM, Murphy EA, Carmichael MD, Davis B. Quercetin increases brain and muscle mitochondrial biogenesis and exercise tolerance. *American Journal of Physiology: Regulatory, Integrative and Comparative Physiology*. 2009;65:1071R-1077R.

71 MacRae HSH, Mefferd KM. Dietary antioxidant supplementation combined with quercetin improves cycling time trial performance. *International Journal of Sport Nutrition and Exercise Metabolism*. 2006;16(4):405-419.

72 Quindry JC, McAnulty SR, Hudson MB, Hosick P, Dumke C, McAnulty LS, Henson D, Morrow JD, Nieman D. Oral quercetin supplementation and blood oxidative capacity in response to ultramarathon competition. *International Journal of Sport Nutrition and Exercise Metabolism*. 2008;18:601-616.

73 Utter AC, Nieman DC, Kang J, Dumke CL, Quindry JC, McAnulty SR, McAnulty LS. Quercetin does not affect rating of perceived exertion in athletes during the Western States Endurance Run. *Research in Sports Medicine*. 2009;17:71-83.

74 Dumke CL, Nieman DC, Utter AC, Rigby MD, Quindry JC, Triplett NT, McAnulty SR, McAnulty LS. Quercetin's effect on cycling efficiency and substrate utilization. *Applied Physiology, Nutrition and Metabolism*. 2009;34:993-1000.

75 Wade N. Red wine ingredient increases endurance, study shows. *New York Times*. NYTimes.com. Accessed November 17, 2006.

76 Lagouge M, Argmann C, Gerhart-Hines Z, Meziane H, Lerin C, Daussin F, Messadeq N, Milne J, Lambert P, Elliott P, Geny B, Laakso M, Puigserver P, Auwerx J. Resveratrol improves mitochondrial function and protects against metabolic disease by activating SIRT1 and PGC-1a. *Cell*. 2006;127(6):1109-1122.

77 Baur JA, Sinclair DA. Therapeutic potential of resveratrol: The in vivo evidence. *Nature Reviews: Journal of Drug Discovery*. 2006;5(6):493-506.

78 Wallerath T, Deckert G, Ternes T, Anderson H, Li H, Witte K, Förstermann U. Resveratrol, a polyphenolic phytoalexin present in red wine, enhances expression and activity of endothelial nitric oxide synthase. *Circulation*. 2002;106(13):1652-1658.

79 Stervbo U, Vang O, Bonnesen C. A review of the content of the putative chemopreventive phytoalexin resveratrol in red wine. *Food Chemistry*. 2007;101(2):449-457.

80 Farina A, Ferranti C, Marra C. An improved synthesis of resveratrol. *Natural Product Research*. 2006;20(3):247-252.

81 Trantas E, Panopoulos N, Ververidis F. Metabolic engineering of the complete pathway leading to heterologous biosynthesis of various flavonoids and stilbenoids in Saccharomyces cerevisiae. *Metabolic Engineering*. 2009;11(6):355-366.

82 Pervaiz S. Resveratrol: From grapevines to mammalian biology. *FASEB Journal*. 2003;17:1975-1985.

83 Elmali N, Baysal O, Harma A, Esenkaya I, Mizrak B. Effects of resveratrol in inflammatory arthritis. *Inflammation*. 2007;30(1/2):1-6.

84 WADA. World Anti-Doping Code, 2010. www.wada-ama.org. (Accessed 8-6-2011)

Chapter 5

1 Shi X, Bartoli W, Horn M, Murray R. Gastric emptying of cold beverages in humans: Effect of transportable carbohydrates. *International Journal of Sport Nutrition and Exercise Metabolism*. 2000;10:394-403.

2 Maughan RJ, Leiper JB. Limitations to fluid replacement during exercise. *Canadian Journal of Applied Physiology*. 1999;24(2):173-187.

3 Gorham ED, Garland CF, Garland FC, Grant WB, Mohr SB, Lipkin M, Newmark HL, Giovannucci E, Wei M, Holick MF. Optimal vitamin D status for colorectal cancer prevention: A quantitative meta analysis. *American Journal of Preventive Medicine*. 2007;2(3):210-216.

4 Fasano A, Berti I, Gerarduzzi T, Not T, Colletti RB, Drago S, Elitsur Y, Green PHR, Guandalini S, Hill ID, Pietzak M, Ventura A, Thorpe M, Kryszak D, Fornaroli E, Wasserman SS, Murray JA, Horvath K. Prevalence of celiac disease in at-risk and not-at-risk groups in the United States. *Archives of Internal Medicine*. 2003;163(3):268-292.

5 Van der Windt D, Jellema P, Mulder CJ, Knupkins CMF, van der Horst HE. Diagnostic testing for celiac disease among patients with abdominal symptoms. *Journal of the American Medical Association*. 2010;203(17);1738-1746.

6 Rothstein M. Running over medical obstacles. *The Journal Gazette*. 2008; August 9.

7 Leone JE, Gray KA, Massie JE, Rossi JM. Celiac disease symptoms in a female collegiate tennis player: A case report. *Journal of Athletic Training*. 2005;40(4):365-369.

8 Eberman LE, Cleary MA. Celiac disease in an elite female collegiate volleyball athlete: A case report. *Journal of Athletic Training*. 2005;40(4):360-364.

9 Lomer MCE, Parkes GC, Sanderson JD. Review article: Lactose intolerance in clinical practice—Myths and realities. *Alimentary Pharmacology and Therapeutics*. 2008;27:93-103.

10 Mathews SB, Waud JP, Roberts AG, Campbell AK. Systemic lactose intolerance: A new perspective on an old problem. *Postgraduate Medicine Journal*. 2005;81:167-173.

11 Wells RW, Blennerhassett MG. The increasing prevalence of Crohn's disease in industrialized societies: The price of progress? *Canadian Journal of Gastroenterology*. 2005;19(2):89-95.

12 Nayar M, Rhodes JM. Management of inflammatory bowel disease. *Postgraduate Medical Journal*. 2004;80(942):206-213.

13 Ikeuchi H, Yamamura T, Nakano H, Kosaka T, Shimoyama T, Fukuda Y. Efficacy of nutritional therapy for perforating and non-perforating Crohn's disease. *Hepatogastroenterology*. 2004;51(58):1050-1052.

14 Faloon WW, Paes IC, Woolfolk D, Nankin H, Wallace K, Haro EN. Effect of neomycin and kanamycin upon intestinal absorption. *Annals of the New York Academy of Sciences*. 1966;132(2):879-887.

15 Mahan LK, Escott-Stump S, eds. *Krause's Food, Nutrition, and Diet Therapy*. Philadelphia: Saunders; 2000:403.

16 Faucheron JL, Parc R. Non-steroidal anti-inflammatory drug induced colitis. *International Journal of Colorectal Disease*. 1996;11:99.

17 Haber P. Magnesium update. *Acta Medica Austriaca*. 2004;31(2):37-39.

18 El-Sayed MS, Ali N, El-Sayed Ali Z. Interaction between alcohol and exercise: Physiological and haematological implications. *Sports Medicine*. 2005;35(3):257-269.

19 Leo A and Lieber CS. Review article: Alcohol, vitamin A, and beta-carotene: Adverse interactions, including hepatotoxicity and carcinogenicity. *American Journal of Clinical Nutrition*. 1999;69(6):1071-1085.

20 Peretti-Watel P, Guagliardo V, Verger P, Pruvost J, Mignon P, Obadia Y. Sporting activity and drug use: Alcohol, cigarette and cannabis use among elite student athletes. *Addiction*. 2003;98(9):1249-1256.

21 Miller KE, Hoffman JH, Barnes GM, Farrell MP, Sabo D, Melnick MJ. Jocks, gender, race, and adolescent problem drinking. *Journal of Drug Education*. 2003;33(4):445-462.

22 Lorente FO, Souville M, Griffet J, Grelot L. Participation in sports and alcohol consumption among French adolescents. *Addictive Behaviors*. 2004;29(5):941-946.

23 Keefe EB, Lowe DK, Goss JR, Wayne R. Gastrointestinal symptoms of marathon runners. *West Journal of Medicine*. 1984;141:481-484.

24 Wilhite J, Mellion MB. Occult gastrointestinal bleeding in endurance cyclists. *Physician and Sportsmedicine.* 1990;18(8):75-78.

25 Strauss RH, Lanese RR, Leizman DJ. Illness and absence among wrestlers, swimmers, and gymnasts at a large university. *American Journal of Sports Medicine.* 1988;16:653-655.

26 McCabe ME 3d, Peura DA, Kadakia SC, Bocek Z, Johnson LF. Gastrointestinal blood loss associated with running a marathon. *Digestive Disease Science.* 1986;31:1229-1232.

27 Butcher JD. Runner's diarrhea and other intestinal problems of athletes. *American Family Physician.* 1993;Sept:623-627.

28 Mündel T, Jones DA. The effects of swilling an L(--)-menthol solution during exercise in the heat. *European Journal of Applied Physiology.* 2010;109:59-65.

29 Ho GWK. Lower gastrointestinal distress in endurance athletes. *Current Sports Medicine Reports.* 2009;8(2):85-91.

Chapter 6

1 Ziegler PJ, Jonnalagadda SS, Nelson JA, Lawrence C, Baciak B. Contribution of meals and snacks to nutrient intake of male and female elite figure skaters during peak competitive season. *Journal of the American College of Nutrition.* 2002;21(2):115-119.

2 Burke LM. Energy needs of athletes. *Canadian Journal of Applied Physiology.* 2001;26(suppl):202S-219S.

3 Hubbard RW, Szlyk PC, Armstrong LE. Influence of thirst and fluid palatability on fluid ingestion during exercise. In: Gisolfi CV, Lamb DR, eds. *Perspectives in Exercise Science and Sports Medicine, Volume 3: Fluid Homeostasis During Exercise.* Carmel, IN: Benchmark Press; 1990:39-95.

4 Hawley JA, Burke LM. Meal frequency and physical performance. *British Journal of Nutrition.* 1997;77:91S-103S.

5 Deutz B, Benardot D, Martin D, Cody M. Relationship between energy deficits and body composition in elite female gymnasts and runners. *Medicine and Science in Sports and Exercise.* 2000;32(3):659-668.

6 Iwao S, Mori K, Sato Y. Effects of meal frequency on body composition during weight control in boxers. *Scandinavian Journal of Medicine and Science in Sports.* 1996;6(5):265-272.

7 Dulloo AG, Girardier C. Adaptive changes in energy expenditure during refeeding following low-calorie intake: Evidence for a specific metabolic component favoring fat storage. *American Journal of Clinical Nutrition.* 1990;52:415-420.

8 Saltzman E, Roberts SB. The role of energy expenditure in regulation: Findings from a decade of research. *Nutrition Reviews.* 1995;53(8):209-220.

9 Benardot D, Thompson WR. Energy: The importance of getting enough and getting it on time. *ACSM's Health and Fitness Journal.* 1999;3(4):14-18.

10 Heshka S, Yank M-U, Wang J, Burt P, Pi-Sunyer FX. Weight loss and change in resting metabolic rate. *American Journal of Clinical Nutrition.* 1990;52:981-986.

11 Bishop NC, Blannin AK, Walsh NP, Robson PJ, Gleeson M. Nutritional aspects of immunosuppression in Athletes. *Sports Medicine.* 1999;3:151-176.

12 Nieman DC, Johansen LM, Lee JW. Infectious episodes in runners before and after the Los Angeles Marathon. *Journal of Sports Medicine and Physical Fitness.* 1990;30:316-328.

13 Chandra RK. Nutrition and the immune system: An introduction. *American Journal of Clinical Nutrition.* 1997;66:460S-463S.

14 Richter EA, Kiens B, Raben A, Tvede N, Pedersen BK. Immune parameters in male athletes after a lacto-ovo vegetarian diet and a mixed Western diet. *Medicine and Science in Sports and Exercise.* 1991;23(5):517-521.

15 Coggan AR. Plasma glucose metabolism during exercise in humans. *Sports Medicine.* 1991;11(2):102-124.

16 Gleeson M, Bishop NC. Elite athlete immunology: Importance of nutrition. *International Journal of Sports Medicine.* 2000;21(suppl 1):44S-50S.

17 Cunningham-Rundles S, McNeeley DF, Moon A. Mechanisms of nutrient modulation of the immune response. *Journal of Allergy and Clinical Immunology.* 2005;115:1119-1128.

18 Costa RJS, Oliver SJ, Laing SJ, Walters R, Bilzon JLJ, Walsh NP. *International Journal of Sport Nutrition and Exercise Metabolism.* 2009;19(4):366-484.

19 Burke L. Fasting and recovery from exercise. *British Journal of Sports Medicine.* 2010;44:502-508.

20 Walsh NP, Gleeson M, Pyne DB, Nieman DC, Dhabhar FS, Shephard RJ, Oliver SJ, Bermon S, Kajeniene A. Position statement. Part two: Maintaining immune health. *Exercise Immunology Review.* 2011;17:64-103.

21 Symons T, Sheffield-Moore M, Wolfe R, Paddon-Jones D. A moderate serving of high-quality protein maximally stimulates protein synthesis in young and elderly subjects. *Journal of the American Dietetic Association.* 2009;109:1582-1586.

22 Benardot D. Timing of energy and fluid intake: New concepts for weight control and hydration. *American College of Sports Medicine Health and Fitness Journal.* 2007;11:13-19.

23 Farshchi HR, Taylor M, MacDonald, I. Decreased thermic effect of food after an irregular compared with a regular meal pattern in healthy lean women. *International Journal of Obesity.* 2004;28:653-660.

24 LeBlanc J, Diamond P. Effect of meal size and frequency on postprandial thermogenesis in dogs. *American Physiological Society.* 1986;250:144-147.

25 Hawley JA, Burke LM. Meal frequency and physical performance. *British Journal of Nutrition.* 1997;77:91S-103S.

26 Jenkins DJA, Wolever TM, Vuksan V, Brighenti F, Cunnane SC, Rao AV, Jenkins AL, Buckley G, Patten R, Singer W, Corey P, Josse RG. Nibbling versus gorging: Metabolic advantages of increased meal frequency. *New England Journal of Medicine.* 1989;321(14):929-934.

27 Metzner HL, Lamphiear DE, Wheeler NC, Larkin FA. The relationship between frequency of eating and adiposity in adult men and women in the Tecumseh Community Health Study. *American Journal of Clinical Nutrition.* 1977;30:712-715.

28 Steen SN, Oppliger RA, Brownell KD. Metabolic effects of repeated weight loss and regain in adolescent wrestlers. *Journal of the American Medical Association.* 1988;260(1):47-50.

29 Benardot D, Martin DE, Thompson WR, Roman S. Between-meal energy intake effects on body composition, performance, and total caloric consumption in athletes. *Medicine and Science in Sports and Exercise.* 2005;37(5):339S.

30 deCastro JM. Genetic influences on daily intake and meal patterns of humans. *Physiology and Behavior.* 1993;53(4):777-782.

31 LeBlanc J, Mercier I, Nadeau A. Components of postprandial thermogenesis in relation to meal frequency in humans. *Canadian Journal of Physiology and Pharmacology.* 1993;71(12):879-883.

32 Luke A, Schoeller DA. Basal metabolic rate, fat-free mass, and body cell mass during energy restriction. *Metabolism.* 1992;41(4):450-456.

33 Tuschl RJ, Platte P, Laessle RG, Stichler W, Pirke KM. Energy expenditure and everyday eating behavior in healthy young women. *American Journal of Clinical Nutrition.* 1990;52(1):81-86.

34 Heshka S, Yang MU, Wang J, Burt P, Pi-Sunyer FX. Weight loss and change in resting metabolic rate. *American Journal of Clinical Nutrition.* 1990;52(6):981-986.

35 Kassab SE, Abdul-Ghaffar T, Nagalla DS, Sachdeva U, Nayar U. Serum leptin and insulin levels during chronic diurnal fasting. *Asia Pacific Journal of Clinical Nutrition.* 2003;12(4):483-487.

36 Friel AJ, Benardot D. The relationship between within-day energy balance and menstrual status in active females. *Medicine and Science in Sports and Exercise*. 2011;43(5):47S-48S.

37 Sandor RP. Heat illness: On-site diagnosis and cooling. *The Physician and Sportsmedicine*. 1997;25(6).

38 Benardot D. *Nutrition for Serious Athletes: An Advanced Guide to Foods, Fluids, and Supplements for Training and Performance*. Champaign, IL: Human Kinetics; 2000:77-78.

39 Williams MH. *Nutrition for Health, Fitness and Sport*. 5th ed. Boston: WCB McGraw-Hill; 1999: 276-277.

40 Maughan RJ, Noakes TD. Fluid replacement and exercise stress: A brief review of studies on fluid replacement and some guidelines for the athlete. *Sports Medicine*. 12:16-31.

41 Levey JM. Runner's diarrhea. *American Medical Association Quarterly*. 2000;14(1):6-7.

42 Blom PCS, Hostmark AT, Vaage O, Kardel KR, Maehlum S. Effect of different post-exercise sugar diets on the rate of muscle glycogen synthesis. *Medicine and Science in Sports and Exercise*. 1987;19:491-496.

43 Welsh RS, Davis JM, Burke JR, Williams HG. Carbohydrates and physical/mental performance during intermittent exercise to fatigue. *Medicine and Science in Sports and Exercise*. 2002;34:723-731.

44 Walberg-Rankin J, Ocel JV, Craft LL. Effect of weight loss and refeeding diet composition on anaerobic performance in wrestlers. *Medicine and Science in Sports and Exercise*. 1996;28:1292-1299.

45 Conley M, Stone M. Carbohydrate ingestion/supplementation for resistance exercise and training. *Sports Medicine*. 1996;21:7-17.

46 Jeukendrup A, Brouns F, Wagenmakers AJ, Saris WH. Carbohydrate-electrolyte feedings improve 1 h time trial cycling performance. *International Journal of Sports Medicine*. 1997;18(2):125-129.

47 Davis JM, Jackson DA, Broadwell MS, Queary JL, Lambert CL. Carbohydrate drinks delay fatigue during intermittent, high-intensity cycling in active men and women. *International Journal of Sport Nutrition*. 1997;7:261-273.

48 Kimber N, Ross JJ, Mason SL, Speedy DB. Energy balance during an Ironman triathlon in male and female triathletes. *International Journal of Sport Nutrition and Exercise Metabolism*. 2002;12:47-62.

49 Sherman WM, Costill DL, Fink W, Hagerman F, Armstrong L, Murray T. Effect of a 42.2-km footrace and subsequent rest or exercise on muscle glycogen and enzymes. *Journal of Applied Physiology*. 1983;55:1219-1224.

50 Bergstrom J, Hermansen L, Hultman E, Saltin B. Diet, muscle glycogen and physical performance. *Acta Physiologica Scandinavica*. 1967;71:140-150.

Chapter 7

1 Maughan RJ. Role of micronutrients in sport and physical activity. *British Medical Bulletin*. 1999;55(3):683-690.

2 Weiler JM, Metzger WJ, Donnelly AL, Crowley ET, Sharath MD. Prevalence of bronchial hyperresponsiveness in highly trained athletes. *Chest*. 1986;90(1):23-28.

3 Larsson K, Ohlsen P, Larsson L, Malmberg P, Rydstrom PO, Ulriksen H. High prevalence of asthma in cross country skiers. *British Medical Journal*. 1993;307(6915):1326-1329.

4 Columbini L. Exercise-induced asthma in children. *Canadian Journal of Continuing Medical Education*. 1998;10(8):67-81.

5 Carlsen KH, Anderson SD, Bjermer L, Bonini S, Brusasco V, Canonica W, Cummiskey J, Delgado L, DelGiacco SR, Drobnic F, Haahtela T, Larsson K, Palange P, Popov T, van Cauwenberge P. Exercise-induced asthma, respiratory and allergic disorders in elite athletes: Epidemiology, mechanisms and diagnosis: Part I of the report from the Joint Task Force of the European Respiratory Society (ERS) and the European Academy of Allergy and Clinical Immunology (EAACI) in cooperation with GALEN. *Allergy*. 2008;63:387-403.

6 Schumacher YO, Schmid A, Grathwohl D, Bultermann D, Berg A. Hematological indices and iron status in athletes of various sports and performances. *Medicine and Science in Sports and Exercise*. 2002;34(5):869-875

7 Beard J, Tobin B. Iron status and exercise. *American Journal of Clinical Nutrition*. 2000;72(2):594S-597S.

8 Portal S, Epstein M, Dubnov G. Iron deficiency and anemia in female athletes: Causes and risks. *Harefuah*. 2003;142(10):698-703, 717.

9 Lukaski HC. Vitamin and mineral status: Effects on physical performance. *Nutrition*. 2004;20(7/8):632-644.

10 Jones GR, Newhouse I. Sport-related hematuria: A review. *Clinical Journal of Sport Medicine*. 1997;7(2):119-125.

11 Fallon KE, Bishop G. Changes in erythropoiesis assessed by reticulocyte parameters during ultralong distance running. *Clinical Journal of Sport Medicine*. 2002;12(3):172-178.

12 Shaskey DJ, Green GA. Sports haematology. *Sports Medicine*. 2000;29(1):27-38.

13 Opara EC. Oxidative stress, micronutrients, diabetes mellitus and its complications. *Journal of the Royal Society of Health*. 2002;122(1):28-34.

14 Shephard RJ, Shek PN. Immunological hazards from nutritional imbalance in athletes. *Exercise Immunology Review*. 1998;4:22-48.

Chapter 8

1 Cleary MA, Sweeney LA, Kendrick ZV, Sitler MR. Dehydration and symptoms of delayed-onset muscle soreness in hyperthermic males. *Journal of Athletic Training*. 2005;40(4):288-297.

2 Parr JJ, Yarrow JF, Garbo CM, Borsa PA. Symptomatic and functional responses to concentric-eccentric isokinetic versus eccentric-only isotonic exercise. *Journal of Athletic Training*. 2009;44(5):462-468.

3 Frey-Law LA, Evans S, Knudston J, Nus S, Scholl K, Sluka K. Massage reduces pain perception and hyperalgesia in experimental muscle pain: A randomized, controlled trial. *Journal of Pain*. 2008;9(8):714-721.

4 Mayer JM, Mooney V, Matheson LN, Erasala GN, Verna JL, Udermann BE, Leggett S. Continuous low-level heat wrap therapy for the prevention and early phase treatment of delayed-onset muscle soreness of the low back: A randomized controlled trial. *Archives of Physical Medicine and Rehabilitation*. 2006;87(10):1310-1317.

5 Cheung K, Hume P, Maxwell L. Delayed onset muscle soreness: Treatment strategies and performance factors. *Sports Medicine*. 2003;33(2):145-164.

6 Prasartwuth O, Taylor JL, Gandevia SC. Maximal force, voluntary activation and muscle soreness after eccentric damage to human elbow flexor muscles. *Journal of Physiology*. 2005;567(1):337-348.

7 Ayilavarapu S, Kantarci A, Fredman G, Turkoglu O, Omori K, Liu H, Iwata T, Yagi M, Hasturk H, Van Dyke TE. Diabetes-induced oxidative stress is mediated by Ca2+-independent phospholipase A2 in neutrophils. *Journal of Immunology*. 2010;184(3):1507-1515.

8 Allen DG, Whitehead NP, Yeung EW. Mechanisms of stretch-induced muscle damage in normal and dystrophic muscle: Role of ionic changes. *Journal of Physiology*. 2005;567(3):723-735.

9 Erikson L. Does dietary supplementation of cod liver oil mitigate musculoskeletal pain? *European Journal of Clinical Nutrition* 1996; 50:689-693.

10 Lenn J, Uhl T, Mattacola C, Boissonneault G, Yates J, Ibrahim W, and Bruckner G. The effects of fish oil and isoflavones on delayed onset muscle soreness. *Medicine & Science in Sports & Exercise* 2002; 34(10): 1605-1613.

11 Tartibian B, Maleki BH, Abbasi A. The effects of ingestion of omega-3 fatty acids on perceived pain and external symptoms of delayed onset muscle soreness in untrained men. *Clinical Journal of Sport Medicine.* 2009;19(2):115-119.

12 Stupka N, Lowther S, Chorneyko K, Bourgeois JM, Hogben C, and Tarnopolsky MA. Gender differences in muscle inflammation after eccentric exercise. *Journal of Applied Physiology* 2000; 89: 2325-2332.

13 Benson J, Wilson A, Stocks N, Moulding N. Muscle pain as an indicator of vitamin D deficiency in an urban Australian Aboriginal population. *Medical Journal of Australia.* 2006;85(2):76-77.

14 Houston DK, Cesari M, Ferrucci L, Cherubini A, Maggio D, Bartali B, Johnson MA, Schwartz GG, and Kritchevsky SB. Association between vitamin D and physical performance: The InCHIANTI study. *Journal of Gerontology, Series A, Biological Sciences and Medical Sciences,* 2007; 62(4):440-446.

15 Silva LA, Pinho CA, Silveira PCL, Tuon T, De Souza, CT, Dal-Pizzol F, Pinho RA. Vitamin E supplementation decreases muscular and oxidative damage but not inflammatory response induced by eccentric contraction. *Journal of Physiological Sciences.* 2010;60(1):51-57.

16 Bryer SC, Goldfarb AH. Effect of high dose vitamin C supplementation on muscle soreness, damage, function, and oxidative stress to eccentric exercise. *International Journal of Sport Nutrition and Exercise Metabolism.* 2006;16(3):270-280.

17 Connolly DA, Lauzon C, Agnew J, Dunn M, Reed B. The effects of vitamin C supplementation on symptoms of delayed onset muscle soreness. *Journal of Sports Medicine and Physical Fitness.* 2006;46(3):462-467.

18 Shimomura Y, Murakami T, Nakai N, Nagasaki M, Harris RA. Exercise promotes BCAA catabolism: Effects of BCAA supplementation on skeletal muscle during exercise. *Journal of Nutrition.* 2004;134:1583S-1587S.

19 Shimomura Y, Yamamoto Y, Bajotto G, Sato J, Murakami T, Shimomura N, Kobayashi H, Mawatari K. Nutraceutical effects of branched-chain amino acids on skeletal muscle. *Journal of Nutrition.* 2006;136(suppl 1):529S-532S.

20 Evans WJ. Muscle damage: Nutritional considerations. *International Journal of Sport Nutrition.* 1991;1(3):214-224.

21 Dugan KM, McAdams M, Lewing M, Foster C, Wilborn C, Taylor LW IV. The effects of pre-and post-exercise whey vs. casein protein consumption on body composition and performance measures in collegiate female athletes. *International Journal of Exercise Science: Conference Abstract Submissions.* 2010;2(2): Article 24.

22 Pritchett K, Bishop P, Pritchett R, Green M, Katica C. Acute effects of chocolate milk and a commercial recovery beverage on postexercise recovery indices and endurance cycling performance. *Applied Physiology, Nutrition, and Metabolism.* 2009;34(6):1017-1022.

23 Ferguson-Stegall L, McCleave E, Doerner PG, Ding Z, Dessard B, Kammer L, Wang B, Liu Y, Ivy JL. Effects of chocolate milk supplementation on recovery from cycling exercise and subsequent time trial performance. *International Journal of Exercise Science: Conference Abstract Submissions.* 2010;2(2): Article 25.

24 Zamboanga BL, Rodriguez L, Horton NJ. Athletic involvement and its relevance to hazardous alcohol use and drinking game participation in female college athletes: A preliminary investigation. *Journal of American College Health.* 2008;56(6):651-656.

25 Yusko DA, Buckman JF, White HR, Pandina RJ. Alcohol, tobacco, illicit drugs, and performance enhancers: A comparison of use by college student athletes and nonathletes. *Journal of American College Health.* 2008;57(3):281-290.

26 Shirreffs SM, Maughan RJ. The effect of alcohol on athletic performance. *Current Sports Medicine Reports.* 2006;5:192-196.

27 Clarkson PM, Reichman F. The effect of ethanol on exercise-induced muscle damage. *Journal of Studies on Alcohol.* 1990;51:19-23.

28 Burke LM, Collier GR, Broad EM, Davis PG, Martin DT, Sanigorski AJ, Hargreaves M. Effect of alcohol intake on muscle glycogen storage after prolonged exercise. *Journal of Applied Physiology.* 2003;95:983-990.

29 Shirreffs SM, Maughan RJ. Restoration of fluid balance after exercise-induced dehydration: Effects of alcohol consumption. *Journal of Applied Physiology.* 1997;83:1152-1158.

30 Bloomer RJ. The role of nutritional supplements in the prevention and treatment of resistance exercise-induced skeletal muscle injury. *Sports Medicine.* 2007;37(6):519-532.

Chapter 9

1 Gayton WF, Broida J, Elgee L. An investigation of coaches' perceptions of the causes of home advantage. *Perceptual Motor Skills.* 2001;92(3):933-936.

2 Nevill AM, Holder RL. Home advantage in sport: An overview of studies on the advantage of playing at home. *Sports Medicine.* 1999;28(4):221-236.

3 Loat E, Rhodes EC. Jet-lag and human performance. *Sports Medicine.* 1989;8(4):226-238.

4 Pace A, Carron AV. Travel and the home advantage. *Canadian Journal of Sport Sciences.* 1992;17(1):60-64.

5 Bishop D. The effects of travel on team performance in the Australian national netball competition. *Journal of Science and Medicine in Sport.* 2004;7(1):118-122.

6 Reilly T, Atkinson G, Waterhouse J. Travel fatigue and jet-lag. *Journal of Sports Sciences.* 1997;15(3):365-369.

7 Atkinson G, Reilly T. Circadian variation in sports performance. *Sports Medicine.* 1996;21(4):292-312.

8 Hill DW, Hill CM, Fields KL, Smith JC. Effects of jet lag on factors related to sport performance. *Canadian Journal of Applied Physiology.* 1993;18(1):91-103.

9 Straub WF, Spino MP, Alattar MM, Pfleger B, Downes JW, Belizaire MA, Heinonen OJ, Vasankari T. The effect of chiropractic care on jet lag of Finnish junior elite athletes. *Journal of Manipulative and Physiological Therapeutics.* 2001;24(3):191-198.

10 Nieman DC. Current perspective on exercise immunology. *Current Sports Medicine Reports.* 2003;5:239-242.

11 So SC, Ko J, Yuan YW, Lam JJ, Louie L. Severe acute respiratory syndrome and sport: Facts and fallacies. *Sports Medicine.* 2004;34(15):1023-1033.

12 Gatorade Sports Nutrition Advisory Board. *Eating on the Road.* Chicago, IL: Gatorade Sports Science Institute; 1996.

13 Klein K, Wegmann H. The resynchronization of human circadian rhythms after transmeridian flights as a result of flight direction and mode of activity. In: Scheving LE, ed. *Chronobiology.* Tokyo: Igaku-Shoin; 1974:564-570.

14 Mielcarek J, Kleiner S. Time zone changes. In: Benardot D, ed. *Sports Nutrition: A Guide for Professionals Working With Active People.* Chicago: American Dietetic Association; 1993.

15 Scurr J, Machin S, Bailey-King S, Mackie I, McDonald S, Smith P. Frequency and prevention of symptomless deep-vein thrombosis in long-haul flights: A randomised trial. *The Lancet.* 357(9267):1485-1489.

16 Herxheimer A, Petrie KJ. Melatonin for the prevention and treatment of jet lag. Cochrane Review. *The Cochrane Library.* 2003;2. Oxford: Update Software.

17 Beaumont M, Batejat D, Pierard C, Van Beers P, Denis JB, Coste O, Doireau P, Chauffard F, French J, Lagarde D. *Journal of Applied Physiology.* 2004;96:50-58.

18 Manfredini R, Manfredini F, Fersini C, Conconi F. Circadian rhythms, athletic performance, and jet lag. *British Journal of Sports Medicine.* 1998;32:101-106.

Chapter 10

1 Levine BD, Stray-Gundersen J. The effects of altitude training are mediated primarily by acclimatization, rather than by hypoxic exercise. *Advances in Experimental medicine and Biology.* 2001;502:75-88.

2 Wilber RL, Stray-Gundersen J, Levine BD. Effect of hypoxic "dose" on physiologic responses and sea-level performance. *Medicine and Science in Sports and Exercise.* 2007;39(9):1590-1599.

3 Gallagher SA,Hackett PH. High-altitude illness. *Emergency Medicine Clinics of North America.* 2004;22:329-55.

4 Derby R, deWeber K. The athlete and high altitude. *Current Sports Medicine Reports.* 2010:79-85.

5 Cooper CE. The biochemistry of drugs and doping methods used to enhance aerobic sport performance. *Essays in Biochemistry.* 2008;44:63-83.

6 Marriott BM, Carlson SJ, eds. *Nutritional Needs in Cold and High-Altitude Environments: Applications for Military Personnel in Field Operations.* Washington DC: National Academy Press; 1996:9.

7 Horvath SM. Exercise in a cold environment. *Exercise Sport Science Review.* 1981;9:221-263.

8 Webb P. Temperature of skin, subcutaneous tissue, muscle and core in resting men in cold, comfortable and hot conditions. *European Journal of Applied Physiology.* 1992;64:471-476.

9 Vallerand AL, Jacobs I. Rates of energy substrates utilization during human cold exposure. *European Journal of Applied Physiology.* 1989;58:873-878.

10 Young AJ, Muza SR, Sawka MN, Gonzalez RR, Pandolf KB. Human thermoregulatory responses to cold air are altered by repeated cold water immersion. *Journal of Applied Physiology.* 1986;60:1542-1548.

11 Febbraio MA. Exercise in climatic extremes. In: Maughan RJ, ed. *Nutrition in Sport.* London: Blackwell Science; 2000:498.

12 Young AJ. Effects of aging on human cold tolerance. *Experimental Aging Research.* 1991;17(3):205-213.

13 Freund BJ, Sawka MN. Influence of cold stress on human fluid balance. In: Marriott BM, Carlson SJ, eds. *Nutritional Needs in Cold and High Altitude Environments.* Washington DC: National Academy Press; 1996.161.

14 Jefferson JA, Simoni J, Escudero E, Hurtado ME, Swenson ER, Wesson DE, Schreiner GF, Schoene RB, Johnson RJ, Hurtado A. Increased oxidative stress following acute and chronic high altitude exposure. *High Altitude Medicine and Biology.* 2004;5(1):61-69.

15 Altitude illness. NOLS Wilderness First Aid. www.elbrus.org/engl/high_altitude1.htm. Accesses March 21, 2005

16 Askew EW. Nutrition at high altitude. Wilderness Medical Society. www.wms.org/news/altitude.asp. Accessed July 12, 2011.

17 Rodway GW, Hoffman LA, Sanders MH. High-altitude-related disorders, part I: Pathophysiology, differential diagnosis, and treatment. *Heart Lung.* 2003;32(6):353-359.

18 Leppk JA, Icenogle MV, Maes D, Riboni K, Hinghofer-Szalkay H, Roach C. Early fluid retention and severe acute mountain sickness. *Journal of Applied Physiology.* 2005;98(2):591-597.

19 Talbot TS, Townes DA, Wedmore IS. To air is human: Altitude illness during an expedition length adventure race. *Wilderness and Environmental Medicine.* 2004;15(2):90-94.

20 Gallagher SA, Hackett PH. High-altitude illness. *Emergency Medicine Clinics of North America.* 2004;22(2):329-355.

21 Hackett PH, Roach RC. High altitude cerebral edema. *High Altitude Medicine and Biology.* 2004;5(2):136-146.

22 High altitude medicine guide. www.ismmed.org/np_altitude_tutorial.htm . Accessed August 8, 2011

23 Shephard RJ. The athlete at high altitude. *Canadian Medical Association Journal.* 1973;109:207-209.

24 Ri-Li G, Chase PJ, Witkowski S, Wyrick BL, Stone JA, Levine BD, Babb TG. Obesity: Associations with acute mountain sickness. *Annals of Internal Medicine.* 2003;139(4):253-257.

25 Beidleman BA, Muza SR, Fulco CS, Cymerman A, Ditzler D, Stulz D, Staab JE, Skrinar GS, Lewis SF, Sawka MN. Intermittent altitude exposures reduce acute mountain sickness at 4300 m. *Clinical Science.* 2004;106(3):321-328.

26 Dumont L, Lysakowski C, Tramer MR, Junod JD, Mardirosoff C, Tassonyi E, Kayser B. Magnesium for the prevention and treatment of acute mountain sickness. *Clinical Science.* 2004;106(3):269-277.

27 Bartsch P, Bailey DM, Berger MM, Knauth M, Baumgartner RW. Acute mountain sickness: Controversies and advances. *High Altitude Medicine and Biology.* 2004;5(2):110-124.

28 Rose MS, Houston CS, Fulco CS, Coates G, Sutton JR, Cymerman A. Operation Everest II: Nutrition and body composition. *Journal of Applied Physiology.* 1988;65:2545.

29 Butterfield GE. Maintenance of body weight at altitude: In search of 500 kcal/day. In: Marriott BM, Carlson SJ, eds. *Nutritional Needs in Cold and High Altitude Environments.* Washington DC: National Academy Press; 1996:357.

30 Reynolds RD, Lickteig JA, Deuster PA, Howard MP, Conway JM, Pietersma A, deStoppelaar J, Deurenberg P. Energy metabolism increases and regional body fat decreases while regional muscle mass is spared in humans climbing Mt. Everest. *Journal of Nutrition.* 1999;129(7):1307-1314.

31 Westerterp-Plantenga MS. Effects of extreme environments on food intake in human subjects. *Proceedings of the Nutrition Society.* 1999;58(4):791-798.

32 Nutrition for Health and Performance: Nutritional Guidance for Military Operations in Temperate and Extreme Environments. (pp 24-39) www.dtic.mil/dtic/tr/fulltext/u2/a261392.pdf. Accessed August 8, 2011

33 Reynolds RD, Lickteig JA, Howard MP, Deuster PA. Intakes of high fat and high carbohydrate foods by humans increased with exposure to increasing altitude during an expedition to Mt. Everest. *Journal of Nutrition.* 1998;128(1):50-55.

34 Askew EW. Environmental and physical stress and nutrient requirements. *American Journal of Clinical Nutrition.* 1995;61(3):632S-637S.

35 Chao WH, Askew EW, Roberts DE, Wood SM, Perkins JB. Oxidative stress in humans during work at moderate altitude. *Journal of Nutrition.* 1999;129(11):2009-2012.

36 Kupper T, Schoffl V, Milledge JS. Traveller's diarrhea: Prevention and treatment in the mountains. *Medicina Sportiva.* 2010;14(3):157 160.

37 Murray R. Fluid needs in hot and cold environments. *International Journal of Sport Nutrition.* 1995;5:62S-73S.

Chapter 11

1 Unnithan VB, Goulopoulou S. Nutrition for the pediatric athlete. *Current Sports Medicine Reports.* 2004;3(4):206-211.

2 Casazza K, Thomas O. Do dietary modifications made prior to pubertal maturation have the potential to decrease obesity later in life? A developmental perspective. *Infant, Child, and Adolescent Nutrition.* 2009;1:271-281.

3 Petrie HJ, Stover EA, Horswill CA. Nutritional concerns for the child and adolescent competitor. *Nutrition.* 2004;20(7/8):620-631.

4 Bass M, Turner L, Hunt S. Counseling female athletes: Application of the stages of change model to avoid disordered eating, amenorrhea, and osteoporosis. *Psychological Reports.* 2001;88(3), pt. 2:1153-1160.

5 Warren MP, Perlroth NE. The effects of intense exercise on the female reproductive system. *Journal of Endocrinology.* 2001;170(1):3-11.

6 Korpelainen R, Orava S, Karpakka J, Siira P, Hulkko A. Risk factors for recurrent stress fractures in athletes. *American Journal of Sports Medicine.* 2001;29(3):304-310.

7 Nattiv A. Stress fractures and bone health in track and field athletes. *Journal of Science and Medicine in Sport.* 2000;3(3):268-279.

8 Tarnopolsky LJ, MacDougall JD, Atkinson SA, Tarnopolsky MA, Sutton JR. Gender differences in substrate for endurance exercise. *Journal of Applied Physiology.* 1990;68:302-308.

9 Gabel KA. The female athlete. In: Maughan RJ, ed. *Nutrition in Sport.* London: Blackwell Science; 2000:417-428.

10 Burke LM, Cox GR, Culmmings NK, Desbrow B. Guidelines for daily carbohydrate intake: Do athletes achieve them? *Sports Medicine.* 2001;31(4):267-299.

11 Lemon PWR. Do athletes need more dietary protein and amino acids? *International Journal of Sport Nutrition.* 1995;5:39S-61S.

12 Perry AC, Crane LS, Applegate B, Marquez-Sterling S, Signorile JF, Miller PC. Nutrient intake and psychological and physiological assessment in eumenorrheic and amenorrheic female athletes: A preliminary study. *International Journal of Sport Nutrition.* 1996;6:3-13.

13 Manore MM. Vitamin B_6 and exercise. *International Journal of Sport Nutrition.* 1994;4:89-103.

14 Huang YC, Chen W, Evans MA, Mitchell ME, Shultz TD. Vitamin B-6 requirement and status assessment of young women fed a high-protein diet with various levels of vitamin B-6. *American Journal of Clinical Nutrition.* 1998;67:208-220.

15 Pate RR, Miller BJ, Davis JM, Slentz CA, Kling-Shirn LA. Iron status of female runners. *International Journal of Sport Nutrition.* 1993;6:3-13.

16 Fogelholm M. Indicators of vitamin and mineral status in athletes' blood: A review. *International Journal of Sport Nutrition.* 1995;5:267-284.

17 Dueck CA, Manore MM, Matt KS. Role of energy balance in athletic menstrual dysfunction. *International Journal of Sport Nutrition.* 1996;6(2):165-190.

18 Van de Loo DA, Johnson MD. The young female athlete. *Clinical Sports Medicine.* 1995;14(3):687-707.

19 Nelson Steen S. Nutrition for the school-aged child athlete. In: Bar-Or O, ed. *The Child and Adolescent Athlete.* Oxford: Blackwell Science; 1996:260-273.

20 Chumlea WC, Schubert CM, Roche AF, Kulin HE, Lee PA, Himes JH, Sun SS. Age at menarche and racial comparisons in US girls. *Pediatrics.* 2003;111(1):110-113.

21 American Academy of Pediatrics, Committee on Sports Medicine and Fitness. Intensive training and sports specialization in young athletes. *Pediatrics.* 2000;106(1):154-157.

22 Kurz KM. Adolescent nutritional status in developing countries. *Proceedings of the Nutrition Society.* 1996;55:321-331.

23 Beard J, Tobin B. Iron status and exercise. *American Journal of Clinical Nutrition.* 2000;72(2):594S-597S.

24 Hebestreit H, Meyer F, Htay-Htay, Heigenhauser GJF, Bar-Or O. Plasma metabolites, volume and electrolytes following 30-s high-intensity exercise in boys and men. *European Journal of Applied Physiology.* 1996;72:563-569.

25 Martinez LR, Haymes EM. Substrate utilization during treadmill running in prepubertal girls and women. *Medicine and Science in Sports and Exercise.* 1992;24:975-983.

26 Eliakim A, Beyth Y. Exercise training, menstrual irregularities, and bone development in children and adolescents. *Journal of Pediatric and Adolescent Gynecology.* 2003;16(4):201-206.

27 Bompa T. *From Childhood to Champion Athlete.* Toronto: Veritas; 1995.

28 Bar-Or O, Dotan R, Inbar O, Rothstein A, Zonder H. Voluntary hypohydration in 10- to 12-year-old boys. *Journal of Applied Physiology.* 1980;48:104-108.

29 Bar-Or O. Nutrition for child and adolescent athletes. *Sports Science Exchange.* 2000;13(2): #77.

30 Campbell WW, Geik RA. Nutritional considerations for the older athlete. *Nutrition.* 2004; 20(7/8):603-608.

31 Miller KK. Mechanisms by which nutritional disorders cause reduced bone mass in adults. *Journal of Women's Health.* 2003;12(2):145-150.

32 Kenney WL. The older athlete: Exercise in hot environments. *Sports Science Exchange.* 1993;6(3): #44.

33 Kenney WL, Hodgson JL. Heat tolerance, thermoregulation and aging. *Sports Medicine.* 1987;4:446-456.

34 Kenney WL, Tankersley CG, Newswanger DL, Hyde DE, Turner NL. Age and hypohydration independently influence the peripheral vascular response to heat stress. *Journal of Applied Physiology.* 1990;68:1902-1908.

35 Kenney WL, Fowler SR. Methylcholine-activated eccrine sweat gland density and output as a function of age. *Journal of Applied Physiology.* 1988;65:1082-1086.

36 Thompson J, Manore M. *Nutrition: An Applied Approach.* New York: Pearson-Benjamin Cummings; 2005:600.

37 Nieman DC. Exercise immunology: Future directions for research related to athletes, nutrition, and the elderly. *International Journal of Sports Medicine.* 2000;21(suppl 1):61S-68S.

Chapter 12

1 Williams MH. *Nutrition for Health, Fitness, and Sport.* New York: WCB McGraw-Hill; 1999:317-318.

2 Okely AD, Booth ML, Chey T. Relationships between body composition and fundamental movement skills among children and adolescents. *Research Quarterly for Exercise and Sport.* 2004;75(3):238-247.

3 Augestad LB, Saether B, Gotestam KG. The relationship between eating disorders and personality in physically active women. *Scandinavian Journal of Medicine and Science in Sports.* 1999;9:304-312.

4 Rivier C, Rivest S. Effect of stress on the activity of the hypothalamic-pituitary-gonadal axis: Peripheral and central mechanisms. *Biology of Reproduction.* 1991;45:523-532.

5 Loucks AB. Energy availability, not body fatness, regulates reproductive function in women. *Exercise and Sport Sciences Reviews.* 2003;31(3):144-148.

6 Hilton LK, Loucks AB. Low energy availability, not exercise stress, suppresses the diurnal rhythm of leptin in healthy young women. *American Journal of Physiology-Endocrinology and Metabolism.* 2000;278:43E-49E.

7 Moriguti JC, Das SK, Saltzman E, Corrales A, McCrory MA, Greenberg AS, Roberts SB. Effects of a 6-week hypocaloric diet on changes in body composition, hunger, and subsequent weight regain in healthy young and older adults. *The Journals of Gerontology: Series A: Cognition, Health, and Aging.* 2000;55(12): B580-B587.

8 Saltzman E & Roberts SB. The role of energy expenditure in energy regulation: findings from a decade of research. *Nutrition Reviews.* 1995;53 209-220.

9 Das SK, Moriguti JC, McCrory MA, Saltzman E, Mosunic C, Greenberg AS, Roberts SB. An underfeeding study in healthy men and women provides further evidence of impaired regulation of energy expenditure in old age. *The Journal of Nutrition.* 2000; 131:1833-1838.

10 Forbes GF, Brown MR, Welle SL, Lipinski BA. Deliberate overfeeding in women and men: Energy cost and composition of the weight gain. *British Journal of Nutrition.* 1986;56:1-9.

11 Roberts SB, Fuss P, Dallal GE, Atkinson A, Evans WJ, Joseph L, Fiatarone MA, Greenberg AS, Young VR. Effects of age on energy expenditure and substrate oxidation during experimental overfeeding in healthy men. *Journal of Gerontology.* 1996;51A:B148-B157.

12 Roberts SB, Young VR, Fuss P, Fiatarone MA, Richard B, Rasmussen H, Wagner D, Joseph L, Holehouse E, Evans

WJ. Body weight regulation in young men: effects of overfeeding on energy expenditure and subsequent nutrient intakes. *American Journal of Physiology*. 1990; 259:R461-R469.

13 Diaz EO, Prentice AM, Goldberg GR, Murgatroyd PR, Coward WA. Metabolic response to experimental overfeeding in lean and overweight healthy volunteers. *American Journal of Clinical Nutrition*. 1992;56:641-655.

14 Leibel RL, Rosenbaum M, Hirsch J. Changes in energy expenditure resulting from altered body weight. *New England Journal of Medicine*. 1995;332:621-628.

15 McCrory MA, Fuss PJ, Saltzman E, Roberts SB. Dietary determinants of energy intake and weight regulation in healthy adults. *The Journal of Nutrition*. 2000;130: 276S-279S.

16 Irving BA, Davis CK, Brock DW, Weltman JY, Swift D, Barrett EJ, Gaesser GA, Weltman A. Effect of exercise training intensity on abdominal visceral fat and body composition. *Medicine and Science in Sports and Exercise*. 2008;40(11):1863-1872.

17 Meyer NL, Shaw JM, Manore MM, Dolan SH, Subudhi AW, Shultz BB, Walker JA. Bone mineral density of Olympic-level female winter sport athletes. *Medicine and Science in Sports and Exercise*. 2004;36(9):1594-1601.

18 Misra M, Prabhakaran R, Miller KK, Tsai P, Lin A, Lee N, Herzog DB, Klibanski A. Role of cortisol in menstrual recovery in adolescent girls with anorexia nervosa. *Pediatric Research*. 2006;59:598-603.

19 Archimedes was a Greek mathematician, engineer, and physicist. He developed formulas for determining the density off different shapes and determined that buoyancy equals the weight of the displayed fluid. This is the principle used to determine body density via both hydrodensitometry and air displacement plethysmography.

20 Yu O-K, Rhee Y-K, Park T-S, Cha Y-S. Comparisons of obesity assessments in over-weight elementary students using anthropometry, BIA, CT, and DEXA. *Nutrition Research and Practice*. 2010;4(2):128-135.

21 Neovius M, Hemmingsson E, Freyschuss B, Udden J. Bioelectrical impedance underestimates total and truncal fatness in abdominally obese women. *Obesity*. 14(10):1731-1738.

22 Position of the American Dietetic Association, Dietitians of Canada, and the American College of Sports Medicine. Nutrition and Athletic Performance. *Journal of the American Dietetic Association*. 2009;109:509-527.

23 Collins MA, Millard-Stafford ML, Sparling PB, Snow TK, Rosskopf LB, Webb SA, Omer J. Evaluation of the Bod Pod for assessing body fat in collegiate football players. *Medicine and Science in Sports and Exercise*. 1999;31(9):1350-1356.

24 Fields DA, Wilson GD, Gladden LB, Hunter GR, Pascoe DD, Goran MI. Comparison of the Bod Pod with the four-compartment model in adult females. *Medicine and Science in Sports and Exercise*. 2001;33(9):1605-1610.

25 Dixon CB, Deitrick RW, Pierce JR, Cutrufello PT, Drapeau LL. Evaluation of the Bod Pod and leg-to-leg bioelectrical impedance analysis for estimating percent body fat in National Collegiate Athletic Association Division III collegiate wrestlers. *Journal of Strength and Conditioning Research*. 2005;19(1):92-97.

26 Maddalozzo GF, Cardinal BJ, Snow CM. Concurrent validity of the Bod Pod and dual energy X-ray absorptiometry techniques for assessing body composition in young women. *Journal of the American Dietetic Association*. 2002;102:1677-1679.

27 Ziomkiewicz A, Ellison PT, Lipson SF, Thune I, Jasienska G. Body fat, energy balance and estradiol levels: A study based on hormonal profiles from complete menstrual cycles. *Human Reproduction*. 2008;23(11):2555-2563.

28 Lovejoy JC, Champagne CM, de Jonge L, Xie H, Smith SR. Increased visceral fat and decreased energy expenditure during the menopausal transition. *International Journal of Obesity*. 2008;32:949-958.

29 Rhea DJ. Eating disorder behaviors of ethnically diverse urban female adolescent athletes and non-athletes. *Journal of Adolescence* 1999; 22(3): 379-388.

30 Sundgot-Borgen J, Torstveit MK. Prevalence of eating disorders in elite athletes is higher than in the general population. *Clinical Journal of Sport Medicine*. 2004;14(1):25-32.

31 Stafford DEJ. Altered hypothalamic-pituitary-ovarian axis function in young female athletes: Implications and recommendations for management. *Treatments in Endocrinology*. 2005;4(3):147-154.

32 Laughlin GA, Yen SSC. Nutritional and endocrine-metabolic aberrations in amenorrheic athletes. *Journal of Clinical Endocrinology and Metabolism*. 1996;81(12):4301-4309.

33 Loucks AB, Verdun M, Heath EM. Low energy availability, not stress of exercise alters LH pulsatility in exercising women. *Journal of Applied Physiology*. 1998;84(1):37-46.

34 Loucks AB, Callister R. Induction and prevention of low-T3 syndrome in exercising women. *Journal of Applied Physiology*. 1993;264:924R-930R.

35 Loucks AB, Heath EM. Dietary restriction reduces luteinizing hormone (LH) pulse frequency during waking hours and increases LH pulse amplitude during sleep in young menstruating women. *Journal of Clinical Endocrinology and Metabolism*. 1994;78:910-915.

36 Weimann E. Gender-related differences in elite gymnasts: The female athlete triad. *Journal of Applied Physiology*. 2002;92(5):2146-2152.

37 Ramsay R, Wolman R. Are synchronized swimmers at risk of amenorrhoea? *British Journal of Sports Medicine*. 2001;35(4):242-244.

38 Hinton PS, Sanford TC, Davidson MM, Yakushko OF, Beck NC. Nutrient intakes and dietary behaviors of male and female collegiate athletes. *International Journal of Sport Nutrition and Exercise Metabolism*. 2004;14(4):389-405.

39 Sundgot-Borgen J. Eating disorders in athletes. In: Maughan RJ, ed. *Nutrition in Sport*. London: Blackwell Science; 2000:510-522.

40 Warren MP, Goodman LR. Exercise-induced endocrine pathologies. *Journal of Endocrinology Investigation*. 2003;26(9):873-878.

41 Thompson RA, Trattner-Sherman R. *Helping Athletes With Eating Disorders*. Champaign, IL: Human Kinetics; 1993.

42 Brownell KD, Rodin J. Prevalence of eating disorders in athletes. In: Brownell KD, Rodin J, Wilmore JH, eds. *Eating, Body Weight and Performance in Athletes: Disorders of Modern Society*. Philadelphia: Lea & Febiger; 1992:128-143.

43 Manore MM. Dietary recommendations and athletic menstrual dysfunction. *Sports Medicine*. 2002;32(14):887-901.

44 Fogelholm GM, Koskinen R, Lasko J. Gradual and rapid weight loss: Effects on nutrition and performance in male athletes. *Medicine and Science in Sports and Exercise*. 1993;25(3):371-377.

45 Fogelholm M. Effects of bodyweight reduction on sports performance. *Sports Medicine*. 1994;18(4):249-267.

46 Reading KJ, McCarger LI, Harber VJ. Energy balance and luteal phase progesterone levels in elite adolescent aesthetic athletes. *International Journal of Sport Nutrition and Exercise Metabolism*. 2002;12(1):93-104.

Chapter 13

1 Robinson-O'Brien R, Perry CL, Wall MM, Story M, Neumark-Sztainer D. Adolescent and young adult vegetarianism: Better dietary intake and weight outcomes but increased risk of disordered eating behaviors. *Journal of the American Dietetic Association*. 2009;109:648-655.

2 Burns RD, Schiller MR, Merrick MA, Wolf KN. Intercollegiate student athlete use of nutritional supplements and the role of athletic trainers and dietitians in nutrition counseling. *Journal of the American Dietetic Association*. 2004;104:246-249.

3 Croll JK, Neumark-Sztainer D, Story M, Wall M, Perry C, Harnack L. Adolescents involved in weight-related and power team sports have better eating patterns and nutrient intakes than non-sport-involved adolescents. *Journal of the American Dietetic Association.* 2006;106:707-717.

4 Jelzberg JH, Waeckerle JF, Camilo J, Selden MA, Tang F, Joyce SA, Browne JE, O'Keefe JH. Comparison of cardiovascular and metabolic risk factors in professional baseball players versus professional football players. *American Journal of Cardiology.* 2010;106(5):664-667.

5 Grivetti LE, Applegate EA. From Olympia to Atlanta: A cultural-historical perspective on diet and athletic training. *Journal of Nutrition.* 1997;127(5):860S-868S.

6 Halberstam, David. *Summer of '49.* New York: W. Morrow; 1989.

7 Recht LD, Lew RA, Schwartz WJ. Baseball teams beaten by jet lag. *Nature.* 1995;377(6550):583.

8 Bonci L. Performance eating for baseball. *Strength and Conditioning Journal.* 2009;31(2):59-63.

9 YenHsuan C, YuLin S, LingYu T. Nutrition knowledge and dietary practices of female softball players. *Nutritional Sciences Journal.* 2009;34(4):133-141.

10 Whitley JD, Terrio T. Changes in peak torque arm-shoulder strength of high school baseball pitchers during the season. *Perceptual Motor Skills.* 1998;86:1361-1362.

11 MacWilliams BA, Choi T, Perezous MK, Chao EY, McFarland EG. Characteristic ground-reaction forces in baseball pitching. *American Journal of Sports Medicine.* 1998;26:66-71.

12 Palumbo CM, Clark N. Case problem: Nutrition concerns related to the performance of a baseball team. *Journal of the American Dietetic Association.* 2000;100(6):704-707.

13 Yoshida T, Nakai S, Yorimoto A, Kawabata T, Morimoto T. Effect of aerobic capacity on sweat rate and fluid intake during outdoor exercise in the heat. *European Journal of Applied Physiology.* 1995;71:235-239.

14 Bast SC, Perry JR, Poppiti R, Vangsness CT, Weaver FA. Upper extremity blood flow in collegiate and high school baseball pitchers: A preliminary report. *American Journal of Sports Medicine.* 1996;24(6):847-851.

15 Schulz R, Curnow C. Peak performance and age among superathletes: Track and field, swimming, baseball, tennis, and golf. *Journal of Gerontology.* 1988;43(5):113-120.

16 van der Ploeg GE, Brooks AG, Withers RT, Dollman J, Leaney F, Chatterton BE. Body composition changes in female bodybuilders during preparation for competition. *European Journal of Clinical Nutrition.* 2001;55(4):268-277.

17 Morrison LJ, Gizis F, Shorter B. Prevalent use of dietary supplements among people who exercise at a commercial gym. *International Journal of Sport Nutrition and Exercise Metabolism.* 2004;14(4):481-492.

18 Hickson JF, Johnson TE, Lee W, Sidor RJ. Nutrition and the precontent preparations of a male bodybuilder. *Journal of the American Dietetic Association.* 1990;90(2):264-267.

19 Britschgi F, Zund G. Bodybuilding: Hypokalemia and hypophosphatemia. *Schweiz Med. Wochenschr.* 1991;121(33):1163-1165.

20 Vertalino M, Eisenberg M, Story M, Neumark-Sztainer D. Participation in weight-related sports is associated with higher use of unhealthful weight-control behaviors and steroid use. *Journal of the American Dietetic Association.* 2007;107:434-440.

21 Barron RL, Vanscoy GJ. Natural products and the athlete: Facts and folklore. *Annals of Pharmacotherapy.* 1993;27(5):607-615.

22 Kleiner SM, Bazzarre TL, Litchford MD. Metabolic profiles, diet, and health practices of championship male and female bodybuilders. *Journal of the American Dietetic Association.* 1990;90(7):962-967.

23 New York City Department of Consumer Affairs. *Magic muscle pills! Health and fitness quackery in nutrition supplements.* New York: New York City Department of Consumer Affairs; 1992.

24 Short SH. Health quackery: Our role as professionals. *Journal of the American Dietetic Association.* 1994;94(6):607-611.

25 Bosselaers I, Buemann B, Victor OJ, Astrup A. Twenty-four hour energy expenditure and substrate utilization in body builders. *American Journal of Clincial Nutrition.* 1994;59:10-12.

26 Lambert CP, Frank LL, Evans WJ. Macronutrient considerations for the sport of bodybuilding. *Sports Medicine.* 2004;34(5):317-327.

27 Andersen RE, Barlett SJ, Morgan GD, Brownell KD. Weight loss, psychological, and nutritional patterns in competitive male body builders. *International Journal of Eating Disorders.* 1995;181(1):49-57.

28 Jonnalagadda SS, Rosenbloom CA, Skinner R. Dietary practices, attitudes, and physiological status of collegiate freshman football players. *Journal of Strength and Conditioning Research.* 2001;15(4):507-513.

29 Akers JA, Wagner TL, Brevard PB, Flohr JA, Yesilcay Y. Health risks associated with nutritional ergogenic aid use in high school football players. *Journal of the American Dietetic Association.* 2003;103(suppl 9):107-108.

30 Vanata DF, Sanders GJ, Peacock SC. Nutritional knowledge relating to actual caloric intake of NCAA Division II collegiate football players. *Journal of the American Dietetic Association.* 2009;109(suppl 9):95A.

31 Kreider RB, Ferreira M, Wilson M, Grindstaff P, Plisk S, Reinardy J, Cantler E, Almada AL. Effects of creatine supplementation on body composition, strength, and sprint performance. *Medicine and Science in Sports and Exercise.* 1998;30(1):73-82.

32 Stone MH, Sanborn K, Smith LL, O'Bryant HS, Hoke T, Utter AC, Johnson RL, Boros R, Hruby J, Pierce KC, Stone ME, Garner B. Effects of in-season (5 weeks) creatine and pyruvate supplementation on anaerobic performance and body composition in American football players. *International Journal of Sport Nutrition.* 1999;9(2):146-165.

33 Mayhew DL, Mayhew JL, Ware JS. Effects of long-term creatine supplementation on liver and kidney functions in American college football players. *International Journal of Sport Nutrition and Exercise Metabolism.* 2002;12(4):453-460.

34 Clancy SP, Clarkson PM, DeCheke ME, Nosaka K, Freedson PS, Cunningham JJ, Valentine B. Effects of chromium picolinate supplementation on body composition, strength, and urinary chromium loss in football players. *International Journal of Sport Nutrition.* 1994;4(2):142-153.

35 Burke LM, Hawley JA. Fluid balance in team sports: Guidelines for optimal practices. *Sports Medicine.* 1997;24(1):38-54.

36 Criswell D, Powers D, Lawler J, Tew J, Dodd S, Iryiboz Y, Tulley R, Wheeler K. Influence of a carbohydrate-electrolyte beverage on performance and blood homeostasis during recovery from football. *International Journal of Sport Nutrition.* 1991;1(2):178-191.

37 Parks PS, Read MH. Adolescent male athletes: Body image, diet, and exercise. *Adolescence.* 1997;32(127):593-602.

38 Wang MQ, Downey GS, Perko MA, Yesalis CE. Changes in body size of elite high school football players: 1963-1989. *Perceptual Motor Skills.* 1993;76(2):379-383.

39 Gomez JE, Ross SK, Calmbach WL, Kimmel RB, Schmidt DR, Dhanda R. Body fatness and increased injury rates in high school football linemen. *Clinical Journal of Sport Medicine.* 1998;8(2):115-120.

40 Kaplan TA, Digel SL, Scavo VA, Arellana SB. Effect of obesity on injury risk in high school football players. *Clinical Journal of Sport Medicine.* 1995;5(1):43-47.

41 Huddy DC, Nieman DC, Johnson RL. Relationship between body image and percent body fat among college male varsity athletes and nonathletes. *Perceptual Motor Skills.* 1993;77(3):851-857.

42 DePalma MT, Koszewski WM, Case JG, Barile RJ, DePalma BF, Oliaro SM. Weight control practices of lightweight football players. *Medicine and Science in Sports and Exercise.* 1993;25(6):694-701.

43 Hickson JF Jr., Duke MA, Risser WL, Johnson CW, Palmer R, Stockton JE. Nutritional intake from food sources of high school football athletes. *Journal of the American Dietetic Association.* 1987;87(12):1656-1659.

44 Jehue R, Street D, Huizenga R. Effect of time zone and game time changes on team performance: National Football League. *Medicine and Science in Sports and Exercise.* 1993;25(1):127-131.

45 Springer RL, Dodson WL, Chromiak JA, Byrd SH. Food compostion and nutrient analysis of diets of pre-selected football players. *Journal of the American Dietetic Association.* 2003;103(suppl 9):14A.

46 Maddux GT. *Men's Gymnastics.* Pacific Palisades, CA: Goodyear; 1970:9.

47 Weimann E, Blum WF, Witzel C, Schwidergall S, Bohles HJ. Hypoleptinemia in female and male elite gymnasts. *European Journal of Clinical Investigation.* 1999;29(10):853-860.

48 Weimann E, Witzel C, Schwidergall S, Bohles HJ. Peripubertal perturbations in elite gymnasts caused by sport specific training regimes and inadequate nutritional intake. *International Journal of Sports Medicine.* 2000;21(3):210-215.

49 Constantini NW, Eliakim A, Zigel L, Yaaron M, Falk B. Iron status of highly active adolescents: Evidence of depleted iron stores in gymnasts. *International Journal of Sport Nutrition and Exercise Metabolism.* 2000;10(1):62-70.

50 Houtkooper LB, Going SB. Body composition: How should it be measured? Does it affect sport performance? *Sports Science Exchange.* 1994;52:7(5S).

51 Bortz S, Schoonen JC, Kanter M, Kosharek S, Benardot D. Physiology of anaerobic and aerobic exercise. In: Benardot D, ed. *Sports Nutrition: A Guide for the Professional Working With Active People.* Chicago: American Dietetic Association; 1993.

52 Benardot D, Czerwinski C. Selected body composition and growth measures of junior elite gymnasts. *Journal of the American Dietetic Association.* 1991;91(1):29-33.

53 Benardot D, Schwarz M, Heller DW. Nutrient intake in young, highly competitive gymnasts. *Journal of the American Dietetic Association.* 1989;89:401-403.

54 Benardot D. Working with young athletes: Views of a nutritionist on the sports medicine team. *International Journal of Sport Nutrition.* 1986;6(2):110-120.

55 Loosli AR. Reversing sports-related iron and zinc deficiencies. *The Physician and Sportsmedicine.* 1993;21(6):70-78.

56 Burns J, Dugan L. Working with professional athletes in the rink: The evolution of a nutrition program for an NHL team. *International Journal of Sport Nutrition.* 1994;4(2):132-134.

57 Akermark C, Jacobs I, Rasmussen M, Karlsson J. Diet and muscle glycogen concentration in relation to physical performance in Swedish elite ice hockey players. *International Journal of Sport Nutrition.* 1996;6(3):272-284.

58 Davis JM, Welsh RS, Alerson NA. Effects of carbohydrate and chromium ingestion during intermittent high-intensity exercise to fatigue. *International Journal of Sport Nutrition and Exercise Metabolism.* 2000;10(4):476-485.

59 Houston ME. Nutrition and ice hockey performance. *Canadian Journal of Applied Sport Science.* 1979;4(1):98-99.

60 Ferguson NL. An assessment of the dietary habits of college hockey players. *Journal of the American Dietetic Association.* 1999;99(suppl 9):39A.

61 Tegelman R, Aberg T, Pousette A, Carlstrom K. Effects of a diet regimen on pituitary and steroid hormones in male ice hockey players. *International Journal of Sports Medicine.* 1992;13(5):424-430.

62 Glycogen synthetase is a hormone that is elevated as glycogen storage becomes depleted. After a game or training session, the higher-circulating glycogen synthetase enables an efficient replacement of glycogen if carbohydrate and fluids are consumed.

63 Horswill CA, Hickner RC, Scott JR, Costill DL, Gould D. Weight loss, dietary carbohydrate modifications, and high intensity, physical performance. *Medicine and Science in Sports and Exercise.* 1990;22(4):470-476.

64 Sugiura K, Suzuki I, Kobayashi K. Nutritional intake of elite Japanese track-and-field athletes. *International Journal of Sport Nutrition.* 1999;9(2):202-212.

65 Nattiv A. Stress fractures and bone health in track and field athletes. *Journal of Science and Medicine in Sport.* 2000;3(3):268-279.

66 Grediagin MA, Cody M, Rupp J, Benardot D, Shern R. Exercise intensity does not effect body composition change in untrained, moderately overfat women. *Journal of the American Dietetic Association.* 1995;(95)6:661-665.

67 Kreider RB, Ferreira M, Wilson M, Grindstaff P, Plisk S, Reinardy J, Cantler E, Almada AL. Effects of creatine supplementation on body composition, strength, and sprint performance. *Medicine and Science in Sports and Exercise.* 1998;30(1):73-82.

68 Chwalbinska-Moneta J. Effect of creatine supplementation on aerobic performance and anaerobic capacity in elite rowers in the course of endurance training. *International Journal of Sport Nutrition and Exercise Metabolism.* 2003;13(2):173-183.

69 Nevill ME, Williams C, Roper D, Slater C, Nevill AM. Effect of diet on performance during recovery from intermittent sprint exercise. *Journal of Sports Science.* 1993;11(2):119-126.

70 Sherman WM, Doyle JA, Lamb DR, Strauss RH. Dietary carbohydrate, muscle glycogen, and exercise performance during seven days of training. *American Journal of Clincial Nutrition.* 1993;57(1):27-31.

71 Berning JR, Troup JP, VanHandel PJ, Daniels J, Daniels N. The nutritional habits of young adolescent swimmers. *International Journal of Sport Nutrition.* 1991;1(3):240-248.

72 Braun WA, Flynn MG, Carl DL, Carroll KK, Brickman T, Lambert CP. Iron status and resting immune function in female collegiate swimmers. *International Journal of Sport Nutrition and Exercise Metabolism.* 2000;10(4):425-433.

73 Guinard JX, Seador K, Beard JL, Brown PL. Sensory acceptability of meat and dairy products and dietary fat in male collegiate swimmers. *International Journal of Sport Nutrition.* 1995;5(4):315-328.

74 Lamb DR. Basic principles for improving sport performance. 1995. *Sports Science Exchange.* 8(2): #55.

75 Microsoft. Wrestling. Encarta 97 Encyclopedia. CD-ROM: Microsoft Corporation; 1993-1996.

76 Oppliger RA, Case HS, Horswill CA, Landry GL, Shelter AC. American College of Sports Medicine position stand: Weight loss in wrestlers. *Medicine and Science in Sports and Exercise.* 1996;28(6):ix-xii.

77 National Collegiate Athletic Association. 2010 and 2011 NCAA Wrestling Rules Book. www.ncaapublications.com. Accessed August 9, 2011.

78 Oppliger RA, Steen SA, Scott JR. Weight loss practices of college wrestlers. *International Journal of Sport Nutrition and Exercise Metabolism.* 2003;13(1):29-46.

79 Kiningham RB, Gorenflo DW. Weight loss methods of high school wrestlers. *Medicine and Science in Sports and Exercise.* 2001;33(5):810-813.

80 Roemmich JN, Sinning WE. Weight loss and wrestling training: Effects on growth-related hormones. *Journal of Applied Physiology.* 1997;82(6):1760-1764.

81 Roemmich JN, Sinning WE. Weight loss and wrestling training: Effects on nutrition, growth, maturation, body composition, and strength. *Journal of Applied Physiology.* 1997;82(6):1751-1759.

82 Rankin JW, Ocel JV, Craft LL. Effect of weight loss and refeeding diet composition on anaerobic performance in wrestlers. *Medicine and Science in Sports and Exercise.* 1996;28(10):1292-1299.

83 Choma CW, Sforzo GA, Keller BA. Impact of rapid weight loss on cognitive function in collegiate wrestlers. *Medicine and Science in Sports and Exercise.* 1998;30(5):746-749.

84 Wroble RR, Moxley DP. Weight loss patterns and success rates in high school wrestlers. *Medicine and Science in Sports and Exercise.* 1998;30(4):625-628.

85 Wroble RR, Moxley DP. Acute weight gain and its relationship to success in high school wrestlers. *Medicine and Science in Sports and Exercise.* 1998;30(6):949-951.

86 Lambert C, Jones B. Alternatives to rapid weight loss in U.S. wrestling. *International Journal of Sports Medicine.* 2010;31(8):523-528.

87 Horswill CA. Weight loss and weight cycling in amateur wrestlers: Implications for performance and resting metabolic rate. *International Journal of Sport Nutrition.* 1993;3:245-260.

88 Oppliger RA, Harms RD, Herrmann DE, Streich CM, Clark RR. The Wisconsin wrestling minimum weight project: A model for weight control among high school wrestlers. *Medicine and Science in Sports and Exercise.* 1995;27(8):1220-1224.

89 Pollock ML, Foster C, Anholm J, Hare J, Farrell P, Maksud M, Jackson AS. Body composition of Olympic speed skating candidates. *Research Quarterly.* 1982;53:150-155.

90 Castellani JW, Young AJ, Ducharme MB, Giesbrecht GG, Glickman E, Sallis RE. ACSM position stand: Prevention of cold injuries during exercise. *Medicine and Science in Sports and Exercise.* 2006;38(11):2012-2029.

91 Webster BL, Barr SI. Calcium intakes of adolescent female gymnasts and speed skaters: Lack of association with dieting behavior. *International Journal of Sport Nutrition.* 1995;5(1):2-12.

92 Erdman KA, Fung TK, Reimer RA. Influence of performance level on dietary supplementation in elite Canadian athletes. *Medicine and Science in Sports and Exercise.* 2006;38(2):349-356.

93 de Hon O, Coumans B. The continuing story of nutritional supplements and doping infractions. *British Journal of Sports Medicine.* 2007;41:800-805.

94 Snyder AC, Foster C. Skating. In: Maughan RJ, ed. *Nutrition in Sport: Volume VII of the Encyclopedia of Sports Medicine.* Blackwell Science: London; 2000:647.

95 van Ingen Schenau GJ, Bakker FC, de Groot G, de Loning JJ. Supramaximal cycle tests do not detect seasonal progression in performance in groups of elite speed skaters. *European Journal of Applied Physiology.* 1992;64:292-297

96 Pauls DW, van Duijnhoven H, Stray-Gundersen J. Iron insufficient erythropoiesis at altitude-speed skating. *Medicine and Science in Sports and Exercise.* 2002;34(5):252S.

97 Snyder AC, Foster C. Physiology and nutrition for skating. In: Lamb DR, Knuttgen HG, Murray R, eds. *Perspectives in Exercise Science and Sports Medicine, Volume 7. Physiology and Nutrition for Competitive Sport.* Cooper Publishing: Carmel Indiana; 1994:181-219.

98 Snyder AC, Schulz LO, Foster C. Voluntary consumption of a carbohydrate supplement by elite speed skaters. *Journal of the American Dietetic Association.* 1989;89:1125-1127.

99 McBride JM, Triplett-McBride T, Davie A, Newton RU. A comparison of strength and power characteristics between power lifters, Olympic lifters, and sprinters. *Journal of Strength and Conditioning Research.* 1999;13(1):58-66.

100 Mettler S, Mitchell N, Tipton KD. Increased protein intake reduces lean body mass loss during weight loss in athletes. *Medicine and Science in Sports and Exercise.* 2010;42(2):326-337.

101 Abbate M, Zoja C, Remuzzi G. How does proteinuria cause progressive renal damage? *Journal of the American Society of Nephrology.* 2006;17:2974-2984.

102 Cribb PJ, Williams AD, Hayes A. A creatine-protein-carbohydrate supplement enhances responses to resistance training. *Medicine and Science in Sports and Exercise.* 2007;39(11):1960-1968.

103 Cribb PJ, Williams AD, Stathis CG, Carey MF, Hayes A. Effects of whey isolate, creatine, and resistance training on muscle hypertrophy. *Medicine and Science in Sports and Exercise.* 2007;39(2):298-307.

104 Hoffman JR, Ratamess NA, Kang J, Falvo MJ, Faigenbaum AD. Effects of protein supplementation on muscular performance and resting hormonal changes in college football players. *Journal of Sports Sciences and Medicine.* 1007;6:85-92.

105 Duncan MJ, Oxford SW. The effect of caffeine ingestion on mood state and bench press performance to failure. *Journal of Strength and Conditioning Research.* 2011;25(1):178-185.

106 Hoffman JR, Ratamess NA, Kang J, Rashti SL, Faigenbaum AD. Examination of a pre-exercise, high energy supplement on exercise performance. *Journal of the International Society of Sports Nutrition.* 2009;6:7.

107 Schaefer MP, Smith J, Dahm DL, Sorenson MC. Ephedra use in a select group of adolescent athletes. *Journal of Sports Science and Medicine.* 2006;5:407-414.

108 Burke LM, Read RSD. Food use and nutritional practices of elite Olympic weightlifters. In: Truswell AS, Wahlqvist ML, eds. *Food Habits in Australia.* Melbourne: Rene Gordon; 1988:112-121.

109 Siahkouhian M, Hedaatneja M. Correlations of anthropometric and body composition variables with the performance of young elite weightlifters. *Journal of Human Kinetics.* 2010;25:125-131.

110 Burke DG, Silver S, Holt LE, Smith Palmer T, Culligan CJ, Chilibeck PD. The effect of continuous low dose creatine supplementation on force, power, and total work. *International Journal of Sport Nutrition and Exercise Metabolism.* 2000;10(3):235-244.

111 Ronsen O, Sundgot-Borgen J, Maehlum S. Supplement use and nutritional habits in Norwegian elite athletes. *Scandinavian Journal of Medicine and Science in Sports.* 1999;9(1):28-35.

112 Juzwiak CR, Ancona-Lopez F. Evaluation of nutrition knowledge and dietary recommendations by coaches of adolescent Brazilian athletes. *International Journal of Sport Nutrition and Exercise Metabolism.* 2004;14(2):222-235.

113 Coyle EF. Fluid and fuel intake during exercise. *Journal of Sports Sciences.* 2004;22(1):39-55.

Chapter 14

1 Katch FI, Katch VL, McArdle WD. *Introduction to Nutrition, Exercise, and Health.* 4th ed. Philadelphia: Lea & Febiger; 1993: 179.

2 Sizer F, Whitney E. *Nutrition: Concepts and Controversies.* 7th ed. Albany, NY: West/Wadsworth; 1997:383.

3 Penry JT, Manore MM. Choline: An important micronutrient for maximal endurance-exercise performance? *International Journal of Sport Nutrition and Exercise Metabolism.* 2008;18(2):191-203.

4 Rodriguez NR, Vislocky LM, Courtney GP. Dietary protein, endurance exercise, and human skeletal-muscle protein turnover. *Current Opinion in Clinical Nutrition and Metabolic Care.* 2007;10(1):40-45.

5 Millard-Stafford M, Childers WL, Conger SA, Kampfer AJ, Rahnert JA. Recovery nutrition: Timing and composition after endurance exercise. *Current Sports Medicine Reports.* 2008;7(4):193-201.

6 Campbell B, Kreider RB, Ziegenfuss T, LaBounty P, Roberts M, Burke D, Landis J, Lopez H, Antonio J. International Society of Sports Nutrition position stand: Protein and exercise. *Journal of the International Society of Sports Nutrition.* 2007;4(8):1-7.

7 Position of the American Dietetic Association, Dietitians of Canada, and the American College of Sports Medicine: Nutrition and athletic performance. *Journal of the American Dietetic Association.* 2009;109:509-527.

8 Smith AE, Walter AA, Graef JL, Kendall KL, Moon JR, Lockwood CM, Fukuda DH, Beck TW, Cramer JT, Stout JR. Effects of β-alanine supplementation and high-intensity interval training on endurance performance and body composition in men: A double-blind trial. *Journal of the International Society of Sports Nutrition.* 2009;6(5):1-9.

9 Lee JKW, Maughan RJ, Shirreffs SM, Watson P. Effects of milk ingestion on prolonged exercise capacity in young, healthy men. *Nutrition.* 2008;24:340-347.

10 Jeukendrup A, Tipton KD. Legal nutritional boosting for cycling. *Current Sports Medicine Reports.* 2009;8(4):186-191.

11 Chen Y-J, Wong SH-S, Wong C-K, Lam C-W, Huang Y-J, Siu PM-F. The effect of a pre-exercise carbohydrate meal on immune responses to an endurance performance run. *British Journal of Nutrition.* 2008;100:1260-1268.

12 Hawley JA, Burke LM. Carbohydrate availability and training adaptation: Effects on cell metabolism. *Exercise and Sport Science Reviews.* 2010;38(4):152-160.

13 Fudge BW, Easton C, Kingsmore D, Kiplamai FK, Onywera VO, Westerterp KR, Kayser B, Noakes TD, Pitsiladis YP. Elite Kenyan endurance runners are hydrated day-to-day with ad libitum fluid intake. *Medicine and Science in Sports and Exercise.* 2008;40(6):1171-1179.

14 Gomez-Cabrera M-C, Domenech E, Romagnoli M, Arduini A, Borras C, Pallardo FV, Sastre J, Viña J. Oral administration of vitamin C decreases muscle mitochondrial biogenesis and dampers training-induced adaptations in endurance performance. *American Journal of Clinical Nutrition.* 2008;87:142-149.

15 Barrack MT, Rauth MJ, Barkai H S, Nichols JF. Dietary restraint and low bone mass in female adolescent endurance runners. *American Journal of Clinical Nutrition.* 2008;87:36-43.

16 Fontana L, Klein S. Holloszy JO. Effects of long-term caloric restriction and endurance exercise on glucose tolerance, insulin action, and adipokine production. *Age.* 2010;32:97-108.

17 Zimberg IZ, Crispim CA, Juzwiak CR, Antunes HKM, Edward D, Waterhouse J, Tufik S, deMello MT. Nutritional intake during a simulated adventure race. *International Journal of Sport Nutrition and Exercise Metabolism.* 2008;18:152-168.

18 Robins A. Nutritional recommendations for competing in the Ironman triathlon. *Current Sports Medicine Reports.* 2007;6:241-248.

19 Havemann L, Goedecke JH. Nutritional practices of male cyclists before and during an ultraendurance event. *International Journal of Sport Nutrition and Exercise Metabolism.* 2008;18:551-566.

20 Pyruvate has been studied as an ergogenic aid to determine if supplemental doses improve performance. Since pyruvate infusion is a self-limiting pathway, it has not been found to be ergogenic. [Juhn MS. Ergogenic aids in aerobic activity. *Current Sports Medicine Reports.* 2002;1(4):233-238.]

21 The tricarboxylic acid cycle is commonly referred to as the Krebs cycle, named for Hans Krebs, who first described the oxidative metabolic reactions. It is also referred to as the citric acid cycle because citric acid is required for one of the first reactions. Therefore, the tricarboxylic acid cycle, Krebs cycle, and citric acid cycle are all referring to the same energy-yielding reactions.

22 Uusitalo AL, Valkonen-Korhonen M, Helenius P, Vanninen E, Bergström KA, Kuikka JT. Abnormal serotonin reuptake in an overtrained, insomniac and depressed team athlete. *International Journal of Sports Medicine.* 2004;25(2):150-53.

23 American College of Sports Medicine. Overtraining: Consensus statement. *Sports Medicine Bulletin.* 1999;31(1):29.

24 Asp S, Rohde T, Richter EA. Impaired muscle glycogen resynthesis after a marathon is not caused by decreased muscle GLUT-4 content. *Journal of Applied Physiology.* 1997;83(5):1482-1485.

25 Naughton G, Farpour-Lambert NJ, Carlson J, Bradney M, Van Praagh E. Physiological issues surrounding the performance of adolescent athletes. *Sports Medicine.* 2000;30(5):309-325.

26 Farber HW, Schaefer EJ, Franey R, Grimaldi R, Hill NS. The endurance triathlon: Metabolic changes after each event and during recovery. *Medicine and Science in Sports and Exercise.* 1991; 23(8):959-965.

27 Dressendorfer RH, Wade CE. Effects of a 15-d race on plasma steroid levels and leg muscle fitness in runners. *Medicine and Science in Sports and Exercise.* 1991;23(8):954-958.

28 Sherman WM, Maglischo EW. Minimizing chronic athletic fatigue among swimmers: Special emphasis on nutrition. *Sports Science Exchange.* 1991:4(35): 1-5

29 Niekamp RA, Baer JT. In-season dietary adequacy of trained male cross-country runners. *International Journal of Sport Nutrition.* 1995;5:45-55.

30 Butterworth DE, Nieman DC, Butler JV, Herring JL. Food intake patterns of marathon runners. *International Journal of Sport Nutrition.* 1994;4(1):1-7.

31 Houtkooper L. Food selection for endurance sports. *Medicine and Science in Sports and Exercise.* 1992;24(9):349S-359S.

32 Hickner RC, Fisher JS, Hansen PA, Racette SB, Mier CM, Turner MJ, Holloszy JO. Muscle glycogen accumulation after endurance exercise in trained and untrained individuals. *Journal of Applied Physiology.* 1997;83(3):897-903.

33 Helmich P, Christensen SW, Darre E, Jahnsen F, Hartvig T. Non-elite marathon runners: Health, training, and injuries. *British Journal of Sports Medicine.* 1989;23(3):177-178.

34 Fogelholm M, Tikkanen H, Naveri H, Harkonen M. High-carbohydrate diet for long distance runners: A practical view-point. *British Journal of Sports Medicine.* 1989;23(2):94-96.

35 Nieman DC, Gates JR, Butler JV, Pollett LM, Dietrich SJ, Lutz RD. Supplementation patterns in marathon runners. *Journal of the American Dietetic Association.* 1989;89(11):1615-1619.

36 Rokitzki L, Hinkel S, Klemp C, Cufi D, Keul J. Dietary, serum, and urine ascorbic acid status in male athletes. *International Journal of Sports Medicine.* 1994;15(7):435-440.

37 Rokitzki L, Sagredos AN, Reuss F, Buchner M, Keul J. Acute changes in vitamin B_6 status in endurance athletes before and after a marathon. *International Journal of Sport Nutrition.* 1994;4(2):154-165.

38 Terblanche S, Noakes TD, Dennis SC, Marais D, Eckert M. Failure of magnesium supplementation to influence marathon running performance or recovery in magnesium-replete subjects. *International Journal of Sport Nutrition.* 1992;2(2):154-164.

39 Barnett DW, Conlee RK. The effects of a commercial dietary supplement on human performance. *American Journal of Clinical Nutrition.* 1984;40(3):586-590.

40 Zaryski C, Kin M, Smith DJ. Training principles and issues for ultra-endurance athletes. *Current Sports Medicine Reports.* 2005;4:165-170.

41 Wein D. Nutrition for ultra endurance events: Energy and macronutrient guidelines. *NSCA's Performance Training Journal.* 2011;6(4):17-18.

42 Francescato MP, Di Prampero PE. Energy expenditure during an ultra-endurance cycling race. *Journal of Sports Medicine and Physical Fitness.* 2002;42:1-7.

43 American College of Sports Medicine Position Statement. Nutrition and athletic performance. *Medicine and Science in Sports and Exercise.* 2009;709-731.

44 McCowan KA, Edelstein S. Are female ultra-endurance triathletes getting a sufficient daily carbohydrate intake? *Topics in Clinical Nutrition.* 2006;21(2):139-144.

45 Linderman J, Demchak T, Dallas J, Buckworth J. Ultra-endurance cycling: A field study of human performance during a 12-hour mountain bike race. *Journal of Exercise Physiology.* 2003;6(3):10-19.

46 Sloniger MA, Cureton KJ, O'Bannon PJ. One-mile run-walk performance in young men and women: Role of anaerobic metabolism. Can. *Journal of Applied Physiology.* 1997;22(4):337-350.

47 Penn IW, Wang ZM, Buhl KM, Allison DB, Burastero SE, Heymsfield SB. Body composition and two-compartment model assumptions in male long-distance runners. *Medicine and Science in Sports and Exercise.* 1994;26:392-397.

48 Reeder MT, Dick BH, Atkins JK, Pribis AB, Martinez JM. Stress fractures: Current concepts of diagnosis and treatment. *Sports Medicine.* 1996;22(3):198-212.

49 Deuster PA, Kyle SB, Moser PB, Vigersky RA, Singh A, Schoomaker EB. Nutritional intakes and status of highly trained amenorrheic and eumenorrheic women runners. *Fertility and Sterility.* 1986;46(4):636-643.

50 Beidleman BA, Puhl JL, DeSouza MJ. Energy balance in female distance runners. *American Journal of Clinical Nutrition.* 1995;61:303-311.

51 Rontoyannis GP, Skoulis T, Pavlou KN. Energy balance in ultramarathon running. *American Journal of Clinical Nutrition.* 1989;49:976-979.

52 Eden BD, Abernethy PJ. Nutritional intake during an ultraendurance running race. *International Journal of Sport Nutrition.* 1994;4:166-174.

53 Millard-Stafford ML, Sparling PB, Rosskopf LB, DiCarlo LJ. Carbohydrate-electrolyte replacement improves distance running performance in the heat. *Medicine and Science in Sports and Exercise.* 1992;24(8):934-940.

54 Hedley AM, Climstein M, Hansen R. The effects of acute heat exposure on muscular strength, muscular endurance, and muscular power in the euhydrated athlete. *Journal of Strength and Conditioning Research.* 2002;16(3):353-358.

55 Noakes TD, Adams BA, Myburgh KH, Greeff C, Lotz T, Nathan M. The danger of an inadequate water intake during prolonged exercise: A novel concept re-visited. *European Journal of Applied Physiology.* 1988;57(2):210-219.

56 Dennis SC, Noakes TD. Advantages of a smaller body mass in humans when distance-running in warm, humid conditions. *European Journal of Applied Physiology.* 1999;79(3):280-284.

57 Schumacher YO, Schmid A, Grathwohl D, Bultermann D, Berg A. Hematological indices and iron status in athletes of various sports and performances. *Medicine and Science in Sports and Exercise.* 2002;34(5):869-875.

58 Lamanca JJ, Haymes EM, Daly JA, Moffatt RJ, Waller MF. Sweat iron loss of male and female runners during exercise. *International Journal of Sports Medicine.* 1988;9(1):52-55.

59 Selby GB, Eichner ER. Endurance swimming, intravascular hemolysis, anemia, and iron depletion: New perspective on athlete's anemia. *American Journal of Medicine.* 1986;81(5):791-794.

60 Ehn L, Carlmark B, Hoglund S. Iron status in athletes involved in intense physical activity. *Medicine and Science in Sports and Exercise.* 1980;12(1):61-64.

61 Noakes T. *Lore of Running.* Champaign, IL: Human Kinetics; 1991:695.

62 Bentley DJ, Wilson GJ, Davie AJ, Zhou S. Correlations between peak power output, muscular strength, and cycle time trial performance in triathletes. *Journal of Sports Medicine and Physical Fitness.* 1998;38(3):201-207.

63 Laurenson NM, Fulcher KY, Korkia P. Physiological characteristics of elite and club level female triathletes during running. *International Journal of Sports Medicine.* 1993;14(8):455-459.

64 Gulbin JP, Gaffney PT. Ultraendurance triathlon participation: Typical race preparation of lower-level triathletes. *Journal of Sports Medicine and Physical Fitness.* 1999;39(1):12-15.

65 Banister EW, Carter JB, Zarkadas PC. Training theory and taper: Validation in triathlon athletes. *European Journal of Applied Physiology.* 1999;79(2):182-191.

66 Guezennec CY, Chalabi H, Bernard J, Fardellone P, Krentowski R, Zerath E, Meunier PJ. Is there a relationship between physical activity and dietary calcium intake? A survey in 10,373 young French subjects. *Medicine and Science in Sports and Exercise.* 1998;30(5):732-739.

67 Kerr CG, Trappe TA, Starling RD, Trappe SW. Hyperthermia during Olympic triathlon: Influence of body heat storage during the swimming stage. *Medicine and Science in Sports and Exercise.* 1998;30(1):99-104.

68 Rogers G, Goodman C, Rosen C. Water budget during ultra-endurance exercise. *Medicine and Science in Sports and Exercise.* 1997;29(11):1477-1481.

69 O'Toole ML, Douglas PS, Laird RH, Hiller DB. Fluid and electrolyte status in athletes receiving medical care at an ultradistance triathlon. *Clinical Journal of Sport Medicine.* 1995;5(2):116-122

70 Speedy DB, Faris JG, Hamlin M, Gallagher PG, Campbell RG. Hyponatremia and weight changes in an ultradistance triathlon. *Clinical Journal of Sport Medicine.* 1997;7(3):180-184.

71 Speedy DB, Noakes TD, Kimber NE, Rogers IR, Thompson JM, Boswell DR, Ross JJ, Campbell RG, Gallagher PG, Kuttner JA. Fluid balance during and after an Ironman triathlon. *Clinical Journal of Sport Medicine.* 2001;11(1):44-50.

72 Rehrer NJ, van Kemenade M, Meester W, Brouns F, Saris WH. Gastrointestinal complaints in relation to dietary intake in triathletes. *International Journal of Sport Nutrition.* 1992;2(1):48-59.

73 Clark N, Tobin J Jr., Ellis C. Feeding the ultraendurance athlete: Practical tips and a case study. *Journal of the American Dietetic Association.* 1992;92(10):1258-1262.

74 Frentsos JA, Baer JT. Increased energy and nutrient intake during training and competition improves elite triathletes' endurance performance. *International Journal of Sport Nutrition.* 1997;7(1):61-71.

75 Ribeiro JP, Cadavid E, Baena J, Monsalvete E, Barna A, DeRose EH. Metabolic predictors of middle-distance swimming performance. *British Journal of Sports Medicine.* 1990;24(3):196-200.

76 Lee EJ, Long KA, Risser WL, Poindexter HB, Gibbons WE, Goldzieher J. Variations in bone status of contralateral and regional sites in young athletic women. *Medicine and Science in Sports and Exercise.* 1995;27(10):1354-1361.

77 Berning JR, Troup JP, VanHandel PJ, Daniels J, Daniels N. The nutritional habits of young adolescent swimmers. *International Journal of Sport Nutrition.* 1991;1(3):240-248.

78 Saris WH, Schrijver J, van Erp Baart MA, Brouns F. Adequacy of vitamin supply under maximal sustained workloads: The Tour de France. *International Journal for Vitamin and Nutrition Research.* 1989;30:205-212.

79 Brouns F, Saris WH, Stroecken J, Beckers E, Thijssen R, Rehrer JN, ten Hoor F. Eating, drinking, and cycling: A controlled Tour de France simulation study, Part II. Effect of diet manipulation. *International Journal of Sports Medicine.* 1989;10(supp 1):41S-48S.

80 Weiler JM, Layton T, Hunt M. Asthma in United States Olympic athletes who participated in the 1996 Summer Games. *Journal of Allergy and Clinical Immunology.* 1998;102(5):722-726.

81 Hoffman MD, Clifford PS. Physiological aspects of competitive cross-country skiing. *Journal of Sports Sciences.* 1992;10(1):3-27.

82 McArdle WD, Katch FI, Katch VL. *Exercise Physiology: Energy, Nutrition and Human Performance.* 5th ed. Philadelphia: Lippincott, Williams & Wilkins; 2006.

83 Coulston AM, Boushey CJ, eds. *Nutrition in the Prevention and Treatment of Disease.* 2nd ed. London: Elsevier; 2008.

84 Bilodeau B, Roy B, Boulay MR. Effect of drafting on work intensity in classical cross-country skiing. *International Journal of Sports Medicine.* 1995;16(3):190-195.

85 Larsson P, Henriksson-Larsen K. Body composition and performance in cross-country skiing. *International Journal of Sports Medicine.* 2008;29(12):971-975.

86 Diaz E, Ruiz F, Hoyos I, Zubero J, Gravina L, Gil J, Irazusta J, Gil SM. Cell damage, antioxidant status, and cortisol levels related to nutrition in ski mountaineering during a two-day race. *Journal of Sports Science and Medicine.* 2010;9:338-346.

87 Haymes EM, Puhl JL, Temples TE. Training for cross-country skiing and iron status. *Medicine and Science in Sports and Exercise.* 1986;18(2):162-167.

88 Francescato MP, Puntil I. Does a pre-exercise carbohydrate feeding improve a 20-km cross-country ski performance? *Journal of Sports Medicine and Physical Fitness.* 2006;46(2):248-256.

89 Seifert JG, Luetkemeier MJ, White AT, Mino LM. The physiological effects of beverage ingestion during cross country ski training in elite collegiate skiers. *Canadian Journal of Applied Physiology.* 1998;23(1):66-73.

90 Rowing Classifications. www.usrowing.org/About/Rowing101/RowingClassifications.aspx Accessed August 8, 2011.

91 Kyparos A, Vrabas I, Nikolaidis MG, Riganas C, Kouretas D. Increased oxidative stress blood markers in well-trained rowers following two-thousand-meter rowing ergometer race. *Journal of Strength and Conditioning Research.* 2009;23(5):1418-1426.

92 Martins AN, Artioli GG, Franchini E. Sodium citrate ingestion increases glycolytic activity but does not enhance 2000 m rowing performance. *Journal of Human Sport and Exercise.* 2010;5(3):411-417.

93 Henson DA, Nieman DC, Nehlsen-Cannarella SL, Fagoaga OR, Shannon M, Bolton MR, Davis JM, Gaffney CT, Kelln WJ, Austin MD, Hjertman JM, Schilling BK. Influence of carbohydrate on cytokine and phagocytic responses to 2 h or rowing. *Medicine and Science in Sports and Exercise.* 2000;32(8):1384-1389.

94 Sellar CM, Syrotuik DG, Field CJ, Bell GJ. The effect of dietary control and carbohydrate supplementation on the immune and hormonal responses to rowing exercise. *Applied Physiology and Nutrition Metabolism.* 2006;31:588-596.

95 Xia G, Chin MK, Girandola RN, Liu RY. The effects of diet and supplements on a male world champion lightweight rower. *Journal of Sports Medicine and Physical Fitness.* 2001;41(2):223-228.

96 Simonsen JC, Sherman WM, Lamb DR, Dernbach AR, Doyle JA, Strauss R. Dietary carbohydrate, muscle glycogen, and power output during rowing training. *Journal of Applied Physiology.* 1991;70(4):1500-1505.

97 Burge CM, Carey MF, Payne WR. Rowing performance, fluid balance, and metabolic function following dehydration and rehydration. *Medicine and Science in Sports and Exercise.* 1993;25(12):1358-1364.

98 Bruce CR, Anderson ME, Fraser SF, Stepto NK, Klein R, Hopkins WG, Hawley JA. Enhancement of 2000-m rowing performance after caffeine ingestion. *Medicine and Science in Sports and Exercise.* 2000;32:1958-1963.

99 Anderson ME, Bruce CR, Fraser SF, Stepto NK, Klein R, Hopkins WG, Hawley JA. Improved 2000-meter rowing performance in competitive oarswomen after caffeine ingestion. *International Journal of Sport Nutrition and Exercise Metabolism.* 2000;10:464-475.

100 Skinner TL, Jenkins DG, Coombes JS, Taaffe DR, Leveritt MD. Dose response of caffeine on 200 m rowing performance. *Medicine and Science in Sports and Exercise.* 2003;3:571-576.

101 Mikulic P. Anthropometric and metabolic determinants of 6,000-m rowing ergometer performance in internationally competitive rowers. *Journal of Strength and Conditioning Research.* 2009; 23(6):1851-1857.

102 Cosgrove MJ, Wilson J, Watt D, Grant SF. The relationship between selected physiological variables of rowers and rowing performance as determined by a 2000 m ergometer test. *Journal of Sports Sciences.* 1999;17(11):845-852.

103 Izquierdo-Gabarren M, Gonzalez de Txabarri Exposito R, de Villarreal ESS, Izquierdo M. Physiological factors to predict on traditional rowing performance. *European Journal of Applied Physiology.* 2010;108:83-92.

104 Morris FL, Payne WR. Seasonal variations in the body composition of lightweight rowers. *British Journal of Sports Medicine.* 1996;30(4):301-304.

105 Brown RC. Nutrition for optimal performance during exercise: Carbohydrate and fat. *Current Sports Medicine Reports.* 2002;1(4):222-229.

106 Miller SL, Wolfe RR. Physical exercise as a modulator of adaptation to low and high carbohydrate and low and high fat intakes. *European Journal of Clinical Nutrition.* 1999;53(suppl 1):112S-119S.

107 Graham TE. Caffeine and exercise: Metabolism, endurance and performance. *Sports Medicine.* 2001;31(11):785-807.

108 Hunter AM, St. Clair Gibson A, Collins M, Lambert M, Noakes TD. Caffeine ingestion does not alter performance during a 100-km cycling time-trial performance. *International Journal of Sport Nutrition and Exercise Metabolism.* 2002;12(4):438-452.

Chapter 15

1 Maughan RJ, Sherriffs SM. Nutrition for soccer players. *Current Sports Medicine Reports.* 2007;6:279-280.

2 Montain SJ. Hydration recommendations for sport 2008. *Current Sports Medicine Reports.* 2008;7(4):187-192.

3 Heikkinen A, Alaranta A, Helenius I, Vasankari T. Use of dietary supplements in Olympic athletes is decreasing: A follow-up study between 2002 and 2009. *Journal of the International Society of Sports Nutrition.* 2011;8:1. www.jissn.com/content/8/1/1. Accessed August 9, 2011.

4 Van der Merwe PJ, Grobbelaar E. Unintentional doping through the use of contaminated nutritional supplements. *South African Medical Journal.* 2005;95:510-511.

5 Tscholl P, Junge A, Dvorak J. The use of medication and nutritional supplements during FIFA World Cups 2002 and 2006. *British Journal of Sports Medicine.* 2008;42:725-730.

6 Bangsbo J. Team sports. In: Maughan R, ed. *Nutrition in Sport.* London: Blackwell Science; 2000:574-587.

7 Davis M. Repeated sprint work is enhanced with consumption of a carbohydrate-electrolyte beverage. *Medicine and Science in Sports and Exercise.* 1995;27:223S.

8 Nicholas CW, Williams C, Phillips G, Nowitz A. Influence of ingesting a carbohydrate-electrolyte solution on endurance capacity during intermittent, high intensity shuttle running. *Journal of Applied Sports Science Research.* 1996;13:282-290.

9 Below PR, Mora-Rodrigues R, Gonzalez-Alonso J, Coyle EF. Fluid and carbohydrate ingestion independently improve performance during one hour of intense exercise. *Medicine and Science in Sports and Exercise.* 1995;27(2):200-210.

10 Murray R, Paul GL, Seifert JG, Eddy DE. Responses to varying rates of carbohydrate ingestion during exercise. *Medicine and Science in Sports and Exercise.* 1991;23(6):713-718.

11 Gisolfi CV, Summers RW, Schedl HP, Bleiler TL. Intestinal water absorption from select carbohydrate solutions in humans. *Journal of Applied Physiology.* 1992;73:2142-2150.

12 Lambert CP. Effects of carbohydrate feeding on multiple-bout resistance exercise. *Journal of Applied Sports Science Research.* 1991;5:192-197.

13 Ryan AJ, Lambert GP, Shi X, Chang RT, Summers RW, Gisolfi CV. Effect of hypohydration on gastric emptying and intestinal absorption during exercise. *Journal of Applied Physiology.* 1998;84(5):1581-1588.

14 Horswill CA. Effective fluid replacement. *International Journal of Sport Nutrition.* 1998;8:175-195.

15 American College of Sports Medicine. Position stand on exercise and fluid replacement. *Medicine and Science in Sports and Exercise.* 1996;28:i-vii.

16 Corley G, Demarest-Litchford M, Bazzarre TL. Nutrition knowledge and dietary practices of college coaches. *Journal of the American Dietetic Association.* 1990;90(5):705-709.

17 Dubnov G, Constantini NW. Prevalence of iron depletion and anemia in top-level basketball players. *International Journal of Sport Nutrition and Exercise Metabolism.* 2004;14(1):30-37.

18 Nowak RK, Knudsen KS, Schulz LO. Body composition and nutrient intakes of college men and women basketball players. *Journal of the American Dietetic Association.* 1988;88(5):575-578.

19 Schroder H, Navarro E, Mora J, Galiano D, Tramullas A. Effects of alpha-tocopherol, beta-carotene and ascorbic acid on oxidative, hormonal and enzymatic exercise stress markers in habitual training activity of professional basketball players. *European Journal of Nutrition.* 2001;40(4):178-184.

20 Schroder H, Navarro E, Tramullas A, Mora J, Galiano D. Nutrition antioxidant status and oxidative stress in professional basketball players: Effects of a three compound antioxidative supplement. *International Journal of Sports Medicine.* 2000;21(2):146-150.

21 Maughan R. Contamination of supplements: An interview with professor Ron Maughan by Louise M. Burke. *International Journal of Sport Nutrition and Exercise Metabolism.* 2004;14(4):493.

22 Mannix ET, Healy A, Farber MO. Aerobic power and supramaximal endurance of competitive figure skaters. *Journal of Sports Medicine and Physical Fitness.* 1996;36(3):161-168.

23 Delistraty DA, Reisman EJ, Snipes M. A physiological and nutritional profile of young female figure skaters. *Journal of Sports Medicine and Physical Fitness.* 1992;32(2):149-155.

24 Ziegler PJ, Nelson JA, Jonnalagadda SS. Use of dietary supplements by elite figure skaters. *International Journal of Sport Nutrition and Exercise Metabolism.* 2003;13(3):266-276.

25 Ziegler P, Hensley S, Roepke JB, Whitaker SH, Craig BW, Drewnowski A. Eating attitudes and energy intakes of female skaters. *Medicine and Science in Sports and Exercise.* 1998;30(4):583-586.

26 Ziegler PJ, Jonnalagadda SS, Nelson JA, Lawrence C, Baciak B. Contribution of meals and snacks to nutrient intake of male and female elite figure skaters during peak competitive season. *Journal of American Collegiate Nutrition.* 2002;21(2):114-119.

27 Smith AD, Ludington R. Injuries in elite pair skaters and ice dancers. *American Journal of Sports Medicine.* 1989;17(4):482-488.

28 Kjaer M, Larsson B. Physiological profile and incidence of injuries among elite figure skaters. *Journal of Sports Science.* 1992;10(1):29-36.

29 Ziegler PJ, Nelson JA, Jonnalagadda SS. Nutritional and physiological status of U.S. national figure skaters. *International Journal of Sport Nutrition.* 1999;9(4):345-360.

30 Tumilty D. Physiological characteristics of elite soccer players. *Journal of Sports Medicine.* 1993;16(2):80-96.

31 Wittich A, Mautalen CA, Oliveri MB, Bagur A, Somoza F, Rotemberg E. Professional football (soccer) players have a markedly greater skeletal mineral content, density, and size than age- and BMI-matched controls. *Calcified Tissue International.* 1998;63(2):112-117.

32 Duppe H, Gardsell P, Johnell O, Ornstein E. Bone mineral density in female junior, senior, and former football players. *Osteoporosis International.* 1996;6(6):437-441.

33 Rico-Sanz J. Body composition and nutritional assessments in soccer. *International Journal of Sport Nutrition.* 1998;8(2):113-123.

34 Maughan RJ. Energy and macronutrient intakes of professional football (soccer) players. *British Journal of Sports Medicine.* 1997;31(1):45-47.

35 Clark K. Nutritional guidance to soccer players for training and competition. *Journal of Sports Science.* 1994;12:43S-50S.

36 Kirkendall DT. Effects of nutrition on performance in soccer. *Medicine and Science in Sports and Exercise.* 1993;25(12):1370-1374.

37 Clark M, Reed DB, Crouse SF, Armstrong RB. Pre- and post-season dietary intake, body composition, and performance indices of NCAA Division I female soccer players. *International Journal of Sport Nutrition and Exercise Metabolism.* 2003;13(3):303-319.

38 Hargreaves M. Carbohydrate and lipid requirements of soccer. *Journal of Sports Science.* 1994;12:13S-16S.

39 Davis JM, Welsh RS, Alerson NA. Effects of carbohydrate and chromium ingestion during intermittent high-intensity exercise to fatigue. *International Journal of Sport Nutrition and Exercise Metabolism.* 2000;10(4):476-485.

40 Ostojic SM. Creatine supplementation in young soccer players. *International Journal of Sport Nutrition and Exercise Metabolism.* 2004;14(1):95-103.

41 Maughan RJ, Merson SJ, Broad NP, Shirreffs SM. Fluid and electrolyte intake and loss in elite soccer players during training. *International Journal of Sport Nutrition and Exercise Metabolism.* 2004;14(3):333-346.

42 MacLeod H, Sunderland C. Fluid balance and hydration habits of elite female field hockey players during consecutive international matches. *Journal of Strength and Conditioning Research.* 2009;23(4):1245-1251.

43 Moore DR, Robinson MJ, Fry JL, Tang JE, Glover EI, Wilkinson SB, Prior T, Tarnopolsky MA, Phillips SM. Ingested protein dose response of muscle and albumin protein synthesis after resistance exercise in young men. *American Journal of Clinical Nutrition.* 2009;89:161-168.

44 Saltin B. Metabolic fundamentals in exercise. *Medicine and Science in Sports.* 1973;5:137-146.

45 Krustrup P, Mohr M, Steensberg A, Bencke J, Kjaer M, Bangsbo J. Muscle and blood metabolites during a soccer game: Implications for sprint performance. *Medicine and Science in Sports and Exercise.* 2006;38:1165-1174.

46 Bangsbo J, Norregaard L, Thorsoe F. The effect of carbohydrate diet on intermittent exercise performance. *International Journal of Sports Medicine.* 1992;13:152-157.

47 Zehnder M, Rico-Sanz J, Kuhne G, Boutellier U. Resynthesis of muscle glycogen after soccer specific performance examined by 13C-magnetic resonance spectroscopy in elite players. *European Journal of Applied Physiology.* 2001;84:443-447.

48 Van Wyk DV, Lambert MI. Recovery strategies implemented by sport support staff of elite rugby players in South Africa. Unpublished thesis. Department of Human Biology, University of Cape Town, South Africa. 2008.

49 Baar K, McGee SL. Optimizing training adaptations by manipulating glycogen. *European Journal of Sport Science.* 2008;8:97-106.

50 Burke LM, Hawley JA. Fluid balance in team sports. Guidelines for optimal practices. *Sports Medicine.* 1997;24:38-54.

51 Maughan RJ, Merson SJ, Broad NP, Shirreffs SM. Fluid and electrolyte intake and loss in elite soccer players during training. *International Journal of Sport Nutrition and Exercise Metabolism.* 2004;14:333-346.

52 Maughan RJ, Watson P, Evans GH, Broad N, Shirreffs SM. Water balance and salt losses in competitive football. *International Journal of Sport Nutrition and Exercise Metabolism.* 2007;17:583-594.

53 Broad EM, Burke LM, Cox GR, Heeley P, Riley M. Body weight changes and voluntary fluid intakes during training and competition sessions in team sports. *International Journal of Sports Nutrition.* 1996;6:307-320.

54 Cox G, Mujika I, Tumilty D, Burke L. Acute creatine supplementation and performance during a field test simulating match play in elite female soccer players. *International Journal of Sport Nutrition and Exercise Metabolism.* 2002;12:33-46.

55 Ostojic SM. Creatine supplementation in young soccer players. *International Journal of Sport Nutrition and Exercise Metabolism.* 2004;14:95-103.

56 Cameron SL, McLay-Cooke RT, Brown RC, Gray AR, Fairbairn KA. Increased blood pH but not performance with sodium bicarbonate supplementation in elite rugby union players. *International Journal of Sport Nutrition and Exercise Metabolism.* 2010;20(4):307-321.

57 Zinn C, Schofield G, Wall C. Evaluation of sports nutrition knowledge of New Zealand premier club rugby coaches. *International Journal of Sport Nutrition and Exercise Metabolism.* 2006;16(2):214-225.

58 Mujika I, Burke LM. Nutrition in team sports. *Annals of Nutrition and Metabolism.* 2010;57(suppl 2):26-35.

59 Groppel JL, Roetert EP. Applied physiology of tennis. *Journal of Sports Medicine.* 1992;14(4):260-268.

60 Bergeron MF, Maresh CM, Kraemer WJ, Abraham A, Conroy B, Gabaree C. Tennis: A physiological profile during match play. *International Journal of Sports Medicine.* 1991;12(5):474-479.

61 Vergauwen L, Brouns F, Hespel P. Carbohydrate supplementation improves stroke performance in tennis. *Medicine and Science in Sports and Exercise.* 1998;30(8):1289-1295.

62 Bergeron MF, Maresh CM, Armstrong LE, Signorile JF, Castellani JW, Kenefick RW, LaGasse KE, Riebe DA. Fluid-electrolyte balance associated with tennis match play in a hot environment. *International Journal of Sport Nutrition.* 1995;5(3):180-193.

63 Baxter-Jones AD, Helms P, Baines-Preece J, Preece M. Menarche in intensively trained gymnasts, swimmers, and tennis players. *Annals of Human Biology.* 1994;21(5):407-415.

64 Harris MB. Weight concern, body image, and abnormal eating in college women tennis players and their coaches. *International Journal of Sport Nutrition and Exercise Metabolism.* 2000;10(1):1-15.

65 Martinovic J, Dopsaj MJ, Kotur-Stevuljevic J, Vujovic A, Stefanovic A, Nesic G. Long-term effects of oxidative stress in volleyball players. *International Journal of Sports Medicine.* 2009;30(12):851-856.

66 Eliakim A, Portal S, Zadik Z, Rabinowitz J, Adler-Portal D, Cooper DM, Zaldivar F, Memet D. The effect of a volleyball practice on anabolic hormones and inflammatory markers in elite male and female adolescent players. *Journal of Strength and Conditioning Research.* 2009;23(5):1553-1559.

67 Malaguti M, Baldini M, Angeloni C, Biagi P, Hrelia S. High-protein-PUFA supplementation, red blood cell membranes, and plasma antioxidant activity in volleyball athletes. *International Journal of Sport Nutrition and Exercise Metabolism.* 2008;18(3):301-312.

68 Peerkhan N, Srinivasan V. Nutrition knowledge, attitude, and practice of college sportsmen. *Sport, Exercise, Medicine.* 2010;1(2):93-100.

69 Anderson DE. The impact of feedback on dietary intake and body composition of college women volleyball players over a competitive season. *Journal of Strength and Conditioning Research.* 2010;24(8):2220-2226.

70 Beals KA. Eating behaviors, nutritional status, and menstrual function in elite female adolescent volleyball players. *Journal of the American Dietetic Association.* 2002;102(9):1293-1296.

71 Hassapidou MN, Manstrantoni A. Dietary intakes of elite female athletes in Greece. *Journal of Human Nutrition and Dietetics.* 2001;14:391-396.

72 Papadopoulou SK, Papadopoulou SD, Gallos GK. Macro- and micro-nutrient intake of adolescent Greek female volleyball players. *International Journal of Sport Nutrition and Exercise Metabolism.* 2002;12(1):73-80.

73 Ahmadi A, Enayatizadeh N, Akbarzadeh M, Asadi S, Tabatabaee SHR. Iron status in female athletes participating in team ball-sports. *Pakistan Journal of Biological Sciences.* 2010;13(2):93-96.

74 Heffner JL, Ogles BM, Gold E, Marsden K, Johnson M. Nutrition and eating in female college athletes: A survey of coaches. *Eating Disorders.* 2003;11:209-220.

75 de Hoyo M. Sanudo B, Carrasco L. Body composition and prevalence of overweight in young volleyball players. *International Journal of Medicine and Science of Physical Activity and Sport.* 2008;8:32:256-269.

76 Martin M, Schlabach G, Shibinski K. The use of nonprescription weight loss products among female basketball, softball, and volleyball athletes from NCAA Division I institutions: Issues and concerns. *Journal of Athletic Training.* 1998;33(1):41-44.

77 Zetou E, Giatsis G, Mountake F, Kominakidou A. Body weight changes and voluntary fluid intakes of beach volleyball players during an official tournament. *Journal of Science and Medicine in Sport.* 2008;11(2):139-145.

78 Associated Press release. Golf, rugby make Olympic roster for 2016, 2020. 2009; October 9, 2009.

79 Stevenson EJ, Hayes PR, Allison SJ. The effect of a carbohydrate-caffeine sports drink on simulated golf performance. *Applied Physiology, Nutrition, and Metabolism.* 2009;34(4):681-688.

80 Chen SC, Davis JM, Nguyen RM, Smith SH. *Medicine and Science in Sports and Exercise.* 2005;37(5):445S-446S.

81 Hogervorst E, Bandelow S, Schmitt J, Jentjens R, Oliveira M, Allgrove J, Carter T, Gleeson M. Caffeine improves physical and cognitive performance during exhaustive exercise. *Medicine and Science in Sports and Exercise.* 2008;40(10):1841-1851.

82 Ng CP, Chung CH. Golf-related injuries: Case series and reports. *Hong Kong Journal of Emergency Medicine.* 2004;11:220-225.

83 Brandon B, Pearch PZ. Training to prevent golf injury. *Current Sports Medicine Reports.* 2009;8(3):142-146.

84 Lee AD. Golf-related stress fractures: A structured review of the literature. *Journal of the Canadian Chiropractic Association.* 2009;53(4):290-299.

85 Wells GD, Collier D. Golf nutrition: What to eat before and after you practice and play. Royal Canadian Golf Association National Player Development Program. www.rcga.org/_uploads/documents/Greg%20Wells%20-%20Golf%20Nutrition.pdf. Accessed August 9, 2011.

Index

Note: The italicized *f* and *t* following page numbers refer to figures and tables, respectively.

A

absorption of nutrients 140-145. *See also specific nutrients*
acclimatization
    heat 92-93, 93*t*, 200
    high altitude 209-210
acute mountain sickness (AMS) 211, 213
adaptation
    fat burning 293
    high altitude 209
    hydration and 92-93, 93*t*
    train low, compete high 325
adenosine diphosphate (ADP) 14
adenosine triphosphate (ATP) 10-11, 11*t*, 115, 115*f*, 189, 261, 261*t*, 293-295
aerobic glycolysis 11, 11*t*
aerobic metabolism 11*t*, 293-295, 295*f*. *See also* endurance sports
age
    body composition changes and 247-248
    gastritis and 134
    older athletes 227-230, 228*t*
    young athletes 222-227, 223*t*, 225*t*, 251, 259
air displacement plethysmography 246-247, 246*f*
alcoholic beverages 134, 145-146, 146*t*, 195, 203, 215, 327, 331-332
alcoholic energy drinks 216
allergies 141
amenorrhea. *See* menstrual disorders
American College of Sports Medicine (ACSM) 279, 281, 317
amino acids
    absorption 137
    branched-chain 15, 161, 194
    as ergogenic aid 118-119
    essential/nonessential 30-31, 31*t*
    in gluconeogenesis 12, 15
    structure and function 29-30, 29*f*, 30*t*, 32, 32*t*
    in vegetarian diets 41
anabolic steroids 44, 112, 114
anaerobic glycolysis 11-12, 11*t*, 261
anaerobic maximum 261

anaerobic metabolism 260-261, 261*t*, 294-295, 295*f*. *See also* power sports
anemia 52, 73, 76, 134, 144, 183-185, 185*f*
anorexia athletica 252-253, 253*t*
anorexia nervosa 155, 252-253, 254*t*
antibiotics 137, 138, 145, 152, 319
antioxidants 187, 187*t*, 215, 329. *See also specific antioxidants*
appetite loss 138-140, 139*t*
asthma 181, 306
athletic performance
    alcohol and 145-146, 146*t*
    body composition and 240-242, 241*f*
    dehydration and 99, 100*t*
    eating disorders and 254-255
    hydration and 102-105, 103*f*, 104*t*

B

banned substances
    anabolic steroids 44, 112
    diuretics 117
    EPO 186, 210
    in ergogenic aids 44, 112, 114
    glycerol 12, 23-24, 101, 101*f*, 117, 216
    WADA code 129
baseball 262-264
basketball 317-320, 320*t*
beta-carotene 58-59
beta-oxidative metabolic pathway 23
bicarbonate 118
bile 136
bioelectrical impedance analysis (BIA) 244-245, 245*f*
biotin 55, 55*t*
blood sugar levels
    carbohydrate metabolism and 8-9, 9*f*
    exercise intensity and 240
    fatigue and 3-4, 10
    meal frequency and 156, 226
    muscle breakdown and 12
    school food programs and 226
Bod Pod 246-247, 246*f*
bodybuilding 111, 265-267
body composition

in anorexia nervosa 155, 254*t*
assessment issues 239, 249-250
body weight and 235-238
changes in 247-249
energy balance and 154-156, 156*f*, 238, 238*f*
estimating 242-247
meal frequency and 157-158, 238, 238*f*, 239*f*
normal percentages 233
performance and 240-242, 241*f*
water in 83, 84*t*, 233
weight loss and 232-234
body weight
    body composition and 235-238
    body mass index 235, 236*t*
    desirable 235
    hydration status and 99-100
    making weight 258, 279-283, 334-335
    weight loss 232-234
    weight management 236-238, 237*t*
    weight tables 223*t*
bone health
    calcium and 65-67
    endurance athletes 299, 301-302, 305-306
    female athletes 219, 221
    older athletes 228-229
    vitamins and 61, 63
    young athletes 225-226
branched-chain amino acids (BCAAs) 15, 161, 194
bulimia nervosa 253
B vitamins
    B1 (thiamin) 46-48, 48*t*
    B2 (riboflavin) 48, 49*t*
    B3 (niacin) 49, 50*t*
    B6 50-51, 52*t*, 221
    B12 52, 53*t*, 134, 137, 144, 184, 185, 229

C

caffeine
    common sources 119*t*
    as ergogenic aid 119-120, 310, 330-331
    at high altitude 215
    hydration and 102

jet lag and 202, 204
in sports gels 108
calcium 60, 64-67, 67*t*, 221
calorie (term) 2
carbohydrate loading 163, 163*f*
carbohydrate polymers 5*t*, 108
carbohydrates
    for endurance athletes 41, 289, 291, 293, 297-298, 298*t*, 308, 311-312
    as ergogenic aid 114-115, 129
    during exercise 12-14, 161-162
    exercise intensity and 4, 6*f*, 13
    female consumption 219, 220*t*
    food sources 18
    functions 4*t*
    glycemic index, glycemic load 19, 20*t*
    at high altitude 214
    importance of 3-4, 14
    intake, by sport 17, 17*t*
    intake adequacy 19-21
    metabolism 8-10, 9*f*
    postexercise 41, 162
    for power/endurance athletes 332
    preexercise 161
    protein-sparing effect 36
    requirements 15-18, 18*t*
    in sports beverages 91, 93-94, 104*t*, 105, 148
    terms 5*t*
    types 6-8, 7*t*
carbonated beverages 92
carnitine (L-carnitine) 120-121
Celiac disease 141-143, 142*t*, 143*t*, 151
central nervous system fatigue 10, 14-15
ceruloplasmin 183
child development 222-226, 223*t*, 225*t*, 251
chloride 71, 71*t*
cholesterol 22, 23, 136
choline 290-291, 290*t*, 291*t*
chromium 81, 81*t*
circadian rhythms 199, 202, 204
competition days 177-178
compression hose 203-204
conditioning
    fat burning and 26-27, 27*f*
    hydration and 92-93
    sweat rate and 90
copper 79, 79*t*, 183
Cori cycle 12
cortisol 10, 162, 308
creatine monohydrate 40-41, 115-116, 115*f*, 261, 279

Crohn's disease 144
cross-country skiing 307-309
cycling 306-307, 354-355*t*

D
dehydration 94-95, 99, 100*t*, 195, 202, 210-211. *See also* hydration
dental health 133, 138-139
dietary reference intake (DRI) 44, 45*t*
dietary restrictions 203
dietary supplements 43-44, 114, 151, 152, 299, 313. *See also specific nutrients*
dieting 140
digestion 140-145. *See also* gastrointestinal tract
digestive enzymes 136-137
dilutional pseudoanemia (sports anemia) 76, 185, 185*f*
disaccharides 5*t*, 6, 8*t*
distance running 98, 101, 301-303, 360-361*t*
distance swimming 305-306
diuretics 117
DOMS (delayed-onset muscle soreness) 122, 189-195, 190*t*
dual-energy X-ray absorptiometry (DEXA) 65, 245-246

E
eating disorders 40, 250-255, 251*t*, 252*f*, 253*f*, 253*t*, 254*t*
eating plans
    endurance sports 351, 352-361*t*
    gluten-free 354-355*t*
    power/endurance sports 363, 364-373*t*
    power sports 335, 336-349*t*
    taper plan 163-165, 166-177*t*
    vegetarian 352-353*t*
electrolytes 86, 86*t*, 104*t*
endurance sports
    aerobic metabolism 293-295, 295*f*
    cross-country skiing 307-309
    cycling 306-307
    dietary adequacy 297-300, 298*t*
    distance running 98, 101, 301-303
    distance swimming 305-306
    eating plans 351, 352-361*t*
    fat burning and 26-27, 27*f*
    hydration 293, 300
    nutrition tactics 41, 288-293
    overtraining 296-297
    overuse injuries 297
    rowing 309-312

    sports beverages 93
    triathlon 303-305
    ultra events 299-300
energy balance
    body composition and 154-156, 156*f*, 238, 238*f*
    meal frequency in 157-159., 225, 226, 238
    in taper plan 164, 166-177*t*
energy intake. *See also* eating plans; *specific sports*
    body composition and 248-249
    endurance athletes 297-300, 298*t*
    energy balance 154-157, 156*f*
    during exercise 161-162
    factors affecting 138-139
    GI distress and 149-152
    at high altitude 214-215
    immune system and 155
    inadequate 154, 250, 251*t*
    nutrient adequacy and metabolism 146-147
    postexercise 149-152, 162
    preexercise 134-135, 149, 150-151, 160-161
energy substrates. *See* carbohydrates; fats (lipids); protein
energy thermodynamics 236
epinephrine 10
ergogenic aids. *See also* banned substances; *specific substances*
    bicarbonate 118
    caffeine 119-120
    carbohydrate as 114-115, 129
    carnitine 120-121
    choosing to use 113-114, 129
    creatine monohydrate 115-116, 115*f*
    defined 110
    false claims 110-112
    ginseng 122
    glycerol 12, 23-24, 101, 101*f*, 117
    history 112
    MCTs 121-122
    omega-3 fatty acids as 121
    proteins and amino acids as 118-119
    quercetin 122-123
    resveratrol 123
    summary of 124-128*t*
    types 112-113, 113*t*
erythropoietin (EPO) 186, 210
esophagus 133-134
essential fatty acids. *See* omega-3 fatty acids

essential/nonessential amino acids 30-31, 31*t*
exercise intensity
  ATP production and 11, 11*t*
  blood sugar levels and 240
  carbohydrate and 4, 6*f*, 13
  fat burning and 13-14, 14*f*, 26, 240, 248
  gastric emptying and 92
  glucose release and 9

F
fatigue 3-4, 10, 12-15
fat mass 233, 249-250. *See also* body composition
fats (lipids). *See also* omega-3 fatty acids; omega-6 fatty acids; triglycerides
  athlete conditioning and 26-27, 27*f*
  digestion 136, 137
  for endurance athletes 298*t*
  exercise intensity and 13-14, 14*f*, 26, 240, 248
  fatigue and 15
  functions 4*t*, 22
  glucogenic 12
  metabolism 26-28
  requirements 21-22, 25-26
  types and structure 22-23
female athletes 219-221, 220*t*
female athlete triad 234, 234*f*, 251
fiber
  defined 5*t*, 6
  food sources 20*t*
  GI distress and 19, 151
  GI health and 137, 138
  glycemic index 19
  requirements 15-16
field hockey 323
figure skating 321-323, 340-341*t*, 356-357*t*, 370-371*t*
fish oil supplements 24, 189, 328
fluids. *See* hydration
folate (folic acid) 53-54, 54*t*, 184, 185
food consumption. *See* energy intake
food sensitivities 141, 148-149
football (American) 267-270, 348-349*t*
foot-strike hemolysis 75, 185, 186
free radicals 62, 122, 187, 319
fructose 6, 7, 105, 149, 162

G
galactose 6
gallbladder 136
gastric emptying 91-92, 134-135
gastritis 134
gastrointestinal tract
  age-related changes in 229

concerns for athletes 147-151
digestion 140-145
function 132
healthy 137-138
intestines 135-138
mouth and esophagus 133-134
nutrient absorption 140-145
pH ranges 134*t*
stomach 134-135
gender differences 146, 219, 248. *See also* female athletes
genetics 247
GI distress
  bicarbonate and 118
  causes 147
  fiber and 19
  food and fluid timing and 149-152
  intestinal problems 138, 141-145, 142*t*
  sports beverages and 105, 148-149, 162
  strategies for reducing 150-151
  travel and 205
ginseng 122
glucagon 8-9, 9*f*
gluconeogenesis 5*t*, 9, 12, 15
glucose 3, 5*t*, 6
glucose polymers 5*t*, 114-115, 162
gluten, gluten-free foods 143*t*
gluten-free eating plan 354-355*t*
gluten intolerance 141-143, 142*t*, 143*t*, 151
glycemic index, glycemic load 19, 20*t*
glycerol 12, 23-24, 101, 101*f*, 117, 216
glycogen stores
  capacity and use 3-4, 8, 10, 12-13, 294*t*
  defined 5*t*
  in female athletes 219
  loading during taper 160, 163, 163*f*
  replenishing 162
glycolysis 5*t*, 10-12, 261
glycolytic system 261
golf 330-332
gymnastics 101, 270-272

H
heart rate, hydration and 103*f*
heat balance 94, 94*f*
heat cramps 95, 95*t*, 328*t*
heat exhaustion 95-96, 102, 228, 328*t*
heat index 88, 89*t*
heatstroke 96, 96*t*, 228, 328*t*
heat tolerance 93, 228, 228*t*
hematuria 186
hemolysis 75, 185, 186
hiatal hernias 133
high altitude

acclimatization 209-210
definitions 210*t*
energy needs 214-215
fluid needs 215-216
training paradigms 208
high-altitude illness (HAI) 211-214, 212*t*
high-fructose corn syrup 6, 149
hockey 273-274
hunger 179
hydration. *See also specific sports*
  adaptations and 92-93, 93*t*
  aerobic performance and 99, 100*t*
  air travel and 201-202
  DOMS and 195
  in endurance sports 293, 300
  during exercise 99, 102-105, 103*f*, 104*t*, 106*t*, 109, 149, 159
  fluid absorption 93-94
  fluid balance 83-88, 85*t*
  fluid intake factors 90-91
  fluid loss factors 88-90
  fluid-related problems 94-99, 100*t*
  gastric emptying of fluids 91-92
  GI distress and 149-152, 205
  glycogen replenishment and 17
  at high altitude 210-211, 214, 215-216
  lactic acid and 12
  postexercise 107-109, 149-152
  preexercise 100-102
  status tests 84, 95, 99-100, 102
  during taper 160
  terms 83
  in young athletes 226
hydrostatic weighing (hydrodensitometry) 242-243
hyponatremia 97-99, 304

I
immune function 155, 188, 229
inflammation 24
insulin 8-9, 9*f*, 158
intestinal problems 138, 141-145, 142*t*
intestines 135-138
intrinsic factor 52-53, 134, 137
iodine 78, 78*t*
iron
  for endurance athletes 303, 308, 309, 311
  female requirements 221
  food sources 224*t*
  function and requirements 73-74, 74*t*
  high altitude and 210, 215
  iron status terms 182*t*
  in oxygen uptake 181-183

in vegetarian diet 73, 74, 74*t*
  youth requirements 223-224
iron-deficiency 73-76, 75*t*, 183-185
iron supplements 76-77, 152
irritable bowel syndrome (IBD) 144

J
jet lag 200, 202-204

K
kilocalorie (term) 2

L
lacrosse 323
lactic acid 11-12. *See also* anaerobic
  metabolism
lactose 6, 8*t*, 143-144, 149
lactose intolerance 10, 143-144, 151,
  162
large intestine 137-138
L-carnitine 120-121
lean mass 233. *See also* body
  composition
lipids. *See* fats (lipids)
liver function 136, 145-146

M
macronutrients. *See* carbohydrates; fats
  (lipids); protein
magnesium 68-69, 69*f*, 69*t*, 145, 152,
  185
maltodextrins 105
maltose 6, 8*t* .
manganese 80, 80*t*
meal frequency 157-159, 225, 226, 238
meal timing 160-162
medications 97, 113, 145, 152
medium-chain triglycerides (MCT) 27-
  28, 121-122
melatonin 204
menarche 222-234, 227, 272
menopause 248
menstrual disorders
  bone health and 65-67, 219
  in endurance athletes 299, 301-
    302
  energy deficits and 158, 255
  in female athlete triad 234, 234*f*
  low body fat and 233-234
  terms 234*t*
  in vegetarians 40
  in young athletes 227
metabolism. *See also specific systems*
  of carbohydrate 8-10, 9*f*
  factors affecting 145-147
  of fats (lipids) 26-28
  of protein 30-32, 32*f*
  systems of 11*t*

vitamins and 47*f*
metric conversions 84*t*
micronutrients. *See* minerals; vitamins
minerals. *See also specific minerals*
  absorption 135, 137, 145
  excessive 43-44
  functions 43, 64
  GI distress and 152
  macrominerals 64-72
  microminerals 73-81
monosaccharides 5*t*, 6, 8*t*, 137
mouth, in digestion 133-134
mouth and tongue problems 138-139
muscle fatigue. *See* fatigue
muscles
  blood sugar levels and 12
  DOMS 122, 189-195, 190*t*
  protein and 38-39, 41
  vitamins and 47*f*
Mutai, Geoffrey 288

N
nandrolone 44, 114
National Collegiate Athletic
  Association (NCAA) 280
niacin (vitamin B3) 49, 50*t*
nonnutritional ergogenic aids 110. *See
  also* ergogenic aids
NSAIDs 97, 134, 145, 152
nutritional ergogenic aids. *See*
  ergogenic aids

O
older athletes 227-230, 228*t*
oligomenorrhea. *See* menstrual
  disorders
Olympic weightlifting 285-287
omega-3 fatty acids
  description and function 22, 24-25
  DOMS and 189, 191-192
  as ergogenic aid 113, 121
omega-6 fatty acids 22, 24-25
overtraining 140, 147, 150, 296-297
overuse injuries 297
oxalic acid 65, 80
oxidative stress 122, 187-188, 215,
  328, 329
oxygen system. *See* aerobic metabolism
oxygen uptake 180-186

P
pancreas 8, 9*f*, 136
pantothentic acid 55, 56*t*
phase shifts 202-203
phosphocreatine (phosphagen) system
  11*t*, 261
phosphorus 60, 67-68, 68*t*
pH ranges, in GI tract 134*t*

phytochemicals 66
polysaccharides 5*t*, 6, 7*t*
postexercise intake
  energy intake 41, 149-152, 162
  hydration 107-109, 149-152
  protein 17, 37, 37*f*, 41
potassium 72, 72*t*
power/endurance sports
  basketball 317-320, 320*t*
  eating plans 363, 364-373*t*
  energy sources 314-315, 315*f*
  field hockey 323
  figure skating 321-323
  fluid intake guidelines 317*t*
  golf 330-332
  lacrosse 323
  nutrition tactics 314-317, 318*t*
  rugby 325-327
  soccer 323-324, 324*t*
  tennis 327
  volleyball 328-330
power sports
  anaerobic metabolism 260-261,
    261*t*
  baseball 262-264
  bodybuilding 111, 265-267
  eating plans 335, 336-349*t*
  football (American) 267-270
  gymnastics 101, 270-272
  hockey 273-274
  nutrition tactics 260
  Olympic weightlifting 285-287
  protein requirements 28, 286
  softball 262-264
  speedskating 283-285
  swimming 276-279, 277*t*
  track and field 274-275
  wrestling 101, 279-283
preexercise intake
  energy intake 134-135, 149, 150-
    151, 160-161
  hydration 100-102
protein
  DOMS and 194-195
  for endurance athletes 28, 291-
    293, 292*f*, 298*t*
  as ergogenic aid 118-119
  excessive 28, 35, 111
  female consumption 219-220
  functions 4*t*, 29-30, 30*t*
  jet lag and 203
  metabolism 30-32, 32*f*
  muscle development and 38-39
  plant sources 35*t*
  postexercise 17, 37, 37*f*, 41
  for power athletes 28, 286
  quality 32-33
  requirements 33-37, 36*t*
  in sample meal plan 34*t*

protein *(continued)*
    in sports beverages 37
    in vegetarian diets 40-41

Q

quercetin 122-123

R

Randle effect 120
reactive oxygen species (ROS) 122,
    187, 189
recovery nutrition. *See* postexercise
    intake
rest, inadequate 147, 150
restaurant food 205-206, 206*t*
resveratrol 123
riboflavin (vitamin B2) 48, 49*t*
rowing 309-312
rugby 325-327
runner's diarrhea 147
running 98, 101, 301-303, 360-361*t*

S

school food programs 226
selenium 78, 79*t*
skinfold caliper tests 243-244
small intestine 135-137
soccer 323-324
sodium
    fluid balance and 85, 86, 86*t*
    on food labels 71*t*
    function and requirements 70, 70*t*
    low blood sodium 97-99
    in sports beverages 70, 93, 104*t*,
        148
softball 262-264
speedskating 283-285
sports anemia 76, 185, 185*f*
sports beverages
    carbohydrates in 91, 93-94, 104*t*,
        105, 148
    digestive enzymes and 136-137
    GI distress and 105, 148-149, 162
    for power/endurance sports 315-
        317
    protein in 37
    sodium in 70, 93, 104*t*, 148
    swilling 148
sports gels 108
stomach 134-135
strength-to-weight ratio. *See* body
    composition

stress 92, 147
stress fracture risks 219, 220*t*, 301-302
sucrose 6, 7, 8*t*
sugars 6-8, 7*t*, 8*t*
sunstroke 96, 96*t*, 228, 328*t*
superhydration 101, 102
supplements. *See* dietary supplements;
    specific nutrients
sweat rate 85-86, 90, 99-100, 159, 214
swimming 276-279, 277*t*, 305-306

T

taper (seven-day)
    eating and exercise plan 163-165,
        166-177*t*
    goals of 160-161
    overview 178-179
taste testing 134
team sports. *See* power/endurance
    sports
temperature regulation 86-88, 87*f*, 88*f*,
    103*f*, 159, 210
tennis 327, 368-369*t*
thiamin (vitamin B1) 46-48, 48*t*
thirst sensation 90-91, 95, 102, 149,
    159, 179
timing, of foods and fluids
    for energy balance 154-157, 156*f*
    fluid intake 159
    GI distress and 149-152
    immune system and 155
    meal frequency 157-159, 225,
        226, 238
    seven-day taper 160-162
track and field 274-275
transferrin 182*t*, 183
travel
    disease risk 200
    eating guidelines 200-202, 201*t*,
        205-206, 206*t*
    foreign locations 205-206
    jet lag 200, 202-204
    planning for 198-199
triathlon 303-305
triglycerides
    medium-chain 27-28, 121-122
    metabolism 12, 23-24
    structure 23*f*
tryptophan 15, 32, 49

U

ultra events 299-300

urine
    blood in 186
    dehydration and 84, 95, 102
UV light therapy 61

V

vegetables, as calcium source 65
vegetarian athletes
    carnitine and 120
    eating plans 352-353*t*
    iron absorption 73, 74, 74*t*
    making weight 258
    protein and health risks in 40-41
    vitamin deficiency risk 48, 52, 53,
        184
vitamin A 58-59, 59*t*, 146
vitamin C 56-57, 57*t*, 152, 193-194
vitamin D 59-61, 60*f*, 61*t*, 65, 67, 138,
    192-193
vitamin E 61-62, 62*t*, 187-188, 193
vitamin K 63, 63*t*
vitamins. *See also specific vitamins*
    appetite loss and 138-140, 140*t*
    excessive 43-44
    fat-soluble 58-63, 137
    functions 43, 45, 47*f*
    GI distress and 152
    maximizing intake 46*t*
    storage capacity 46
    vegetarians and 48, 52, 53
    water-soluble 46-57
volleyball 328-330, 372-373*t*
voluntary dehydration 95, 216, 226

W

water, in body composition 83, 84*t*,
    233. *See also* hydration
weightlifting 285-287
weight loss. *See* body weight
World Anti-Doping Agency (WADA)
    129
wrestling 101, 279-283

Y

Yoder Begley, Amy 141
yogurt 138
young athletes 222-227, 223*t*, 225*t*,
    259

Z

zinc 77, 77*t*

About the Author

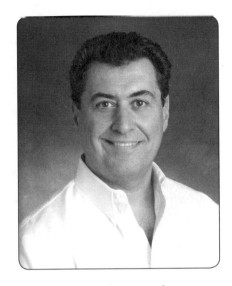

Dan Benardot, **PhD, RD, LD, FACSM,** is full professor at Georgia State University (GSU). He received his doctorate in human nutrition and health planning from Cornell University in 1980 and is a registered and licensed dietitian. Benardot's primary area of expertise is sports nutrition, with a research emphasis in energy balance and nutrition issues related to young athletes. He cofounded and directs the Laboratory for Elite Athlete Performance at GSU.

As the national team nutritionist and a founding member of the Athlete Wellness Program for USA Gymnastics, Benardot worked with the gold-medal-winning women's gymnastics team at the 1996 Atlanta Olympic Games and the medal-winning U.S. marathoners at the 2004 Athens Olympic Games. He also worked with the marathoners selected to represent the United States at the 2008 Beijing Olympic Games. He has served as an officer of the USA Figure Skating Sports Medicine Society and continues to work regularly with national team figure skaters. His research has been funded by several organizations, including the United States Olympic Committee, the Gatorade Sports Science Institute, and the American Cancer Society.

Benardot has received a doctor of humane letters, *honoris causa*, from Marywood University and is a fellow of the American College of Sports Medicine (ACSM). Born in Salonika, Greece, Benardot gained his love for sports while growing up in the Lake Placid region of northern New York. He now lives in Atlanta, Georgia, where he enjoys cello, tennis, and photography.

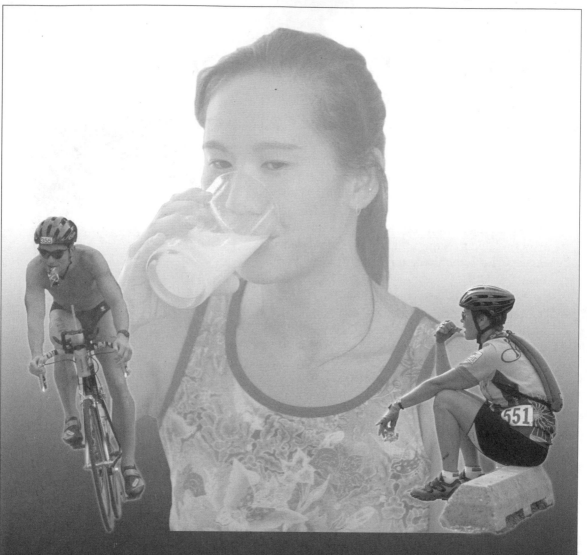

You'll find other outstanding sports nutrition resources at

www.HumanKinetics.com/nutritioninsport

In the U.S. call 1-800-747-4457

Australia 08 8372 0999 • Canada 1-800-465-7301
Europe +44 (0) 113 255 5665 • New Zealand 0800 222 062

HUMAN KINETICS
The Premier Publisher for Sports & Fitness
P.O. Box 5076 • Champaign, IL 61825-5076 USA

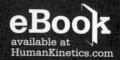

eBook
available at
HumanKinetics.com